T0227328

A CLINICAL GUIDE
to BLENDING
LIQUID HERBS

A CLINICAL GUIDE to BLENDING LIQUID HERBS

Herbal Formulations for the Individual Patient

Kerry Bone

MediHerb Pty Ltd
Warwick, Qld, Australia

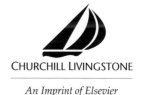

CHURCHILL LIVINGSTONE

An Imprint of Elsevier

**CHURCHILL
LIVINGSTONE**

An Imprint of Elsevier

11830 Westline Industrial Drive
St. Louis, Missouri 63146

NOTICE

Complementary and Alternative Medicine is an ever-changing field. Standard safety precautions must be
followed, but as new research and clinical experience broaden our knowledge, changes in treatment and drug
therapy may become necessary or appropriate. Readers are advised to check the most current product
information provided by the manufacturer of each drug to be administered to verify the recommended dose,
the method and duration of administration, and contraindications. It is the responsibility of the licensed
prescriber, relying on experience and knowledge of the patient, to determine dosages and the best treatment
for each individual patient. Neither the Publisher nor the author assumes any liability for any injury and/or
damage to persons or property arising from this publication.

THE PUBLISHER

ISBN-13: 978-0-443-06632-0
ISBN-10: 0-443-06632-9

Publishing Director: Linda Duncan
Acquisitions Editor: Kellie White
Sr. Developmental Editor: Kim Fons
Publishing Services Manager: Linda McKinley
Project Manager: Ellen Kunkelmann
Designer: Julia Dummitt

When Simon Mills and I published *Principles and Practice of Phytotherapy* (PPP) in 1999, it was hailed as the first textbook of modern herbal practice. Since then, several other herbal texts have been released for the professional reader. However, most of these publications contain only herbal monographs and seem to be based on the assumption that knowing about the properties of herbs is all that is necessary to understand herbal practice. Furthermore, many of these materia medica textbooks are not written by practicing herbalists and, rather than acting as working manuals or references for the herbal clinician, are quite negative about the worth and safety of many herbal treatments (under the guise of an evidence-based evaluation).

Very few, if any, modern texts reflect the current core activity of most western herbal practitioners: namely arriving at an individual prescription after an extensive consultation and then dispensing this prescription as a compounded liquid formulation. Herbalists in the U.K., Australia, and the U.S. have functioned in this way for more than 100 years, yet this mode of practice is regarded by many as on the fringe of medicine. This contrasts strongly with traditional Chinese medicine where the textbooks do reflect current practice and draw strongly from the traditional knowledge base. No one in China belittles the traditional basis of their herbal practice, unlike many western herbal texts.

For some time now, I have felt the need for a text reflecting the western herbalist's art of formulating liquids for the individual patient. This need, coupled with the common criticism that PPP contained too few herbs, led to the development of this book. In one sense, this text is an appendage to and update of PPP; this is particularly reflected in the way the monographs are written.

This book contains three main sections. The first section deals with all the practical issues involved in prescribing and dispensing liquid herbal products. The second section outlines, with many worked examples, the rationale and thought processes behind using individual prescribing with liquid herbs for the treatment of a variety of health issues. In the third section the reader will find up-to-date monographs on more than 100 herbs. In particular, these monographs are written from the perspective of a prescribing herbal clinician and contain indications from both traditional sources and scientific investigations. (One feature of the monographs is that the level of evidence behind each indication is clearly stated.)

This book was written for both herbal students (who may find PPP rather daunting early on in their studies) and any clinician who wishes to understand and apply in a modern scientific context the fascinating, flexible, and (in my experience) clinically effective methodology of the traditional western herbalist.

Kerry Bone, Warwick, Australia, 2003

Foreword

*M*any herbal texts are currently available. However, well-written guidelines to the actual practice of herbal medicine are extremely rare. In most books, herbs are described in general terms, reflecting their use in mass marketing. Those who are required in their work to give herbal advice to individuals soon learn that the information in monographs only goes part way to help make the right decisions in practice.

There is nothing more fascinating than the individual story. Even succumbing to illness is a personal passage that requires a unique resolution. Each case of migraine or arthritis is unprecedented. Those who find themselves using herbs to help people through their illnesses find themselves in wonderfully rewarding work, but in an area that is barely charted.

In our book *Principles and Practice of Phytotherapy*, Kerry Bone provided many illuminating case histories to indicate how the general herbal information could be applied to the particular need. In *A Clinical Guide to Blending Liquid Herbs*, he goes much further. He combines many years of herbal research and a personal commitment to producing the highest-quality herbal remedies with an equal experience in the consulting room with real patients. With this combination of skills, he has produced the most important guide to herbal prescription so far.

He introduces each medical condition with broad treatment strategies and goals, and links this with relevant herbal activity. Examples of formulations that might be used are given. However, it is clear that this is not a book of recipes. What Kerry has provided are tools for individual adaptation. The key is the choice of liquid preparations. Liquid extracts of herbs are the most suitable for blending to individual needs. Among other advantages, liquids are compact and convenient, involve minimal processing, and truly reflect the chemical spectrum of the original herb. Unlike solid forms, a liquid has all these phytochemical constituents already in solution and does not need to be dissolved or subjected to the digestive processes to be available for absorption.

To make the clinical guidelines particularly useful, no less than 125 herb monographs are provided. Each includes full prescribing information and references.

The book is an essential prescribing reference for all serious herbal clinicians, including physicians, naturopaths, pharmacists, and others who wish to use herbs productively in their works. This book will serve as an excellent text for herbal students.

Simon Mills
University of Exeter, U.K.
May 2003

Acknowledgments

Michelle Morgan, assisted by Janice McMillan, Allan Keith Baldock, Mark Walker, and Rob Santich, made a substantial contribution to the monograph section of this book. Their assistance with literature research and drafting is gratefully acknowledged. Thanks also to Jan Frousheger and Petra Moroney for typing and corrections and to Amanda Williams and Berris Burgoyne for proofreading.

Contents

Appendices

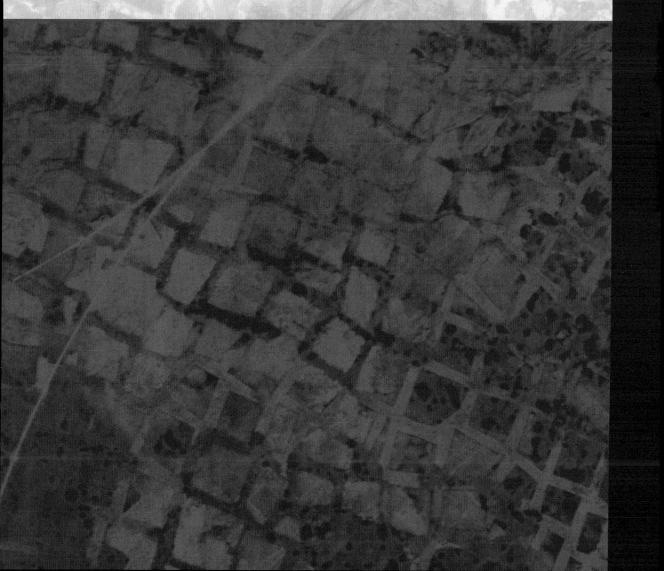

SECTION

I

OVERVIEW

Fundamental Concepts

1

CHAPTER

WHY USE HERBAL LIQUIDS?

*I*f a person walks into any retail outlet that sells herbal products, from supermarkets to health food stores, simple observation will reveal that the vast majority of products offered are in solid-dose form, mainly as tablets and hard-shell capsules. Clearly the contemporary consumer of self-prescribed herbal supplements prefers these modern dose forms. In contrast, health care professionals trained in herbal therapy generally emphasize traditional liquid preparations.

This preference is not an anachronism. Herbal liquid preparations confer considerable advantages. The main advantage, which will be emphasized in this book, is the easy preparation of a unique formulation according to the needs of each patient (extemporaneous dispensing). Another considerable advantage of liquids is that, if properly prepared, they involve minimal processing during their manufacture and thereby truly reflect the chemical spectrum of the original herb in a compact and convenient form.

Superior bioavailability is also an underresearched advantage of herbal liquids. When a solid-dose preparation is ingested, it must first disintegrate. The plant's phytochemicals need to dissolve in digestive juices (and the water that is simultaneously imbibed with the tablet or capsule) to be absorbed by the body. Research has demonstrated that a relationship exists between the rate and degree of dissolution of the phytochemicals in a solid-dose preparation and their ultimate absorption into the bloodstream. The advantage of herbal liquids is that the all-important phytochemical constituents are already in solution.

Herbal liquids confer considerable dose flexibility, which is especially relevant when prescribing low doses for small children. Additionally, children generally find liquids easier to take, although the taste can sometimes be a challenge for them.

TASTE ISSUE

A perceived disadvantage of herbal liquids is their taste, although in the case of bitters, the taste is an essential factor in the therapeutic response. The taste issue can be somewhat exaggerated by a minority of practitioners and patients. This author has found that only a minor percentage of patients actually cannot cope with the taste of herbal liquids. Asking each patient before prescribing if they mind taking strong-tasting liquids is helpful. This practice will draw a commitment from people who say the taste issue is not a problem. The health care provider should prescribe tablets or capsules to patients who say they do mind.

Most patients will grow accustomed to the taste of their mixture, and the feedback is that some even grow to like it. Flavoring preparations are available that are particularly useful for children.

The way an herbal liquid is taken can minimize the experience of any unpleasant taste. The most important factors are the contact time of the remedy in the mouth and the intensity of the contact. Some practitioners claim that absorption from the oral cavity is often part of the activity of herbal preparations, thus prolonging the contact time may in fact be preferable. However, from the point of view of taste, contact time in the mouth should be minimized.

To reduce the intensity of the contact, the herbal liquid must be diluted. However, if the liquid is diluted too much, the contact time will be too long. Thus a trade-off exists between intensity and contact time. The recommendation is that a 5-ml dose be diluted with approximately 10 ml of water or fruit juice. This mixture can be easily swallowed in one go, making the contact time minimal. Another way to further reduce the intensity of the contact is to suck on some ice beforehand, which deadens the taste buds and the olfactory nerve. Chilling the medicine beforehand and adding chilled water is another way to reduce the taste intensity.

Contact time can be further reduced by immediately rinsing the mouth with water or fruit juice. Approximately 50 ml should be quickly consumed immediately after the liquid is taken. To best achieve this effect, the diluted liquid should be in one hand and the rinse in the other. The two liquids are then consumed in a one-two action, as quickly as possible. Using this technique, taste can be dramatically minimized, and few patients complain of any problem. For herbs with a lingering aftertaste, eating something afterwards will help.

Another option to avoid the taste of an herbal liquid is to put the liquid (undiluted) into a hard gelatin capsule using a dropper. The capsule will soften slowly over the next hour, thus it can be conveniently consumed well before this happens.

HOW HERBAL LIQUIDS ARE MADE

Some of the factors involved in the preparation of herbal liquids are useful to consider in detail.

STRENGTH OR RATIO

The strength of an herbal liquid preparation is usually expressed as a ratio. For example, 1:2 means that 2 ml of the final preparation is equivalent to 1 g of the dried herb from which the preparation was made. When fresh herbs are used, the ratio can be based on the fresh weight, in which case, this information should be additionally specified. Herbal liquid preparations weaker than 1:2 are usually called tinctures, whereas 1:1 and 1:2 preparations are called extracts. Tinctures are usually made by a soaking process known as maceration, whereas extracts are best made using percolation. However, tinctures can also be adequately manufactured by a percolation process. These days, 1:1 liquid extracts are often made by reconstituting soft or powdered concentrates and as a result can be of inferior quality.

SOLVENT USED

Ethanol (or alcohol) has been used for hundreds of years to prepare herbal liquid preparations, and ethanol-water mixtures do appear to be quite efficient for the extraction of the wide variety of phytochemicals found in medicinal plants. Old texts describe steeping herbs in wine for long periods and then using the resultant liquid.

A number of studies have highlighted the importance of the correct choice of the ethanol percentage in terms of maximizing the quality of herbal liquid preparations. A Swiss study found that 55% ethanol was the optimum percentage for the extraction of the essential oil from chamomile (*Matricaria chamomilla*).[1] Higher percentages of ethanol did not extract any additional oil, and the solids content of the extract was decreased, indicating that other components were being less efficiently extracted. More recently, Meier found that 40% to 60% ethanol was the optimum range for achieving the highest extraction efficiency for the active components of a variety of herbs.[2] For example, at 25% ethanol, none of the saponins in ivy leaves (*Hedera helix*) were extracted, but at 60% ethanol, they were maximally extracted. Similarly, the alkylamides, which give the oral tingling sensation from Echinacea, are better extracted at higher ethanol percentages. Extracts of milk thistle (*Silybum marianum*) prepared in 25% ethanol will not contain any silymarin because it is insoluble at this concentration.

Practitioners should keep this consideration in mind when assessing a high-ethanolic extract of an herb. In many cases, the product may be more active (because of the correct choice of a high ethanol percentage), thus less liquid needs to be prescribed for an effective dose. The patient's ethanol intake may actually be lower than when prescribed a higher quantity of a low-ethanol extract of the same herb.

Higher ethanol percentages do not always confer higher activity. French researchers found that *Viburnum prunifolium* bark extracted at 30% ethanol was five times more spasmolytic compared with a 60% extract.[3]

The basic guidelines for the choice of the ethanol percentage to optimize the activity of the final liquid extract are as follows:

- 25%: Water-soluble constituents such as mucilage, tannins, and some glycosides (including some flavonoids and a few saponins)
- 45% to 60%: Essential oils, alkaloids, most saponins, and some glycosides
- 90%: Resins and oleoresins

Glycetracts or glycerites are herbal liquid preparations made using glycerol and water instead of ethanol and water. Glycetracts are useful preparations when the active components are water soluble, for example, marshmallow root (*Althaea officinalis*), because they do not contain alcohol, and the sweetness of the glycerol gives them a better taste. However, the importance of these preparations should not be overrated. Glycerol is a poor solvent for many of the active components found in herbs, and glycetracts are less stable compared with alcoholic extracts (see the later discussion). Moreover, because of the viscosity of glycerol, concentrated preparations are difficult to make by percolation. The manufacture of 1:1 or 1:2 glycetracts therefore invariably requires the use of a concentration step involving the application of heat or vacuum, which risks deterioration of the product.

Some practitioners are concerned about possible exposure of their patients to the toxic effects of ethanol, such as during pregnancy. However, these toxic effects are dose related and do not occur for the small quantities of alcohol involved. For adverse effects to arise after ethanol intake, the blood alcohol level must rise to a certain level. A 5-ml dose of herbal extract contains as much ethanol as does approximately one sixth of a standard glass of beer or wine. The liver rapidly metabolizes such a small intake of ethanol, and consequently its effect on the blood alcohol level might not even be measurable. Only a much higher intake of ethanol will overload the liver's metabolizing capacity and lead to significant blood alcohol levels. Moreover, the body is naturally conditioned to a small exposure to ethanol from ripe fruit and the natural fermentation of food. Refrigeration has minimized this exposure in industrialized countries. However, human beings, be they children or adults, have evolved and adapted to levels of ethanol intake through food that are similar to those from herbal extracts.

Only a small minority of patients are genuinely sensitive to ethanol. In other individuals, a presumed sensitivity is only an exaggerated reflex response to the medicine, which can usually be alleviated by prescribing lower doses at a greater frequency, taken with food or water. Recovering alcoholics and Muslims are advised to take tablet preparations. Patients with mild liver conditions should not be adversely affected by a small ethanol intake.

Herbal liquid preparations based on alcohol can exhibit superior bioavailability. Results of a double-blind, placebo-controlled, crossover study on children with chronic obstructed airways were reported in the "Industry News" section of the *Zeitschrift für Phytotherapie*.[4] The therapeutic effects of ethanolic and ethanol-free galenical extracts of ivy leaves (*Hedera helix*) were compared. Spirometric testing showed a significant improvement in lung function for both products, which was superior to conventional bronchodilators. However, results indicated that the addition of alcohol to the preparation yielded an increase in the bioavailability of active components. The dose of the alcohol-free preparation needed to be adjusted to a higher level to obtain the same effect.

GLYCEROL-WATER COMBINATIONS

Recently, glycerol-water preparations have become popular, resulting from some perceived disadvantages of ethanol-water combinations (see the previous discussion). A less important reason in real terms is that glycerol is seen to be less toxic than is ethanol. However, glycerol is chemically classified as an alcohol and is also toxic at high levels. The 26th edition of *Martindale's Extra Pharmacopoeia* states that large doses of glycerol by mouth can exert systemic effects such as headache, thirst, and nausea. The injection of large doses may induce convulsions, paralysis, and hemolysis. A 2.6% solution of glycerol will cause 100% hemolysis of red blood cells. Glycerol has an irritant effect on the gastric mucosa when given at concentrations greater than 40%, and large oral doses of glycerol caused signs that were misdiagnosed as cardiac arrest in one elderly patient with hypertension.[5] The authors concluded that these elderly patients were liable to be dehydrated and that the effects from glycerol ingestion on an empty stomach may be acute.[5]

However, it must be stressed that, similar to ethanol, the low intake of glycerol involved in using herbal preparations will not cause negative health effects.

Most importantly, glycerol or glycerol-water combinations are poor solvents for many of the active components found in herbs. For example, essential oil components, resins, and many saponins will not extract well into glycerol-water combinations. Some companies have developed a special process to overcome this problem. The herb is first extracted with an ethanol-water mixture. The ethanol is then removed and replaced with glycerol. However, quantitative and qualitative analyses have been initiated using high-performance liquid chromatography (HPLC), which show that if this process is not performed correctly, considerable losses of activity can result. The removal of the ethanol may cause loss of volatile components and may also cause precipitation of active components because they are no longer soluble once the ethanol is removed or the glycerol is added. These problems can sometimes be overcome but only with great care in manufacture, dealing with each problem on a case-by-case basis.

Glycerol is a poor preservative. Several instances of homemade or commercial herbal preparations have developed bacteria or mold growths. Additionally, few studies have been conducted on the long-term chemical stability of glycerol-based herbal products.

MACERATION

As previously mentioned, the two most common extraction methods used to prepare herbal liquid products are maceration and percolation. With either technique, the solvent is termed the menstruum, and the inert, fibrous, or other insoluble material remaining after the menstruum has done its work is called the marc.

With maceration:

- The menstruum is usually an ethanol-water mixture.
- The herb is maintained in contact with the menstruum for a relatively long period.
- The process is conducted at ordinary room temperature.
- After straining, the liquid remaining in the marc is pressed out and mixed with the strained liquid. (The marc often soaks up a considerable quantity of menstruum that can only be satisfactorily recovered by pressing.)

The form of the herb varies. Although the whole herb is sometimes used, the cut herb and in some cases the powdered herb are more often used. The required amount of herb (say 1 kg) is placed in a vessel; the required amount of menstruum is also put in the vessel (say 5 L, to make a 1:5 tincture); and the vessel is closed to prevent the loss of alcohol. The vessel is shaken and the contents turned regularly, preferably daily, for a length of time that depends on the herb, but is usually from 7 to 10 days. The direction to shake or stir daily must be strictly adhered to so as to disperse the saturated layer of menstruum that surrounds the marc, thereby allowing fresh liquid to come into contact with the marc. After the prescribed time, the liquid is drained from the residue or marc. When draining is completed, the marc is put in a press to obtain that part of the menstruum that the marc absorbed.

The pressing of the marc can be done in various ways. One of the most basic is to enclose the marc in a cloth and then to manually squeeze out the menstruum. The best way of exerting pressure is to put the marc into a press. The expressed liquid is mixed with the strained liquid and the mixture left to stand until it is clear, whereupon it is filtered. Normally, no final adjustment to a definite volume is required. The reason for this omission is that the final volume of liquid extract depends on the type and efficiency of the press. Additionally, the liquid retained in the marc is of the same concentration as is the liquid that was strained off. Thus the act of making the volume up to a set amount, for example, the same amount of menstruum that was originally used, would give a final product of varying concentration, depending on the amount of menstruum left in the marc after pressing. Moreover, any adjustment would destroy the ratio of the tincture, which must be preserved for dose consistency.

PERCOLATION

In the majority of instances, percolation is considered the best method for obtaining a solution of the active principles of herbs. Briefly, percolation consists of allowing a liquid, the menstruum, to trickle slowly through a column of the herb that has been previously ground into a more or less fine powder. The liquid is carried out in a vessel called a percolator in such a way that every solid particle is, in turn, submitted to the solvent action of the gravitating fluid.

The process of percolation, as laid down in various pharmacopeias, is carried out as follows: the crude herb is reduced to a degree of fineness, which is specified for each case, and it is moistened with an amount of the menstruum, again specified for each case. The herb is evenly moistened with this amount of menstruum and then placed in a closed vessel for 4 to 24 hours. This procedure is used to allow the particles of the herb to absorb the menstruum and to swell to a certain degree. If dried herb was placed directly into the percolator and then brought into contact with the menstruum, it may in some cases swell sufficiently to completely obstruct the flow of the menstruum through the percolator. After the designated time, the moist powder is passed through a coarse sieve to break up any masses formed.

Before the percolator is packed, the bottom of the percolator must be loosely plugged with a wad of some material such as glass wool to prevent the powder from falling through the outlet and blocking it. The moist herb is now introduced into the percolator, each layer of 2 to 3 cm in thickness being lightly pressed down by means of a suitable implement. The technique of packing the percolator is fundamental to the quality of extract at the end. The percolator is now placed in position, and a sufficient quantity of the menstruum is poured on. If all the conditions have been properly observed, the menstruum will penetrate the wetted powder equally until it has passed to the bottom of the percolator.

The outlet is closed, and the percolator is now covered to prevent evaporation and left to stand (usually for 24 hours) to allow the herb to macerate in the menstruum. This maceration facilitates the extraction process. Percolation is then commenced by opening the outlet to such a degree that the liquid drops from it at a rate of 10 to 30 drops per minute. A layer of menstruum must be constantly maintained above the powder. Percolation is continued until three quarters of the volume of finished product has been collected or until the herb is exhausted. The fluid collected from the percolator is called the percolate. When the percolation is finished, the marc is often removed from the percolator and pressed, the expressed liquid is then mixed with the percolate, and a sufficient amount of menstruum is added to produce the required volume. In the case in which the marc is completely exhausted by percolation, pressing the marc is not required. The resulting percolate is then filtered.

This percolation process is sometimes described as cold percolation because it is conducted at room temperature without the application of heat.

WHY ARE 1:2 HERBAL LIQUIDS GENERALLY RECOMMENDED?

Even using percolation, manufacturing a 1:1 liquid extract (1 kg of dried herb extracted into 1 L of liquid) is difficult without using some form of concentration step. This problem occurs because the bulky nature of most herbs means that the volume of 1 kg generally far exceeds the volume of 1 L of liquid. Additionally, many manufacturers are not interested in the labor-intensive and costly requirements of doing percolation properly. Hence 1:1 liquid extracts are produced inefficiently because phytochemicals are lost or changed during a concentration step, or the herb is poorly extracted in a vain attempt to produce a highly concentrated product by limiting the amount of solvent, or both.

This problem was the main reason why herbalists throughout the world in the 1970s moved to adopt tinctures as their preferred liquid products. However, because traditional dose information was typically based on high-quality 1:1 extracts, the use of these more dilute preparations resulted in a reduction of the actual dose given to patients.

Approximately 20 years ago the author of this text chose 1:2 liquid extracts made by cold percolation as a preferred preparation because they represented the best of both worlds. Similar to tinctures, liquid extracts do not need heating or a concentration step in their manufacture, thus no risk occurs to the delicate balance of the phytochemical spectrum of the original herb. However, liquid extracts are sufficiently concentrated to allow the convenient use of pharmacologically effective doses. A true, well-extracted 1:1 liquid extract cannot be made without using a concentration step (meaning that at least 2 L of percolate needs to be produced for every 1 kg of herb, which is then concentrated back to 1 L). In contrast, 1:2 extracts can achieve high-extraction efficiencies.

The argument holds that 1:2 extracts are relatively new, are not mentioned in the British Herbal Pharmacopoeia 1983 (BHP) or other pharmacopeias, and therefore should not be used. In fact, 1:2 extracts are mentioned in nineteenth century texts[6,7] and are described in the seventh edition of the German pharmacopeia (Deutsches Arzneibuch [DAB], published in 1968).[8] The seventh edition of the DAB actually defines a liquid extract as a 1:2 extract.[9] Therefore the precedent for their use is ample.

FRESH PLANT TINCTURES

In recent times, the use of tinctures made from the fresh plant has become popular among some herbalists. The belief is often that a fresh plant tincture better reflects the plant's "vitality" or "energy" and therefore will be a more therapeutic preparation. Other practitioners believe that a fresh plant tincture will better preserve the delicate active components of the plant.

On the other hand, the following observations need to be considered:

- The evidence from phytochemical analysis that fresh plant tinctures contain better levels of active components than do dried plant tinctures is generally lacking. In fact, fresh plant tinctures are usually prepared in a low-alcohol environment (see later discussion), which means that some less polar (more lipophilic) components may be only poorly extracted. Furthermore, the enzymatic activity of the plant material may not be inhibited in this low-alcohol environment, meaning that key phytochemicals may actually be decomposed during the maceration process. This fact was dramatically illustrated by Bauer, who found that cichoric acid in fresh plant preparations of Echinacea purpurea was largely decomposed by enzymatic activity.[10] Therefore what can be found in the living Echinacea plant was not preserved in the fresh plant tincture.

- Fresh plant tinctures were never official. Although fresh plant preparations were included in homeopathic pharmacopeias (which is understandable, given the energetic considerations in homeopathy), they were never listed in conventional pharmacopeias other than a few entries for stabilized fresh juices known as succi (singular: succus). Hence the use of a wide range of fresh plant tinctures is travel into unknown territory.

- Because of the water content of fresh plant tinctures, making preparations that are stronger than a 1:5 on a dry-weight basis is difficult. This problem can be readily illustrated by the following example. A leafy, fresh plant material typically contains 80% moisture. Therefore 100 g of this material represents 20 g of dried herb. To make a 1:5 tincture, this 20-g equivalent of dried herb must be mixed with 100 ml of liquid menstruum. However, 80 ml of water already exists from the herb itself. Therefore to preserve the 1:5 ratio, only 20 ml of 96% ethanol can be added. This 20 ml of ethanol is not enough to physically extract the bulky 100 g of fresh plant material. However, what is probably just as detrimental is that the effective ethanol percentage is only 20% (20 ml of ethanol and 80 g [or ml] of water from the fresh plant). This amount is too low to extract lipophilic components and barely enough to preserve the tincture. Some authors suggest using multiple maceration to overcome this problem, whereby the resultant tincture is macerated with a new batch of fresh herb, but this only makes the situation worse, diluting the alcohol to below the level that can stabilize the final tincture.

In summary:

- 100 g of a fresh plant containing 80% moisture is macerated in 20 ml of solvent (alcohol-water).
- The dried herb weight is 20 g.
- The amount of liquid is 80 ml (moisture from the fresh plant) + 20 ml (solvent) = 100 ml.
- Hence the result is equivalent to a 1:5 tincture on a dry-weight basis (20-g dried herb:100-ml liquid).
- However, the result may be even weaker because of the enzymatic decomposition and the low effective ethanol percentage.

Clearly from the previous discussion, given that the water content of fresh leafy plant material varies from 75% to 90%, the only practical way to make a reliable fresh plant tincture is to work on an equivalent dried herb ratio of 1:10. (Perhaps a 1:5 ratio can be achieved for roots, barks, and seeds that contain less moisture.) However, because the use of 1:10 or even 1:5 tinctures makes therapeutic doses of most herbs difficult, the herbal practitioner who endorses pharmacologic dosing will generally find little advantage in using fresh plant tinctures. Some exceptions occur based on traditional use or instances when the herb is so potent that it is normally used as a tincture (e.g., poke root, Thuja), but these are few.

From the previous discussion, a fresh plant tincture will never be as strong as will a 1:1 or 1:2 liquid extract, provided that:

a. The liquid extract has been made from carefully harvested and dried raw material of high quality.

b. The correct ethanol percentage was used to extract the dried herb.

c. No steps were used in manufacturing (e.g., exposure to high temperatures) that will damage the delicate active component spectrum of the plant.

Dried plant preparations made in such a way will still preserve the "vitality" or "energy" of the original plant, which is embodied in its chemical complexity. Fig. 1-1 gives a visual comparison of a dried plant extract **(A)** with a fresh plant tincture **(B)** using a paper chromatography technique known as vertical capillary dynamolysis. Adherents to the anthroposophy movement believe this technique can demonstrate the "vitality" of a preparation under test. Although the analysis of the chromatograms is subjective, the

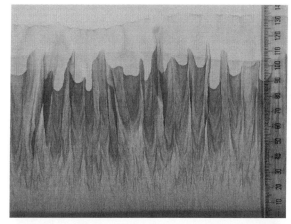

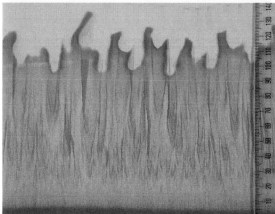

Fig. 1-1 A visual comparison of a dried plant extract **(A)** and fresh plant tincture **(B)** obtained by a paper chromatography technique (vertical capillary dynamolysis).

figure does show that a "vitality" to dried plant extracts exists.

Some practitioners use fresh plant preparations that are 1:3 or 1:5 (or even 1:10) based on fresh weight in the mistaken belief that they are using highly active preparations. However, a simple mathematical calculation shows that these practitioners are deceiving themselves. Taking a 1:5 fresh weight ratio as an example and assuming again that the herb contains 80% moisture, the following calculations can be made. If 100 g of fresh herb is macerated in 500 ml of menstruum, the dry-weight equivalent of herb is 20 g, and the total amount of liquid is 500 ml plus the 80 ml from the plant, which equals 580 ml. Hence the so-called 1:5 tincture is actually 1:29 on a dry-weight basis—completely unsuitable for therapeutic herbal doses.

GALENICAL EXTRACTS AND THE CONCEPT OF SYNERGY

A galenical extract is a traditional pharmacopeial extract of an herb. Guidelines were laid down in the various pharmacopeias (e.g., earlier versions of the British Pharmaceutical Codex) that defined the method of preparation, the extracting solvent (which was usually a combination of ethanol and water), and the ratio of the starting material (the herb) to finished product (the extract). Galenical extracts are usually in liquid form, typically the tinctures and liquid extracts already described in this chapter. However, with the modern trend to solid-dose forms, quite often, a galenical extract is dried to its solid residue and incorporated into a tablet or capsule.

Herbalists often regard galenical extracts as "whole" extracts in that they extract a comprehensive spectrum of the phytochemical content of the plant. Although this practice is generally the case, the reader should keep in mind that alcohol-water mixtures are still selective solvents and do not equally extract everything from the plant that is extractable. Something will always be left behind, depending on the percentage of ethanol that is chosen for the solvent. The ethanol percentages laid down in the pharmacopeias therefore represent what was thought to be the optimum solvent for extracting the widest activity from the herb in question. As mentioned previously, the percentages were often chosen with regard to the particular phytochemical classes known to occur in the plant; for example, a higher ethanol percentage was chosen for herbs containing resins or essential oils and so on as already mentioned.

The main reason why herbalists prefer "whole" or galenical extracts is their belief that the active component is the herb itself. In other words, all of the phytochemicals in the plant act together to confer the therapeutic benefit. According to Sharma:[11]

> ... the active ingredient model does not stem from a strength of the scientific method, as often supposed; rather it stems from a weakness—from the inability of the reductionist methods to deal with complex systems.

One of the underlying motivations for using galenical extracts is the concept of synergy. Synergy is an important concept in herbal pharmacology. In the context of a mixture of chemicals (e.g., an herbal extract), synergy applies if the therapeutic action of the chemical mixture is greater than the arithmetic sum of the actions of the mixture's components. In other words, the whole is greater than the sum of the individual parts. A well-known example of synergy is exploited in the use of insecticidal pyrethrins. A chemical synergist known as piperonyl butoxide, which has little insecticidal activity of its own, interferes with the insect's ability to break down the pyrethrins, thereby substantially increasing their toxicity. This example emphasizes what is probably an important mechanism behind the synergy observed for medicinal plant components: increased or prolonged levels of key components at the active site. In other words, components of plants that are not active themselves can act to improve the stability, solubility, bioavailability, or half-life of the active components. Hence a particular chemical might, in pure form, have only a fraction of the pharmacologic activity that it has in its plant matrix. This important example of synergy therefore has a pharmacokinetic basis.

An excellent discussion of synergy in the context of herbal therapy was provided by E. M. Williamson.[12] According to the author, "It is almost inescapable that these interactions between ingredients will occur; however, whether the effects are truly synergistic or merely additive is open to question..." In other words, the more likely interaction between the components of a galenical extract is an addition of their pharmacologic effects, rather than true synergy. Even in this case, the "whole" will still be better than a selection of the parts.

As previously inferred, one area in which synergistic interactions probably apply is that of the enhanced bioavailability of key components. Eder and Mehnert discussed the basic issues, and examples can be found in the scientific literature.[13] The isoflavone glycoside daidzin given in crude extract of *Pueraria lobata* achieves much greater concentrations in plasma than does equivalent doses of pure daidzin.[14] Ascorbic acid in a citrus extract was more bioavailable than was ascorbic acid alone.[15] Coadministration of procyanidins from *Hypericum perforatum* (St. John's wort) significantly increased the *in vivo* antidepressant effects of hypericin and pseudohypericin. This effect was attributed to the observed enhanced solubility of hypericin and pseudohypericin in the presence of procyanidins. The result also indicates that pure hypericin and pseudohypericin have considerably less antidepressant activity than do their equivalent amounts in St. John's wort extract.[16]

However, synergy can also have a pharmacodynamic basis. One example is the antibacterial activity of major components of lemon grass essential oil. Although geranial and neral individually elicit antibacterial action, the third main component, myrcene, did not show any activity. However, myrcene enhanced antibacterial activities when mixed with either of the other two main components.[17] Sennoside A and sennoside C from senna have similar laxative activities in mice. However, a mixture of these compounds in the ratio 7:3 (which somewhat reflects the relative levels found in senna leaf) has almost double the laxative activity.[18]

Additional examples of synergy for galenical extracts are provided by Williamson and include kava, valerian, dragon's blood, and *Artemisia annua*.[12]

QUALITY ISSUES FOR HERBAL LIQUIDS

NECESSITY FOR PHARMACEUTICAL GOOD MANUFACTURING PRACTICE

In a number of countries, including those in Europe, as well as Japan and Australia, all herbal products must, by law, be made according to the code of pharmaceutical good manufacturing practice (GMP). This code is a fail-safe system of quality assurance and quality control that defines a number of procedures and observances, including:

- Validation of equipment and processes
- Documented standard operating procedures covering every aspect of manufacture
- Documented cleaning and calibration logs for equipment
- Control of the manufacturing environment, air, and water
- Quarantining and unique identification and testing of raw materials, labels, and packaging
- Discrete batch identification
- Comprehensive batch record documentation
- Reconciliation of raw materials, product, packaging, and labels
- Quarantining and testing of finished products
- Documented release for sale procedures
- Testing of stability of finished product
- Documentation of customer complaints and recall procedures

Although some large herbal medicine manufacturers in the United States voluntarily comply with close to full pharmaceutical GMP, the recently proposed legal requirement is that less than full GMP (the smaller GMPs) will need to be adhered to (at the time of writing, not yet law in the United States). The smaller GMPs are a series of quality requirements that, taken together, do not amount to full pharmaceutical GMP. Currently, most herbal companies in the United States operate under food GMP, which is an even lower quality standard.

In practice, herbal manufacturing under pharmaceutical GMP is probably more complex than it is for conventional drugs because an herb is biologically defined and:

- May be incorrectly identified
- May vary in chemical content and hence efficacy
- Carries with it a history (e.g., may be contaminated with unwanted substances)
- Processing of herbs may enhance or impair their safety and efficacy
- Stability may be difficult to define and measure

Nevertheless, all of these considerations point strongly to the importance of herbal products being made under appropriate pharmaceutical GMP. However, a specialized phytochemical knowledge is also required to deal with these issues.

As part of pharmaceutical GMP, herbal raw materials should be subjected to a battery of tests to ensure their quality and purity. These tests are outlined in Box 1-1. The BHP provides a useful guide to the British and European standards in these areas.[19]

Thin-layer chromatography (TLC) is a particularly useful technique for the identification of plant material. TLC can also be used to quantify plant constituents. The process of performing TLC is outlined in Box 1-2.

Finished herbal products also need to undergo testing before their release. Box 1-3 provides examples of possible testing protocols for finished herbal liquids.

MARKER COMPOUNDS AND ACTIVE CONSTITUENTS

In Boxes 1-1 and 1-3, reference is made to active or marker compounds. The opinion of this author holds that producing a galenical liquid extract that is set to

---

BOX 1-1

Herbal Raw Material Testing

- Identity and quality with thin-layer chromatography (TLC)
- Microscopic analysis
- Macroscopic analysis and organoleptic assessment
- Pesticide residues
- Microbial levels
- Aflatoxins
- Heavy metals
- Foreign material
- Infestation
- Radiation levels
- Active or marker compounds (quantitative)

contain a minimum level of a carefully chosen marker compound or group of marker compounds is often advantageous. In fact, setting this minimum level is more than just advantageous; it is a positive step in the development of herbal quality, provided that the considerations discussed later are observed. Serious herbal clinicians should prefer such quantified activity liquid extracts.

Marker compounds are characteristic phytochemicals found in a plant that are chosen to represent a standard for quality. Hence in the case of say passion flower (*Passiflora incarnata*), the marker compound is often chosen to be the flavonoid isovitexin. Marker compounds are not necessarily active compounds (see later discussion). However, if well chosen, marker compounds do serve a useful function in terms of quality, such as the

BOX 1-2

Thin-Layer Chromatography (TLC)

- An extract of an herb is spotted at the bottom of a thin layer of silica gel on a glass plate.
- The plate is dipped in a solvent mixture.
- The solvent draws up the layer and carries the components in the herb for different distances.
- Sprays, ultraviolet light, or both are used to view the components, giving a characteristic pattern of spots.
- Each spot corresponds to a component in the herb.
- Different solvent systems draw out different classes of components in the herb.

BOX 1-3

Quality Considerations for Finished Herbal Liquid Products

- Extraction efficiency
- Identity
  a. Organoleptic assessment
  b. TLC or HPLC fingerprint
- Active or marker components
- Microbial testing
  a. Total count
  b. Pathogens
  c. Yeast and mold
- Pesticides

purposes of identification and ensuring appropriate drying, handling, and extraction of the herbal starting material.

To achieve a consistent level of a marker compound (or compounds) in a liquid extract, the starting herbal raw material will usually need to contain a minimum acceptable level. This measure implies consistent quality practices in terms of harvesting, drying, and storage of the herb. Additionally, the way in which the herb is processed, such as extraction conditions and choice of solvent, will need to be carefully controlled. As a consequence, fixing a galenical extract to a consistent level of marker compound or compounds will also likely render the extract more or less consistent in terms of other phytochemical components, at least for that particular manufacturer. This aspect underpins much of the utility of such extracts as consistent products.

Active constituents are phytochemicals, which are important for a given therapeutic effect of an herbal extract. Although this issue is highly complex, one proposition is simple and clear: marker compounds are not necessarily active compounds. Hence when *Ginkgo biloba* leaf standardized extract (GBE) was originally manufactured to contain 24% ginkgo flavone glycosides, no unequivocal evidence existed that these compounds conferred the various and exciting therapeutic activities that had been discovered for the extract. Later research suggested that a different group of phytochemicals, the ginkgolides and bilobalide, were more important, and GBE is now standardized for these as well. However, in terms of, for example, its effects in Alzheimer's disease, results did not show which are the active compounds in GBE. Even if the ginkgolides and bilobalide were found to be important (this might be achieved by a clinical trial comparing two Ginkgo extracts with high and low levels of these compounds which were otherwise identical), it would be unlikely that they were the only compounds important for activity.

Such a dilemma supports the basic premise of herbalists that the true active component is the herbal extract itself. Nonetheless, also likely is that an extract low in marker compounds, which from pharmacologic experiments have been found to have some relevant activity, will be less likely to confer a therapeutic effect and hence be of poorer quality.

This last point underlies an important issue with marker compounds: they should be chosen carefully. Preference must be given to phytochemicals that (on the basis of current knowledge) are likely to have pharmacologic activity, which is relevant to the proposed clinical use of the extract. On the other hand, if a marker compound is chosen that has no known useful pharmacologic activity, it should not be optimized in the extract at the expense of other phytochemicals. For example, selecting for and optimizing echinacoside levels in *Echinacea angustifolia* at the expense of alkylamides is likely to lead to a less active product. When the marker compound is inactive (on current knowledge), the safest approach to take is to produce a normal galenical extract using the marker as a quality guide only. However, selecting a different marker is preferable.

The great body of pharmacologic and clinical evidence that researchers have for an herb sometimes relates only to the use of one isolated, purified constituent. Good examples are ephedrine from Ephedra and berberine from *Berberis* species. Clearly, believing that extracts of these herbs should be quantified for these compounds makes sense. On the other hand, the temptation to regard the herbal extract in question as merely a carrier of this constituent should be resisted. The whole extract will confer matrix effects, which might modify the activity of these key compounds.

STANDARDIZED EXTRACTS

In the herbal context, a standardized extract is an herbal extract that is made to a consistent standard. This standard can be quite simple, such as the ratio of the starting herbal raw material to the finished extract. Hence a 4:1 extract, whereby 4 kg of dried herb is extracted to yield 1 kg of final extract, can technically be called a standardized extract. Generally however, the term has a more specific meaning: a standardized extract is one that is manufactured to contain a consistent level of one or more phytochemical constituents that are derived from the original starting material.

The aim of standardized extracts is to achieve consistent activity of an herbal product from batch to batch. Depending on the circumstances, this consistency is not always the case. If compounds other than the chosen marker compounds are important for activity, and these are not also fixed at consistent levels by the manufacturing process, then a standardized extract will not achieve consistent activity. If the analytical method chosen is not specific enough towards the desired marker compounds, the result will be failure of batch-to-batch consistency, even though the certificate of analysis of the extract will provide data to suggest the same "activity" for each batch.

Standardized extracts are not a guarantee of quality, as they are often represented. Inappropriate choice of marker compounds, poor design or execution of analytical methods, spiking with pure phytochemicals or other substances, or failure to demonstrate phytoequivalence (that is, containing the equivalent phytochemical

spectrum) can mean that the standardized extract is poorer in quality or less effective compared with a well-made galenical extract. Only the manufacturers who practice good science and have a comprehensive understanding of the many complex issues that affect herbal quality will be able to produce meaningful standardized extracts.

Many standardized extracts are nothing more than "improved" galenical extracts. Provided these extracts are produced carefully from good quality starting herb and the ethanol percentage, marker compounds, and analytical methodology are appropriately chosen, this development is positive in herbal therapy, which is to be commended.

Standardized extracts other than the galenical type include selective phytochemical extracts (in which one particular phytochemical group is selectively extracted from the herb) and highly concentrated extracts (usually greater than 10:1). Both of these extracts are made by processes different from those used in the manufacture of galenical type standardized extracts. They may involve extraction with solvents different than ethanol-water mixtures (e.g., acetone, chloroform, liquid carbon dioxide), multiple solvent extraction steps, and standard chemical isolation techniques (e.g., chromatography columns, ion exchange resins, precipitation).

Selective phytochemical extracts and highly concentrated extracts are also covered by the general term of "standardized extracts"; but these products are quite different from standardized galenical extracts. In a few cases, whether these products can even be called herbal products is arguable. However, provided these extracts are supported by sound clinical and safety data, they do have a role in modern phytotherapy. The temptation among scientists and physicians is to regard these products as true "herbal therapy" when, in fact, they are only a minor part of a therapeutic system that draws from many hundreds, if not thousands, of galenical extracts.

ADVANCED METHODS FOR QUALITY CONTROL OF HERBAL LIQUIDS

The accurate determination of active or marker compounds requires advanced methods of chemical analysis. Chromatography, particularly HPLC, is ideally suited to the analysis of herbal liquids; but gas chromatography can also be a valuable technique.

High Performance Liquid Chromatography. Chromatographic techniques incorporate a means of separating the chemical components of a mixture and a means of detecting these components. In the case of HPLC, the separation technique is a narrow column packed with a suitable chemical through which a liquid (mixture of solvents) containing the test mixture is driven at high pressure. As the separated chemical components of the mixture emerge from the column one by one, they are detected using an appropriate technique. The results are displayed graphically: each peak on the graph corresponds to a component of the mixture (e.g., an herbal extract). The area of each peak is proportional to the amount of chemical component present. This test can be used to measure each chemical compound, provided a suitable chemical reference material (which is often the compound itself) is available. Under the same chromatographic conditions, a given compound will take the same time to travel through the column. This characteristic is known as the retention time and provides information about the identity of the compound.

The most common detection system used in HPLC is the absorption of light by the compound as it passes a detector. This light can cover a wide spectrum from ultraviolet to visible wavelengths, referred to as UV-VIS in the jargon. In more sophisticated modern machines, the complete UV-VIS spectrum of the compound can be determined as it passes the detector. The detection system capable of performing this task is called a diode array detector. This spectrum also provides valuable information about the identity of the compound.

Other detection systems used in HPLC that can also provide information about the amount of the compound present and its identity as well include mass spectrometry and, in highly expensive and sophisticated equipment, nuclear magnetic resonance.

Gas Chromatography. In the case of gas chromatography (GC), the chemical mixture is driven through a long glass capillary column by an inert gas such as nitrogen. This technique is suitable only for volatile substances, such as essential oils. Alternatively, nonvolatile substances can be made volatile by first reacting them with another chemical, a technique known as derivatization.

The detection system often used in GC is flame ionization detection (FID). As each compound emerges from the column, it is combusted in a flame, which generates ions that are transformed into an electrical signal. Again, the results are displayed graphically (often referred to as the trace) with each peak on the graph corresponding to a compound in the mixture (e.g., an essential oil).

FID does not provide any information about the identity of each compound peak in the trace (other than that provided by the individual retention times). Therefore a more sophisticated technique that is capable of providing this additional information is being increasingly used. This technique is known as gas chromatography with mass spectrometry detection (GC-MS).

EXAMPLES OF COMMONLY ENCOUNTERED QUALITY PROBLEMS

Substitution. The issue of substitution is the most significant quality issue for herbal medicine today, and some relatively common problems for herbal liquids are discussed here.

Arnica. *Arnica montana* is becoming increasingly rare in the wild; hence substitution with *Arnica chamissonis* is now permitted in the pharmacopeias. The therapeutic properties are quite similar. However, another substitution is more widespread, presumably because of the high cost of authentic *Arnica* species. This substitution is with *Heterotheca inuloides* (Mexican arnica), which resembles Arnica very closely in the dried form. The *German Pharmacopeia* (DAB 10) provides methods for the ready differentiation between authentic and Mexican arnica. *Heterotheca inuloides* contains the flavonoids rutin and hyperoside, whereas authentic Arnica does not.[20]

Brahmi. Both *Centella asiatica* (gotu kola) and *Bacopa monnieri* have the same common name of Brahmi in India, and they are often interchanged.[20] Detection of gotu kola's characteristic compounds is readily achieved by HPLC, which allows easy differentiation between the two herbs (Fig. 1-2).

Devil's claw. *Harpagophytum procumbens* (devil's claw) is a slow-growing tuber from southwest Africa, traditionally wild crafted, but cultivation is now underway. Substitution with the related species *Harpagophytum zeyheri* has been widespread, with most of the pre-1990s clinical work apparently being performed on a variable mixture of the two species. The substitution is made during harvesting when the tubers are collected from the wild. A proposal to allow this admixture was put forth in the literature but was rejected. HPLC using diode array detection enables ready differentiation between the two mixtures and detection of admixtures. The compound 8-para-coumaryl harpagide (8-PCHG) is present in only small amounts in *H. procumbens*, but in larger amounts in *H. zeyheri*. The key marker compound harpagoside is present in both species. If a ratio of harpagoside to 8-PCHG of greater than 10 is set as a quality standard for *H. procumbens*, then substitution with or admixture with *H. zeyheri* is readily detected. Analysis of liquid products on the Australian market indicated the presence of products containing significant amounts of *H. zeyheri*.[21]

Golden seal. Golden seal root (*Hydrastis canadensis*) is a very expensive and endangered herb. Responsible practitioners should use this herb only from cultivated sources. The expense and the environmental issue has naturally led to the search for substitutions, some openly stated and others not. Common substitutions

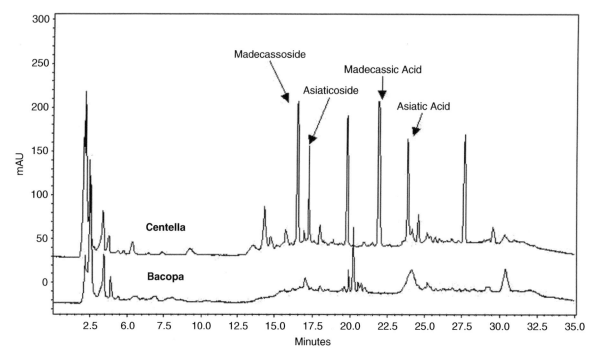

Fig. 1-2 HPLC trace of Bacopa *(Bacopa monnieri)* and gotu kola *(Centella asiatica)* extracts showing the peaks of the major active constituents in gotu kola.

for golden seal are golden thread (*Coptis chinensis*), barberry (*Berberis vulgaris*), Indian barberry (*Berberis aristata*), and Oregon grape (*Berberis aquifolium*). All of the varieties have the intense yellow color of golden seal because of their berberine content but are lacking the key and characteristic alkaloid of golden seal, namely hydrastine.[20] In fact, hydrastine is probably found only in golden seal.

Authentic liquid extract or tincture of golden seal is readily differentiated from its substitutes (or admixtures with them, which is also common) by HPLC using diode array detection (Fig. 1-3). A small peak for a berberine-related compound appears before berberine in the substitutes. If this peak is present, then golden seal has been mixed with a substitute herb. If hydrastine is absent, then the substitution is 100%.

A recent survey of eight golden seal root samples and two products in the United States found that only five of the eight root samples and neither of the products contained hydrastine.[22] Surprisingly, one of the eight root samples contained no berberine. Hence, of the 10 "golden seal" products or root samples, only five were authentic. Some of the authentic five might have also been mixed with substitute herbs, which was not determined in the study.

One enterprising company has suggested that it can supply Indian golden seal (*Hydrastis mamira*) as an alternative to *Hydrastis canadensis*. However, *Hydrastis mamira* does not exist botanically. In fact, there is only one other species of Hydrastis, a Japanese species, Hydrastis jezoensis. A species of Coptis (*Coptis teeta*) is found in India, which has the Hindi name mamira. The product in question was found to contain berberine but not hydrastine.

Skullcap. Skullcap (*Scutellaria lateriflora*) is a widely used but poorly investigated herb (Fig. 1-4). Until quite recently, its characteristic flavonoid profile was unknown. Now, skullcap has been shown that baicalin (also the main flavonoid in Baical skullcap—*Scutellaria baicalensis*) is the main flavonoid in *S. lateriflora*, not scutellarin, which is reported in the traditional literature.[23] The Australian Therapeutic Goods Administration (TGA) recognized adulteration problems with skullcap and enforced product recalls on several manufacturers in the 1990s. Substitution is often with other species of *Scutellaria*. However, a more sinister substitution is that with *Teucrium chamaedrys* (germander) and other species of Teucrium. This is a significant issue because germander has been linked to rare but fatal liver damage.

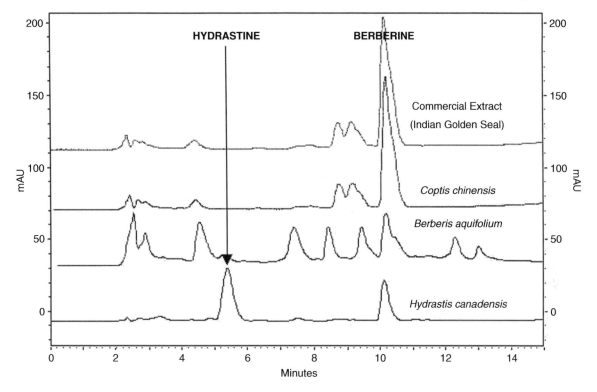

Fig. 1-3 HPLC trace of golden seal, golden thread, Oregon grape, and an adulterated commercial herbal extract. The constituent hydrastine is contained only in the authentic golden seal extract.

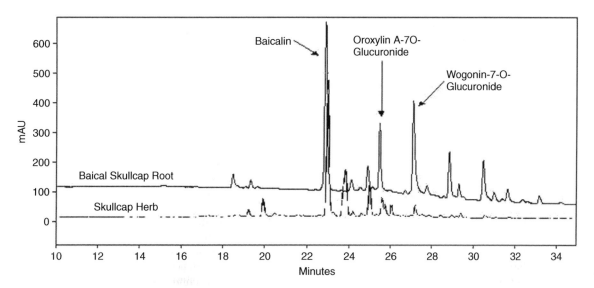

Fig. 1-4 HPLC trace of skullcap and Baical skullcap showing the main flavonoids present in each herbal extract.

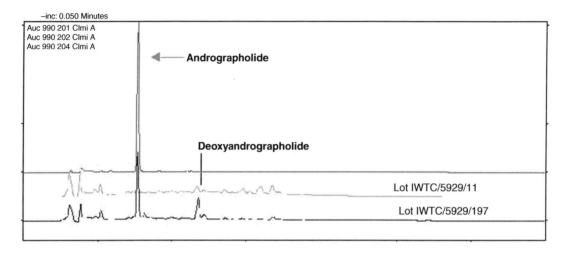

Fig. 1-5 HPLC trace showing key marker compounds present and absent in two herbal extracts of *Andrographis paniculata*.

Stephania or Aristolochia. Aristolochia is commonly substituted for several Chinese herbs, but particularly *Stephania tetrandra*. The problem with this substitution is that Aristolochia is highly toxic and can cause renal failure. Aristolochia contains aristolochic acid, whereas *Stephania* contains tetrandrine, which allows ready differentiation by HPLC using diode array detection. A survey of eight products sold as *Stephania tetrandra* by Chinese herb wholesalers in Australia and Hong Kong found that only one was authentic.[24] Authorities such as the U.S. Food and Drug Administration (FDA), the Australian TGA, and the British Medicines Control Agency (MCA) have issued high-level warnings about this widespread substitution. Other Chinese herbs such as Asarum are also substituted with *Aristolochia* species.

Valerian. European valerian (*Valeriana officinalis*) is substituted with cheaper forms of valerian such as Indian valerian (*Valeriana wallichii*). Only European valerian contains valerenic acid, which allows the positive identification of this species.[20]

Key Marker Compounds Absent from the Herb. Key marker compounds that are known to occur in an herb at significant levels are sometimes absent in a product made from that herb. This absence may be a result of poor raw material or inappropriate processing. For example, as shown in Fig. 1-5, an Andrographis extract (lot IWTC/5929/11) supposedly standardized to andrographolide (by an inappropriate gravimetric technique) was found by HPLC to contain virtually no andrographolide.[24]

The species *Coleus forskohlii* exhibits varieties that do not contain the important marker compound forskolin.

Some Echinacea products on the market lack the presence of alkylamides (which are often lost in processing). The Chinese herb *Paeonia lactiflora* (white peony) contains the important marker compound paeoniflorin. However, depending on how the herb is processed (according to traditional dictates), all the paeoniflorin can be lost (Fig. 1-6).[24]

Wide Variations in Marker Compounds. This problem is typically common in the galenical extracts that are not quantified activity extracts. The problem also exists in other products manufactured from galenical extracts such as tablets and capsules.

One example has been chosen from the literature. The following is a survey of *Echinacea purpurea* products on the Australian market carried out by Professor R. Wills and D. Stuart. These researchers tested for alkylamides and caffeoyl phenols (mainly cichoric acid) and found a huge variation in the levels of these compounds (Table 1-1).[25]

STABILITY ISSUES FOR HERBAL LIQUIDS

Some educators have suggested that herbal liquids are a less desirable dose form because they are less stable than are solid-dose preparations. However, objective evidence to back up this assertion is scarce. Some companies now undertake stability studies on their herbal liquids as a requirement of pharmaceutical GMP, and this author's experience in this field indicates that most liquids maintain their phytochemical profiles within the normal shelf-life requirements of 2 to 3 years.

Therefore provided herbal liquids are purchased through an herbal manufacturer that operates under

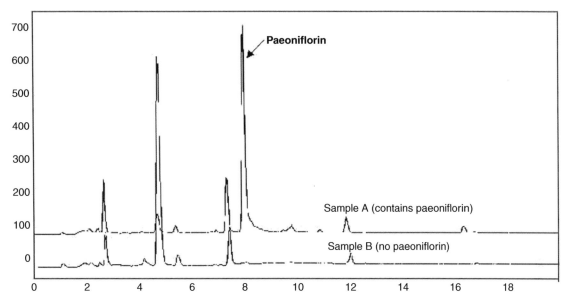

Fig. 1-6 HPLC trace of two white peony *(Paeonia lactiflora)* extracts indicating the presence or absence of the marker compound paeoniflorin.

TABLE 1-1

Alkylamide and Caffeoyl Phenol Levels (mg) in Different Types of Manufactured Echinacea Products[25]

	No. of Products	ALKYLAMIDES		CAFFEOYL PHENOLS	
		Mean	Range	Mean	Range
		CONCENTRATION PER g (ml) OF PRODUCT			
Tablets, capsules	14	0.49	0.0-1.4	2.39	0.2-6.0
Liquid extracts					
Retail	9	0.45	0.0-1.6	1.19	0.0-3.9
Naturopath	9	0.80	0.0-1.9	1.91	0.1-4.7
		CONCENTRATION PER g ADDED ECHINACEA			
Tablets, capsules	14	0.47	0.0-1.7	3.04	0.4-5.7
Liquid extracts					
Retail	9	1.29	0.0-3.8	2.91	0.0-7.1
Naturopath	9	1.25	0.0-1.9	3.19	0.1-4.7

pharmaceutical GMP and has a comprehensive stability program in place, keeping to within expiry dates is sufficient to ensure retained activity, provided of course that the manufacturer's recommended storage conditions are observed. Sunlight is particularly damaging to the phytochemicals in an herbal liquid, thus they must be stored in amber glass bottles away from direct sunlight. Temperature is also an important factor.

Generally, storage below 30°C (86°F) is recommended (temperatures occasionally above 30°C (86°F) will not cause a problem, provided that the average is below this level). Additionally, a minimal storage temperature of 10°C (50°F) should be maintained. Some herbal liquids such as celery and wild yam will form into a gel if they become too cold. Although gentle reheating will generally make these gels liquid again, irreversible changes may occur if the cold conditions are prolonged.

Many herbal liquids develop a sediment over time. Provided that the extract has not been heated during its manufacture, sedimentation is a natural occurrence that generally has only a minor impact on quality. A common question among practitioners is whether this sediment should be rejected or redispersed into the liquid (for mixtures of several herbal liquids, the sediment should always be redispersed; see later discussion). Although no hard and fast rules exist here, a general guide is that if the sediment has tended to aggregate or concrete into a hard mass, then it should be rejected. If, however, the sediment is fine and easily redispersed, then the bottle should be shaken to do this before dispensing.

If decanting is used to avoid dispensing any sediment, this can lead to wastage of liquid, because a small but significant amount of liquid in association with the sediment will be rejected when the bottle is almost empty. One way to avoid this wastage is to instead filter the dregs to recover the last amount of liquid. This procedure need not be done using a fine filter paper. A fine clean cloth will often suffice, and the rate of filtration will be much quicker than that through a filter paper.

Whether to reject or redisperse a sediment is really at the discretion of the practitioner. However, the following list can serve as a guide. The herbs listed are those for which the author believes the sediment should be rejected. Although this list is not comprehensive, it does include several herbs that are not covered in this text.

Product	Botanical Name
Albizia	*Albizia lebbeck*
Angelica	*Angelica archangelica*
Baical skullcap	*Scutellaria baicalensis*
Bayberry	*Myrica cerifera*
Bearberry	*Arctostaphylos uva-ursi*
Beth root	*Trillium erectum*
Blood root	*Sanguinaria canadensis*
Cascara	*Rhamnus purshiana*
Cranesbill	*Geranium maculatum*
Elder flower	*Sambucus nigra*
Ephedra	*Ephedra sinica*
Globe artichoke	*Cynara scolymus*
Goat's rue	*Galega officinalis*
Jambul	*Syzygium jambolanum*
Ladies mantle	*Alchemilla vulgaris*
Marshmallow leaf	*Althaea officinalis*
Phyllanthus	*Phyllanthus amarus*
Pinellia	*Pinellia ternata*

Raspberry leaf	*Rubus idaeus*
Rhubarb root	*Rheum palmatum*
Rosemary	*Rosmarinus officinalis*
Rue	*Ruta graveolens*
Sage	*Salvia officinalis*
Senna pods	*Cassia spp*
Skullcap	*Scutellaria lateriflora*
St. John's wort	*Hypericum perforatum*
White peony	*Paeonia lactiflora*
Wild cherry	*Prunus serotina*
Yellow dock	*Rumex crispus*

DOSAGE ISSUES FOR HERBAL LIQUIDS

The dosage flexibility offered by using herbal liquids has led to considerable disparity over what is considered to be a therapeutic dose. This problem is generally not the case for solid-dose forms such as tablets for which a minimum possible dose exists (one half or one tablet), and the manufacturer usually provides specific dose recommendations.

This disparity can be illustrated by the example of St. John's wort. The effective dose of St. John's wort in tablet form for depression has been established by clinical trials at three doses of 300 mg of dry extract per day. The dry extract is standardized to 0.3% hypericin and usually represents at least a five times the concentration of the original dried herb. Hence the clinically effective dose of St. John's wort equates to approximately 4.5 g of herb (900 mg of extract) per day. Now, the corresponding amount of 1:5 dried herb tincture per day is 5×4.5 g, which equals 22.5 ml (almost one ounce of tincture). As an aside, this example further illustrates the value of 1:2 extracts, given that the equivalent daily dose is only 9 ml, which is much more achievable.

Despite the fact that the clinically established antidepressant dose for a St. John's wort tincture is in the region of 22.5 ml of tincture per day, some herbalists routinely prescribe 10 to 20 drops, three to four times a day; and some of these practitioners also occasionally use St. John's wort tablets at the correct (clinically established) doses! Clearly, such a difference in dosage approaches is difficult to rationalize.

The previous example highlights another issue with liquid dosing: the use of drops as a dosage measure. Although this method can be valid for highly potent herbs such as Tylophora and Phytolacca, in general, similar to ounces, using drops is an archaic dose measure that should not be used. Recently, a National Aeronautics and Space Administration (NASA) Mars probe missed its target because of an error that was made between the conversion of pounds and feet into kilograms and meters. As in space, anachronisms have no place in modern herbal therapy. Although all solid doses are expressed in metric for both drugs and herbal products, for some reason, this is not the case with some herbal liquids.

This problem is further compounded by the fact that the drop is an inherently imprecise measure of volume. Most herbalists do not have an accurate appreciation of the amount and the variability of the drops per ml of an herbal liquid. Glib calculations are based on 20 drops per ml, but some manufacturers even claim it is as low as 12 drops per ml.

The author of this text conducted a simple experiment. A comparison of the drops per ml for five alcoholic extracts and one glycetract was conducted using two different droppers supplied by manufacturers, one with a larger bore and the other with a smaller bore. The results are summarized in Table 1-2.

These results indicate that the number of drops per ml depends on the alcohol strength of the herbal liquid, which, in turn, influences its viscosity. The approximate difference between the two alcohol extremes is almost twofold, and the drops per ml varies between 28 and 65 drops. For the milk thistle glycetract, which was by far the most viscous liquid tested, the number of drops per ml was nowhere near 12 or 20, even using the dropper with the larger bore. Clearly, there can be no general role for the drop as a reliable and consistent measure of dose.

However, the other important issue is that the use of the drop as a measure encourages low, subtherapeutic doses. How then can people arrive at the right doses of herbal liquids? Coming back to the St. John's wort example, the clinically proven therapeutic dose would equate to approximately 900 drops per day.

The subject of appropriate dose is probably the most controversial aspect of contemporary Western herbal medicine. Among Western herbal practitioners, many different dosage approaches are found from country to country and within countries. Underlying these different approaches are different philosophies about the therapeutic action of medicinal plants.

At one extreme is the assumption that the therapeutic effect relies on a specific dose of the active chemicals contained in each particular plant. At the other extreme, emphasis is often placed on the assumption that an herbal medicine, being derived from a living organism, carries a certain energy or vital force. The quality of this energy confers the therapeutic effect, and hence the amount of actual herb is not as important, as long as some is present. Other practitioners believe that perhaps the active components act as catalysts to restore health and do not need to be present in what would be considered to be pharmacologic quantities in the sensitive patient.

The low-dose approach should not be confused with homeopathy, although it has been influenced by this system. One important difference from homeopathy is that the therapeutic indications are not derived from the principal of similars and mainly come from traditional indications.

Both the high- and low-dose approaches have their adherents who maintain that their respective systems give good results in the clinic. Although labeling one approach as correct and the other incorrect is inappropriate (indeed, even high doses of herbs possibly also act in part through the energy factor or as catalysts), reviewing and contrasting current and historical dosage approaches is useful. By doing so, one can arrive at

---

TABLE 1-2

Comparison of Drop Numbers for Several Extracts Using Small and Large Bore Droppers

Product	Alcohol %	DROPS (PER ml)	
		Large Bore	Small Bore
Milk thistle 1:1 glycetract	5	28.2	33.2
Devil's claw 1:2	25	39.0	43.7
White peony 1:2	45	45.2	50.3
Celery seed 1:2	60	49.9	59.9
Myrrh 1:5	90	50.3	65.1

an appropriate dosage system for modern phytotherapy in that it is consistent with:

- Dose ranges used in other important herbal traditions, such as China and India
- Doses used by important historical movements in Western herbal medicine, such as the Eclectics
- Doses currently recommended in pharmacopeias
- Doses established from pharmacologic and clinical research

In any discussion of herbal doses, the influence of dose form and quality of preparations must also be considered, as should the mechanics of formulation and prescription writing.

REVIEW OF DOSAGE APPROACHES

Traditional Chinese Medicine. The daily dose for individual nontoxic herbs in traditional Chinese medicine (TCM) is usually in the range of 3 to 10 g, given as a decoction, or in pill or powder form.[26] Often, higher doses are prescribed by decoction than for pills, as might be expected given that not all active components readily dissolve in hot water.[27] (Pills generally consist of the powdered herb incorporated into a suitable base.) Herbs are invariably prescribed in formulations. Doses for such formulations in pill or granule form are typically 3 to 9 g taken three times daily but can be much higher in the case of decoctions.

For each individual herb, a wide dose range is usually given in texts and applies for all herbal systems. One reason for this wide range is that if an herb is used by itself, or with just a few other herbs, a larger dose is used than when it is combined with many other herbs.[27] Dose also varies according to the weight and age of patients and the severity or acuteness of their condition. Some herbs, or closely related species, are used in both Chinese and Western herbal medicine. Table 1-3 compares dosages for a few of these herbs.

In general, the similarity in the dose range between the different systems is striking. Discrepancies do exist for ginger and dandelion root, which in the case of ginger can be explained by a higher content of the active components in the alcoholic tincture compared with the decoction and in the case of dandelion may be a reflection of the different species used.

Eclectic Medicine. Eclectic medicine was a largely empirical school of medicine that developed in the United States during the nineteenth century.[28] The movement was most prominent for a brief period from the late nineteenth to the early twentieth centuries, when several teaching universities offered courses and many eminent scholars studied eclectic medicine. Although the Eclectics used simple chemical medicines such as phosphoric acid, they mainly prescribed herbs. The Eclectics' knowledge of materia medica was their greatest contribution to Western herbal therapy. For example, the Eclectics made herbs such as Echinacea and golden seal popular after observing their use by native Americans.

The Eclectics tended to use *higher* doses compared with those recommended in current texts and pharmacopeias, although the ranges tend to overlap. Table 1-4 compares dosages currently used with those found in Eclectic texts[29,30] for alcoholic extracts of herbs.

The British Herbal Pharmacopoeia. The BHP 1983 carries extensive dose information for individual herbs and is generally regarded as an important reference on this

---

TABLE 1-3

Comparison of Dosages Used in Traditional Chinese and Western Herbal Medicine

Herb	Chinese Dosage[26] (g/day)	Western Dosage[28,29] (g/day)
Ephedra sinica	3-9	3-12 (decoction) 3-9 (extract)
Zingiber officinale (ginger)	3-9	0.75-3.0 (decoction) 0.38-0.75 (tincture)
Taraxacum mongolicum (dandelion)	9-30	6-24 (decoction) 3-6 (tincture)
Glycyrrhiza uralensis (licorice)	3-12	3-12 (decoction) 6-12 (extract)
Rheum palmatum (rhubarb)	3-6	2.3-4.5 (decoction) 1.8-6.0 (extract)

Note: For dosages of tinctures and extracts given three times daily, the corresponding amount of dried herb per day has been calculated.

subject for Western herbal practitioners. Doses given in the BHP were derived from earlier texts, such as the *British Pharmacopoeia* (BP) and the *British Pharmaceutical Codex* (BPC), but also resulted from a survey of herbal practitioners. More recently, the *British Herbal Compendium* (BHC) has been published with dose information for the practitioner. Both the BHP and the BHC have been used to derive the doses for 1:2 extracts recommended in this book (via appropriate calculation mainly from tincture doses). In some cases, the 1:2 dose has been derived from the 1:1 dose.

The doses given in the BHP contain some inconsistencies. The main problem is that doses for tinctures often do not correlate to corresponding doses for liquid extracts. For a 1:1 extract and a 1:5 tincture of a particular herb to correlate in terms of dose, the dose range for the tincture should be five times that of the extract, given that the tincture is five times weaker. This problem contrasts with other pharmacopeias such as

the BPC 1934 in which the correlation is generally, but not exactly, observed. Some examples that highlight this problem are provided in Table 1-5.

This poor correlation demonstrated in Table 1-5, which, in the case for *Eupatorium purpureum* (gravel root), the tincture dose is actually *less* than the extract dose, is probably for two reasons:

- As previously stated, the BHP doses were derived in part from a survey of herbal practitioners. That different dose philosophies existed between practitioners using extracts compared with those using tinctures is probable. Hence a correlation should not be expected.
- Tinctures are manufactured using different techniques to 1:1 liquid extracts. This aspect is particularly important. Liquid extracts at that time were often prepared by reconstituting more concentrated extracts, rather than the traditional method of reserved percolation. In either case, the heat or vacuum used in concentration can rob

---

TABLE 1-4

Comparison of Dosages Used by the Eclectics with Modern Dosages

Herb	Eclectic Dosage[31,32] (g/day)	Current Dosage[28,29] (g/day)
Euphorbia hirta	1.8-10.8	0.36-0.90
Echinacea angustifolia	0.9-5.4	0.75-3.00
Hydrastis canadensis (golden seal)	0.9-10.8	0.9-3.0
Passiflora incarnata (passion flower)	1.8-10.8	1.5-3.0
Valeriana officinalis (valerian)	2.1-6.0	0.9-3.0
Rumex crispus (yellow dock)	1.8-10.8	6.0-12.0
Viburnum opulus (cramp bark)	3.6-10.8	6.0-12.0
Sabal serrulata (saw palmetto)	2.7-10.8	1.8-4.5

Note: The corresponding amount of dried herb per day has been calculated from the recommended dosages for liquid extracts.

TABLE 1-5

Comparison of Extract and Tincture Dosages in the BHP 1983

Herb	Dose Range 1:1 Extract[28]	Dose Range 1:5 Tincture[28]	Expected Dose Range for 1:5 Tincture
Agrimonia eupatoria (agrimony)	1-3 ml	2-4 ml	5-15 ml
Achillea millefolium (yarrow)	2-4 ml	2-4 ml	10-20 ml
Eupatorium purpureum (gravel root)	2-4 ml	1-2 ml	10-20 ml
Menyanthes trifoliate (bogbean)	1-2 ml	1-3 ml	5-10 ml

Note: The expected dose range for the 1:5 tincture is calculated by multiplying the dose range for the 1:1 extract by 5.

the preparation of important active chemicals. Tinctures better preserve the activity of the whole plant because they are made without heat or a concentration procedure. Liquid extracts are also often manufactured using lower alcohol strengths compared with tinctures, and important active components may therefore not be extracted from the starting plant material. The result of these considerations is that a 1:1 liquid extract can have an activity that is much less than five times that of a 1:5 tincture. (This again underlines the value of using 1:2 extracts, which offer the best of both worlds.)

Because tinctures better preserve the chemical profile of the dried herb, more credibility should be given to the tincture doses when using the dose ranges in the BHP. (The 1:5 tincture dose multiplied by 0.4 gives the corresponding 1:2 dose.)

COMPARING DOSES

Comparing doses between liquid and solid preparations made with various types of extracts is often difficult for practitioners. The concept of "dried herb equivalent" is a useful way for comparing doses between different strengths of herbal liquids or between liquids and tablets. Using the extract or product ratio, the dried herb equivalent of a given amount of product can be calculated. The extract or product ratio expresses the weight of original dried herb starting material to the volume or weight of finished product (in that order), for example, 5:1, 1:4, 1:1, and so forth.

For example, a dried herb equivalent of 1 g might be:
- 2 ml of a 1:2 liquid extract
- 1 ml of 1:1 liquid extract
- 250 mg of 4:1 soft extract
- 200 mg of a 5:1 spray-dried powder

DOSE INFORMATION SUMMARY

The dose summary chart (see Appendix A) contains a listing of the herbal liquids covered in this book. Listed from left to right is:
- Common name of the herb
- Botanical name of the herb
- Part of the plant used to make the herbal liquid
- Percentage of ethanol recommended in the manufacture of the herbal liquid
- Strength or ratio of the liquid (expressed as dried herb to final liquid)
- Minimum and maximum dose in milliliters to be prescribed per day
- Minimum and maximum dose in milliliters to be prescribed per week

The reader should note that these doses are calculated for adults for long-term use. For short-term use, as in acute conditions, the daily dose may be increased above the maximum for a week or so (but *never* in the case of Tylophora and Phytolacca).

CHILDREN'S DOSES

For calculating doses for children, a number of methods can be used. These values are only approximations, because of the complex metabolic changes that occur during growth and maturation. The author of this text prefers Ausberger's weight rule because it is based on weight rather than age and takes into account the faster metabolism of children. This calculation is as follows:

($1.5 \times$ weight in kg $+ 10$) is the percentage of the adult dose for the child. Expressed in terms of pounds, the formula becomes:

$$\frac{(1.5 \times \text{weight in kg} + 10)}{2.2}$$

Therefore if a child weighs 20 kg (44 lbs), then he or she should receive $(1.5 \times 20) + 10 = 40\%$ of the adult dose. A child weighing 10 kg (22 lbs) would receive 25% of the adult dose and so on. Clark's rule is more basic and is as follows:

$$\frac{\text{weight in kg}}{67} \times \text{adult dose} = \text{child's dose}$$

Various rules based on age have been established. For example, Young's rule is:

$$\frac{\text{age in years}}{(\text{age} + 12)} \times \text{adult dose} = \text{child's dose}$$

For young infants, applying Fried's rule rather than Ausberger's weight rule is sometimes more prudent. This rule is as follows (for infants around 1 to 2 years):

$$\frac{\text{age in months}}{150} \times \text{adult dose} = \text{child's dose}$$

HERBAL LIQUID INCOMPATIBILITIES

Incompatibilities can result when two or more herbal liquids are mixed together. This incompatibility can be either physical or chemical and can affect the efficacy of the resultant formulation. Generally, when mixing herbal liquids, avoiding any precipitation is impossible. For this reason, such liquid mixtures should always carry the directions, "Shake the bottle well before pouring" or words to that effect.

Some simple rules that have been established can be followed:

1. Herbs containing tannins, such as cranesbill root, are incompatible with herbs containing alkaloids, such as golden seal. If the two substances are mixed together, a precipitate will form. Hence tannins and alkaloids should be dispensed separately and taken at different times.
2. Herbs extracted in a high-percentage alcohol, such as ginger and myrrh, often contain resins that precipitate when the extract is mixed with other herbal liquids with low alcohol. One way to minimize this precipitation is to include a small quantity (10%) of licorice in the formula. The saponins in the licorice act as an emulsifying agent and can keep everything in suspension. The licorice should be added first before adding the resinous liquid.
3. Bladderwrack is also not compatible with tannin-containing herbs.
4. Herbal liquids are generally mixed in ascending order in terms of their ethanol content.
5. Mucilaginous herbs, such as marshmallow root and aloe juice concentrate, are not compatible with high ethanol extracts.

PRESCRIPTION RECORDS AND DISPENSING

The following has been adapted from course material from the College of Phytotherapy in the United Kingdom.

PRESCRIPTION RECORDS

Keeping full records of each patient's case is essential. Such records should include the case history and previous treatments, presenting symptoms, signs, diagnosis, prescriptions, progress reports, alterations and adjustments to treatment, and subsequent response. Dating each entry on the card is most important. Although each practitioner will, no doubt, develop his or her own style and system of record keeping after some experience, a tried and tested scheme is a good starting place.

A number of practitioners keep the information of their patients on a record card (A) and on another separate card or sheet (B). The first record card contains the name and address of the patient, including the patient's number. This card serves mainly to hold the information about the prescription.

The diagnosis, case history, and all medical and private information is kept on card or sheet (B), which carries no name but only the patient's number, the same

number as that on the prescription card. The advantages of this system are the following:

- The record card with the prescriptions is kept in the dispensary and filed under name. When the patient phones for repeat prescription, appointment, or advice, the card is easily traced, and all vital information is readily available to the dispenser, telephone operator, or secretary, without revealing any confidential information.
- By not having all the medical information on the card, the card can be kept simple. Sufficient space is provided for several repeat prescriptions, and all information on the card is easily traced.
- By keeping the second card or sheet (B) in the consulting room, filed under number, complete confidentiality is ensured. The data can be added to during each visit, and more cards or sheets can be added as required.

PRESCRIPTION

Using anything but the metric system in dispensing is inappropriate. Consequently, any remedy must be issued in metric. For the herbs, the proper Latin names are best used. If only one species of any genus is in your dispensary, then the generic name will suffice. However, if more than one herb in a genus is used, the specific name should be used as well. Generic names always start with a capital letter, and the specific name always follows with a small letter; for example, with *Rumex crispus* (yellow dock) "Rumex" is the generic name and "crispus" is the specific name. Record the recommended strength of the preparation, such as 1:2, 1:1, 1:5, and so on.

The prescription is divided into several parts:

- The inscription designates ingredients and quantities, such as Hypericum 1:2 30 ml.
- The subscription gives directions to the dispenser as to the form or mode of preparation, quantity to be sent, and the manner in which to be sent.
- Signature, meaning "let it be labeled," includes directions for the patient, method of application or dose, time of administration, vehicle or means of administration, and the part of the body to which it is to be administered.

The prescription is best written for 1 week's supply of medicine. If seeing the patient again in 3 weeks is necessary, then the whole prescription is trebled by the dispenser; this is indicated at the end of the prescription by writing 3 weeks. If the amount of herbal liquid to be dispensed for 1 week is short of 100 ml per week, the bottle is filled with syrup, water, diluted alcohol, or glycerol, as appropriate.

The normal or average dose is 5 ml (1 metric teaspoon), usually 3 times a day (tds or tid). (Note: a normal modern teaspoon is 3 to 4 ml, much smaller than a metric teaspoon.) Dosage can be varied widely according to the needs of each individual case. Including some form of sweetening in a child's medicine (e.g., a flavoring mix) is common, and the dose is then often without water.

DISPENSING PROCEDURES FOR HERBAL LIQUIDS

A set of preferably class A, metric, conical, glass measures are used by dispensing chemists. The sizes available include 10, 50, and 100 ml. These measures can be used for herbal dispensing, although measuring cylinders used in laboratories are also suitable.

The following is the traditional technique for dispensing. The measure is held in the left hand (even if left-handed) around the base. Holding the measure at eye level achieves accurate measuring. The right hand takes the dispensing bottle from the shelf; the stopper is removed and held with the little finger of the left hand. The correct amount of tincture is dispensed into the measure from which it is transferred to the medicine bottle.

The stopper is then replaced in the dispensing bottle and returned to the shelf (the stopper is never put down, but is held all the time by the little finger). Note: this traditional technique requires stoppered bottles. If screw caps are used, then the technique must be modified accordingly.

The surface of a liquid in a vessel is always curved. This property is known as a meniscus. A meniscus is read with the measure horizontal, at eye level, and from the highest point on a convex meniscus and the lowest point on a concave one. (Herbal liquids will generally be concave.)

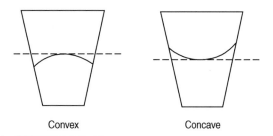

Convex   Concave

Errors in reading a meniscus arise from:
- Dirty or greasy measures
- Liquids poured down the side of a measure instead of into its center; with a viscous liquid, a large proportion can still be crawling down the sides of a measure when the correct meniscus reading has been reached
- A measure not being held or stood horizontally
- The meniscus not being viewed at eye level (parallax effects)

Small volumes can be measured using metric calibrated droppers, pipettes, or syringes. The dropper or pipette should be checked to see if it is made to be completely emptied; some are not.

LABELING

All dispensed medicines must be correctly labeled, giving the patient clear and concise instructions on how to take or use the preparation. Neat and careful labeling is important because this helps reinforce the patient's confidence in the medicine. A badly presented bottle of medicine may give the patient doubts as to the efficacy of the contents.

Information Provided on the Label

1. **Directions for use.** Writing the name of the type of preparation dispensed at the top of the label, such as "The Herbal Mixture," "The Tablets," and so on, is usual practice in dispensing. This practice is not essential in herbal dispensing. Below this information should be written the instructions to the patient, for example, "one 5-ml spoonful to be taken three times daily in a little water before meals," or "two tablets to be taken three times daily after meals." Stating "5 ml" rather than "one teaspoonful" is more precise, particularly if the patient has been supplied with a 5-ml plastic spoon or measure. The words "as directed" may be entered on the label if the patient has been supplied with separate written instructions.
2. **Patient's name.**
3. **Date.** Always writing the date when a medicine is dispensed on the label is good practice. The dates of all medicines dispensed must always be entered on the patient's case history. An expiry date is also a good idea.
4. **Batch code.** The number correlates with a separate record of the batches of individual herbs used in the formulation.
5. **The volume of herbal liquid in the bottle.**
6. **Basic storage information.**
7. **Any other instructions.**

The following is an example of a suitable dispensing label.

THE HERBAL MIXTURE

KEEP OUT OF REACH OF CHILDREN

Name

Directions for Use   drops/ml in water or fruit juice times daily

Other Instructions ▶

Store below 30°C (86°F) and out of direct sunlight

SHAKE WELL BEFORE POURING

Dispensed by ▶

Quantity:

Date of Supply:

Expiry Date:

Practitioner Initials:

Practitioner Code:

REFERENCES

1 Munzel K, Huber K: Extraction procedures in the preparation of chamomile fluid extract, Pharm Acta Helv 36:194, 1961.

2 Meier B: The extraction strength of ethanol/water mixtures commonly used for the processing of herbal drugs, Planta Med 57(suppl 2):A26, 1991.

3 Balansard G et al: Selection criteria for a Viburnum extract, Viburnum prunifolium L., as a function of its veino-tonic and spasmolytic action, Plant Med Phytother 17(3):123, 1983.

4 [No author listed.] Industrie, Z Phytother 18(5):296, 1997.

5 D'Alena P, Ferguson W: Adverse effects after glycerol orally and mannitol parenterally, Arch Ophthalmol 75(2):201, 1966.

6 Lyle TJ: Physio-medical therapeutics, materia medica and pharmacy, London, 1897, reprinted 1932, National Association of Medical Herbalists of Great Britain.

7 Scudder JM: Specific medication and specific medicines, Cincinnati, 1913, Scudder Brothers.

8 Ellingwood F, Lloyd JU: American materia medica, therapeutics and pharmacognosy, Portland, 1983, Eclectic Medical Publications.

9 Bundesministerium des Innern, West Germany: Deutsches Arzneibuch, ausg 7, ed 7, Stuttgart, 1968, Deutscher Apotheker-Verlag.

10 Bauer R et al: Beeinflussung der phagozytose-aktivität durch Echinacea-extrakte, Z Phytother 10:43, 1989.

11 Sharma H: Phytochemical synergism: beyond the active ingredient model, Alt Ther Clin Pract, May/June:91, 1997.

12 Williamson EM: Synergy: myth or reality? In Ernst E, editor: Herbal medicine: a concise overview for professionals, Oxford, 2000, Butterworth-Heinemann.

13 Eder M, Mehnert W: Bedeutung pflanzlicher begleitstoffe in extrakten, Pharmazie 53(5):285, 1998.

14 Keung W et al: Potentiation of the bioavailability of daidzin by an extract of Radix puerariae, Proc Natl Acad Sci USA 93:4284, 1996.

15 Vinson JA, Bose PB: Comparative bioavailability to humans of ascorbic acid alone or in a citrus extract, Am J Clin Nutr 48:601, 1988.

16 Butterweck V et al: Solubilized hypericin and pseudohypericin from Hypericum perforatum exert antidepressant activity in the forced swimming test, Planta Med 64:291, 1998.

17 Onawunmi GO, Yisak W, Ogunlana EO: Antibacterial constituents in the essential oil of Cymbopogon citratus (DC) Stapf, J Ethnopharmacol 12:279, 1984.

18 Kisa K et al: Potentiating effect of sennoside C on purgative activity of sennoside A in mice, Planta Med 42:302, 1981.

19 British Herbal Medicine Association's Scientific Committee: British herbal pharmacopoeia, ed 4, Bournemouth, UK, 1996, BHMA.

20 Lehmann R, Penman K, Halloran K: Information on file (2003). MediHerb Research Laboratory, University of Queensland, St. Lucia, Queensland 4072, Australia.

21 Peltz K, Penman K, Lehmann R: Devil's claw authentication by HPLC. Herbal Medicine: Practice and Science International Conference 1999, Brisbane, September 3-5, 1999.

22 Govindan M, Govindan G: A convenient method for the determination of the quality of goldenseal, Fitoterapia 71:232, 2000.

23 Lehmann R et al: Identification of the major flavonoid from Scutellaria lateriflora. International Congress and 48th Annual Meeting of the Society for Medicinal Plant Research. Sixth International Congress on Ethnopharmacology of the International Society for Ethnopharmacology, September 3-7, 2000, P1E/11.

24 Lehmann R, Penman K: Quality assessment in the herbal industry: as illustrated by Chinese and Ayurvedic herbs. MediHerb Clinical Update: Chinese and Ayurvedic Herbs in Western Clinical Practice, Brisbane, April-May, 2000. Information available from MediHerb Research Laboratory, University of Queensland, St. Lucia, Queensland 4072, Australia.

25 Wills RBH, Stuart DL: Levels of active constituents in manufactured Echinacea products, Chem Aust September:17, 1998.

26 Bensky D, Gamble A: Chinese herbal medicine materia medica, Seattle, 1986, Eastland Press.

27 Yanchi L: The essential book of traditional Chinese medicine, vol 2, Clinical Practice, New York, 1988, Columbia University Press.

28 British Herbal Medicine Association's Scientific Committee. *British Herbal Pharmacopeia*. Bournemouth, 1983, BHMA.

29 Pharmaceutical Society of Great Britain. *British Pharmaceutical Codex 1934*. London, 1941, The Pharmaceutical Press.

30 Griggs B: *Green pharmacy*, London, 1981, Jill Norman and Hobhouse.

31 Felter HW: *The eclectic materia medica, pharmacology and therapeutics*, Portland, 1922, reprinted 1983, Eclectic Medical Publications.

32 Felter HW, Lloyd JU: *King's American dispensatory*, ed 18, rev 3, Portland, 1905, reprinted 1983, Eclectic Medical Publications.

Formulating for the Individual Patient

2 CHAPTER

A SYSTEMATIC APPROACH

*T*he Western herbal system of prescribing for the individual patient is simpler than that for traditional Chinese and Ayurvedic medicine and does not necessarily require traditional diagnostic techniques such as the pulse and tongue. Nevertheless, the Western system can be powerful, and the author of this text has seen the Western herbal prescription succeed when other approaches have failed. The systematics of the Western herbal approach are summarized here. For a full exposition on this topic, the reader is referred elsewhere.[1]

The goals of Western herbal prescribing for the individual patient are to:

- Raise vitality, which is central to the individual's capacity to resist disease.
- Neutralize the perceived causes that either predispose a person to or provoke the disease process.
- Neutralize the sustaining causes that maintain the disease processes; chronic inflammation can be a sustaining cause.
- Promote and nourish the healthy functioning of bodily tissues, organs, and systems (as appropriate to the conditions being treated).
- Control counterproductive symptoms. For example, an itchy rash can interfere with sleep and debilitate the patient and is therefore counterproductive—thus the itch should be alleviated without excessively suppressing the rash.

Information about the causes of a patient's health problems can come from several sources:

- Clinical experience of the health care professional and their colleagues
- Traditional perspective on the disorder
- Epidemiologic studies, which can provide particular information about the predisposing causes

- Knowledge of the pathologic processes involved in the disorder that can provide particular information about provoking and sustaining causes
- Clinical studies on patients with the disorder, which might provide information about a link with a particular pathogen, an abnormality in bowel flora, or an association with another condition, such as the link between asthma and sinusitis

This information needs to be filtered according to the individual case history. Using the example given, if a patient with asthma does not exhibit signs and symptoms of sinusitis, then focusing treatment on his or her sinus is pointless. Once the processing of the information that an extensive case history provided is done, a series of treatment goals can be established. These treatment goals are then linked to the chosen herbs via the required actions.

The actions are traditional herbal concepts, but scientific research also yields information about the actions of an herb. The stepwise process in linking the treatment goals to the choice of herbs for the prescription is then as follows.

1. Treatment goals should be decided based on:
   - Traditional herbal concepts
   - The orthodox medical understanding of the disorder and the patient's case
   - The history and needs of the individual patient
2. The goals should be individualized to the requirements of the individual case (after taking an extensive case history).
3. The immediate priorities of treatment should be determined.
4. Required actions are determined are based on the immediate treatment goals.
5. Reliable herbs that have these actions are determined, with as much overlap of actions as possible. For example, if antiinflammatory and antispasmodic actions are

required for the gut, chamomile can effectively cover both of these requirements. These herbs are matched to the patient's constitution and general condition.

6. If a particular action needs to be reinforced, more than one herb with this action is chosen, or an effective herb is used in a higher dose.

7. The liquid herbs are combined in a formula with appropriate doses. Choosing too many herbs should be avoided because this will compromise the patient's individual doses in the formula and may lead to undefined interactions.

To facilitate this process, the practitioner needs a clear understanding of herbs in terms of their reliable, well-established actions. For this reason, an actions index is included as an important part in this book. The reader will also find the system of prescribing in weekly doses to be a convenient adjunct to this process. (See later discussion.)

The remaining part of this chapter then sets out examples of the process previously described for a number of common disorders under the following headings:

- Background (each disorder is briefly described as appropriate in terms of possible causes, counterproductive symptoms, and sustaining causes and organs or tissues requiring optimization of function)
- Treatment Strategy: Goals, Actions, and Herbs
- Example Formula
- Case History (presented for some disorders)

This approach is missing one important element: the case history of the individual patient. Therefore these examples are designed to illustrate the process and are not intended to provide a definitive statement about how a particular disorder should be treated. The needs of the individual are paramount.

HOW TO PREPARE A FORMULATION ACCORDING TO WEEKLY DOSES

The herbal formulation or prescription is an important aspect of herbal therapy; it allows the health care professional to make up a mixture using herbs that are specific to the patient. Arriving at a formulation can be done in many ways; one of the simplest ways is to use weekly doses.

If the patient is to take 5 ml of a formulation three times a day (15 ml per day), the total amounts to 105 ml per week, which can be rounded down to 100 ml. The herbs in the formulation can then be assigned appropriate doses by referring to their weekly dose ranges in the dosage table provided in Appendix A or in the individual monographs. The total should add up to 100 ml. The patient is then advised to take 5 ml three times per day, thereby automatically receiving the required amount of each herb.

When prescribing for children, the practitioner can still work on the 100-ml-per-week approach and still include the full adult weekly doses in the formulation. Adjustment is then made to the formulation dose; for example, it may become 2 ml three times per day rather than 5 ml. The way in which this adjustment can be made for children has already been outlined.

An example prescription for 1 week might be similar to that shown in Table 2-1.

In this example, the herbs were selected, and then the appropriate dose of each herb was chosen by considering the weekly dose range in conjunction with the purpose of the herb in the formula. Each of the herbs selected falls within its dose range, and the total also adds up to 100 ml. If the total turns out to be greater than 100 ml, then the formula would normally be adjusted (by lowering the dose of individual herb or herbs—but not below the minimum in the dose range—or by

TABLE 2-1

Common Name	Ratio	Dose (Range)	Selected Dose
Elder flower	1:2	15-40 ml	20 ml
Echinacea root (E. angustifolia)	1:2	20-40 ml	25 ml
Licorice	1:1	15-40 ml	20 ml
White horehound	1:2	15-40 ml	25 ml
Ginger	1:2	5-15 ml	10 ml
Total			100 ml

Dosage: 5 ml with water, three times per day.

reducing the number of herbs or by substituting an herb that has a lower dose range). Alternatively, the total might be adjusted to 105 or 110 ml without compromising the doses of individual herbs.

The previous sample prescription provides enough formula for 1 week. When dispensing for more than 1 week, the weekly doses are multiplied by the number of weeks required. For example, see Table 2-2.

Generally, formulations should not contain more than six or seven herbs. If using 1:5 tinctures, fewer herbs must be used in the formulation to ensure that no less than the minimum weekly dose is prescribed for each herb. Prescribing herbs below the minimum in the dose range, for example, at less than 5 ml per week of ginger 1:2 (dose range: 5 to 15 ml per week), means that a therapeutic effect may not be achieved.

When preparing formulations for patients that are to be taken over extended periods, the maximum dose is usually not exceeded for safety reasons. When prescribing for acute conditions, the maximum dose may need to be exceeded, but usually not for long (1 to 2 weeks). Following the normal weekly dose system and increasing the frequency of the 5 ml dose to say 5 or 6 times per day achieves this goal.

If more than six or seven herbs are required in a formulation, then the total may be set at 150 ml. The dosage for the patient then becomes 7.5 ml (or 8 ml) three times a day.

THERAPEUTICS

ACUTE BRONCHITIS

Background. Acute bronchitis, a bacterial infection of the trachea and bronchi, commonly follows the common cold, influenza, measles, or whooping cough.

Patients with chronic bronchitis are particularly prone to developing episodes of acute bronchitis (when their sputum turns from gray or white to yellow or green). Other factors that can predispose a person to this kind of bacterial infection include cold, damp, and dusty conditions, as well as cigarette smoking.

Initially, an irritating, unproductive cough occurs, which eventually progresses over a few days to copious, mucopurulent sputum. Infection usually starts in the trachea and progresses to the bronchi accompanied by a general febrile disturbance with temperatures of 38° to 39°C (100° to 102°F). Gradual recovery should occur over the next 4 to 8 days. However, the condition may progress to bronchiolitis or bronchopneumonia.

Treatment Strategy: Goals, Actions, and Herbs

- Immune function can be improved with immune enhancing herbs such as Echinacea root and Andrographis, and respiratory infection can be controlled with respiratory antiseptic herbs such as elecampane and thyme. These herbs should be prescribed throughout the course of the infection and preferably should be continued 1 week into recovery to prevent relapse.
- During the dry, unproductive cough phase, reflex demulcents such as marshmallow root should be prescribed to alleviate the resultant irritation and debilitation from an unproductive cough.
- Diaphoretic herbs are indicated during the febrile phase, particularly pleurisy root, which is almost a specific for acute lower respiratory tract infections. The herb is often combined with ginger to enhance its effectiveness. Other diaphoretics such as lime flowers and yarrow can also be prescribed.
- Expectorant herbs, which include elecampane, thyme, licorice, fennel, and white horehound, can help clear mucous secretions and alleviate cough.

TABLE 2-2

Common Name	Ratio	Dose (Range)	Selected Dose	Dose for 4 Weeks
Elder flower	1:2	15-40 ml	20 ml	80 ml
Echinacea root *(E. angustifolia)*	1:2	20-40 ml	25 ml	100 ml
Licorice	1:1	15-40 ml	20 ml	80 ml
White horehound	1:2	15-40 ml	25 ml	100 ml
Ginger	1:2	5-15 ml	10 ml	40 ml
Total			100 ml	400 ml

Dosage: 5 ml with water, three times per day.

TABLE 2-3

Echinacea root (*E. angustifolia* or *E. purpurea*)	1:2	25 ml
Pleurisy root	1:2	20 ml
Ginger	1:2	5 ml
Elecampane	1:2	20 ml
Licorice	1:1	15 ml
Fennel	1:2	20 ml
Total		105 ml

Dosage: 5 ml with 40 ml warm water five to six times a day.

These herbs can be prescribed throughout the course of the disorder. Pleurisy root will also act as an expectorant.

- Anticatarrhal herbs, especially mullein and golden seal, may be indicated when the sputum is particularly copious or if the productive cough lingers beyond the acute stage.
- Antitussive herbs such as Bupleurum and licorice should be used to help the cough, especially at night, and wild cherry is particularly indicated to allay cough if tracheitis predominates.

Example Formula. See Table 2-3.

ALLERGIC RHINITIS

Background. Allergic rhinitis is triggered by inhaled allergens and may be perennial or seasonal (hay fever). In the herbal treatment of rhinitis, identifying whether inhaled allergens are involved is important because this determines the approach to treatment.

Allergic rhinitis is usually characterized by sneezing, itching, nasal discharge, conjunctivitis, and nasal congestion. A family history of allergy is usually present, and secretions are often copious, clear, and thin. A positive skin prick test or radioallergosorbent test (RAST) to aeroallergens confirms the diagnosis.

The acute allergic response in rhinitis results from the interaction of inhaled allergen with a specific immunoglobulin E antibody on the surface of mast cells and basophils. This interaction leads to the release of histamine and other factors, which causes the acute symptoms.

Although allergens involved in seasonal allergic rhinitis are usually grass pollens, pollens from other plants, including trees, may be implicated. In perennial allergic rhinitis, house dust mite, molds, cockroaches, and cats are common sources of allergen.

Treatment Strategy: Goals, Actions, and Herbs. The approach to the herbal treatment of rhinitis is to control symptoms and remove causes. Avoidance measures to reduce exposure to aeroallergens should be part of this treatment.

Dietary exclusions should be trialed for both allergic and nonallergic rhinitis. Herbalists believe that diet can create a state of hypersensitivity and catarrh of the mucous membranes, which predisposes the individual to rhinitis. Importantly, the dietary components that contribute to this process do not necessarily give a positive reaction on the RAST or skin prick test. These components include dairy products, wheat, salt, and refined carbohydrates. Patients with rhinitis should avoid excessive consumption of these dietary components, and complete exclusion of one component (e.g., dairy) should be trialed for at least 3 months.

The goals of herbal treatment include the following:

- Immune system can be balanced with immune modulating herbs, especially Echinacea root.
- Integrity of mucous membranes can be improved with mucous membrane trophorestoratives (golden seal) and anticatarrhal herbs (eyebright, golden rod), which will help prevent the allergen from reaching the mast cells that are deeper in the mucous membranes.
- Allergic response can be toned down with antiallergic herbs such as Albizia and Baical skullcap.
- Effects of stress (which can exacerbate rhinitis) can be alleviated with adaptogens (ashwaganda, Eleutherococcus), anxiolytics (valerian, kava, passion flower), and nervine tonics (St. John's wort, skullcap).
- Treatment of rhinitis at a deeper level may involve the use of depuratives, particularly blue flag, burdock, cleavers, sarsaparilla, and yellow dock.
- When treating seasonal allergic rhinitis (hay fever), treatment must be commenced 6 weeks before the season starts and continued throughout the season. Any helpful dietary exclusions should also follow this time pattern.

Example Formula. See Table 2-4.

The reader should note that the tannins in Albizia are not compatible with the alkaloids in golden seal, hence it has not been used in this particular example.

ANXIETY

Background. Anxiety disorders can be classified as follows:

- Panic disorder, which is characterized by the presence of recurrent and unpredictable panic attacks
- Phobic disorders, which involve marked and persistent fear of objects or situations, exposure to which results in anxiety, such as claustrophobia

TABLE 2-4

Echinacea root (*E. angustifolia* or *E. purpurea*)	1:2	35 ml
Eyebright	1:2	20 ml
Golden seal	1:3	20 ml
Baical skullcap	1:2	30 ml
Total		105 ml

Dosage: 5 ml with water three times a day before meals.

- Generalized anxiety disorder in which the patient suffers persistent and often unrealistic worry together with symptoms such as muscle tension, impaired concentration, restlessness, and disturbed sleep
- Posttraumatic stress disorder, which follows extreme trauma such as a life-threatening event

Patients with anxiety should be treated as a whole. Aspects of lifestyle and diet should be considered and extremes corrected when possible, for example excessive use of alcohol, recreational drugs, sexual indulgence, imbalanced diet, excessive tea and coffee intake, and cigarette smoking. Such corrections will need to be carefully considered because patients often use these factors to allay anxiety, and their abrupt withdrawal might exacerbate symptoms.

Appropriate professional guidance and counseling, with the introduction of simple techniques for relaxation, can be beneficial.

Treatment Strategy: Goals, Actions, and Herbs

- Anxiolytic and sedative herbs such as kava, valerian, and passion flower can help dampen symptoms of anxiety.
- Other herbs in these categories that can provide valuable assistance are California poppy, spiny jujube (*Zizyphus jujuba* var. *spinosa*), and Corydalis.
- Nervine tonic herbs also have a role (these herbs are calming, but also lift mood) in the treatment of anxiety. These herbs include St. John's wort, vervain, lemon balm, skullcap, oats, and damiana.
- Spasmolytic herbs can be used to alleviate spasm. Cramp bark and chamomile may be useful for any visceral symptoms associated with the anxiety, and hawthorn berry can be prescribed when cardiac symptoms are present.
- Anxious patients stress their bodies and deplete their adrenal reserves, which can create a vicious cycle. Hence tonic and adaptogenic herbs may be required. The herb of choice in this context is ashwaganda because of its calming properties.

TABLE 2-5

Valerian	1:2	20 ml
Passion flower	1:2	20 ml
Ashwaganda	1:2	35 ml
St. John's wort	1:2	25 ml
Total		100 ml

Dosage: 5 ml with water three times a day.

Example Formula. See Table 2-5.

ASTHMA

Background. Asthma has been defined as the occurrence of dyspneic bronchospasmodic crises that are linked to a bronchial hyperreactivity (BH).[2] Similar to autoimmune disease, asthma is a chronic disturbance of immunologic function, which can be controlled to some extent but not eradicated by modern drug therapy. In other words, asthma is *not* just the attacks (crises). Asthma is a chronic disturbance of the immune system. The attacks are the "tip of the iceberg." Hence any treatment aimed only at relaxing airways and relieving symptoms, be it orthodox or herbal, is superficial and will not change the chronicity of the disease.

Recent research has identified many factors that may contribute to the causes and morbidity of asthma. Traditional herbal medicine also recognizes the role of inefficient digestion, poor immunity, stress, inadequate diet, and unhealthy mucous membranes in the development of the disease. Contributing factors identified from research on patients with asthma include inhaled allergens (exposure to which contributes to the chronicity of the disease, not just the attacks), dietary allergens, poor air quality, concurrent sinusitis,[3,4] poor hydrochloric acid production,[5] gastroesophageal reflux (GER),[6,7] coexisting or episodic infections,[8-10] excessive salt intake,[11] poor immunity,[12,13] stress,[14,15] and antioxidant status.[16-18] Platelet-activating factor (PAF) may be involved in the inflammatory response. (Ginkgo has anti-PAF activity.)

Treatment Strategy: Goals, Actions, and Herbs. Tables 2-6 and 2-7 outline the treatment strategy for asthma.

Example Formulas

- For both symptomatic treatment and dealing with underlying factors when concurrent sinusitis is involved (see Table 2-8)

TABLE 2-6

Treating the Underlying Factors That Created the Asthmatic Condition

Goal	Required Actions	Herbs
Control the allergic response	Antiallergic	Baical skullcap, Albizia
Treat sinusitis	Anticatarrhal, antiallergic, immune enhancing	Eyebright, Andrographis
Increase gastric acid	Bitter tonic, digestive	Gentian, Andrographis
Control reflux	Antispasmodic, demulcent, antacid, mucoprotective	Meadowsweet, marshmallow root, licorice
Eliminate infection	Immune enhancing, antiviral, antibacterial	Echinacea root, Andrographis
Reduce the physical effects of stress	Adaptogen	Astragalus, Eleutherococcus
Reduce anxiety and tension	Sedative and nervine tonic	Valerian, St. John's wort
Boost the hypothalamic-pituitary-adrenal axis	Tonic, adrenal tonic	Ashwaganda, Rehmannia
Balance immunity	Immune modifying, immune depressant	Echinacea root, Hemidesmus, Tylophora
Improve antioxidant status	Antioxidant	Ginkgo, rosemary
Improve the health of mucous membranes	Anticatarrhal, mucous membrane trophorestorative, lymphatic, depurative	Eyebright, golden seal

TABLE 2-7

Treating the Symptoms and Sustaining Causes of Asthma, Such as Inflammation

Goal	Required Actions	Herbs
Control the allergic response	Antiallergic	Baical skullcap, Albizia
Control acute respiratory infection	Diaphoretic, immune enhancing	See information for common cold and influenza
Reduce inflammation	Antiinflammatory, reflex demulcent	Ginkgo, Bupleurum, marshmallow root
Clear the airways	Expectorant	Elecampane, fennel
Relax bronchial smooth muscle	Bronchospasmolytic	Elecampane, Grindelia, Coleus
Allay debilitating cough	Expectorant, demulcent, antitussive	Elecampane, marshmallow root, Bupleurum, licorice

- For night cough and GER (Table 2-9)
- When stress and anxiety are significant factors (Table 2-10)

BENIGN PROSTATIC HYPERPLASIA

Background. Benign prostatic hyperplasia (BPH) is an androgen-dependent disorder within the prostate. (Androgen is a male hormone.) As men age, significant changes in hormone levels occur:

- Testosterone and particularly free testosterone is decreased.
- Prolactin, estradiol, sex hormone–binding globulin, luteinizing hormone (LH), and follicle-stimulating hormone (FSH) are increased.

The ultimate effect is increased dihydrotestosterone (DHT) within the prostate. New generation drugs for

TABLE 2-8

Baical skullcap	1:2	30 ml
Ginkgo (standardized extract)	2:1	25 ml
Eyebright	1:2	15 ml
Echinacea root blend	1:2	30 ml
Total		100 ml

Dosage: 5 ml with water three to four times a day.

TABLE 2-9

Licorice	1:1	15 ml
Meadowsweet	1:2	20 ml
Marshmallow root glycetract	1:5	65 ml
Total		100 ml

Dosage: 3 to 5 ml undiluted as required up to six times a day.

TABLE 2-10

Astragalus	1:2	30 ml
Valerian	1:2	15 ml
Rehmannia	1:2	30 ml
Ashwaganda	1:2	35 ml
Total		110 ml

Dosage: 5 ml with water three to four times a day.

TABLE 2-11

Saw palmetto	1:2	30 ml
Nettle root	1:2	30 ml
Crataeva	1:2	40 ml
Total		100 ml

Dosage: 5 ml with water three times a day.

BPH such as Proscar (finasteride) inhibit the enzyme 5-alpha-reductase, which converts testosterone into DHT.

Many other factors are likely involved in BPH, including increased DHT receptors in the prostate (which may result from the increased estradiol), reduced metabolism of testosterone and DHT, accumulation of cholesterol, and inflammatory changes in the prostate.

A dynamic component to the symptoms of urethral obstruction is also present, which is known as "prostatism."[19] Alpha-adrenergic (sympathetic) nerve fibers innervate the smooth muscle of the prostatic urethra and bladder neck. Some of the symptoms of BPH are related to the state of contraction of this smooth muscle, which explains why symptoms can vary in severity at any given time for a man with BPH. Alpha-adrenergic blocking drugs such as Minipress (prazosin hydrochloride) are often prescribed to alleviate the symptoms of prostatism.

Treatment Strategy: Goals, Actions, and Herbs
- Prostate function can be improved with antiprostatic herbs, which act by various mechanisms and include saw palmetto, nettle root, and willow herb.
- Male hormonal function can be corrected with male tonics such as Korean ginseng.

- Compromised bladder function can be improved with the bladder tonic Crataeva.
- Prostatism can be alleviated with spasmolytic herbs, especially cramp bark, kava, and valerian.

Example Formula. See Table 2-11.

CHRONIC FATIGUE SYNDROME

Background[20]. Chronic fatigue syndrome (CFS) can be viewed as a subtle immune dysfunction possibly resulting from a complex interaction among emotional, infectious, and environmental stressors. This immune dysfunction leads to a state of autotoxicity, which can be further exacerbated by previous or current exposure to environmental toxins. For each patient, the particular factors that may be contributing to this interaction need to be identified and dealt with through the therapeutic regime. In addition, the abnormalities that are now known to occur in CFS should be countered or corrected.

Patients with CFS were usually devitalized before they contracted the disorder. This condition might have been the result of emotional pressures, work pressures, family pressures, ambition, toxins, pregnancy, or even a bad diet; but the end result is the same. The finding that stress is a significant predisposing factor in CFS supports this observation.[21] Any stressor, be it chemical, physical, biologic, or emotional, then acts to aggravate the condition. This reduced capacity to cope with stress is a key factor in creating the vicious cycle, which perpetuates the syndrome.

The devitalization then leads to weakened immunity and finally to an abnormal immune response to a viral infection. A stalemate is reached when the resultant hyperimmune state causes autotoxicity but is not sufficiently focused to resolve a viral presence, or any other cause, and to restore health. Devitalization is a curious state in which some compartments of the immune system are overactive, but other compartments are deficient.

Other causative factors might add either to the immune dysfunction or to the autotoxicity, or they may act as stressors to increase devitalization. These factors include:

- Intestinal dysbiosis, endotoxemia, or similar syndromes
- Allergies or food intolerances
- Toxins (e.g., dental amalgam, hair dyes, pesticides)
- Chronic inflammation or infection

These additional factors will not apply in every patient; it is a matter of individualization and appropriate treatment.

Possible factors identified in the cause or progression of CFS include viruses, immune abnormalities, circulatory abnormalities (including reduced blood flow to some parts of the brain), brain abnormalities, pituitary abnormalities, and sleep disorders, as well as muscle, metabolic, and biochemical abnormalities.[20] Depression is a common feature that is to be expected given the morbidity of this disorder and its association with poor vitality.

Treatment Strategy: Goals, Actions, and Herbs

- Energy levels can be revitalized with tonics such as Korean ginseng, ashwaganda, and Astragalus; the response to stress can be improved with adaptogens such as Eleutherococcus.
- Depleted adrenal reserves can be restored with adrenal tonics, specifically licorice and Rehmannia.
- Immune function can be balanced with immune modulators, specifically Echinacea root and, when necessary, immune-depressing agents such as Hemidesmus and even Tylophora.
- Any viral association can be managed with antiviral herbs such as St. John's wort and Thuja.
- Mood and vitality can be boosted with nervine tonics such as St. John's wort, oats, Bacopa, and skullcap.
- Cerebral blood flow and general tissue perfusion can be improved with Ginkgo.
- Bacopa and Ginkgo will also improve memory.

TABLE 2-12

Korean ginseng	1:2	10 ml
Ashwaganda	1:2	35 ml
St. John's wort (high hypericin)	1:2	15 ml
Ginkgo (standardized extract)	2:1	20 ml
Astragalus	1:2	30 ml
Total		110 ml

Dosage: 5 ml with water three times a day.

- Sleep patterns can be improved and restorative sleep can be reestablished with hypnotic herbs such as valerian, spiny jujube, and kava.

Example Formula. See Table 2-12.

COMMON COLD AND INFLUENZA

Background. The common cold (acute rhinitis) is a benign viral infection of the upper respiratory tract that usually occurs in the winter months. Viruses commonly involved are rhinovirus, adenovirus, influenza virus, and parainfluenza virus. Acute rhinitis usually begins with a sore throat, nasal congestion, sneezing with clear discharge, and mild fever. After a few days, a mucopurulent discharge occurs resulting from secondary bacterial infection. A few days of bed rest may be necessary, and full recovery usually occurs 7 to 10 days after onset. Complications or sequelae include acute sinusitis, sore throat, tonsillitis, and otitis media.

In contrast, influenza is often a more severe respiratory infection that can result in loss of life. The main viruses that cause influenza are enveloped viruses known as influenza A and B.[22] These viruses are capable of mutating, and new strains constantly appear. Influenza is also mainly a winter disease. The influenza virus can produce a range of disease states, from a mild common cold to fatal pneumonia (especially in older adults or people who are severely debilitated). True influenza is usually differentiated from other "flulike" illnesses by its marked systemic symptoms, with high fever, malaise, and muscle pain. Bed rest is usually always required.

Treatment Strategy: Goals, Actions, and Herbs

- Immune function can be improved with immune-enhancing herbs such as Echinacea root and Andrographis.

TABLE 2-13

Echinacea root (*E. angustifolia* or *E. purpurea*)	1:2	35 ml
Ginger	1:2	5 ml
Lime flowers	1:2	20 ml
Eyebright	1:2	20 ml
Elder flower	1:2	20 ml
Total		100 ml

Dosage: 5 ml with 40 ml hot water five to six times a day.

- Fever can be modified to optimize its fight against the invading pathogen. Diaphoretics are used for this effect and include elder flower, lime flowers, peppermint, and yarrow. These agents work best when administered hot (hot water is added to the herbal liquid) and in conjunction with ginger, acting as a diffuse circulatory stimulant. Chamomile is a good diaphoretic for children.
- Excessive discharge of mucus and upper respiratory congestion can be reduced with anticatarrhal herbs such as elder flower, eyebright, and golden seal. Traditional writers say that golden seal was contraindicated in the acute stage of infection,[23] thus its use may be best in the later stages of the secondary bacterial infection, when a thick yellowish nasal discharge occurs.
- The virus can be controlled with antiviral herbs, especially St. John's wort, which is active against the enveloped viruses that are often involved.

Example Formula. See Table 2-13.

DEPRESSION

Background. Unipolar depressive disorders (depression without a manic or hypomanic phase) that are not associated with medical illness are classified as follows:

- Major depression, which can be characterized by sadness, apathy, irritability, disturbed sleep, disturbed appetite, weight loss, fatigue, poor concentration, guilt, and thoughts of death
- Dysthymic disorder, which consists of a pattern of chronic, ongoing mild depressive symptoms that are less severe than are those of major depression
- Seasonal affective disorder (SAD), which is more common in women and related to seasonal changes; prevalence increases with increasing latitude and can be treated by light therapy; symptoms include

lack of energy, weight gain, and carbohydrate craving

Depression may be associated with prolonged anxiety or stress. Hypersecretion of adrenocorticotropin hormone (ACTH) from the pituitary is often a feature. Some writers theorize that this excess of ACTH may be related to a conditioned response resulting from traumatic events in childhood.[24]

Impaired circulation to the brain, especially in elderly patients, is a cause of depression. Low systolic blood pressure was also associated with a poor perception of well being in 50-year-old men[25] and depression in men aged 60 to 89 years.[26]

The general considerations outlined in the treatment of anxiety also apply here. Patients with depression should be treated as a whole with due attention to lifestyle, diet, drug use, and mental hygiene (productive attitudes for coping with life events). Professional guidance and counseling is often appropriate, rather than regulating depression to just a biochemical imbalance to be corrected with pharmacologic agents.

Treatment Strategy: Goals, Actions, and Herbs. Herbal treatment is most appropriate for mild to moderate episodes of depression, dysthymic disorder, and SAD. Episodes of major depression may require the more strident therapy that conventional drugs can offer, although herbs can have a supportive role, especially in terms of boosting vitality. Herbs can also be relevant when the patient improves and wishes to discontinue drug therapy.

- The nervine tonic herbs are the mainstay of treatment, especially St. John's wort, which is a well-proven treatment for mild to moderate depression. Other important herbs in this category include vervain, damiana, oats, and skullcap.
- Patients who are also anxious should be prescribed anxiolytic herbs. Kava combines well with St. John's wort. Valerian is also useful, but hop is contraindicated.
- Depressed patients are low in vitality, thus adrenal tonic (licorice and Rehmannia), tonic, and adaptogenic herbs are often indicated. Korean ginseng may have antidepressant activity, but it should be used cautiously if anxiety is present. Ashwaganda or Eleutherococcus are preferred choices in these cases. Licorice and Schisandra also have exhibited some antidepressant activity in animal models. Such herbs will also help correct the adverse long-term effects of stress on the physiology of the stress response.
- If required, herbs that improve circulation to the brain should be prescribed, especially Ginkgo.

Example Formula. See Table 2-14.

TABLE 2-14

Valerian	1:2	20 ml
St. John's wort	1:2	25 ml
Skullcap	1:2	20 ml
Damiana	1:2	20 ml
Licorice	1:1	15 ml
Total		100 ml

Dosage: 5 ml with water three times a day.

ECZEMA (ATOPIC DERMATITIS)

Background. Eczema, or dermatitis, is a pruritic inflammatory skin reaction that demonstrates with variable clinical pictures. Atopic dermatitis is a dermatitis that is linked to the atopic state. The patient is much troubled by itching skin, and a history of chronic or chronically relapsing dermatitis, worse on the flexures (elbows, back of knees), and a family or personal history of atopy (e.g., asthma, hay fever, urticaria) is present.

Factors involved in the cause or pathogenesis of atopic dermatitis are discussed here.

Family History. Atopic syndrome is genetically determined and is associated with high plasma levels of immunoglobulin E (IgE). When both parents have the same atopic disease, their child has approximately a 70% risk of expressing this disease. However, the increasing prevalence of atopic dermatitis is difficult to explain based on genetics alone.[27]

Biochemical Abnormalities. The skin of patients with atopic dermatitis is typically dry, which may be linked to an abnormality of essential fatty acid metabolism. Some research has proposed that a deficiency in the enzyme δ-6 desaturase may imbalance the essential fatty acid content of the skin and reduce the production of important antiinflammatory prostaglandins. These postulates underpin the use of oral and topical evening primrose oil in the treatment of atopic dermatitis.

Allergen Exposure. A long-standing controversy exists as to whether allergy is a major pathogenic factor in atopic dermatitis. In some patients, studies have associated food allergy, inhalant allergens, and skin contact with airborne allergens with atopic dermatitis.[28]

Even in the absence of specific IgE for house dust mites, infants with atopic dermatitis have proliferative T-cell responses to these antigens.[28] A double-blind, controlled trial found that measures to avoid house dust mite greatly reduced the activity of atopic dermatitis, especially in children.[29] Responses to this therapy varied considerably, despite the fact that allergic reactivity to house dust mite antigens can be established by prick-test challenge in virtually all patients with atopic dermatitis.

These observations highlight a potential misconception concerning allergen exposure in this disorder: a positive skin prick test (which tests for an IgE-based response) does not necessarily identify the particular allergens that might be contributing to the underlying immunologic disturbance. Some patients with a positive skin reaction to dust mite do not respond to reduced exposure. A corollary is that food allergens are not necessarily identified by a prick test challenge, although it can be a useful guide.

Immunologic Abnormalities. For atopic dermatitis, a definite defect is present in cell-mediated immunity within the skin and increased susceptibility to cutaneous viral and fungal infections, yet patients are not systemically immunosuppressed.[28]

Although many types of inflammatory cells are present in skin lesions, the major abnormality is thought to involve hyperstimulatory T cells.[28] Much interest has focused on the shift in T-helper-cell activity toward a T-helper 2 (Th-2) type response. Both Th-1 and Th-2 cells can induce B cells to produce immunoglobulins, but only Th-2 cells induce IgE.[28]

Link to Infection or Abnormal Microflora. The cutaneous microbial flora of patients with atopic dermatitis show striking differences in terms of the presence of *Staphylococcus aureus*. The relative rarity of colonization on normal skin is in sharp contrast to the high rate found in patients with atopic dermatitis, ranging from 76% on unaffected areas up to 100% on acute, weeping lesions.[30] *Staphylococcus aureus* can induce inflammatory reactions via a range of activities, including toxin and protein secretion. Among these toxins and secretions are the superantigens, which have potent inflammatory and immunologic effects.[30] (Superantigens bind directly to macrophages without antigen processing, which can have profound pathologic effects caused by the release of cytokines by these cells or via the subsequent activation of T cells.[31])

The superantigen *S. aureus* enterotoxin B (SEB) induces the expansion of Th-2 cells, leading to increased IgE synthesis.[30] In addition, several alternative mechanisms have been proposed for the pathogenic role of bacterial superantigens in atopic dermatitis.[31] Some conventional approaches to atopic dermatitis are now advocating oral and topical antibiotic therapy aimed against *S. aureus*, with improved results being claimed.[30]

Digestive Function. Some early studies found a low gastric production of hydrochloric acid was correlated with incidence of atopic dermatitis, for example Ayers in 1929[32] and Brown and co-workers in 1935.[33] Therapy with hydrochloric acid resulted in a dramatic improvement in some cases.[32] A Russian study found markedly reduced activity of membrane-bound small-intestinal enzymes in 346 patients with atopic dermatitis. Correction of this dysfunction results in improvements in both digestion and skin.[34] A related study found a similar problem in infants with atopic dermatitis. Reduction of disaccharide intake (e.g., lactose, sucrose, maltose) was instituted.[35]

Treatment Strategy: Goals, Actions, and Herbs

- The immune response can be balanced with immune modifiers, particularly Echinacea root. Experience shows that the herb does not aggravate atopic dermatitis (and may even shift responses away from Th-2 type to Th-1). Boosting the immune response with Echinacea root, Astragalus, and Andrographis, may help control S. aureus infection.
- The allergic and inflammatory responses can be controlled with antiallergic herbs (e.g., Albizia, Baical skullcap, nettle leaf) and antiinflammatory herbs (e.g., licorice, gotu kola, Bupleurum).
- Bitter herbs and aromatic digestives will improve digestion (if indicated).
- Long-term treatment with depuratives such as burdock, nettle leaf, cleavers, yellow dock, and sarsaparilla is aimed at correcting the metabolic imbalances underlying this disorder.
- Bacterial colonization of the skin can be corrected and inflammation allayed by topical treatment with antiinflammatory and antiseptic herbs. The antiseptic herbs will help control skin microflora imbalance and infection with S. aureus. Calendula has both antiseptic and antiinflammatory properties. Myrrh has antiseptic properties, and topical treatment with myrrh and Echinacea root may improve the cutaneous immune response. Golden seal contains antimicrobial alkaloids (it should not be combined with tannins).
- In severe cases, Tylophora can be used to suppress the Th-2 cell response. Tylophora should be used cautiously in children (with appropriate low doses) and in adults only after experience has been gained with its application.

Case Histories

Case History 1. An 8-year-old girl had eczema that started approximately 4 years earlier. The condition was worse each summer, perhaps as a result of swimming in the local pool. The mother had tried removing dairy products from her diet, without much success. The girl seemed to be eating quite a few sweet biscuits, thus it was suggested that these be reduced. The child's physician had prescribed a topical steroid. On examination, the lesions on her face showed signs of a secondary infection.

See Table 2-15 for the prescribed formula and dosage (based on her weight of 25 kg).

Topical application of a chickweed cream was also recommended for the lesions, and one capsule of evening primrose oil was to be broken and taken internally or applied topically (on the abdomen where the skin is thinner, for dermal absorption) twice a day.

On review after 4 weeks, the rash had improved substantially, and her face was clear. Using the local swimming pool did not seem to aggravate the condition as it did previously. Treatment was continued for several months, and improvement was maintained.

Case History 2. A woman, age 23 years, had severe atopic dermatitis. The skin was itchy and infected, and her hands, legs, scalp, face (around the lips), and chest were affected. The condition started approximately 6 years ago and was currently being treated with topical steroids. The condition was worse premenstrually, and she had a family history of atopy and suffered herself from asthma.

The subject was prescribed the formula in Table 2-16, which included feverfew for antiallergic and antiinflammatory effects:

In addition, the woman was advised to avoid all dairy products, take 2 ml of chaste tree 1:2 liquid (because of

TABLE 2-15

Echinacea root blend	1:2	50 ml
Baical skullcap	1:2	25 ml
Nettle leaf	1:2	25 ml
Total		100 ml

Dosage: 3 ml with water twice a day.

TABLE 2-16

Astragalus	1:2	25 ml
Echinacea root blend	1:2	25 ml
Gotu kola	1:2	20 ml
Feverfew	1:5	10 ml
Bupleurum	1:2	20 ml
Total		100 ml

Dosage: 5 ml with water three times a day.

the premenstrual aggravation) with water on rising each morning, and 3×1000 mg evening primrose oil capsules per day. A chickweed cream was prescribed for topical application.

Four weeks later, her condition was about the same. She had made a decision (without seeking advice) to completely stop her steroid cream, and her rash grew much worse (a characteristic rebound effect). Since then, the condition had stabilized, but did not improve. Treatment was continued (but not the steroid cream).

After another 8 weeks of treatment, her skin condition showed a significant improvement. Treatment was continued over several more months, after which her atopic dermatitis had more or less subsided.

GASTROESOPHAGEAL REFLUX

Background. Major factors thought to be involved in the cause of gastroesophageal reflux (GER) are:[36]
- Inappropriate relaxation of the lower esophageal sphincter (LES), perhaps triggered by gastric distension
- Poor functioning of the LES through low basal sphincter tone, a factor that applies particularly in patients who also have irritable bowel syndrome[37]
- Increased acidity or irritant effect from the contents of the stomach
- Delayed esophageal clearance
- Delayed gastric emptying
- Poor saliva output and poor mucosal resistance

The previously recognized association between hiatus hernia and GER is downplayed in modern thinking.

Treatment Strategy: Goals, Actions, and Herbs
Practical Measures
- The head of the bed is elevated by 10 to 15 cm, which improves esophageal clearance at night.
- Regular meal times are adhered to, and eating on the run or during stressful situations is avoided.
- Foods that reduce LES tone, including chocolate, carminatives (e.g., peppermint, spearmint), fatty foods, coffee, tomato concentrates, and onions, are avoided; these foods will vary from individual to individual. Spicy foods may also aggravate the condition.
- Individual intolerance to certain foods (e.g., dairy products) may aggravate reflux and should be avoided.
- Drugs that reduce LES tone, such as theophylline, calcium channel blockers, and progesterone, are avoided.
- The patient should give up smoking and excessive alcohol intake (these reduce LES tone).

- The patient should refrain from overeating.
- The patient should avoid eating at bedtime.
- The patient should lose weight, if overweight.

Herbal Treatment
- Mucosal resistance can be improved with demulcent herbs such as licorice and marshmallow root. These herbs are best taken after meals and before bedtime. Additional supplementation with slippery elm powder can be useful. For best mucoprotective effect, a licorice liquid high in glycyrrhizin is used.
- LES tone can be increased and gastric emptying and saliva output can be improved with bitter herbs at low doses. However, gastric acid can also increase, thus caution should be used. Gentian and wormwood are the strongest bitters. If the use of these herbs aggravates the condition, then gentler bitters such as dandelion root, globe artichoke, or yarrow might be tried. Golden seal as a mucous membrane trophorestorative and bitter can be useful.
- Inappropriate levels of gastric acid can be reduced using antacid herbs—the best is meadowsweet.
- Healing can be enhanced and inflammation can be allayed with vulnerary herbs (e.g., Aloe juice concentrate, Calendula, chamomile, gotu kola) and antiinflammatory herbs (particularly chamomile). For best results, chamomile liquid high in bisabolol is used.
- Effects of stress on the functioning of the autonomic nervous system can be alleviated with anxiolytic herbs (e.g., passion flower, valerian, and kava) and nervine tonics (especially skullcap and St. John's wort).
- Any associated dyspepsia can be treated with low doses of carminatives given before food (because high doses will aggravate GER). Fennel and peppermint are among the best carminatives.

Example Formula. See Table 2-17.

TABLE 2-17

Passion flower	1:2	20 ml
Chamomile	1:2	25 ml
Meadowsweet	1:2	25 ml
Licorice	1:1	15 ml
Yarrow	1:2	15 ml
Total		100 ml

Dosage: 5 ml with water three times a day after meals. An extra dose can be taken before retiring in the evening.

HERPES SIMPLEX

Background. Herpes simplex skin outbreaks are characteristic mucocutaneous lesions that are caused by new infection with herpes simplex virus 1 (HSV1) or 2 (HSV2) or by reactivation of latent virus residing in the nervous system. Typically, HSV1 affects the face, lips, or mouth, and HSV2 affects the genitals, although either virus can infect either location.

HSV is a double-stranded, deoxyribonucleic acid (DNA), enveloped virus. HSV infection of some neuronal cells does not result in cell death. Instead, the cell maintains the viral genomes in a repressed state that is compatible with survival and normal activities of the cell, a condition known as latency.

Treatment Strategy: Goals, Actions, and Herbs

- Immune-enhancing herbs will assist the fight against the virus in acute outbreaks and will prevent reactivation of latent virus. Key herbs include Echinacea root, Andrographis, and Astragalus. Astragalus should not be used in acute outbreaks.
- Internal treatment with St. John's wort preparations that are high in hypericin appears to exert a significant activity against the virus (which is enveloped).
- Debilitated patients with recurrent outbreaks may benefit from adrenal tonics, tonics, adaptogenic herbs, and nervine tonics between outbreaks. Key herbs in these categories include Rehmannia, ashwaganda, Eleutherococcus, and St. John's wort.
- Topical treatment of lesions includes Calendula extract (applied neat to the lesions) and lemon balm and licorice in ointment or cream form. Clinical studies have shown that using lemon balm ointment on lesions helps prevent future outbreaks.

Example Formula. For acute outbreaks, the formula in Table 2-18 has helped several patients in conjunction with topical application of Calendula extract.

HYPERTHYROIDISM

Background. Graves' disease (hyperthyroidism) is an inflammatory, autoimmune disease affecting the thyroid gland. Thyroid-stimulating antibodies are present. Symptoms include weight loss, tremor, tachycardia, heat intolerance, palpitations, restlessness, and irritability.

Treatment Strategy: Goals, Actions, and Herbs

- Thyroid function can be dampened with thyroid-stimulating hormone (TSH) antagonists, specifically bugleweed.
- Cardiac symptoms such as tachycardia and palpitations can be controlled with antiarrhythmic herbs, particularly motherwort, which reputedly has antithyroid activity as well.
- Immune system function can be balanced with immune-modifying herbs such as Echinacea root and immune depressing herbs such as Hemidesmus and Tylophora.
- Inflammation can be reduced with antiinflammatory herbs such as Rehmannia and Bupleurum.
- Any suspected viral cause can be treated with antiviral herbs such as St. John's wort (active only against enveloped viruses) and Thuja.

Example Formula. See Table 2-19.

MALE IMPOTENCE

Background. Impotence is the failure to achieve erection, ejaculation, or both. A variety of complaints may be demonstrated, including low libido, inability to initiate or maintain an erection, inability to ejaculate, and premature ejaculation. Although previous beliefs concluded that psychologic causes predominated, possible organic or functional problems occupy current thinking. Thus a multifactorial approach to assessment and treatment is required.

TABLE **2-18**

Echinacea root blend	1:2	70 ml
St. John's wort (high hypericin)	1:2	30 ml
Total		100 ml

Dosage: 5 ml with water four to five times a day until the lesions heal.

TABLE **2-19**

Bugleweed	1:2	20 ml
Motherwort	1:2	20 ml
Echinacea root (E. angustifolia or E. purpurea)	1:2	20 ml
Bupleurum	1:2	25 ml
St. John's wort (high hypericin)	1:2	20 ml
Total		105 ml

Dosage: 5 to 8 ml with water three times a day.

Androgen deficiency, lowered vitality, psychologic disturbance (particularly anxiety and depression), and prescribed or recreational drugs may cause a loss of desire. Failure of erection may be the result of these factors or factors beyond herbal treatment such as penile diseases and neurologic damage. In contrast, a number of herbs can help impotence related to circulatory problems.

Treatment Strategy: Goals, Actions, and Herbs

- Anxiety can be treated with anxiolytic herbs such as kava and valerian. Nervine tonics are often required, particularly damiana, skullcap, and St. John's wort.
- Devitalization is often a factor that can be attenuated by tonic herbs such as Korean ginseng, ashwaganda, and Eleutherococcus. If the devitalization is chronic, then adrenal tonics will be required, such as licorice and Rehmannia.
- Male hormone levels can be improved with male tonics: saw palmetto and Korean ginseng.
- Improving circulation will always provide a benefit to maintain erection, and circulatory herbs, particularly ginger, Ginkgo, and prickly ash, will assist this treatment goal. Hawthorn berry and Astragalus may be required if heart function is poor.

Example Formula. See Table 2-20.

MENOPAUSE

Background. Not all women who undergo menopause experience symptoms. This fact highlights that menopause is a normal event in a woman's life. Approximately 70% of women experience hot flashes, and 40% suffer from depression. Other symptoms such as sweating, fatigue, irregular menstruation, and insomnia occur in 20% to 40% of perimenopausal women.

The aim of herbal treatment is to:
- Assist the adjustment to this important change.
- Provide symptomatic alleviation of the effects of estrogen withdrawal.

Herbal treatment should not be prescribed indefinitely, although it may be required for several years.

In recent tradition (the last 60 or so years), herbalists have emphasized herbs containing steroidal saponins or similar compounds (e.g., false unicorn root, wild yam, black cohosh) for managing menopausal symptoms. To regard these herbs as overtly estrogenic in the postmenopausal woman is a mistake. Such phytochemicals possibly act by interacting with hypothalamic estrogen receptors, thereby allaying the effects of estrogen withdrawal.

The oral use of wild yam is therefore related more to its subtle estrogenic properties and not to any reputed progesterogenic properties. In fact, no evidence exists that wild yam, the herbal extract, can produce progesterone in the body. Any link between wild yam and progesterogenic effects is a confusing coincidence derived from the fact that progesterone can be made (in a factory or laboratory) from wild yam.

Treatment Strategy: Goals, Actions, and Herbs. The main aims of herbal assistance with the menopausal change are to:

- Assist the body to adapt to the new hormonal levels by reducing the effects of estrogen withdrawal. Prescribing saponin-containing herbs such as false unicorn root, wild yam, and black cohosh achieves this goal. Korean ginseng is a tonic saponin-containing herb with some evidence for estrogenic activity. However, irritability and insomnia may be aggravated, thus Korean ginseng should be used cautiously and at lower doses.
- The nervous system can be supported with tonic and nervine tonic herbs. St. John's wort is almost a specific for menopausal depression; skullcap and oats are also popular.
- The intensity of the hot flashes or sweating should be abated. The important herb here is sage, although cardiovascular herbs such as hawthorn berry and motherwort can also be useful.

Chaste tree has a role to play for the perimenopausal woman who experiences PMS-like symptoms (which may or may not be premenstrual resulting from menstrual irregularity). Some herbalists are of the opinion that chaste tree also helps allay other menopausal symptoms such as hot flashes. The influence of chaste tree on pituitary function might be the key here.

Example Formula. See Table 2-21.

OSTEOARTHRITIS

Background. Despite being the most common disorder affecting the human species, osteoarthritis (OA) is

TABLE 2-20

Ginkgo (standardized extract)	2:1	20 ml
Korean ginseng	1:2	15 ml
Saw palmetto	1:2	25 ml
Damiana	1:2	20 ml
Eleutherococcus	1:2	20 ml
Total		100 ml

Dosage: 5 ml with water three times a day.

TABLE 2-21

Wild yam	1:2	20 ml
False unicorn root	1:2	20 ml
Sage	1:2	20 ml
St. John's wort	1:2	25 ml
Chaste tree	1:2	15 ml
Total		100 ml

Dosage: 5 ml with water three times a day.

still poorly understood. Approximately 60% of men and 70% of women who died in their 60s and 70s had signs of OA.[38] The prevalence of radiographic OA increases with age for all joints.[38] Up to 35% of men and 49% of women over the age of 65 report disability related to arthritis.[38]

Aging and genetic factors can lead to abnormalities in cartilage, which, in conjunction with obesity, trauma, and poor joint alignment, leads to abnormal stress on joints. These abnormalities result in inflammation and cartilage remodeling. Cells in the synovial lining release cytokines, which, in complex and poorly understood reactions, lead to cartilage degradation, synovitis, and changes in bone (thickening and osteophyte formation).[38]

Conventional medicine now recognizes that diet may play a role in developing OA. In particular, antioxidant vitamins and vitamin D may play a role in slowing the progression of the disease.[39]

Although OA is a slowly progressive disease, some patients can improve. The correlation between radiologic findings and the patient's symptoms is often poor—indicating that the disorder is related to more than just the mechanical functioning of the joint.[38,40]

A number of distinct subsets of patients with OA have been identified, including those with[40]:

- Mechanical joint derangement, for example, postinjury
- Unilateral hip OA
- Generalized nodal OA (Heberden's and Bouchard's nodes), seen most commonly in women with symptoms starting around menopause

Pain is the earliest and most consistent manifestation of early OA and tends to be associated with joint activity. Cartilage has no nerve endings, thus the pain must come from other sources, such as ischemia in bone, psychologic stress, inflammation in ligaments, and pressure on nerves.[41]

Treatment Strategy: Goals, Actions, and Herbs. Antirheumatic herbs are generally prescribed for the treatment of arthritis and rheumatism.

- Herbs that make the body more alkaline are a key part of the treatment for OA, and the main herb in this category is celery. Celery is considered by some herbalists to increase the excretion of acidic metabolites in the urine. Celery probably also has antiinflammatory activity. Other herbs used for OA in this category include dandelion leaf and meadowsweet.
- Depuratives, which are believed to aid in the clearance of metabolic waste from the body, are also often prescribed. These herbs include burdock and yellow dock; but the key herb is nettle leaf, which has recently been found to also have antiinflammatory activity in arthritis.
- Bladderwrack is used for obese patients with arthritis because of its thyroid-stimulating activity, but it may also have other effects.
- St. John's wort is prescribed when nerve entrapment is present. Because of its positive effect on the nervous system, particularly in cases of depression, St. John's wort can also help compensate for negative psychosocial factors and improve sleep quality.
- Antiinflammatory herbs are often used, and these include devil's claw, black cohosh, willow bark, feverfew, ginger, and turmeric.
- Herbalists have long recognized the importance of improving the circulation to affected joints, and traditional treatments such as prickly ash and cayenne can be supplemented with modern treatments such as Ginkgo.
- Although cramp bark, kava, and valerian are sometimes used to relax the muscles around an arthritic joint, whether they can really act in this way is debatable. The value of these herbs may be more in their ability to relax the patient and improve sleep quality.
- Analgesic herbs may be useful and include California poppy and Jamaica dogwood.

Example Formula. See Table 2-22.

Case History. A 66-year-old man had been diagnosed with spinal stenosis, with a tendency to calcification in his body, for example, the lower aorta. He was experiencing pain in the left side (referred pain) and also pain in his left hip (OA of the hip was confirmed by x-ray diagnosis). He was taking nonsteroidal antiinflammatory drug (NSAID) pain-killers and was previously a long-term smoker.

He was prescribed the formulation in Table 2-23.

Nettle leaf and birch leaf decoction of one to two heaped metric teaspoons per dose, twice a day was also prescribed.

After 7 months of treatment, he was not experiencing any symptoms and was no longer taking the

TABLE **2-22**

Celery seed	1:2	30 ml
Devil's claw	1:2	40 ml
Ginger	1:2	10 ml
Nettle leaf	1:2	25 ml
Total		105 ml

Dosage: 5 ml with water three times a day.

TABLE **2-23**

Ginkgo standardized extract	2:1	20 ml
St. John's wort	1:2	25 ml
Celery seed	1:2	35 ml
Dandelion leaf	1:1	20 ml
Total		100 ml

Dosage: 8 ml with water twice a day.

NSAID. He continued with the treatment at one half the initially prescribed doses for another 6 months, after which he discontinued herbal treatment because he was pain free. He remains free of pain 4 years later.

Nettle leaf and birch leaf were prescribed for the arthritis and calcification tendency. Ginkgo was to improve microcirculation to joints and nerves (history of smoking), and St. John's wort was for nerve entrapment pain.

PREMENSTRUAL SYNDROME

Background. Recent experiments have examined the relationship between premenstrual syndrome (PMS) and hormones.[42-44] Inhibition of the luteal phase with a progesterone-receptor antagonist does not alter symptoms of PMS.[42] However, ovarian suppression usually reduces PMS.[43]

Taken together, this finding implies that PMS is triggered by hormone-related events in the follicular or periovulatory phases. Ovarian suppression under double-blind conditions in women with PMS decreased the severity and eliminated the cyclicity of symptoms in approximately 50% of women.[44] Symptoms returned when either progesterone or estradiol were replaced at physiologic levels in these women. Unfortunately, the study does not elaborate on whether estrogen and progesterone (not taken at the same time) returned symptoms in the same women.

The most striking finding in this study is that although women with PMS had few symptoms during ovarian suppression and recurrence of symptoms during ovarian steroid hormone replacement, normal women had no perturbation of mood during either manipulation. These observations suggest that normal plasma concentrations of gonadal steroids can trigger an abnormal response—deterioration in mood state—in susceptible women. This finding highlights the importance in PMS of treating the nervous system, as well as the endocrine system. (The current use of antidepressant drugs to treat PMS underlines this consideration.)

Elevated levels of prolactin may be involved, for example, causing breast tenderness. Prolactin may not be raised all the time: with the condition known as latent hyperprolactinemia, it is only elevated during stress. This theory may have particular relevance to the use of chaste tree in PMS.

Until recently, the way chaste tree acted in the body was poorly understood. Some theories suggested that chaste tree acted on the pituitary to regulate a relative progesterone deficiency, but this was based on 40-year-old research. Modern studies have found that some chaste tree extracts are dopaminergic (prolactin from the pituitary is inhibited by dopamine). Hence chaste tree may act in PMS by treating the presence of latent hyperprolactinemia. A chaste tree extract optimized for dopaminergic phytochemicals was effective in a double-blind, placebo-controlled, clinical trial in women with PMS.[45]

Treatment Strategy: Goals, Actions, and Herbs

- Any hormonal imbalance can be corrected with chaste tree and is usually prescribed throughout the cycle on a long-term basis. Usual dose is 2 ml of a 1:2 extract taken with water on rising.
- Treating emotional disturbances, which can often be the most important part of the therapy, should be a priority. Treatment is usually maintained throughout the cycle. For depression, nervine tonics such as St. John's wort are used, and for anxiety or insomnia, mild sedatives such as kava or valerian are used.
- The main physical symptoms should be treated as they occur: fluid retention can be treated with diuretics such as dandelion leaf, aches and pains with an herbal analgesic such as California poppy, and sweats with sage. Ginkgo throughout the cycle was found to be useful for breast symptoms. Sometimes symptomatic treatment will not be necessary if the other aims are addressed.

TABLE 2-24

St. John's wort	1:2	20 ml
Schisandra	1:2	25 ml
Ashwaganda	1:2	30 ml
Skullcap	1:2	25 ml
Total		100 ml

Dosage: 8 ml with water twice a day.

TABLE 2-25

Gentian	1:2	10 ml
Cinnamon	1:2	25 ml
Coleus	1:1	40 ml
Ginger	1:2	25 ml
Total		100 ml

Dosage: 20 drops (approximately 0.5 ml) with water 20 minutes before meals.

- The adverse effects of stress on the body can be relieved by using adaptogenic herbs such as Eleutherococcus and ashwaganda.
- The liver should be treated if signs of sluggishness are apparent (e.g., difficulty digesting fats, tendency to constipation, history of liver disease, tendency to nausea, preference for light or no breakfasts). The liver is the site of the breakdown of female hormones, and a sluggish liver may contribute to hormonal imbalance. Herbs to use include Schisandra and milk thistle.
- If the previous protocol is unsuccessful, estrogen-modulating herbs containing steroidal saponins such as false unicorn root and wild yam may be included in the treatment.

Example Formula. Chaste tree 1:2, 2 ml with water on rising (see Table 2-24).

If fluid retention is present as a predominating symptom, dandelion leaf at 8 ml once a day may be included in the second half of the cycle.

POOR DIGESTIVE FUNCTION

Background. Poor upper gastrointestinal function may be the result of inefficient functioning of the salivary glands, stomach, pancreas, liver or gallbladder, or a combination of these. Symptoms include anorexia, a prolonged sensation of fullness or stagnation after eating, undigested food in stools, belching or flatulence, intolerance of fatty foods, and nausea.

However, although poor upper digestive function may be largely asymptomatic in itself, it may contribute to other conditions such as food intolerance or allergies, intestinal dysbiosis (abnormal bowel flora), constipation, nutrient deficiencies, and migraine headaches. Herbalists believe that many chronic diseases begin with poor digestive function and that good upper digestive function is a prerequisite for a healthy digestive system.

Poor upper digestive function can also be a consequence of prolonged or serious illness or can occur with convalescence. The condition is also reflected in children by their failure to thrive, anemia, and susceptibility to infections. Digestive function also deteriorates with age, particularly gastric acid and pancreatic enzyme output.

Treatment Strategy: Goals, Actions, and Herbs

- All aspects of upper digestive function can be improved with bitters such as gentian.
- Saliva and gastric acid output can be improved with aromatic digestives, including cinnamon and Coleus, and pungent herbs, especially ginger.
- Bile production by the liver can be improved with choleretic herbs such as dandelion root, milk thistle, and globe artichoke.
- Gallbladder function can be improved with cholagogue herbs, especially fringe tree, peppermint, and greater celandine.
- In debilitated patients, or in children failing to thrive, tonic herbs, especially ashwaganda, are included.

Example Formula. An example formula for improving upper digestive function is found in Table 2-25.

The reader should note that when using a dropper, it must be a pharmaceutically calibrated dropper.

POOR LIVER FUNCTION

Background. Symptoms that may be caused by poor liver function include sluggish digestion, fat intolerance, nausea, and chronic constipation, as well as chemical, food, or drug intolerances. A poorly functioning liver may also contribute to a number of disease states, such as psoriasis, autoimmune disease, irritable bowel syndrome, allergies, and cancer. Patients might reveal a history of past liver infection, infestation or damage, alcohol or drug abuse, or exposure to medical drugs or environmental pollutants such as pesticides. Drug side effects are more likely to occur in patients with poor liver function.

Treatment Strategy: Goals, Actions, and Herbs

- Hepatoprotective and hepatic trophorestorative herbs can improve the liver's capacity to withstand toxic insult and can help alleviate previous toxic damage, especially if a history of liver damage or exposure to toxins is present. Principal herbs include milk thistle and globe artichoke. Schisandra is particularly useful because it also enhances the detoxifying capacity of the liver. These herbs will assist in cases of nausea and intolerances from any cause.
- Choleretic herbs boost bile production, hence the digestive role of the liver are particularly indicated if digestive symptoms are predominant. Choleretic herbs will also boost detoxification via the bile and therefore can be valuable in conditions such as psoriasis and cancer. The hepatoprotective herbs previously listed possess a gentle choleretic activity as does dandelion root, but strongly choleretic herbs include golden seal, barberry, greater celandine, and bitter herbs. These strongly choleretic herbs will cause nausea and irritability in a patient who has some history of liver damage. Therefore choleretic herbs should be avoided at first in these circumstances and only introduced after prior treatment with hepatic trophorestoratives and gentle choleretics.
- Depurative herbs are also indicated in cases in which hepatic detoxification may be inadequate. Herbs that act principally via the liver and digestive tract include burdock, yellow dock, fringe tree, and Oregon grape.
- Liver phase I and phase II detoxification can be treated with Schisandra, rosemary, and turmeric.

Example Formula. See Table 2-26.

Case History. A female patient, age 38, wished to take the contraceptive pill. She found that even a low-dose pill still caused symptoms of female hormone excess such as abdominal bloating, weight gain, nausea, and depression. She had a history of liver damage caused by hydatid cysts during childhood.

See Table 2-27 for the treatment.

The patient found that she was able to take the pill without any adverse effects as long as she also took the herbal treatment.

REACTIVE HYPOGLYCEMIA (DYSGLYCEMIA)

Background. Reactive hypoglycemia is a controversial syndrome that is not acknowledged as a true hypoglycemic condition in conventional medical literature.[46] Reactive hypoglycemia is characterized by hunger and autonomic symptoms such as anxiety, trembling, and sweating, as well as those that may be related to low blood sugar, such as dizziness and poor concentration. These symptoms typically occur in the mid to late

TABLE 2-26		
Milk thistle	1:1	30 ml
Globe artichoke	1:2	25 ml
Schisandra	1:2	25 ml
Fringe tree	1:2	20 ml
Total		100 ml

Dosage: 5 ml with water three times a day before meals.

TABLE 2-27		
Milk thistle	1:1	30 ml
Dandelion root	1:2	35 ml
Schisandra	1:2	35 ml
Total		100 ml

Dosage: 5 ml with water twice a day.

mornings and afternoons and are relieved by eating. Other terms to describe this syndrome have been suggested, such as dysglycemia or idiopathic postprandial syndrome.[46]

What may be at work is that these individuals are more sensitive to a drop in blood sugar, perhaps from the effects of caffeine, stress, poor cerebral blood flow, or any combination. The effect of caffeine intake on recognition of and physiologic responses to hypoglycemia was studied in patients with insulin-dependent diabetes mellitus (IDDM).[47] For the patient with diabetes, hypoglycemia unawareness is potentially dangerous. The study looked at the effect of ingestion of 250 mg of caffeine (2 to 3 cups of coffee) on the hypoglycemic response at 3.8 and 2.8 mmol/L (68 and 50 mg/dl) blood glucose under double-blind conditions.

Caffeine caused an immediate and sustained fall in cerebral blood flow. At a blood glucose of 3.8 mmol/L (68 mg/dl), plasma epinephrine (adrenaline) levels were twice as high after caffeine compared with placebo. When glucose was lowered to 2.8 mmol/L (50 mg/dl), caffeine was associated with a greater awareness of hypoglycemia with significantly more intense autonomic and neurologic symptoms (for example, hunger, palpitations, sweating, irritability, and dizziness). Levels of epinephrine, cortisol, and growth hormone were also raised.

The same research group previously found that if blood glucose levels fall into the "low-normal" range in individuals without diabetes, prior caffeine intake augments both the symptomatic and hormonal responses to a modest reduction in blood glucose.[48] This finding is of particular interest. The medical orthodoxy considers true reactive hypoglycemia to be rare. However, some health care professionals maintain that hypoglycemia is relatively common. The confounding factors may be caffeine intake, given that it strongly accentuates the symptoms of even mild hypoglycemia, or just a greater sensitivity to low blood sugar. Patients with symptoms of reactive hypoglycemia should certainly avoid caffeine in all its forms.

In true hypoglycemia, glucose counter-regulatory mechanisms are activated when blood sugar falls below 3.75 mmol/L. These mechanisms comprise the release of the hormones glucagon, epinephrine, growth hormone, and cortisol. The release of epinephrine causes many of the symptoms of true hypoglycemia. In reactive hypoglycemia, some of these mechanisms may also be inappropriately activated, which underlies the role of adrenal support in the herbal treatment of the condition.

Treatment Strategy: Goals, Actions, and Herbs

Diet. Refined carbohydrates should be avoided because they can overstimulate insulin release (which may be one aspect of the syndrome). Intake of caffeine should also be avoided. Meals should ideally be smaller and more often, and substantial protein intake should be part of each meal (protein stimulates gluconeogenesis, which results in a consistent output of glucose from the liver).

Herbal Treatment

- Adrenal gland function can be supported with adrenal restorative herbs such as licorice and Rehmannia. Only Rehmannia should be used if the patient has high blood pressure.
- Detrimental effects of stress on the adrenal glands can be reduced with adaptogens such as ashwaganda, Korean ginseng, and Eleutherococcus.
- Adrenal function can be boosted with tonics such as Korean ginseng.
- Cerebral circulation can be improved with rosemary and Ginkgo.
- Lower doses of Gymnema in liquid preparations (10 ml of 1:1 extract per 100 ml formula) can help control reactive hypoglycemia and sugar craving, as can bitter herbs such as gentian.

TABLE 2-28

Rehmannia	1:2	30 ml
Licorice	1:1	15 ml
Gymnema	1:1	10 ml
Schisandra	1:2	25 ml
Eleutherococcus	1:2	25 ml
Total		105 ml

Dosage: 5 ml with water three times a day before meals.

- Liver function can be supported with Schisandra and milk thistle because the liver also has a role in regulating blood sugar.

Example Formula. See Table 2-28.

VARICOSE VEINS

Background. In varicose veins (VV), the valves do not function properly, which results in dilated, tortuous superficial veins in the legs. Primary VV originate in the superficial vein system and are more common in women. Approximately one half of these patients have a family history of VV. Secondary VV result from venous insufficiency in the deep veins and indicate more serious venous reflux (compromise of venous return).

Symptoms include a dull ache or pressure sensation in the legs, especially after prolonged standing, and restless leg syndrome (restless legs in bed). Signs, other than the veins themselves, include atrophic changes in the skin of the foot and ankle, mild ankle edema, and discoloration of the skin caused by the rupture of a varicosity. Complications include skin ulceration and superficial vein thrombosis.

VV can occur during pregnancy because of hormonal changes and increased pressure caused by the expanding uterus. Obesity, menopause, aging, and repeated abdominal strain, as with heavy lifting or constipation, may contribute. Long periods of standing or sitting with the legs bent or crossed should be avoided.

Weakness of the vein wall and poor venous tone can lead to valves becoming incompetent, and natural treatments stress the need to maintain good venous and connective tissue tone.

Treatment Strategy: Goals, Actions, and Herbs. No known herbal treatment has been found that will return VV to normal veins. However, herbal treatment can correct symptoms and prevent further deterioration or complications.

TABLE **2-29**

Horsechestnut	1:2	30 ml
Ginkgo (standardized extract)	2:1	20 ml
Bilberry	1:1	30 ml
Hawthorn leaf	1:2	20 ml
Total		100 ml

Dosage: 5 ml with water three times a day.

- Venous return, vein function, and connective tissue tone can be improved with venotonic herbs, particularly horsechestnut, collagen-stabilizing herbs (hawthorn berry), and vasoprotective herbs (bilberry).
- Circulatory function can be improved with circulatory stimulants, especially Ginkgo.

Example Formula. See Table 2-29.

TOPICAL USE OF LIQUID HERBS

MAKING HERBAL CREAMS FROM LIQUIDS

Although the topical use of herbs is often an effective means of treatment, the available range of prepared creams and ointments is quite limited. Practitioners who wish to use a wider range to fully tap the healing potential of a variety of herbs can manufacture their own herbal creams by using herbal liquids mixed into a suitable neutral base. An inexpensive and convenient way to make herbal creams is described here.

Although one can have philosophic objections to their use (and sometimes practical objections because they can act as irritants), the cream base should contain adequate levels of a synthetic preservative, largely because:

- Creams are used repeatedly, and each time the patient touches the cream, he or she introduces microbes that can grow and multiply, unless preservatives are present.
- The addition of liquids to a cream base might also introduce microbes that have the potential to spoil the cream or even render it harmful (especially if applied to broken skin).

Aseptic technique*[49] must be used when making herbal creams.

Example Formulations. A few examples of how to make different herbal creams are provided. However, the possibilities are many, and specific formulations containing several herbs can be prepared for individual patients. Information on the topical use of individual herbs is provided in the various monographs provided in this text.

Antiseptic Cream. To make an antiseptic cream, the following ingredients may be combined:

100 g cream base
5 ml thyme 1:2 extract
5 ml myrrh 1:5 tincture
5 ml Calendula 1:2 extract

Cream is stirred thoroughly until a smooth consistency is obtained.

Comment. This method can be used to incorporate small quantities of tinctures or extracts into the cream base. Because the tinctures and extracts are incorporated directly without removal of alcohol, the resultant cream will sting if applied to broken skin.

Herpes Cream. 100 ml of lemon balm extract 1:2 is reduced on low heat (over 1 hour) to 15 to 20 ml. This concentrate is poured while hot onto 100 g of cream base and mixed thoroughly until the resultant cream has an even color. The cream is applied to lesions every few hours.

Comment. This technique is a general method for making creams with high levels of activity by incorporating large quantities of extracts into the cream base. The alcohol is removed during the concentration step. This method is not suitable for herbs containing essential oils (volatile oils) because they will evaporate during the concentration step. (The antiviral activity of lemon balm is not a result of the essential oil.)

In the case of the lemon balm cream, 100 ml of 1:2 extract has been recommended as the initial volume. However, for most other herbs, 30 to 50 ml of 1:2 extract concentrated to 10 to 15 ml is sufficient to make a cream with good activity (see later discussion). Less extract can be used when making up an Arnica cream given that it is quite active.

Varicose Vein Cream. 30 ml of horsechestnut 1:2 is reduced on low heat to approximately 10 ml. This concentrate is poured while hot onto 100 g of cream base and mixed thoroughly until the resultant

---

*Bacteria and mold will grow in a cream if introduced under certain conditions. If fingers are dipped into the cream, or if any water or other contaminant gets into the cream, bacteria and mold may grow. When formulating creams, the following technique is suggested: Hands are washed with soap and warm water and dried thoroughly before using the cream. **A sterile instrument is used to take cream from the jar and transfer it to a sterilized container.** Cream is stored below 30°C (86°F) and away from direct sunlight. In summer, it is stored in a refrigerator. The lid is replaced firmly after each use to ensure the contents are sealed.

cream has an even color. The mixture is applied to varicose veins twice a day. The cream is also beneficial for soft tissue injuries, but it should not be applied to broken skin.

Healing Cream. 10 ml of Calendula 1:2 and 20 ml of gotu kola 1:2 is reduced on low heat to approximately 15 ml; 30 ml of Aloe vera juice concentrate is added to the hot liquid and continued to concentrate until the final mixture is 15 to 20 ml. This concentrate is poured while hot onto 100 g of cream base and mixed thoroughly until the resultant cream has an even color. This cream can be applied to wounds, abrasions, and ulcers.

OTHER EXAMPLES OF THE TOPICAL USE OF LIQUIDS

Throat Syrup

30 ml *Echinacea purpurea* glycetract 1:3
34 ml marshmallow glycetract 1:5
15 ml elecampane 1:2
10 ml wild cherry bark 1:2
10 ml licorice 1:1
1 ml ginger 1:2

Blend ingredients together and take 3 ml up to six times a day.

Feminine Douche

2 cups warm water (or Calendula tea)
1 tbsp apple cider vinegar
2 drops tea tree oil
5 ml Oregon grape
5 ml pau d'arco
3 ml *Echinacea purpurea* or *angustifolia* root 1:2

Mix together and douche using a very slow, gentle flow.

Nasal Rinse or Neti Pot

$\frac{1}{2}$ cup warm water
$\frac{1}{2}$ tsp sea salt
1 ml Baical skullcap 1:2
1 ml eyebright 1:2
1 ml golden seal 1:3
1 ml chamomile 1:2 (optional)

Dissipating the alcohol for this procedure is not necessary, because the alcohol will not irritate the tissue. This solution can be placed in a Neti Pot (similar to a mini-teapot and is designed for nasal rinsing) or inserted into a large dropper and gently poured into one nostril at a time, over a sink, while holding the other nostril closed. The solution will rinse the nasal passageways and run down the back of the throat and into the mouth for discarding.

Mouthwash

$\frac{1}{2}$ cup of water (or peppermint tea for flavor)
3 ml Oregon grape
3 ml sage
3 ml *Echinacea purpurea* or *angustifolia* root 1:2

Ingredients are mixed together and swished and swallowed three times a day after meals.

Saline Nasal Spray

Base:
30 ml purified water
$\frac{1}{4}$ tsp sea salt
5 ml glycerin
Ingredients are mixed together.
The following herbs are added:
2 ml Baical skullcap 1:2
2 ml eyebright 1:2
2 ml golden seal 1:3

The base and herbs are mixed together and poured into a clean, empty, saline, nasal-spray bottle and sprayed into each nostril as needed.

Caution: Potential allergic reaction could occur with use.

Contraindicated in infection or blockage of the sinuses.

Soothing Eyebath

8 drops eyebright 1:2
8 drops chamomile 1:2 (caution if allergy to the daisy family)

Herbs are placed in heat resistant container. Pour $\frac{1}{2}$ cup of boiling water over this mixture to dissipate the alcohol. Mixture is allowed to cool, and eyebath cup is filled. This amount will be enough to fill several eyebath cups. Fresh solution should be used for each eye and should be used within 4 hours. *If a stronger solution is needed, 8 drops of golden seal 1:3 can be used instead of chamomile.*

Note to the reader: Herbal extracts, once diluted in water, will have a limited shelf life. Recommendations suggest that for optimal efficacy, any water-mix formulas used should be as fresh as possible and not stored.

Acknowledgment. The assistance of herbalist Linda Ryan in preparing this section on the topical use of liquids is gratefully acknowledged.

REFERENCES

1 Mills S, Bone K: *Principles and practice of phytotherapy: modern herbal medicine,* Edinburgh, 2000, Churchill Livingstone.
2 Germouty J et al: Does extrinsic asthma exist? *Allerg Immunol* 22(suppl 10):32, 1988.

3 Brugman SM et al: Increased lower airways responsiveness associated with sinusitis in a rabbit model, *Am Rev Respir Dis* 147(2):314, 1993.

4 Friday GA Jr, Fireman P: Sinusitis and asthma: clinical and pathogenetic relationships, *Clin Chest Med* 9(4):557, 1988.

5 Bray GW: The hypochlorhydria of asthma in childhood, *Quart J Med* 24:181, 1931.

6 Barberio G et al: Gastro-esophageal reflux and asthma. Clinical experience, *Minerva Pediatr* 41(7):363, 1989.

7 Giudicelli R et al: Gastroesophageal reflux and respiratory manifestations: diagnostic approach, therapeutic indications and results, *Ann Chir* 44(7):552, 1990.

8 Sly PD, Hibbert ME: Childhood asthma following hospitalization with acute viral bronchiolitis infancy, *Pediatr Pulmonol* 7(3):153, 1989.

9 Szczeklik A: Aspirin-induced asthma as a viral disease, *Clin Allergy* 18(1):15, 1988.

10 Hahn DL, Dodge RW, Golubjatnikov R: Association of Chlamydia pneumoniae (strain TWAR) infection with wheezing, asthmatic bronchitis, and adult-onset asthma, *JAMA* 266(2):225, 1991.

11 Burney P: A diet rich in sodium may potentiate asthma. Epidemiological evidence for a new hypothesis, *Chest* 91(suppl 6):143S, 1987.

12 Lock K et al: Immunoglobulin G subclass deficiency in patients with asthma and chronic obstructive bronchitis, *Immun Infekt* 18(5):157, 1990.

13 Loftus BG et al: IgG subclass deficiency in asthma, *Arch Dis Child* 63(12):1434, 1988.

14 Rumbak MJ et al: Perception of anxiety as a contributing factor of asthma: indigent versus nonindigent, *J Asthma* 30(3):165, 1993.

15 Mrazek DA et al: Early asthma onset: consideration of parenting issues, *J Am Acad Child Adolesc Psych* 30(2):277, 1991.

16 Boljevic S, Daniljak IG, Kogan AH: Changes in free radicals and possibility of their correction in patients with bronchial asthma, *Vojnosanit Pregl* 50(1):3, 1993.

17 Greene LS: Asthma and oxidant stress: nutritional, environmental, and genetic risk factors, *J Am Coll Nutr* 14(4):317, 1995.

18 Hatch GE: Asthma, inhaled oxidants, and dietary antioxidants, *Am J Clin Nutr* 61(suppl 3):625S, 1995.

19 Moul JW: Benign prostatic hyperplasia, *Postgrad Med* 94(6):141, 151, 1993.

20 Bone K: Chronic fatigue syndrome and its herbal treatment, *Modern Phytotherapist* 1(3):12, 1995. MediHerb Pty Ltd, Warwick, Queensland, Australia.

21 Stricklin A, Sewell M, Austad C: Objective measurement of personality variables in epidemic neuromyasthenia patients, *S Afr Med J* 77(1):31, 1990.

22 Harrison TR, Fauci AS, eds: *Harrison's principles of internal medicine*, ed 14, [Compact Disc], New York, 1998, McGraw-Hill.

23 Felter HW, Lloyd JU: *King's American dispensatory*, ed 18, rev 3, Portland, 1905, reprinted 1983, Eclectic Medical Publications.

24 Nemeroff CB: The neurobiology of depression, *Sci Am* 278(6):42, 1998.

25 Rosengren A, Tibblin G, Wilhelmsen L: Low systolic blood pressure and self perceived wellbeing in middle aged men, *BMJ* 306(6872):243, 1993.

26 Barrett-Connor E, Palinkas LA: Low blood pressure and depression in older men: a population based study, *BMJ* 308(6926):446, 1994.

27 Bos JD, Kapsenberg ML, Sillevis Smitt JH: Pathogenesis of atopic eczema, *Lancet* 343(8909):1338, 1994.

28 Rudikoff D, Lebwohl M: Atopic dermatitis, *Lancet* 351(9117):1715, 1998.

29 Tan BB et al: Double-blind controlled trial of effect of house dust-mite allergen avoidance on atopic dermatitis, *Lancet* 347(8993):15, 1996.

30 Abeck D, Mempel M: *Staphylococcus aureus* colonization in atopic dermatitis and its therapeutic implications, *Br J Dermatol* 139(suppl 53):13, 1998.

31 Leung DYM et al: The role of superantigens in human diseases: therapeutic implications for the treatment of skin diseases, *Br J Dermatol* 139(suppl 53):17, 1998.

32 Ayers S: Gastric secretion in psoriasis, eczema and dermatitis herpetiformis, *Arch Dermatol Syphilol* 20:854, 1929.

33 Brown WH, Smith MS, McLachlan AD: Fractional gastric analysis in diseases of the skin. Further observation in 316 cases with special reference to rosacea, *Br J Dermatol Syphilis* 47:181, 1935.

34 Nikitina LS, Shinsky GE, Trusov VV: Contribution of the membranous digestion and the small intestine absorption to the pathogenesis of eczema, *Vestnik Dermatol Venerol* (2):4, 1989.

35 Vasiliev YV: Digestive activity of intestinal disaccharidases in infants suffering from eczema, *Vestnik Dermatol Venerol* 10:16, 1984.

36 Robinson M: Gastroesophageal reflux disease. Selecting optimal therapy, *Postgrad Med* 95(2):88, 1994.

37 Smart HL, Nicholson DA, Atkinson M: Gastro-esophageal reflux in the irritable bowel syndrome, *Gut* 27(10):1127, 1986.

38 Brooks PM, March LM: New insight into osteoarthritis, *Med J Aust* 163(7):367, 1995.

39 McAlindon T, Felson DT: Nutrition: risk factors for osteoarthritis, *Ann Rheum Dis* 56(7):397, 1997.

40 Schnitzer TJ: Osteoarthritis treatment update; minimizing pain while limiting patient risk, *Postgrad Med* 93(1):89, 1993.

41 Altman RD: Osteoarthritis: differentiation from rheumatoid arthritis, causes of pain, treatment, *Postgrad Med* 87(3):66, 1990.

42 Schmidt PJ et al: Lack of effect of induced menses on symptoms in women with premenstrual syndrome, *N Engl J Med* 324(17):1174, 1991.

43 Muse KN et al: The premenstrual syndrome. Effects of "medical ovariectomy," *N Engl J Med* 311(21):1345, 1984.

44 Schmidt PJ et al: Differential behavioral effects of gonadal steroids in women with and in those without premenstrual syndrome, *N Engl J Med* 338(4):209, 1998.

45 Schellenberg R: Treatment for the premenstrual syndrome with agnus castus fruit extract: prospective, randomised, placebo controlled study, *BMJ* 322(7279):134, 2001.

46 Service FJ: Hypoglycemic disorders, *New Engl J Med* 332(17):1144, 1995.

47 Debrah K et al: Effect of caffeine on recognition of and physiological responses to hypoglycemia in insulin-dependent diabetes, *Lancet* 347(8993):19, 1996.

48 Kerr D et al: Effect of caffeine on the recognition of and responses to hypoglycemia in humans, *Ann Intern Med* 119(8):799, 1993.

How to Use the Monographs

*T*hese monographs are aimed at providing the herbal clinician with accessible and clinically relevant information on more than 100 well-known and widely used herbs. The information is presented as 125 herbal monographs that cover 137 liquid herbal extracts.

Each monograph is structured in the following way:
- Information that defines the herb by common names, botanical names, plant family, and plant part used
- Prescribing information that contains a summary of clinically relevant information, including actions, potential indications, contraindications, warnings and precautions, interactions, use in pregnancy and lactation, side effects, and dosage
- Supporting information that provides further detail to support the prescribing information and includes traditional prescribing, pharmacologic research, clinical studies, and references

The information in each monograph is covered under the following headings.

COMMON NAMES

Common names of the herb are used throughout the monographs and are presented in lower case. Exceptions are when the botanical name of the genus is used as a common name in which case it is capitalized, as in Echinacea, or when the common name contains a locality, as in Korean ginseng.

OTHER COMMON NAMES

This section lists other common names of the herb that are frequently used, particularly in the literature.

BOTANICAL NAMES

The botanical name consists of two Latin names: a generic name, which comes first, plus a specific epithet, both of which are italicized, as in *Lycopus virginicus*. The generic name, which is capitalized, defines the genus to which the plant belongs and may be abbreviated to its initial letter (e.g., *L. virginicus*). The members of a species may be grouped into subspecies or varieties, such as *Arnica chamissonis* subsp. *foliosa* or *Viburnum opulus* var. *americanum*.

Botanical names other than the current or preferred botanical name, which may be commonly encountered in the scientific or herbal literature, are also listed. These names are denoted by the superscript symbol # as an alternative name. Botanical nomenclature is being frequently updated, thus species and even genus names may change over time. Taxonomists and botanical authorities often disagree, and the status of a botanical name may change (an "old" name may become the "new" name). The botanical name listed first in this section of the monographs is not necessarily the most current botanical synonym but is usually the most widely used. The monographs do not contain a comprehensive listing of all botanical synonyms. Only the more recent or frequently encountered ones are included.

The American Herbal Products Association (AHPA) has reviewed the taxonomy of the most commonly used and important therapeutic herbs in use in the United States. The Association's findings are reflected in the book *Herbs of Commerce* (2nd edition, October, 2000), a document that may supersede the previous *Herbs of Commerce* document that the U.S. Food and Drug Administration uses for the labeling requirements of the Dietary Supplement Health and Education Act 1994. The recommended changes by AHPA for the herbs featured in this book are listed in Table 1.

Proposed Botanical Name Changes for Common Herbs

Common Name	Old Botanical Name	New Botanical Name
Black cohosh	*Cimicifuga racemosa*	*Actaea racemosa*
Couch grass	*Agropyron repens*	*Elymus repens*
Eyebright	*Euphrasia officinalis*	*Euphrasia rostkoviana, Euphrasia stricta*
Jamaica dogwood	*Piscidia erythrina*	*Piscidia piscipula*
Lavender	*Lavandula officinalis*	*Lavandula angustifolia*
Oregon grape	*Berberis aquifolium*	*Mahonia aquifolium*

Note: *Anemone pulsatilla* has been incorrectly assigned in this publication as *Pulsatilla patens* and *Pulsatilla pratensis* instead of *Pulsatilla vulgaris*.

A medicinally interchangeable species refers to another species, subspecies, or variety of an herb that has very similar therapeutic action or actions and may be clinically used in place of the preferred or official species. This species is denoted by the superscript plus symbol +.

Example: *Lycopus virginicus, Lycopus europaeus*[+]

Lycopus virginicus is the preferred species for the uses described for the herb bugleweed, but *Lycopus europaeus* (gypsywort) can also be used for the same clinical applications.

Occasionally, assigning the status of the species as medicinally interchangeable or as alternative is not easily resolved, and the alternative botanical name is listed with both symbols, for example, eyebright: *Euphrasia officinalis, Euphrasia rostkoviana*[#/+].

FAMILY

The plant family is the higher grouping after the genus in the overall hierarchy of the plant kingdom. When investigating botany, an important aspect is to draw a distinction between nomenclature (naming) and taxonomy (classification in a hierarchical system). Taxonomy in particular is a constantly changing field in which plants are often reclassified into a different genus or family.

For simplicity, one authority was chosen as the primary reference: Mabberley DJ: *The Plant Book*, ed 2, Cambridge, 1997, Cambridge University Press. In this book, the author follows primarily the system of Cronquist (1981), which has been modified by Kubitzki (1990). Although this book is not the most recent source of taxonomic information, it is convenient for searching. (More recent classifications do not allow searching by genus.) Therefore changes in taxonomy that have occurred after the publication of Mabberley (1997) will not necessarily be represented here. Currently, the Scrophulariaceae and Malvaceae are

Family Name	Alternative Family Name
Palmae	Arecaceae
Gramineae	Poaceae
Cruciferae	Brassicaceae
Leguminosae	Fabaceae
Guttiferae	Clusiaceae
Umbelliferae	Apiaceae
Labiatae	Lamiaceae
Compositae	Asteraceae

undergoing revision, which is likely to affect several medicinal plants, especially *Rehmannia glutinosa*.

Mabberley uses the family names recognized by the International Association of Botanical Nomenclature (St. Louis Code, 1999). However, alternative family names are also valid. Mabberley is outlined as follows:

This code indicates that both sets of family names are valid, with "Compositae" not out of date compared with "Asteraceae." The issue of which family name to use comes down to the individual's preference. The family names listed in the first column have been chosen for use in this text.

PLANT PARTS USED

The part or parts of the plant that are used therapeutically are defined.

PRESCRIBING INFORMATION

ACTIONS

This field contains a listing of the most relevant actions of the herb. Herbs have activity on the body either when taken orally or applied topically. This information comes mainly from traditional texts, but sources also include recent clinical use and established pharmacologic actions. A glossary at the end of the book provides definitions for these terms, and the appendix contains two action indexes that are categorized according to either the herb common name or the action.

POTENTIAL INDICATIONS

Recommended potential indications, considering the unique needs of the patient, are listed in an easy-to-read list. At the end of each indication, a number (or series of numbers) is displayed that denotes the level of evidence for that indication. This code is not a reference or citation in the usual sense. (Reference numbers are found throughout the rest of the monograph denoted by superscripted numbers.) The level of evidence code is presented as italic numerals in parentheses.

The aim of the code is to provide the reader with a powerful and concise summary of the supporting evidence for the recommended use of the herb by summarizing at a glance the traditional, pharmacologic, and clinical information contained throughout the rest of the monograph.

Definition	Notes
Level 1 Evidence obtained from a systematic review of all relevant randomized, controlled trials	Includes systematic review (of randomized, controlled trials) and meta-analysis.
Level 2 Evidence obtained from at least one properly designed, randomized, controlled trial	Trials must be controlled but not necessarily placebo controlled. Controls may include a controlled diet, compression stockings, or other physical treatments or conventional medication.
Level 3 • Evidence obtained from well-designed, controlled trials without randomization, or • Evidence obtained from well-designed cohort or case-control analytical studies preferably from more than one center or research group, or • Evidence obtained from multiple time series with or without the intervention (Dramatic results in uncontrolled experiments may also be regarded as being of this level of evidence.)	Includes epidemiologic studies and pharmacologic studies in healthy humans, regardless of whether they were well designed or randomized.
Level 4 Opinions of respected authorities, based on clinical experience, descriptive studies (such as uncontrolled trials, postmarketing studies), or reports of expert committees	Includes: • German Commission E monographs (see "Clinical Studies" section for an explanation) • ESCOP monographs (see "Clinical Studies" section for an explanation) • University level textbooks
Level 4a Clinical trial information of any level, testing a constituent isolated from an herb when the dose and bioavailability are sufficient to be extrapolated to oral use of the herb (Examples include clinical trials using escin, the triterpenoid saponin isolated from *Aesculus hippocastanum*.)	If the constituent is present within the herbal extract at the tested dose, then a higher level of evidence may be assigned, depending on the study design.

Continued

Definition	Notes
Level 5 Well-established traditional use of more than 50 years in a major system, such as Western herbal medicine, Ayurveda, or TCM, which is reflected in current practice	Sources of this information include pharmacopeias and authoritative texts: • Pharmacopoeia Commission of the People's Republic of China: *Pharmacopoeia of the People's Republic of China,* English ed, Beijing, 1997, Chemical Industry Press • British Herbal Medicine Association's Scientific Committee: *British herbal pharmacopoeia,* Bournemouth, UK, 1983, BMHA • British Herbal Medicine Association: *British herbal compendium,* Bournemouth, 1992, BHMA Other traditional Western herbal medicine texts: • Felter HW, Lloyd JU: *King's American dispensatory,* ed 18, rev 3, Portland, 1905, reprinted 1983, Eclectic Medical Publications • Felter HW: *The eclectic materia medica, pharmacology and therapeutics,* Portland, 1922, reprinted 1983, Eclectic Medical Publications • Ellingwood F, Lloyd JU: *American materia medica, therapeutics and pharmacognosy,* ed 11, Portland, 1983, Eclectic Medical Publications • Osol A et al: *The dispensatory of the United States of America,* ed 24, Philadelphia, 1947, JB Lippincott Clinical TCM texts: • Bensky D, Gamble A: *Chinese herbal medicine materia medica,* Seattle, 1986, Eastland Press • Chang HM, But PP: *Pharmacology and applications of Chinese materia medica,* Singapore, 1987, World Scientific Clinical Ayurvedic texts: • Chopra RN et al: *Chopra's indigenous drugs of India,* ed 2, Calcutta, 1958, reprinted 1982, Academic Publishers • Thakur RS, Puri HS, Husain A: *Major medicinal plants of India,* Lucknow, 1989, Central Institute of Medicinal and Aromatic Plants • Kapoor LD: *CRC handbook of Ayurvedic medicinal plants,* Boca Raton, 1990, CRC Press. For other ethnic systems, this level is used when primary references are cited.
Level 6 Other traditional writings, particularly those that are secondary sources; reports of primary traditional use, or not likely to be readily used in modern clinical practice	Includes all other books or sources not covered in level 5.
Level 7 Extrapolation from *in vivo* animal studies, with emphasis on studies using oral administration	

TCM, Traditional Chinese medicine.

These levels of evidence are based on those recommended by the Australian government's Therapeutic Goods Administration for the purposes of registering claims for herbal products. The levels have been extended in this book to further distinguish traditional sources of information and to allow inclusion of clinical trials involving herbal constituents and, in some instances, pharmacologic studies. The level of evidence codes are defined in the table on pages 51-52. This table is best referred to regularly until the reader becomes familiar with its contents.

In most cases, when a higher level of evidence exists for using an herb, any lower levels for the same use are not listed:

- If level 1 evidence for randomized, controlled trials is present, the lower level clinical trial evidence (2,3,4) is not listed beside the indication (and similarly for levels 2 and 3). The exception is that level 4 is still listed with a higher level of evidence when it corresponds to respected authorities and expert committees (e.g., Commission E, European Scientific Cooperative on Phytotherapy [ESCOP]).
- When level 4 evidence from an uncontrolled trial exists for an herb, level 4a (trial information on one of its constituents) is not listed.
- Level 6 traditional information is not listed when level 5 occurs. However, if both traditional and clinical support exists for using an herb, both levels of evidence are noted.
- Level 7 is not listed when clinical evidence exists (levels 1 through 4) because pharmacologic animal studies are usually conducted before clinical trials are begun.

Other points worth noting include the following:

- Only systematic reviews evaluating randomized, controlled trials are included as level 1 evidence. (A review of pharmacologic activity [in vivo studies] does not count as level 1.) A review of uncontrolled trials or trials without randomization would be level 3 or 4 evidence.
- When information regarding the quality of the trial is insufficient, a lower level of evidence has been assigned. For example, a controlled trial not stated as randomized would be listed as level 3, not level 2.

When a clinical trial used specialized extracts, such as standardized extracts that contain a certain amount of marker or active compound or compounds, the level of evidence code reflects the ability of a liquid herbal product to deliver such levels of these phytochemicals. For example, in trials using standardized hawthorn leaf and flower extract, 30 to 45 mg/day of oligomeric procyanidins (OPCs) was administered. This amount of OPC is achievable from a good quality extract in the recommended dose range (3 to 6 ml/day of 1:2 liquid extract delivering 10 mg/ml of OPCs). Hence the indications that clinical trial information established carry the appropriate level of evidence, depending on the quality of the trial or trials. Indications in this example would be cardiac insufficiency, particularly corresponding to New York Heart Association stages I and II, with level 1 evidence. (The reader should note that regular, galenical liquid extracts with lower or unknown amounts of OPCs may not duplicate the trial results, and therefore level 1 evidence would not be appropriate for such products.)

On the other hand, when an extract is unable to deliver the required amount of active or marker constituents, a level 4a code is applied (thus denoting clinical trial information for a constituent). For example, a number of clinical studies have investigated the use of silymarin (a complex of active constituents within milk thistle [*Silybum marianum*]) with 420 mg per day being the most commonly administered dose. A good quality standardized 1:1 ethanolic extract of milk thistle should contain not less than 25 mg/ml of silymarin. With a recommended daily dose range of 4.5 to 8.5 ml, this amount of 420 mg would not be reached (8.5 ml × 25 mg/ml = 212.5 mg silymarin/day). Therefore the potential indications derived from these clinical trials carry a level 4a rating of evidence.

CONTRAINDICATIONS, WARNINGS AND PRECAUTIONS, INTERACTIONS, USE IN PREGNANCY AND LACTATION, SIDE EFFECTS

In general, the safety information contained in these sections is drawn from the text *Principles and Practice of Phytotherapy* or from relevant papers in peer reviewed journals. However, the opinions of expert committees (Commission E, ESCOP) are included when appropriate. If a statement concerning safety is made that is not drawn from any of these sources, it represents the author's subjective evaluation of the available information. Appropriate safety information from traditional sources is also included.

A general principle holds that clinicians should refrain from giving medicines to a pregnant woman unless clearly necessary. Although pregnant women have used some herbs, particular care should be used when prescribing these herbs in the crucial first trimester during fetal organ development. Additional doubt exists as to how secondary plant metabolites, many of which pass easily and even preferentially into breast milk, affect the breast-fed infant. The recommendations listed in the "Use in Pregnancy and Lactation" section are based on an informed evaluation

Dose per day*	Dose per week*
Minimum to maximum ml of x:y liquid extract/ tincture	Minimum to maximum ml of x:y liquid extract/ tincture

of current research and regulatory and traditional sources of information.

DOSAGE

Doses are provided for both daily and weekly intervals. In most cases, the doses are presented in an easy-to-read table, with the minimum and maximum values in ml and the strength of the liquid extract or tincture (x:y).

The weekly dose is convenient when preparing herbal formulations to be dispensed over a period of weeks (see the above box). The daily dose has been calculated from the weekly dose and has been rounded off (hence it is not an "exact" division).

Further information about the literature source of the dose range is listed as a footnote (*) on the same page as is the dose table. The literature sources include traditional texts, clinical studies, expert committees, or other writings.

With regard to traditional sources of dose information, the range given in the monograph is not an exact mathematical extrapolation. Rather, the range is an interpretation of the information available from a variety of traditional sources, recent clinical and scientific studies, and the author's education and clinical experience. Traditional sources for Western herbal medicine include the *British Herbal Pharmacopoeia* (BHP), *British Herbal Compendium*, and some older documents to which authors refer (such as early editions of the *British Pharmacopoeia* and *British Pharmaceutical Codex*).

The discussion on dosage in Chapter 1 (p. 18) indicates that because tinctures better preserve the chemical profile of the dried herb, more credibility should be given to the tincture doses when using the dose ranges outlined in the BHP rather than the liquid extract doses (1:1). (The 1:5 tincture dose multiplied by 0.4 gives the corresponding 1:2 dose. In the absence of a 1:5 tincture dose, the 1:10 tincture dose can be multiplied by 0.2.)

SUPPORTING INFORMATION

The information in this section has been summarized for the reader's convenience. That the reader should wade through extensive and lengthy monographs is not the intention of this book.

TRADITIONAL PRESCRIBING

This section includes information about traditional prescribing covering several traditional systems. Words with specific meaning in Ayurveda and traditional Chinese medicine (TCM) are italicized (e.g., *medharasayan*, *damp heat*). The reader is advised to consult appropriate texts for further understanding of these traditional terms.

The United States Pharmacopeia (USP) was established in 1820, and the National Formulary (NF) was initially published in 1888 as a sister compendium to the Pharmacopeia. The NF has been published with the USP in a single volume since 1980 (USP-NF). The edition published in 2000-2001 is USP24-NF19. Early editions of the USP and NF contained entries on herbs that reflected their use as orthodox medicines at the time. As modern orthodox medicine developed, most herbs were dropped from these official publications. Recently, many herbs have been reinstated with quality standards included. Information has been included in this section from old USP and NF editions, which is deemed to be indicative of traditional professional use.

PHARMACOLOGIC RESEARCH

Pharmacologic research relevant to the major activities and indications of each herb is presented in a concise form, including *in vitro* studies and *in vivo* animal studies (experimental models). All pharmacologic studies conducted involving human volunteers are listed in the "Clinical Studies" section. When available for *in vivo* studies, the route of administration of the herb or constituent has been included, such as orally or by injection.

Extrapolation from animal or *in vitro* studies to humans is fraught with difficulties, and this information is provided mainly to give the reader an indication of what is known about the possible pharmacologic properties of each herb. Given that all the herbs in this book are approved for use in most countries, the most relevant pharmacologic information would be revealed or confirmed by studies involving human volunteers.

CLINICAL STUDIES

The doses administered in clinical trials were generally included when such information was readily available. For concentrated extracts, the dose has been translated into an equivalent amount of herb based on the concentration ratio. Thus 900 mg of a 6:1 extract is listed as "equivalent to approximately 5.4 g/day of dried herb" (900 mg × 6). In the case when the concentrated extract is listed as a range, the dose is calculated from the average of the range. Thus 900 mg of a 3:1 to 6:1 extract is listed as "equivalent to approximately 4 g/day of dried herb" (900 mg × ((3 + 6) ÷ 2)).

The terms "effective" and "efficacious" are defined in the glossary of clinical terms (Appendix C) and are used in the following way in the monographs:

- Efficacious: proven in well-designed, randomized, double-blind, placebo-controlled trials
- Effective: proven in case-control, postmarketing or drug monitoring trials, particularly when a patient's assessment is recorded and in other less well-designed trials such as uncontrolled trials

In addition to clinical or pharmacologic studies in humans, this section includes indications recommended by expert committees, such as the German Commission E and ESCOP (see later description). Indications from the Commission E are listed for its approved herbs only. Because of the regulatory nature of the information, herbs that have been reinstated in the USP-NF are also listed in this section.

German Commission E: In 1978 the German Federal Health Department established an expert committee (Commission E) with a strong clinical background to review and approve the safety and efficacy of selected herbs. The Commission E monographs were based on extensive review of the scientific data and traditional information, as well as the interdisciplinary expertise of the members of the Commission. Each herb investigated was given a positive or negative assessment, and an unpublished justification was attached to each monograph (with the reference material stored at the German Health Department). The Commission was discontinued after the early 1990s, but much of the information remains valid.

ESCOP: The European Scientific Cooperative on Phytotherapy was founded in June 1989 as an umbrella organization representing national phytotherapy associations across Europe, especially for liaison with European medicine regulators. ESCOP's aims are to advance the scientific status of phytomedicines and to assist with the harmonization of their regulatory status at the European level. An important objective of the organization is to produce reference monographs on the therapeutic use and safety of herbal remedies. The ESCOP monographs were prepared in a similar way to that of the Commission E monographs. To date, ESCOP has published a total of 60 monographs. More information is available from the following web page: http://www.escop.com/.

REFERENCES

References are cited to support the information in the monographs, except when the reader is referred to the text: Mills S, Bone K: *Principles and Practice of Phytotherapy: Modern Herbal Medicine*, Edinburgh, 2000, Churchill Livingstone. In monographs when this is the case, only research published subsequent to the *Principles and Practice of Phytotherapy* is referenced.

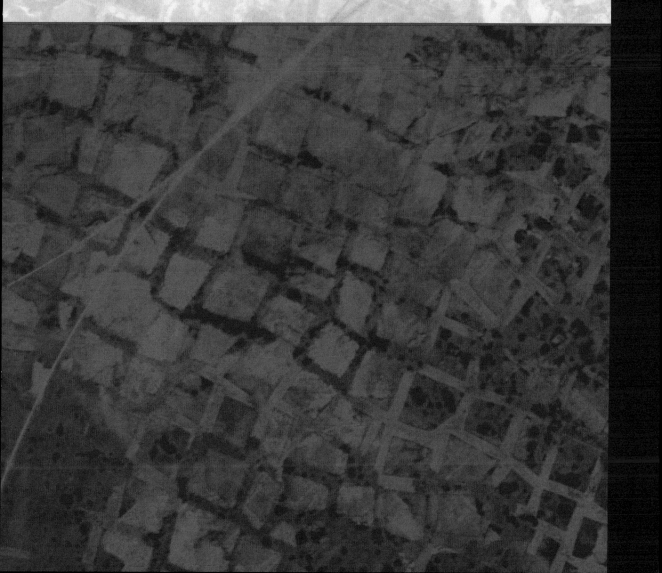

MONOGRAPHS

ALBIZIA

Botanical Names: *Albizia lebbeck, Albizzia lebbeck[#], A. lebbek[#]*
Family: Leguminosae
Plant Part Used: Stem bark

Actions	Antiallergic, hypocholesterolemic, antimicrobial
Potential Indications	Based on appropriate evaluation of the patient, practitioners should consider prescribing Albizia in formulations in the context of: • Allergic rhinitis *(5,7)* • Allergic respiratory disorders especially asthma *(4,5)* • Eczema *(5)* • Possible benefit in hypercholesterolemia *(7)*
Contraindications	None known.
Warnings and Precautions	None required.
Interactions	None known.
Use in Pregnancy and Lactation	No adverse effects expected.
Side Effects	None expected if taken within the recommended dose range.

Dosage

*Dose per day**	*Dose per week**
3.5-8.5 ml of 1:2 liquid extract	25-60 ml of 1:2 liquid extract

SUPPORTING INFORMATION

Traditional Prescribing	Traditional Ayurvedic uses include: • Bronchitis, asthma, allergic disorders, leprosy, eczema, pruritus, paralysis, gum inflammation, worm infestation[1-4] • As an antiinflammatory agent[5]
Pharmacologic Research	• Studies found Albizia to have antiallergic and antianaphylactic activity.[5-7] Early processes of sensitization were inhibited, levels of allergy-inducing antibodies were depressed, as was T-lymphocyte and B-lymphocyte activity. A stabilizing effect on mast cells compared with disodium cromoglycate and prednisolone was exhibited.[3,6] • A protective effect on the adrenal glands was demonstrated for oral administration of Albizia extract or decoction. An increase in adrenal activity was also observed.[3,8,9] • Oral doses of Albizia significantly decreased serum cholesterol *in vivo*.[3,6]

Albizia *continued on page 60*

[#] Alternative name.

* This dose range is extrapolated from traditional Ayurvedic medicine[1] and the author's education and experience.

- Albizia demonstrated antiulcer activity *in vivo* but not in nonsteroidal antiinflammatory drug (NSAID) models of ulcer induction (indomethacin and acetylsalicylic acid).[10]
- Albizia has demonstrated antimicrobial activity[11] and anthelmintic activity[12] *in vitro*.

Clinical Studies

In an uncontrolled study involving 20 patients with asthma, the response to Albizia was excellent for asthma of recent onset (less than 2 years) but less predictable in more chronic cases. Improvement in clinical and biochemical parameters such as plasma cortisol, catecholamine, histaminase, and blood histamine were observed. The significant increase in plasma cortisol levels after treatment suggests that Albizia might provide benefit through supporting the adrenal cortex. Albizia was administered as a decoction (25 ml four times/day) for 3 weeks.[13]

REFERENCES

1 Kapoor LD: *CRC handbook of ayurvedic medicinal plants*, Boca Raton, Fla, 1990, CRC Press.

2 Kirtikar KR, Basu BD: *Indian medicinal plants*, vol 2, Allahabad, India, 1933, SN Basu.

3 Tripathi RM, Sen PC, Das PK: *J Ethnopharmacol* 1(4):385-386, 1979.

4 Thakur RS, Puri HS, Husain A: *Major medicinal plants of India*, Lucknow, India, 1989, Central Institute of Medicinal and Aromatic Plants.

5 Tripathi RM, Das PK: *Indian J Pharmacol* 9:189-194, 1977.

6 Tripathi RM, Sen PC, Das PK: *J Ethnopharmacol* 1:397-406, 1979.

7 Johri RK et al: *Indian J Physiol Pharmacol* 29(1):43-46, 1985.

8 Tripathi SN, Shukla P: *Indian J Exp Biol* 17:915-917, 1979.

9 Tripathi P et al: *Indian J Physiol Pharmacol* 27(2):176-178, 1983.

10 Chatterjee SS, Jaggy H: 4th International Congress on Phytotherapy, Munich, September 10-13, 1992; Abstract SL75.

11 Ganguli NB, Bhatt RM: *Indian J Exp Biol* 31:125-129, 1993.

12 Kaleysa Raj R: *Indian J Physiol Pharmacol* 19:47-49, 1975.

13 Tripathi SN et al: *Quart J Surg Sci* 14:169-176, 1978.

ALOE VERA

Other Common Name: Aloe
Botanical Name: *Aloe* spp.
Family: Asphodelaceae
Plant Part Used: Juice from the leaf

PRESCRIBING INFORMATION

Actions	Immune enhancing, antiviral, vulnerary, antiinflammatory, antitumor
Potential Indications	Based on appropriate evaluation of the patient, practitioners should consider prescribing Aloe juice concentrate in formulations in the context of:

- Non-insulin–dependent diabetes mellitus, hypertriglyceridemia *(3)*
- Adjuvant therapy for the treatment of human immunodeficiency virus (HIV) infection and acquired immunodeficiency syndrome (AIDS) *(4)*
- Improving the response of the immune system *(7)*
- Topical treatment for genital herpes *(2)*
- Topical treatment for psoriasis and seborrheic dermatitis *(3)*
- Topical treatment for chronic leg ulcers *(4)*
- Topical treatment for burns *(4)*
- Topical treatment for mouth ulcers *(4a,6)*
- Topical treatment for wounds and abscesses *(6)*

Contraindications	Individuals with known hypersensitivity should avoid using Aloe juice products.[1,2]
Warnings and Precautions	None required.
Interactions	None known.
Use in Pregnancy and Lactation	No adverse effects expected.
Side Effects	Aloe products have caused hypersensitivity reactions such as dermatitis when used topically and orally.[1,2]
Dosage	25 ml of Aloe juice concentrate (4.5:1) is taken one to four times per day. Aloe juice concentrate can be taken in orange or pineapple juice.* Aloe juice concentrate is best given on its own and not mixed with herbal extracts.

Leaf concentrates providing quantified levels of acemannan are recommended and should ideally contain not less than 11.25 mg/ml of acemannan. Additionally, the safety assessments in this monograph apply only for Aloe liquids that contain low levels of anthraquinones (usually by a removal process).

Aloe Vera *continued on page 62*

*This dose range is extrapolated from pharmacologic and clinical trial data.[3]

Traditional Prescribing

Uses from traditional Ayurvedic and Thai medicine include:
- Peptic ulcers[4]
- Topically for burns, wounds, abscesses, mouth ulcers,[4] and inflamed areas[5]

Pharmacologic Research

- Important constituents in Aloe leaves, apart from the anthraquinone glycosides, are the polysaccharides, in particular, acetylated galactomannan. This long-chain polysaccharide was given the name acemannan.[6]
- Short-term exposure of peritoneal macrophages to acemannan upregulated their respiratory burst, phagocytosis, and killing of *Candida albicans*.[7]
- Several studies have shown acemannan to have a beneficial effect in treating and preventing tumors.[8,9] Injection of Aloe powder (undefined) stimulated cell-mediated responses in an experimental tumor model.[10]
- Oral administration or injection of acemannan was beneficial for treating feline immunodeficiency virus infection *in vivo*.[11] Experimental studies suggest that acemannan has some benefits in the management of HIV.[12-14]
- Acemannan was shown to increase splenic and peripheral blood cellularity and levels of hematopoietic progenitors in the spleen and bone marrow in experimental studies.[15]
- Oral administration of Aloe gel was active as an antiinflammatory agent in several models of inflammation. The activity was said to depend on the presence of anthraquinones.[16]
- In laboratory studies, wounds were treated either by topical application or by oral administration of Aloe gel, with both treatments producing beneficial results.[17-19] Aloe cream demonstrated benefit in first- and second-degree burns,[20] which may be a result of inhibition of thromboxane B_2 and prostaglandin $F_{2\alpha}$ formation, thereby preserving dermal circulation and decreasing burn wound tissue.[21]
- Gastrointestinal treatment with Aloe juice (170 ml/day) resulted in improved gastric and intestinal function.[22]

Clinical Studies

The Aloe leaf yields two products that have medicinal, pharmaceutical, and cosmetic uses: Aloe resin and Aloe gel (often made into a juice). Aloe resin is a solid residue obtained from the latex or sap that exudes from the cut leaf. The resin contains anthraquinone components and is well known for its laxative activity. Aloe gel is a mucilaginous material obtained mainly from the central part of the leaf, known particularly for healing wounds. Both the resin and the gel have been used traditionally. Recently, the Aloe gel in the form of extracts or juices has demonstrated new medical applications. In many of the clinical studies listed here, the Aloe extract is not defined, but assumptions are that the extract does not contain large amounts of anthraquinones.

Aloe Vera *continued on page 63*

- Several clinical studies using acemannan in treating HIV and AIDS have been conducted.[23,24] In an uncontrolled clinical study, 29 patients with AIDS received *Aloe vera* whole leaf juice (containing 1200 mg/day of acemannan), essential fatty acids, and nutrients. Karnofsky scores improved in all of these patients over 180 days.[25]

- Seventy two patients with recently diagnosed non-insulin–dependent diabetes received either Aloe juice or placebo over 6 weeks in an open trial. From day 14, the blood sugar levels of patients treated with Aloe were significantly reduced compared with the control group and continued to fall steadily over the treatment period. Blood triglyceride levels were significantly reduced from day 28. Cholesterol levels were unaffected.[26] In a single-blind, placebo-controlled trial, Aloe juice in combination with glibenclamide significantly reduced levels of fasting blood glucose within 2 weeks and triglycerides within 4 weeks compared with glibenclamide alone. Even after 6 weeks of treatment however, blood sugar levels had not fallen to normal values.[27] In both trials, 1 tablespoon of 80% Aloe juice prepared from gel was taken twice per day.

- Oral administration of an Aloe extract for 6 months demonstrated benefit in patients with chronic asthma. One third of the 33 patients were regarded as effectively treated based on patients' impressions and physicians' observations. Aloe was not beneficial for patients who had previously been administered a steroid drug. The daily dose prescribed was 10 ml of a 20% solution of Aloe extract in saline. The extract was not defined except that it was stored in the dark at 4° C (39° F) for 7 days.[28]

- In a double-blind trial, topical application of Aloe extract (0.5%) in a hydrophilic cream was significantly more beneficial than was the placebo in treating psoriasis.[29] Topical application of an Aloe emulsion (containing 30% Aloe extract) was an efficacious treatment for patients with seborrheic dermatitis in a double-blind, placebo-controlled trial.[30]

- Aloe gel was beneficial in treating partial-thickness burns in a controlled trial compared with gauze containing white petroleum jelly.[31] In an open trial, Aloe was beneficial for treating chronic leg ulcers. Patients received an Aloe drink (60 ml/day of 98% stabilized gel) and applied aloe gel topically.[32]

- Aloe extract (0.5%) in a hydrophilic cream was more efficacious than was placebo in a randomized, double-blind trial involving 60 men with genital herpes. The group treated with Aloe had shorter mean time to healing compared with the placebo group and contained a higher number of healed patients.[33]

- Patients with a history of recurrent aphthous stomatitis (mouth ulcers or canker sores) were treated with an acemannan hydrogel. Patients using the acemannan hydrogel showed a significant reduction in the healing time of mouth ulcers compared with an active over-the-counter preparation.[34]

Aloe Vera *continued on page 64*

REFERENCES

1 Morrow DM, Rapaport MJ, Strick RA: *Arch Dermatol* 116(9):1064-1065, 1980.

2 Hogan DJ: *CMAJ* 138(4):336-338, 1988.

3 Plaskett LG: *The health and medical use of Aloe vera*, Tacoma, Wash, 1996, Life Sciences Press.

4 Farnsworth NR, Bunyapraphatsara N, editors: *Thai medicinal plants*, Bangkok, 1992, Medicinal Plant Information Center.

5 Chopra RN et al: *Chopra's indigenous drugs of India*, ed 2, Calcutta, 1958, reprinted 1982, Academic Publishers.

6 Pelley RP: *Aloe polysaccharides and their measurement*. In *Inside Aloe*, Irving, Tex, 1997, International Aloe Science Council.

7 Stuart RW et al: *Int J Immunopharmacol* 9(2):75-82, 1997.

8 Peng SY et al: *Mol Biother* 3(2):79-87, 1991.

9 King GK et al: *J Am Anim Hosp Assoc* 31(5):439-447, 1995.

10 Corsi MM et al: *Int J Tissue React* 20(4):115-118, 1998.

11 Yates KM et al: *Vet Immunol Immunopathol* 35(1-2):177-189, 1992.

12 McDaniel HR, Rosenberg LJ, McAnalley BH: *Int Conf AIDS* 9(1):498, 1993.

13 Yates KM et al: *Int Conf AIDS* 9(1):196, 1993.

14 Kemp MC et al: *Int Conf AIDS* 6(2):315, 1990.

15 Egger SF et al: *Cancer Immunol Immunother* 43(4):195-205, 1996.

16 Davis RH et al: *J Am Podiatr Med Assoc* 79(6):263-276, 1989.

17 Chithra P, Sajithlal GB, Chandrakasan G: *Mol Cell Biochem* 181(1-2):71-76, 1998.

18 Chithra P, Sajithlal GB, Chandrakasan G: *J Ethnopharmacol* 59(3):195-201, 1998.

19 Chithra P, Sajithlal GB, Chandrakasan G: *J Ethnopharmacol* 59(3):179, 1998.

20 Bunyapraphatsara N et al: *Phytomed* 2(3):247-251, 1996.

21 Heggers JP et al: *J Surg Res* 28(2):110-117, 1980.

22 Bland J: *Prev Med* March/April:1, 1985.

23 Montaner JS et al: *J Acquir Immune Defic Syndr Hum Retrovirol* 12(2):153-157, 1996.

24 *Scrip—World Pharmaceutical News*, issue 1530:23, 1996.

25 Pulse TL, Uhlig E: *J Advancement Med* 3(4):209-230, 1990.

26 Yongchaiyudha S et al: *Phytomed* 3(3):241-243, 1996.

27 Bunyapraphatsara N et al: *Phytomed* 3(3):245-248, 1996.

28 Shida T, Nishimura H: *Proc Symp Wakanyaku* 13:47-51, 1980. Cited in Shida T et al: *Planta Med* 51(3):273-275, 1985.

29 Syed TA et al: *Trop Med Int Health* 1(4):505, 1996.

30 Vardy DA et al: *J Dermatol Treat* 10:7-11, 1999.

31 Visuthikosol V et al: *J Med Assoc Thai* 78(8):403-409, 1995.

32 Atherton P: *Nurs Stand* 12(41):49-52, 54, 1998.

33 Syed TA et al: *J Dermatol Treat* 8(2):99-102, 1997.

34 Plemons JM et al: *Wounds* 6(2):40-45, 1994.

ANDROGRAPHIS

Botanical Name: *Androgr_aphis paniculata*
Family: Acanthaceae
Plant Part Used: Aerial parts

PRESCRIBING INFORMATION

Actions	Bitter tonic, choleretic, immune enhancing, hepatoprotective, antipyretic, antiinflammatory, antiplatelet, antioxidant, anthelmintic
Potential Indications	Based on appropriate evaluation of the patient, practitioners should consider prescribing Andrographis in formulations in the context of:

- Bacterial and viral respiratory tract infections (including the common cold) and reducing associated fever (2,5)
- Preventing the common cold and pharyngotonsillitis (2)
- Preventing urinary tract infections* following shock wave lithotripsy (3)
- Enteric infections (4,5)
- Infective hepatitis (4)
- Loss of appetite, dyspepsia, flatulence, diarrhea, dysentery, gastroenteritis, bowel complaints in children (5)
- Infestation with intestinal worms (5)

Contraindications	Possibly in pregnancy (See "Use in Pregnancy and Lactation.")
Warnings and Precautions	None required.
Interactions	None known.
Use in Pregnancy and Lactation	The antifertility effect in female mice (albeit at high doses) suggests that Andrographis should not be used during human pregnancy, especially in the first trimester.
Side Effects	High doses may cause gastric discomfort, anorexia, and emesis (vomiting), but generally, few side effects associated with its use occur, and it is not toxic. Generally, Andrographis has been well tolerated in clinical trials. Two cases (8% of patients) of urticaria were reported in one trial investigating respiratory infections,[1] and in another trial, one patient in a treatment group of 90 reported adverse effects (unpleasant sensations in the chest and intensified headache).[2] A high incidence of adverse effects was reported in a trial involving patients with HIV,[3] but the dose of pure andrographolide that was administered was very high compared with the normal therapeutic doses of Andrographis extract.

Dosage	Dose per day[†]	Dose per week[†]
	3-6 ml of 1:2 liquid extract	20-40 ml of 1:2 liquid extract

Andrographis *continued on page 66*

---

*Andrographis has also been used in traditional herbal medicine for treating urinary tract infections. (5)
[†]This dose range is extrapolated from traditional Ayurvedic medicine[4] and the author's education and experience.

Up to 12 ml per day of 1:2 liquid extract may be taken during infection. Quantification of andrographolides is preferable to ensure that the liquid extract delivers an adequate level of activity.

Because Andrographis is energetically *cold*, it is preferably taken in combination with *warm* herbs when used during winter as a preventative treatment, especially if the user has a *cold* constitution. Warming herbs include ginger, Astragalus, and holy basil *(Ocimum tenuiflorum)*.

SUPPORTING INFORMATION

Traditional Prescribing

Traditional Ayurvedic uses include:
- Flatulence, loss of appetite, bowel complaints in children, dysentery, dyspepsia,[4,5] diarrhea, sluggish liver,[4] liver disorders[6]
- General debility,[4,5] convalescence after fever, neuralgia[4]
- As a febrifuge, tonic, depurative, anthelmintic[5]

Uses and properties from traditional Chinese medicine (TCM) include:
- Bitter and *cold*, used to clear *heat* from the *blood* and detoxify *fire poison*[7,8]
- Influenza with fever, acute or chronic cough, sore throat, mouth ulcers[8]
- Colitis, dysentery, urinary infection with difficult and painful urination[8]
- Carbuncles, sores, snakebite[8]

Traditional Thai and Indonesian medicine uses include:
- Fever, stomachache, dysentery, typhoid,[9] diarrhea[10]
- Abscesses, herpes simplex, herpes zoster[10]
- As a febrifuge, tonic, diuretic, hypoglycemic[9]
- Topically for snakebite and other poisonous bites and for itching[9]

Pharmacologic Research

The aerial parts of Andrographis contain diterpenoid lactones, collectively referred to as andrographolides and consist of aglycones (such as andrographolide itself) and glucosides (such as neoandrographolide and andrographiside).
- An experimental study demonstrated activity for Andrographis alcoholic extract against an *Escherichia-coli*-enterotoxin–induced secretory response (which causes diarrhea). Andrographis and the enterotoxin were co-administered into isolated ileal tissue. However, several *in vitro* and *in vivo* studies have failed to show any bactericidal activity.
- Andrographis root extract demonstrated strong *in vitro* anthelmintic activity against human *Ascaris lumbricoides,* and subcutaneous administration of a decoction of the leaves reduced nematode larvae in the blood of dogs by 85%.

Andrographis *continued on page 67*

- Oral administration of Andrographis extract and isolated andrographolide stimulated both antigen-specific and nonspecific immune responses in an experimental model. Andrographis decoction and andrographolides have demonstrated an immunostimulant action, especially on phagocytosis, *in vitro*. Andrographolides by injection enhanced phagocytosis in animal models.
- Oral doses of Andrographis extract demonstrated protective activity against chemical- and alcohol-induced toxic liver damage in experimental models. Andrographolide showed hepatoprotective activity in chemical-induced acute hepatitis after oral and intraperitoneal administration.
- Andrographolide increased bile flow, bile salts, and bile acids dose-dependently after oral and intraperitoneal administration in experimental models.
- Andrographis extract reduced mean arterial blood pressure without decreasing heart rate in an experimental model (route unknown) and exhibited a dose-dependent hypotensive effect in both spontaneously hypertensive and normotensive models (intraperitoneal route).
- Andrographis alleviated myocardial ischemia-reperfusion injury and atherosclerotic arterial stenosis in experimental models (route unknown). Andrographis lowered the restenosis rate after experimental angioplasty.
- Oral administration of Andrographis leaf powder to male rats produced an antifertility effect and biochemical changes in the testes and male accessory organs. However, these results were not duplicated in a similar study using a standardized dried ethanolic extract. Pregnancy was prevented in 100% of female mice fed dried Andrographis powder.
- Several studies have shown antipyretic and antiinflammatory effects for andrographolides (by oral administration or injection) in a number of animal models, including adjuvant-induced arthritis. Andrographolide demonstrated antiallergic activity after oral[11] and intraperitoneal administration.[12]
- Andrographis extract reduced fasting serum glucose and increased the activity of antioxidant enzymes in an experimental model of diabetes when given orally. Nondiabetic animals were not affected. Results were comparable to metformin (a hypoglycemic drug).[13]
- Andrographis extract prevented glucose-induced hyperglycemia (route unknown) but failed to prevent glucose absorption from the gut. Oral administration activated intestinal enzymes (lactase, maltase, and sucrase), suggesting Andrographis accelerates intestinal digestion and absorption of carbohydrate (rather than absorption of simple glucose).
- A drug derived from andrographolide (dehydroandrographolide succinic acid [DASM]) has been found to inhibit HIV *in vitro*. However, *in vitro* studies with aqueous extracts of Andrographis showed little or no inhibition of HIV-1. (However, see the pilot study mentioned under "Clinical Studies.")

Andrographis *continued on page 68*

Clinical Studies

- Andrographis and andrographolides have shown immunostimulant activity during the treatment of bacterial and viral respiratory infections in several uncontrolled clinical trials in China. In one study, Andrographis treatment lowered body temperature during the common cold.
- Several uncontrolled Chinese studies assessing oral administration of Andrographis or andrographolides in acute bacillary dysentery and enteritis found a marked benefit. A Thai study found that Andrographis powdered leaf and stem (2 g/day for 2 days) reduced the Shigella population in patients with acute diarrhea but was less beneficial than was tetracycline for cholera.
- A randomized, double-blind study involving 152 patients with pharyngotonsillitis found Andrographis treatment (6 g/day for 7 days) was as efficacious as was acetaminophen (paracetamol) in providing relief of fever and sore throat compared with changes from baseline values.
- Tiredness, sleeplessness, sore throat, and nasal secretions were significantly decreased by the second day of treatment with Andrographis extract (1200 mg/day for 5 days; standardized to 5% andrographolides) compared with placebo in a randomized, double-blind trial involving 158 patients with the common cold. By day 4, all measured symptoms (including headache, earache, expectoration, frequency of cough, and intensity of cough) were significantly decreased compared with placebo.[14]
- Andrographis extract (1200 mg/day for 4 days, standardized to 4% andrographolides) significantly reduced the manifestations of the common cold (strength of disease, tiredness, sweating and shivering, sore throat, and muscular ache) compared with placebo and significantly reduced clinical signs (lymphatic swellings, rhinitis, sinus pain, and headaches) in a double-blind trial.
- Andrographis extract (200 mg/day, standardized to 5.6% andrographolides) given to healthy children for 3 months over the winter season significantly decreased the incidence of the common cold compared with a placebo treatment in a randomized, double-blind trial.
- In a randomized, double-blind, placebo-controlled pilot study, subjective evaluation of outpatients with the common cold demonstrated a significantly reduced number of sick days, improved symptoms, and hastened recovery after therapy with standardized Andrographis extract (1020 mg/day for 5 days; level of andrographolide not stated). Subsequent studies of similar design by the same group found that herbal tablets containing Andrographis extract (1020 mg/day; standardized to 6.2% andrographolides and subtherapeutic levels of Eleutherococcus) significantly improved the total symptom score and total diagnosis score, as rated by patients and physicians respectively, compared with placebo in patients with uncomplicated upper respiratory tract infection. Throat symptoms and signs demonstrated the most significant improvement.[2]

Andrographis *continued on page 69*

- A controlled study found that Andrographis treatment (3 g/day for 5 days) was as beneficial as was the antibiotics cotrimoxazole and norfloxacin for reducing pyuria and hematuria (associated with urinary tract infection) in patients undergoing dissolution of kidney stones (shock wave lithotripsy).
- Eighty percent of cases of infective hepatitis were cured, and 20% were relieved after treatment with Andrographis decoction (40 g of herb/day for 24 days) in an uncontrolled trial. Significant decreases from baseline values of various liver function parameters were also observed.
- Andrographolide (5 mg/kg for 3 weeks, then 10 mg/kg for 3 weeks) significantly increased mean CD4[+] lymphocyte levels from baseline in 13 HIV-positive patients. Mean plasma HIV-1 ribonucleic acid (RNA) levels did not significantly change. Patients did not use the antiretroviral medications during the trial. Twelve of the thirteen patients reported at least one adverse event during the treatment.[3]

REFERENCES

Except when specifically referenced, the following book was referred to in the compilation of the pharmacologic and clinical information: Mills S, Bone K: *Principles and Practice of Phytotherapy: Modern Herbal Medicine*, Edinburgh, 2000, Churchill Livingstone.

1 Melchior J, Palm S, Wikman G: *Phytomed* 3(4):315-318, 1996-1997.
2 Melchior J et al: *Phytomed* 7(5):341-350, 2000.
3 Calabrese C et al: *Phytother Res* 14(5):333-338, 2000.
4 Kapoor LD: *CRC handbook of Ayurvedic medicinal plants,* Boca Raton, Fla, 1990, CRC Press.
5 Chopra RN et al: *Chopra's indigenous drugs of India,* ed 2, Calcutta, 1958, reprinted 1982, Academic Publishers.
6 Bharatiya Vidya Bhavan's Swami Prakashananda Ayurveda Research Centre: *Selected medicinal plants of India,* Bombay, 1992. Chemexcil.
7 Bensky D, Gamble A: *Chinese herbal medicine materia medica,* Seattle, 1986, Eastland Press.
8 Pharmacopoeia Commission of the People's Republic of China: *Pharmacopoeia of the People's Republic of China,* English ed, Beijing, 1997, Chemical Industry Press.
9 Dharma AP: *Indonesian medicinal plants,* Jakarta, 1987, Balai Pustaka.
10 Farnsworth NR, Bunyapraphatsara N, editors: *Thai medicinal plants,* Bangkok, 1992, Medicinal Plant Information Center.
11 Madav S et al: *Indian J Pharm Sci* 60(3):176-178, 1998.
12 Gupta PP, Tandon JS, Patnaik GK: *Pharmaceut Biol* 36(1):72-74, 1998.
13 Zhang XF, Tan BK: *Clin Exp Pharmacol Physiol* 27(5-6):358-363, 2000.
14 Caceres DD et al: *Phytomed* 6(4):217-223, 1999.

ARNICA

Botanical Names: *Arnica montana, Arnica chamissonis* subsp. *foliosa*[+]
Family: Compositae
Plant Part Used: Flower

PRESCRIBING INFORMATION

Actions	Topical only: antiinflammatory, antiecchymotic (against bruises), analgesic, antimicrobial
Potential Indications	Based on appropriate evaluation of the patient, practitioners should consider prescribing Arnica for *external use* in the context of:

- Chronic venous insufficiency, particularly for feelings of heaviness in the legs, edema *(2)*
- Muscle ache *(3,5)*
- Bruises, sprains *(4,5)*
- Inflamed insect bites *(4,5)*
- Hematomas, dislocations, edema resulting from fracture, rheumatic muscle and joint problems, superficial phlebitis *(4)*
- Furunculosis *(4)*
- Painful swellings, unbroken chilblains, alopecia neurotica *(5)*

Contraindications	Not to be taken internally. Arnica should be applied only to unbroken skin and withdrawn on first sign of dermatitis. Contraindicated in people with known allergy to Arnica.
Warnings and Precautions	Not for internal use. Not for prolonged external application. People with known sensitivity to other members of the Compositae family (such as ragweed, daisies, and chrysanthemums) should avoid using Arnica.
Interactions	None known.
Use in Pregnancy and Lactation	Not for internal use. For topical use only.
Side Effects	Topical application of Arnica, mostly the tincture, has been known to cause allergic or irritant contact dermatitis since 1844. Cross-reactivity to other Compositae plants has also been reported. Arnica ointments and plasters are considered to pose a much lower risk compared with other types of applications.
	The Commission E advises that prolonged treatment of damaged skin can cause edematous dermatitis with the formation of pustules. Extended use may cause eczema. In treatments involving higher than normal therapeutic concentrations, primary toxic skin reactions with the formation of vesicles or even necrosis may occur.

Arnica continued on page 71

[+]Medicinally interchangeable species.

After repeated use of Arnica tincture for rosacea, a 66-year-old patient developed acute allergic contact dermatitis after a single application of the tincture to the hand. Patch testing proved contact allergy of the delayed type.[1]

Dosage

Dilute a 1:5 tincture five times water and apply two to three times per day to the affected area. Ointment should contain 10% to 25% tincture applied two to three times per day.*

SUPPORTING INFORMATION

Traditional Prescribing

External uses from traditional Western herbal medicine include:
- Bruises, sprains,[2-4] painful swellings, cuts, lacerations, insect bites[2]
- Muscle soreness, especially from strain and exertion[4]
- Unbroken chilblains, alopecia neurotica[3]

Pharmacologic Research

Arnica flowers contain sesquiterpene lactones of the pseudoguaianolide type (0.2% to 1.5%), including helenalin and $11\alpha,13$-dihydrohelenalin and their esters, flavonoids, and an essential oil.
- Results from *in vitro* studies suggest that several possible mechanisms exist behind the antiinflammatory activity of Arnica:
  1. Uncoupling of oxidative phosphorylation in polymorphonuclear neutrophils
  2. Elevation of cyclic adenosine monophosphate (cAMP) in neutrophils and liver cells
  3. Inhibition of lysosomal enzymatic activity in neutrophils and liver cells
  4. Inhibition of the activation of transcription factor NF-kappa B, which is responsible for the transcription of genes encoding various inflammatory mediators[5]
    - Sesquiterpene lactones from Arnica have demonstrated analgesic and antiinflammatory activities in experimental models, such as carrageenan-induced paw edema and chronic adjuvant arthritis (after intraperitoneal administration).
    - Arnica extracts applied to animal smooth muscle *in vitro* inhibited experimentally induced spasm.
    - Components of the essential oil of Arnica have demonstrated potent activity against gram-positive and gram-negative bacteria and against *Candida* spp, *in vitro*. Helenalin and helenalin acetate were also active *in vitro* against gram-positive bacteria and *Proteus vulgaris*.
    - Arnica extract stimulated phagocytosis *in vitro* and *in vivo* after injection and protected against *Listeria monocytogenes* infection in an experimental model following injection.
    - Sesquiterpene lactones of Arnica inhibited Walker 26 carcinosarcoma and Ehrlich ascites tumor growth *in vivo*.

Arnica *continued on page 72*

*This dose range is extrapolated from clinical trial information.

Clinical Studies

- In a placebo-controlled, double-blind, randomized study of patients with pronounced symptoms of chronic venous insufficiency, Arnica gel (containing 20% Arnica tincture) improved the feeling of heaviness in the legs compared with placebo, improved venous tone, and reduced edema.
- Arnica gel was more effective than was a placebo gel when applied externally for muscle ache in male volunteers.
- In Germany, the Commission E supports the external use of Arnica flower for inflammation of the oral and throat region, furunculosis, inflammation caused by insect bites, superficial phlebitis, hematoma, dislocations, contusions (bruises), edema resulting from fracture, and rheumatic muscle and joint problems.[6]
- The European Scientific Cooperative on Phytotherapy (ESCOP) recommends external use of Arnica flower for treating bruises, sprains, inflammation caused by insect bites, gingivitis, aphthous ulcers, and the symptomatic treatment of rheumatic complaints.[7]

REFERENCES

Except when specifically referenced, the following book was referred to in the compilation of the pharmacologic and clinical information: Mills S, Bone K: *Principles and Practice of Phytotherapy: Modern Herbal Medicine,* Edinburgh, 2000, Churchill Livingstone.

1 Hormann HP, Korting HC: *Phytomed* 4: 315-317, 1995.

2 Felter HW, Lloyd JU: *King's American dispensatory,* ed 18, rev 3, Portland, 1905, reprinted 1983, Eclectic Medical Publications.

3 British Herbal Medicine Association's Scientific Committee: *British herbal pharmacopoeia,* Bournemouth, 1983, BHMA.

4 Felter HW: *The eclectic materia medica, pharmacology and therapeutics,* Portland, 1922, reprinted 1983, Eclectic Medical Publications.

5 Lyb G et al: *Pharm Pharmacol Lett* 9(1):5-8, 1999.

6 Blumenthal M et al, editors: *The complete German Commission E monographs: therapeutic guide to herbal medicines,* Austin, 1998, American Botanical Council.

7 Scientific Committee of European Scientific Cooperative on Phytotherapy [ESCOP]: *ESCOP monographs: Arnicae flos,* European Scientific Cooperative on Phytotherapy, ESCOP Secretariat, Argyle House, Gandy Street, Exeter, Devon, EX4 3LS, UK, July 1997.

ASHWAGANDA

Other Common Names:	Withania, ashwagandha
Botanical Name:	*Withania somnifera*
Family:	Solanaceae
Plant Part Used:	Root

PRESCRIBING INFORMATION

Actions

Tonic, adaptogenic, mild sedative, antiinflammatory, immune modulating, antianemic

Potential Indications

Based on appropriate evaluation of the patient, practitioners should consider prescribing ashwaganda in formulations in the context of:

- Promoting growth in children *(2,5)*
- Conditions associated with aging *(2)*
- Increasing hemoglobin and red blood count in healthy elderly males and increasing hemoglobin and serum iron in children *(2)*
- Alleviating male sexual inadequacy *(2,5)*
- Improving stamina in athletes *(4)*
- Insomnia *(4)*
- Arthritis *(4,5)*
- Adjunctive treatment for non-insulin–dependent diabetes and hyper-cholesterolemia *(3)*
- Inflammatory conditions such as asthma, bronchitis, psoriasis, and rheumatic pains *(5)*
- Senile dementia *(5,7)*
- Promoting learning and memory *(5,7)*
- Conditions exacerbated by stress *(5,7)*
- Convalescence after acute illness, as a general tonic for disease prevention *(5,7)*
- Enhancing immune function and for depressed white blood cell count *(7)*

Contraindications

None known.

Warnings and Precautions

None required.

Interactions

None known.

Use in Pregnancy and Lactation

No adverse effects expected.

Side Effects

None expected if taken within the recommended dose range.

Dosage

*Dose per day**	*Dose per week**
5-13 ml of 1:2 liquid extract	35-90 ml of 1:2 liquid extract

Ashwaganda *continued on page 74*

*This dose range is extrapolated from traditional Ayurvedic medicine[1] and the author's education and experience.

SUPPORTING INFORMATION

Traditional Prescribing

Traditional Ayurvedic uses include:
- Inflammatory conditions such as bronchitis, asthma, psoriasis, and ulcers (undefined)[2]
- Wasting in children, insomnia, senile debility[2]
- Leukoderma, lumbago, arthritis,[2] rheumatism, lumbar pains[3]
- Promoting conception[2]
- Providing fresh energy and vigor for a system worn out by any constitutional disease[1]
- As a nutrient and tonic for pregnant women and older adults[1]
- Regarded as a *medharasayan* or promoter of learning and memory retrieval[4]

According to other traditional systems, such as those of Tibet and the Middle East, uses include:
- As a sedative and hypnotic, taken for rheumatic pains[5]
- As a general tonic in seminal diseases, as a nervine tonic[6]

Ashwaganda is also used in traditional herbal medicine of Southeast Asia to treat headaches and convulsions and to promote lactation.[7]

Pharmacologic Research

Major constituents of ashwaganda root include steroidal compounds (lactones and glycosides). Alkaloids are also present.
- Oral doses of ashwaganda demonstrated significant antistress activity, increased endurance, and enhanced growth and development in experimental models.
- A pharmacologic comparison of ashwaganda and Korean ginseng demonstrated that ashwaganda had similar potency to Korean ginseng in terms of adaptogenic, tonic, and anabolic effects. However, ashwaganda lacks the stimulating effects of Korean ginseng and is therefore ideally suited to the treatment of patients who are overactive but debilitated, for whom Korean ginseng would tend to cause overstimulation.
- Ashwaganda enhanced learning and memory in both young and old rats when given orally.
- Ashwaganda was shown to significantly increase the total white blood cell and neutrophil counts when given orally, both before and after cyclophosphamide treatment, and to reduce leukopenia induced by gamma radiation *in vivo*.
- After oral doses of ashwaganda, hemoglobin concentration, red blood cell count, white blood cell count, platelet count, and body weight were significantly raised in *in vivo* laboratory models of immunosuppression.
- Ashwaganda has immunomodulatory activity. Extracts were shown to increase mobilization, activation, phagocytosis, and secretory activity of macrophages *in vitro* and to significantly inhibit experimentally

Ashwaganda continued on page 75

induced immunosuppression *in vivo* after oral administration. In contrast, ashwaganda lactones have demonstrated immunosuppressive effects *in vitro* and *in vivo*.

- Ashwaganda lactones exhibited antitumor and radiosensitizing activity in several tumor cell models *in vitro* and *in vivo* after intraperitoneal and oral administration.
- Intraperitoneal and subcutaneous administration of ashwaganda produced an antiinflammatory effect in several studies. Furthermore, ashwaganda was shown to be better at decreasing biomarkers of inflammation than were standard antiinflammatory drugs at the relative doses tested.
- Ashwaganda alkaloids demonstrated depressant activity on higher cerebral functions and caused prolonged hypotensive, bradycardic, respiratory stimulant, and sedative effects. Ashwaganda extract exhibited significant antiepileptic action and cognition enhancement when administered orally in models of epilepsy and Alzheimer's disease, respectively.
- Oral and intraperitoneal dosing with ashwaganda suppressed the development of tolerance to morphine-induced analgesia and morphine withdrawal jumps, suggesting that it may be useful in the treatment of morphine withdrawal.

Clinical Studies

- A randomized, double-blind, placebo-controlled trial found that milk fortified with ashwaganda (2 g/day of herb for 60 days) significantly increased mean corpuscular hemoglobin and serum albumin and tended to increase blood hemoglobin, serum iron, body weight, and strength of hand grip in children aged 8 to 12 years. The placebo group did not show any significant change or tendency to change.
- When tested on 101 healthy male patients aged 50 to 59 years, ashwaganda (3 g/day for 1 year) significantly improved hemoglobin, red blood cell count, seated stature, and hair melanin content. Ashwaganda also caused a decrease in serum cholesterol and erythrocyte sedimentation rate and countered decreased nail calcium. The trial was of randomized, double-blind, placebo-controlled design. About 71% of volunteers receiving ashwaganda reported improvement in sexual performance.
- In an uncontrolled trial, ashwaganda (1 g/day for 29 days) improved sleep patterns, responsiveness, alertness, state of awareness, and physical capabilities in trainee mountaineers over a 29-day trek, which included a 5200 m (over 17,000 ft) altitude gain.
- Ashwaganda (3 g/day for 30 days) decreased blood sugar levels from baseline in six patients with non-insulin–dependent diabetes. The hypoglycemic effect was similar to that obtained in the control group treated with glibenclamide. In addition, ashwaganda increased diuresis, as evidenced by decreased serum potassium and increased urinary excretion of sodium and potassium. In a group of six patients with hypercholesterolemia, ashwaganda significantly decreased serum total cholesterol, triglycerides, low-density lipoprotein (LDL), and very

Ashwaganda continued on page 76

low-density lipoprotein (VLDL) cholesterol compared with baseline values. Lipid profiles remained largely unchanged in the untreated control group. The mean calorie and fat intakes of the treatment groups were higher than those of the control groups.[8]

- Ashwaganda (4 to 9 g/day) was beneficial for patients with acute rheumatoid arthritis (and some cases of nonarticular rheumatism and chronic rheumatoid arthritis with acute exacerbations) in an uncontrolled trial conducted in the late 1960s.[9]

REFERENCES

Except when specifically referenced, the following book was referred to in the compilation of the pharmacologic and clinical information: Mills S, Bone K: *Principles and Practice of Phytotherapy: Modern Herbal Medicine*, Edinburgh, 2000, Churchill Livingstone.

1 Kapoor LD: *CRC handbook of Ayurvedic medicinal plants,* Boca Raton, Fla, 1990, CRC Press.
2 Thakur RS, Puri HS, Husain A: *Major medicinal plants of India,* Lucknow, India, 1989, Central Institute of Medicinal and Aromatic Plants.
3 Chopra RN et al: *Chopra's indigenous drugs of India,* ed 2, Calcutta, 1958, reprinted 1982, Academic Publishers.
4 Bhattacharya SK, Kumar A, Ghosal S: *Phytother Res* 9(2):110-113, 1995.
5 Miller AG, Morris M: *Plants of Dhofar. The southern region of Oman. Traditional, economic and medicinal uses,* Diwan of Royal Court Sultanate of Oman, 1988, The Office of the Adviser for Conservation of the Environment.
6 Chauhan NS, Uniyal MR, Sannd BN: *Nagarjun* 22:190-193, 1979.
7 World Health Organization: *The use of traditional medicine in primary health care: a manual for health workers in Southeast Asia,* New Delhi, 1990, WHO Regional Office for Southeast Asia.
8 Andallu B, Radhika B: *Indian J Exp Biol* 38:607-609, 2000.
9 Bector NP, Puri AS, Sharma D: *Indian J Med Res* 56:1581-1583, 1969.

ASTRAGALUS

Botanical Names: *Astragalus membranaceus, Astragalus membranaceus* var. *mongholicus*[+]
Family: Leguminosae
Plant Part Used: Root

PRESCRIBING INFORMATION

Actions	Immune enhancing, tonic, adaptogenic, cardiotonic, diuretic, hypotensive, antioxidant
Potential Indications	Based on appropriate evaluation of the patient, practitioners should consider prescribing Astragalus in formulations in the context of:

- Impaired immunity, prophylaxis of the common cold, chronic viral infections *(4)*
- General debility, excessive sweating, decreased appetite, chronic diarrhea *(5)*
- Leukopenia *(2)*
- Ischemic heart disease, angina pectoris *(3)*
- A tonic for elderly patients, in combination with *Salvia miltiorrhiza* and *Polygonum multiflorum (3)*
- Postpartum fever and recovery from severe loss of blood, uterine bleeding, organ prolapse *(5)*
- Topical adjuvant therapy for chronic viral cervicitis *(3)*

Contraindications	Not advisable in acute infections.
Warnings and Precautions	None required.
Interactions	None known.
Use in Pregnancy and Lactation	No adverse effects expected.
Side Effects	None expected if taken within the recommended dose range.
Dosage	**Dose per day*** **Dose per week*** 4.5-8.5 ml of 1:2 liquid extract 30-60 ml of 1:2 liquid extract

SUPPORTING INFORMATION

Traditional Prescribing	Uses and properties from TCM include:

- Tonifies *qi, blood,* and *spleen*[1]
- Postpartum fever and recovery from severe loss of blood, fatigue linked to decreased appetite, diarrhea, and anemia[1-3]

Astragalus *continued on page 78*

[+]Medicinally interchangeable species.
*This dose range is adapted from dried plant doses administered by decoction in TCM.[3] The author's experience and the fact that ethanol-water is a more effective solvent than is water for many phytochemicals are taken into account.

- Organ prolapse, abnormal uterine bleeding; spontaneous sweating resulting from weakened resistance; promotes urination, tissue healing, the discharge of pus; removes edema[1-3]

Pharmacologic Research

- Astragalus stimulates natural killer cell activity *in vitro*. Positive effects on other aspects of immunity such as thymus weight and protection from immune suppression were noted in experimental models after oral administration of Astragalus.
- The *in vitro* antiviral activity of Astragalus is most likely a result of the positive effects on immune function and possibly follows from enhanced interferon production.
- Enhanced tolerance to stress, better learning ability, increased endurance, and improved energy metabolism have been shown in experimental models.
- *In vivo* studies support the traditional use of Astragalus with organ prolapse and promoting urinary tract function.

Clinical Studies

- Astragalus extract demonstrated a protective effect on erythrocyte deformability *ex vivo* for blood taken from normal volunteers and patients with systemic lupus erythematosus.
- High oral doses of Astragalus decoction given to participants susceptible to the common cold enhanced immune protection. A prophylactic effect for the common cold was observed in another uncontrolled study, as evidenced by decreased incidence and shortened duration of infection after Astragalus treatment.
- Combined treatment of TCM herbs (such as Astragalus, *Panax ginseng* leaf, and others) raised the survival rates in patients with small cell lung cancer undergoing chemotherapy, radiotherapy, and immunotherapy.
- Average white blood cell counts increased significantly in two groups of patients with leukopenia after treatment with concentrated Astragalus preparations (equivalent to 10 g/day and 30 g/day of Astragalus) for 8 weeks. The results were dose-dependent. Patients were randomized to receive either the low or high dose of Astragalus.
- In a comparative clinical study, Korean ginseng-Astragalus injection reduced toxic chemotherapy effects, increased body weight, and increased cellular immune function compared with chemotherapy alone in patients with malignant tumors of the digestive tract.
- Administration of Astragalus (route undefined) to a large number of patients with chronic viral hepatitis resulted in a success rate of 70%. In most cases, elevated serum glutamic-pyruvic transaminase (GPT) levels returned to normal after 1 to 2 months. (In TCM, Astragalus is often administered by injection for the treatment of hepatitis.[4])
- Natural killer cell activity increased significantly in patients with Coxsackie B viral myocarditis who were treated with intramuscular injections of Astragalus for 3 to 4 months.

Astragalus continued on page 79

- In a comparative trial, 92 patients with ischemic heart disease were treated with Astragalus, *Salvia miltiorrhiza*, or the antianginal drug nifedipine. Results were superior for the Astragalus-treated group, as demonstrated by marked relief from angina pectoris and improvement in several objective clinical parameters.
- In a double-blind, placebo-controlled, clinical trial of 507 elderly people, oral administration of Astragalus in combination with *Polygonum multiflorum* and *Salvia miltiorrhiza* demonstrated significant antiaging effects.
- In two double-blind, clinical trials, topical application of Astragalus combined with interferon was beneficial treating chronic cervicitis associated with viral infection.

REFERENCES

Except when specifically referenced, the following book was referred to in the compilation of the pharmacologic and clinical information: Mills S, Bone K: *Principles and Practice of Phytotherapy: Modern Herbal Medicine*, Edinburgh, 2000, Churchill Livingstone.

1 Bensky D, Gamble A: *Chinese herbal medicine materia medica,* Seattle, 1986, Eastland Press.
2 Chang HM, But PP: *Pharmacology and applications of Chinese materia medica,* Singapore, 1987, World Scientific.
3 Pharmacopoeia Commission of the People's Republic of China: *Pharmacopoeia of the People's Republic of China,* English ed, Beijing, 1997, Chemical Industry Press.
4 Han DW, Xu RL, Yeoung SCS: *Abst Chin Med* 2(1):105-134, 1988.

BACOPA

Botanical Names: *Bacopa monnieri, Bacopa monniera#, Herpestis monnieri#*
Family: Scrophulariaceae
Plant Part Used: Aerial parts

Actions

Cognition enhancing, nervine tonic, mild sedative, mild anticonvulsant, anxiolytic, possibly adaptogenic

Potential Indications

Based on appropriate evaluation of the patient, practitioners should consider prescribing Bacopa in formulations in the context of:
- Improving concentration in healthy individuals (4)
- Improving mental performance and memory (3)
- Nervous disorders, nervous debility (5)
- Insomnia (4,6)
- Epilepsy, anxiety (4,5)

Contraindications

None known.

Warnings and Precautions

None required.

Interactions

None known.

Use in Pregnancy and Lactation

No adverse effects expected.

Side Effects

As with all saponin-containing herbs, oral use may cause irritation of the gastric mucous membranes and reflux.

Dosage

*Dose per day**	*Dose per week**
5-13 ml of 1:2 liquid extract	35-90 ml of 1:2 liquid extract

Traditional Prescribing

Traditional Ayurvedic uses include:
- As a nervine tonic for the treatment of nervous disorders, especially nervous breakdown, epilepsy, insanity; debility, aphonia (loss of voice), hoarseness; for a supposed direct cardiac tonic activity,[2-4] for urinary incontinence, particularly accompanied by constipation[1]
- As a tonic for diseases of the skin, nervous system, and blood[2]

Brahmi oil, which consists mainly of brahmi juice, coconut oil, and other medicinal plants, is considered a most effective brain tonic. Brahmi oil is said to strengthen memory and revive hair growth and is used as a cooling remedy instead of ice in epidemic fevers. Brahmi oil is also employed in headache, insomnia, and epilepsy.[3,4]

Bacopa *continued on page 81*

#Alternative name.
*This dose range is extrapolated from traditional Ayurvedic medicine[4] and the author's education and experience.

Pharmacologic Research

- An early study demonstrated Bacopa to have cardiotonic, vasoconstricting, and sedative activities.[5]
- A laboratory study using a formulation containing Bacopa (known as Brahmi Rasayan) found high doses have sedative (without affecting motor coordination), analgesic, and anticonvulsant activities.[6]
- Standardized extract of Bacopa (25% bacoside A) produced an anxiolytic effect *in vivo* that was qualitatively comparable with that of lorazepam (a benzodiazepine drug). Statistically significant results were elicited with higher doses of Bacopa, which, unlike lorazepam, did not produce any significant motor deficit.[7]
- An early study compared the effects of an alcohol extract of Bacopa and the tranquilizer chlorpromazine on the learning process in rats. Both substances reduced errors and improved performance in the learning phase, but the effect of Bacopa was more marked. Chlorpromazine depressed motor efficiency, but no such deleterious effect was observed with Bacopa treatment. In fact, Bacopa improved motor efficiency compared with controls.[8] In later studies, learning and memory retention were improved in rats in a number of experimental models after oral and intraperitoneal administration of Bacopa.[9,10]
- Oral doses of Brahmi Rasayan were found to suppress experimentally induced inflammation in an animal model. The activity was comparable to that of the NSAID indomethacin. The herbal formula did not produce gastric irritation.[11]

Clinical Studies

- In an uncontrolled trial, 35 patients with anxiety neurosis were treated with the equivalent of 12 g per day of dried Bacopa for 1 month. A significant reduction occurred in anxiety, as well as improvements in mental performance and memory. This result was accompanied by a reduction in mental fatigue, a general feeling of enhanced well being, improved sleep and appetite, and an increase in body weight.[12,13]
- Bacopa had a positive effect on concentration, but not on short-term memory, in a small number of volunteers tested in the mid-1960s.[14] Bacopa (1 g/day for 3 months) improved intellectual functions such as visual motor function, short-term memory, and mental reaction times in children. Unlike individuals who were treated with Bacopa, the placebo group did not improve from baseline values.[15]
- An uncontrolled clinical study on 13 patients with epilepsy using a defatted ethanolic extract of Bacopa (2 to 4 mg/kg body weight/day) demonstrated reductions in the frequency of fitting over 2 to 5 months. The onset of epileptic fits was completely checked in five cases.[16]
- An Australian clinical trial examined the long-term effects of a Bacopa extract on cognitive function in 46 healthy human volunteers.[17] The study was of double-blind, placebo-controlled design in which subjects were randomly allocated to receive Bacopa or placebo. Neuropsychologic testing was conducted before treatment and at 5 and 12 weeks after treatment. After 12 weeks, the largest cognitive

Bacopa continued on page 82

change from Bacopa treatment (which was also statistically significant compared with placebo, $p < 0.05$) was a time reduction for the inspection time (IT) test (64.5 ± 16.7 min vs. 75.9 ± 25.3 min). IT is regarded as a measure of the integrity of the early stages of information processing and may act as a rate-limiting factor for cognition. This finding indicates that Bacopa significantly improved the speed of visual information processing. Verbal learning rate and memory consolidation as assessed by the Rey Auditory Verbal Learning Test were also somewhat improved against placebo at 12 weeks ($p < 0.05$). However, the most striking finding was the highly significant ($p = 0.001$) reduction in anxiety in volunteers receiving Bacopa. The percentage of adverse effects was similar for both groups, except that a higher incidence of nausea, dry mouth, and fatigue occurred in the Bacopa group.

REFERENCES

1 Kapoor LD: *CRC handbook of Ayurvedic medicinal plants*, Boca Raton, Fla, 1990, CRC Press.

2 Chopra RN et al: *Chopra's indigenous drugs of India*, ed 2, Calcutta, 1958, reprinted 1982, Academic Publishers.

3 Sandu DV: *Indian therapeutics*, ed 2, Delhi, 1987, Sri Satguru Publications.

4 A Panel of Vaidyas: *Clinical application of Ayurvedic remedies*, ed 4, Delhi, 1998, Sri Satguru Publications.

5 Malhotra CL, Das PK: *Indian J Med Res* 47:294-305, 1959.

6 Shukia B, Khanna NK, Godhwani JL: *J Ethnopharmacol* 21(1):65-74, 1987.

7 Bhattacharya SK, Ghosal S: *Phytomed* 5(2):77-82, 1998.

8 Prakash JC, Sirsi M: *J Sci Ind Res* 21C:93-96, 1962.

9 Singh HK, Dhawan BN: *J Ethnopharmacol* 5:205-214, 1982.

10 Singh HK, Dhawan BN: *Indian J Pharmacol* 10:72, 1978.

11 Jain P et al: *Indian J Exp Biol* 32(9):633-636, 1994.

12 Udupa KN, Singh RH: *Clinical and experimental studies on rasayana drugs and Pancakarma therapy*, ed 2, New Delhi, 1995, Central Council for Research in Ayurveda and Siddha.

13 Singh RH, Singh L: *J Res Ayurveda Siddha* 1:133-148, 1980.

14 Ghosh S, Kar SK: *J Exp Med Sci* 10(1):12-13, 1966.

15 Sharma R, Chaturvedi C, Tewari PV: *J Res Educ Indian Med* 6:1-10, 1987.

16 Mukherjee GD, Dey CD: *J Exp Med Sci* 11(4):82-85, 1968.

17 Stough C et al: *Psychopharmacol* 156(4):481-484, 2001.

BAICAL SKULLCAP

Botanical Name: *Scutellaria baicalensis*
Family: Labiatae
Plant Part Used: Root

PRESCRIBING INFORMATION

Actions

Antiinflammatory, antiallergic, antibacterial

Potential Indications

Based on appropriate evaluation of the patient, practitioners should consider prescribing Baical skullcap in formulations in the context of:
- Chronic inflammatory conditions, allergy, asthma, arthritis *(7)*
- Hypertension *(4,5)*
- Infections, including bronchitis, the common cold, bacillary dysentery, scarlet fever *(4)*
- High fevers, cough with thick sputum, pneumonia *(5)*
- Nausea, vomiting, hemoptysis, jaundice, diarrhea, or dysentery-like diseases *(5)*
- Hepatitis *(6)*
- Adjuvant therapy for cancer *(4)*

Contraindications

Contraindicated in *cold* conditions (Chinese traditional understanding).[1]

Warnings and Precautions

None required.

Interactions

None known.

Use in Pregnancy and Lactation

No adverse effects expected.

Side Effects

None expected if taken within the recommended dose range.

Dosage

Dose per day*	*Dose per week**
4.5-8.5 ml of 1:2 liquid extract	30-60 ml of 1:2 liquid extract

SUPPORTING INFORMATION

Traditional Prescribing

Uses and properties from TCM include:
- Clearing *heat* and draining *damp heat*[1]
- High fevers, cough with thick sputum, pneumonia; nausea, vomiting, hemoptysis, jaundice,[1-3] viral hepatitis[4]
- Diarrhea or dysentery-like diseases, painful urinary dysfunction, hypertension, restless fetus, carbuncles[1-3]

Pharmacologic Research

Baical skullcap root contains a number of flavone derivatives, including baicalin, wogonin, and baicalein.[5]

Baical Skullcap *continued on page 84*

---

*This dose range is adapted from dried plant dose administered by decoction in TCM.[3] The author's experience and the fact that ethanol-water is a more effective solvent than is water for many phytochemicals are taken into account.

- Flavones and flavonols inhibited the release of histamine by mast cells *in vitro*.[6] Baicalin and baicalein demonstrated antiallergic and antiasthmatic activity *in vivo*.[2]
- Oral doses of an extract of Baical skullcap and baicalin, baicalein, and wogonin demonstrated mild antiinflammatory activity and decreased long-term bone destruction in adjuvant-induced arthritis.[7]
- Baicalin and baicalein have demonstrated significant antiplatelet activity after oral doses in an experimental model, but not anticoagulant activity.[8]
- Baicalein demonstrated antioxidant activity *in vitro*.[9] Baicalein demonstrated antiepileptic and neuronal protective effects *in vivo* (by injection), probably because of free radical quenching and antioxidant activity.[10] Baicalein reduced oxidative stress during hypoxia, ischemia, and reperfusion *in vitro*.[11]
- A combination of baicalin and licorice extract dramatically reduced sorbitol levels in red blood cells in experimental models without affecting blood glucose levels.[12] This finding has implications for preventing diabetic complications.
- Baical skullcap reduced the toxicity of anticancer drugs and decreased cancer cell viability in experimental tumors.[13]

Clinical Studies

- Baical skullcap extract promoted an increase in the immunoregulation index (increased immunoglobulin A [IgA] at stable IgG levels) of patients with lung cancer who were receiving antineoplastic chemotherapy.[14]
- Positive results have been demonstrated in uncontrolled trials for acute bronchitis, the common cold, bacillary dysentery, scarlet fever, hepatitis (baicalin; route unknown), and cholecystitis (baicalin; by injection). The daily dose for respiratory disorders ranged from 6 ml to 8 to 10 ml of a 50% decoction depending on the age of the child.[2] A 70% success rate was shown in chronic hepatitis with improvements in symptoms and liver function tests (route and preparation undefined).[15]
- In an uncontrolled trial involving 255 patients in China with allergic rhinitis, Baical skullcap and *Paeonia suffructicosa* were added to the TCM herbal prescription for patients with nasal inflammation.[16]
- An antihypertensive effect was demonstrated in an uncontrolled study involving 51 cases.[2]

REFERENCES

1 Bensky D, Gamble A: *Chinese herbal medicine materia medica,* Seattle, 1986, Eastland Press.
2 Chang HM, But PP: *Pharmacology and applications of Chinese materia medica,* Singapore, 1987, World Scientific.
3 Pharmacopoeia Commission of the People's Republic of China: *Pharmacopoeia of the People's Republic of China,* English ed, Beijing, 1997, Chemical Industry Press.
4 Lu LX: *Shaanxi J Chin Trad Med* 8(5):228-229, 1987.
5 Tang W, Eisenbrand G: *Chinese drugs of plant origin,* Berlin, 1992, Springer-Verlag.
6 Amella M et al: *Planta Med* 51(1):16-20, 1985.
7 Kubo M et al: *Chem Pharm Bull (Tokyo)* 32(7):2724-2729, 1984.
8 Kubo M et al: *Chem Pharm Bull (Tokyo)* 33(6):2411-2415, 1985.

Baical Skullcap *continued on page 85*

9 Hara H et al: *Eur J Pharmacol* 221(2-3):193-198, 1992.

10 Hamada H et al: *Arch Biochem Biophys* 306(1):261-266, 1993.

11 Shao ZH et al: *Acad Emerg Med* 8(5):562-563, 2001.

12 Zhou YP, Zhang JQ: *Chin Med J (Eng)* 102:203-206, 1989.

13 Razina TG et al: *Vopr Onkol* 33(2):80-84, 1987.

14 Smol'ianinov ES et al: *Eksp Klin Farmacol* 60(6):49-51, 1997.

15 Chang HM et al, editors: *Advances in Chinese medicinal materials research,* Singapore, 1985, World Scientific.

16 Lin WS: *Shanghai J Trad Chin Med* 1:22-24, 1987.

BAPTISIA

Other Common Name: Wild indigo
Botanical Name: *Baptisia tinctoria*
Family: Leguminosae
Plant Part Used: Root

PRESCRIBING INFORMATION

Actions

Depurative, antipyretic, immune enhancing

Potential Indications

Based on appropriate evaluation of the patient, practitioners should consider prescribing Baptisia in formulations in the context of:
- Treating and preventing nonspecific upper respiratory tract infections, in combination with a number of herbs, including *Echinacea* spp. root and Thuja (2)
- Sinusitis, in combination with a number of herbs, including *Echinacea* spp. root and Thuja (3)
- Tonsillitis, pharyngitis, pneumonia, fevers, the common cold, influenza (5)
- Septic conditions, boils, mouth ulcers, inflammation of the mouth or teeth (5)

Contraindications

None known.

Warnings and Precautions

None required.

Interactions

None known.

Use in Pregnancy and Lactation

No adverse effects expected.

Side Effects

None expected if taken within the recommended dose range.

Dosage

Dose per day*	Dose per week*
2-6 ml of 1:2 liquid extract	15-40 ml of 1:2 liquid extract

SUPPORTING INFORMATION

Traditional Prescribing

Traditional Western herbal medicine uses include:
- Infections of the upper respiratory tract, particularly tonsillitis, pharyngitis; diphtheria, acute catarrhal infection, lymphadenitis, fevers, pneumonia[1,2]
- Sepsis, furunculosis, typhoid conditions, enfeebled circulation, mouth ulcers, gingivitis, stomatitis[1,2]

Native Americans administered Baptisia to children who seemed drowsy and lifeless and at the point of becoming sick. Externally,

Baptisia *continued on page 87*

*This dose range is extrapolated from the British Pharmaceutical Codex 1934, the British Herbal Pharmacopoeia 1983, and the author's education and experience.

Baptisia was used to bathe wounds and cuts. Baptisia was official in the United States Pharmacopeia (USP) from 1831 to 1842, the National Formulary (NF) from 1916 to 1936, and was used as an emetic, cathartic, stimulant, astringent, and antiseptic.[3]

Pharmacologic Research

- Glycoprotein derivatives from Baptisia root have demonstrated immunomodulating activity *in vitro* by provoking the stimulation of B lymphocytes with a concomitant increase of interferon release.[4]
- Fractions of Baptisia extract have demonstrated immune-enhancing activity *in vitro* and *in vivo* (by injection).[5]

Clinical Studies

No clinical studies have been conducted using Baptisia alone.

- Three herbal formulations containing Baptisia have been used successfully for treating and preventing nonspecific upper respiratory tract infections in randomized, double-blind, placebo-controlled trials.[6,7] These formulations consisted of: (a) Baptisia, *Echinacea* spp. root, and Thuja; (b) these same herbs combined with homeopathic remedies; and (c) *E. angustifolia* aerial parts and root with boneset, Baptisia, and homeopathic Arnica. In most of these trials, the daily dose of herbs was below the normal therapeutic limit (and was similar to a homeopathic protocol). Only in trials conducted with the last formulation did patients receive herbs approaching the normal therapeutic range. The daily dose in these trials ranged from 1.2 to 3.0 g of the total formulation (dry weight equivalent), including homeopathic Arnica, for periods ranging from several days in treatment trials to 8 weeks in a prevention trial.[6,8]
- A controlled trial found combined use of the first formulation previously listed with the antibiotic doxycycline had better success than did doxycycline alone in the treatment of acute sinusitis.[9]

REFERENCES

1 British Herbal Medicine Association's Scientific Committee: *British herbal pharmacopoeia,* Bournemouth, 1983, BHMA.

2 Felter HW, Lloyd JU: *King's American dispensatory,* ed 18, rev 3, Portland, 1905, reprinted 1983, Eclectic Medical Publications.

3 Vogel VJ: *American Indian medicine,* Norman, Okla, 1970, University of Oklahoma Press.

4 Beuscher N et al: *Planta Med* 55:358-363, 1989.

5 Beuscher N et al: *Angewandte Botanik Berichte* 6:46-61, 1997.

6 Barrett B, Vohman M, Calabrese C: *J Fam Prac* 48(8):628-635, 1999.

7 Henneicke-von Zepelin HH et al: *Curr Med Res Opin* 15(3):214-227, 1999.

8 Melchart D et al: *Phytomed* 1:245-254, 1994.

9 Zimmer M: *Therapiewoche* 35:4024-4028, 1985.

BARBERRY AND INDIAN BARBERRY

Common Name:	Barberry
Other Common Names:	Common barberry, European barberry
Botanical Name:	*Berberis vulgaris*
Family:	Berberidaceae
Plant Parts Used:	Root, stem bark, or both

Common Name:	Indian barberry
Botanical Name:	*Berberis aristata*
Family:	Berberidaceae
Plant Parts Used:	Root, stem bark, or both

PRESCRIBING INFORMATION

Actions

Barberry: antimicrobial, cholagogue, choleretic, antiemetic, mild laxative, bitter tonic

Indian barberry: antimicrobial, cholagogue, choleretic, antiemetic, mild laxative, bitter tonic

Potential Indications

Based on appropriate evaluation of the patient, practitioners should consider prescribing barberry or Indian barberry in formulations in the context of:
- Acute infectious diarrhea *(4a,5)*
- Gastritis, peptic ulcer (involving Helicobacter infection), giardiasis, hypertyraminemia *(4a)*
- Adjuvant therapy for non-insulin–dependent diabetes mellitus *(4a)*
- Jaundice *(5)*
- Topical treatment for mouth ulcers *(5)*

Practitioners should also consider prescribing barberry for:
- Improving digestive function (bile production and release) *(5)*
- Gallbladder inflammation, gallstones, intestinal dyspepsia *(5)*
- Topical treatment for lip sores, chronic ophthalmia *(5)*

Practitioners should also consider prescribing Indian barberry for:
- Improving digestive function (bile production and release) *(5)*
- Enlargement of the liver and spleen, colitis *(5)*
- Topical treatment for skin ulcers and abrasions, hemorrhoids, boils, acne *(5)*

Contraindications

Berberine-containing plants are not recommended for use during pregnancy or for jaundiced neonates.

Warnings and Precautions

None required.

Interactions

Berberine may reinforce the effects of other drugs that displace the protein binding of bilirubin. Rather than possible uterine-contracting

Barberry and Indian Barberry *continued on page 89*

effects, this activity might explain the traditional contraindication for berberine-containing herbs in pregnancy.

Use in Pregnancy and Lactation

Contraindicated in pregnancy.

Side Effects

At daily doses higher than 0.5 g, berberine may cause dizziness, nose-bleeds, dyspnea, skin and eye irritation, gastrointestinal irritation, nausea, diarrhea, nephritis, and urinary tract disorders. Such doses of berberine will not be reached using the liquid doses recommended here.

Dosage

It is preferable to use liquid extracts quantified for their berberine content.

Barberry:

*Dose per day**	*Dose per week**
3-6 ml of 1:2 liquid extract	20-40 ml of 1:2 liquid extract

Indian barberry:

Dose per day[†]	*Dose per week*[†]
2.0-4.5 ml of 1:1 liquid extract	15-30 ml of 1:1 liquid extract

For topical use of berberine-containing herbs (such as for treatment of ophthalmia), a solution of about 5 to 6 drops of a 1:2 extract is prepared in an eye bath of recently boiled water or saline. The liquid should be allowed to cool before applying to the eye. (Allowing the alcohol to evaporate through this process is important before applying to the eye.)

SUPPORTING INFORMATION

Traditional Prescribing

Traditional Western herbal medicine uses of barberry root, stem bark, or both include:
- Gallbladder inflammation, gallstones,[1] jaundice,[1,2] chronic diarrhea, dysentery, cholera infantum, intestinal dyspepsia[2]
- Renal calculi, soreness and burning of the urinary tract[2]
- Leishmaniasis, malaria,[1] fever[2]
- As a tea for blood purification, as a tonic[2]
- Topically as a decoction for mouth ulcers and lip sores, chronic ophthalmia[2]

Barberry was used by Native Americans to treat sore throat, ulcerated gums, and ulcerated stomach. Barberry was official in the USP from 1863 to 1882.[3]

Barberry and Indian Barberry *continued on page 90*

---

*This dose range is extrapolated from the British Herbal Pharmacopoeia 1983 and the author's education and experience.
†This dose range is extrapolated from traditional Ayurvedic medicine[4,5] and the author's education and experience.

Traditional Ayurvedic uses of Indian barberry root bark include:
- Debility, remittent and intermittent fever,[4] especially malarial fever[4,6]
- Skin diseases, inflammation[7]
- Neuralgia, dysentery, colitis[4]
- Enlargement of the liver and spleen, jaundice[4]
- Diseases of the eye, ear, and face[4]
- Topically for oriental sores, mouth sores, skin ulcers and abrasions, pimples, boils, affections of the eyelids, chronic ophthalmia, piles,[4] muscular or rheumatic pain[8]

Pharmacologic Research

Key constituents of barberry bark include alkaloids, comprising those of the isoquinoline group: protoberberines (berberine, jateorrhizine, and palmatine) and bisbenzylisoquinolines (including oxyacanthine). The principal alkaloid is berberine. Indian barberry root bark also contains berberine.[9]

The root bark is the preferred plant part for therapeutic use for both barberry and Indian barberry. The root bark has been preferred traditionally and is higher in alkaloids than the stem bark. However, given that the entire plant is killed in the harvesting process, the stem bark is a more environmentally sustainable option. The stem bark also contains the active alkaloids, albeit at lower concentrations, and is a valid therapeutic option. Several other plant parts of Indian barberry have been used in Ayurvedic medicine, including the fruit.

The following information pertains to the root bark (except when the plant part has not been defined in the study, as noted). Pharmacologic information on berberine, the signature component of barberry and Indian barberry, has also been provided when relevant.
- *In vitro* and *in vivo* studies have demonstrated that berberine has antimicrobial activity against a wide variety of microorganisms, including bacteria, fungi, and parasites. Barberry tincture was better than was berberine chloride (0.2%) at inhibiting the growth of various microorganisms *in vitro*. Indian barberry extract (part undefined) displayed inhibitory activity against *Salmonella typhi in vitro*.[10]
- Pustular skin lesions from *Staphylococcus aureus* and *S. pyogenes* infection were healed within 2 weeks when a combination of Indian barberry (part undefined) and *Cedrus deodora* was taken internally and also applied as a gel in an experimental model. The combined treatment was more beneficial than was the topical application alone.[11]
- Berberine combined with Geranium leaf extract (oral doses) significantly inhibited diarrhea. Oral berberine significantly reduced intestinal fluid accumulation triggered by *Escherichia coli* enterotoxin *in vivo*.
- Berberine increased thrombocytes, decreased factor XIII activity, inhibited platelet aggregation and adhesiveness, and inhibited clot retraction *in vivo* (route unknown). Indian barberry root extract inhibited platelet activating factor (PAF) aggregation of platelets in a dose-dependent manner and binding of radiolabeled PAF to platelets *in vitro*.

Barberry and Indian Barberry continued on page 91

- Berberine has demonstrated cytotoxic activity in several *in vitro* models. Indian barberry extract (part undefined) demonstrated anticancer activity against human epidermal carcinoma of the nasopharynx *in vitro*.[12]
- Intraperitoneal administration of barberry extract demonstrated higher antiinflammatory activity than did isolated berberine and three different alkaloidal fractions in experimental models of acute and chronic inflammation.
- Barberry tincture increased contractions in isolated intestinal tissue and demonstrated cholagogue and cholekinetic activity in experimental models. Oral administration of berberine hydrochloride significantly increased bilirubin excretion in experimental hyperbilirubinemia without affecting the functional capacity of the liver.
- Oral pretreatment or posttreatment with berberine (4 mg/kg) prevented chemical-induced liver damage, indicating hepatoprotective activity.[13]
- Berberine prolonged pentobarbital-induced sleeping time and increased strychnine-induced toxicity after oral administration, suggesting an inhibitory effect on liver drug metabolizing enzymes (cytochrome P-450).[13]
- Lipogenesis was suppressed in isolated sebaceous glands by berberine.
- Berberine significantly decreased scopolamine-induced amnesia in an experimental model.
- Indian barberry root extract demonstrated hypoglycemic activity in an experimental model (route unknown).[12]

For more information on the pharmacologic parameters of berberine, see the monograph on golden seal *(Hydrastis canadensis)*.

Clinical Studies

No clinical studies using barberry or Indian barberry have been found. Clinical trials using berberine are outlined here. The berberine doses used in many of these trials were higher than what could be achieved using herbal liquid extracts.

- Berberine (100 mg/day) demonstrated an antidiarrheal action and compared well against standard antidiarrheal drugs in an uncontrolled study involving children with gastroenteritis. In randomized, controlled trials, berberine has exhibited benefit in treating diarrhea caused by *Escherichia coli* infection but was of little value against *Vibrio cholerae* infectious diarrhea (cholera). The trials with positive outcomes for *E. coli* diarrhea were conducted using either untreated controls (active therapy: 400 mg of berberine sulfate as a single dose) or compared rehydration therapy against only rehydration therapy with berberine (200 mg). In another trial, neither berberine (400 mg/day) nor tetracycline exhibited any benefit over placebo in patients with noncholera diarrhea.
- Berberine (900 mg/day) was more efficacious than was ranitidine in clearing *Helicobacter pylori* and improving gastritis in *H. pylori*-associated duodenal ulcer in a randomized, comparative clinical trial. Ranitidine was the superior treatment for ulcer healing.

Barberry and Indian Barberry *continued on page 92*

- In two controlled trials, berberine (5 to 10 mg/kg/day for 6 to 10 days) was superior to placebo and compared favorably with established drugs in treating giardiasis in children.
- In an uncontrolled trial, berberine (600 to 800 mg/day) corrected hypertyraminemia and prevented the elevation of serum tyramine after tyramine stimulation in patients with liver cirrhosis. (Hypertyraminemia [i.e., elevated blood levels of tyramine] is common in hepatic cirrhosis.)
- In an uncontrolled trial berberine (0.9 to 1.5 g/day for 1 to 3 months) in combination with a therapeutic diet improved the major symptoms of patients with non-insulin–dependent diabetes. Berberine treatment improved patients' strength, normalized blood pressure, decreased blood lipids, and in 60% of patients, normalized fasting glycemic levels.
- Berberine bisulfate (15 mg/day for 15 days) increased platelet counts in patients with primary and secondary thrombocytopenia in an uncontrolled clinical trial.
- In a randomized, controlled trial, berberine chloride (1.5 g/day) was more efficacious than were both tetracycline and a sulfamethoxazole-trimethoprim combination in clearing asexual parasitemia in patients with chloroquine-resistant malaria (all agents were used in conjunction with pyrimethamine).
- Weekly intralesional injection of berberine salt solution (1%) healed cutaneous leishmaniasis after 4 to 8 weeks in a small, uncontrolled trial. (Cutaneous leishmaniasis is a protozoal skin infection caused by species of Leishmania.)

REFERENCES

Except when specifically referenced, the following book was referred to in the compilation of the pharmacologic and clinical information: Mills S, Bone K: *Principles and Practice of Phytotherapy: Modern Herbal Medicine*, Edinburgh, 2000, Churchill Livingstone.

1 British Herbal Medicine Association's Scientific Committee: *British Herbal Pharmacopoeia*, Bournemouth, 1983, BHMA.

2 Felter HW, Lloyd JU: *King's American dispensatory*, ed 18, rev 3, Portland, 1905, reprinted 1983, Eclectic Medical Publications.

3 Vogel VJ: *American Indian medicine*, Norman, Okla, 1970, University of Oklahoma Press.

4 Thakur RS, Puri HS, Husain A: *Major medicinal plants of India*, Lucknow, India, 1989, Central Institute of Medicinal and Aromatic Plants.

5 Kapoor LD: *CRC handbook of Ayurvedic medicinal plants*, Boca Raton, Fla, 1990, CRC Press.

6 Chopra RN et al: *Chopra's indigenous drugs of India*, ed 2, Calcutta, 1958, reprinted 1982, Academic Publishers.

7 Kumar S et al: *J Ethnopharmacol* 70(3):191-195, 2000.

8 Joshi AR, Joshi K: *J Ethnopharmacol* 73:175-183, 2000.

9 Chauhan SK, Singh BP, Agrawal S: *Indian Drugs* 35(8):468-470, 1998.

10 Sohni YR, Padmaja K, Bhatt RM: *J Ethnopharmacol* 45(2):141-147, 1995.

11 Chakkrabarti A, Guha C, Sen TB: *Indian Vet J* 76(5):432-434, 1999.

12 Dhar ML et al: *Indian J Exp Biol* 6(4):232-247, 1968.

13 Janbaz KH, Gilani AH: *Fitoterapia* 71:25-33, 2000.

BILBERRY

Botanical Name: *Vaccinium myrtillus*
Family: Ericaceae
Plant Part Used: Fruit

PRESCRIBING INFORMATION

Actions

Vasoprotective, antiedema, antioxidant, antiinflammatory

Potential Indications

Based on appropriate evaluation of the patient, practitioners should consider prescribing bilberry that contains anthocyanins (e.g., fresh or dried fruit, standardized tablets) as part of an overall treatment program in the context of:
- Vision disorders, myopia, retinitis, hemeralopia, simple glaucoma *(4)*
- Venous insufficiency, especially of the lower limbs *(1)*
- Peripheral vascular disorders, diabetic retinopathy *(3)*
- Hypertensive retinopathy, nosebleed caused by capillary fragility *(3)*
- Chronic primary dysmenorrhea *(3)*
- Raynaud's syndrome *(4)*
- Venous disorders during pregnancy, including hemorrhoids *(4)*
- Postoperative complications from nose surgery *(4)*
- Decreased capillary resistance (bruising, petechiae, fecal occult blood) *(4)*
- Nonspecific, acute diarrhea *(4)*
- Topical treatment for mild inflammation of the mouth and throat *(4)*

Based on appropriate evaluation of the patient, practitioners should consider prescribing bilberry that contains no anthocyanins (e.g., liquid extracts) in formulations in the context of digestive disorders, including diarrhea, dyspepsia, gastrointestinal infections, and inflammations; scurvy, urinary complaints, vaginal discharges *(6)*

Contraindications

None known.

Warnings and Precautions

Very high doses of the standardized tablets should be used cautiously in patients with hemorrhagic disorders and in those taking warfarin or antiplatelet drugs. (Inhibition of platelet aggregation was demonstrated from the blood of healthy volunteers after oral administration of an extract containing 173 mg/day of anthocyanins for 30 to 60 days.)

Interactions

Possible interaction may occur with warfarin and antiplatelet drugs but only for very high doses.

Use in Pregnancy and Lactation

No adverse effects expected.

Side Effects

A surveillance study reported mild side effects in a small percentage of patients affecting the gastrointestinal, cutaneous, or nervous systems.

Bilberry *continued on page 94*

Dosage

	*Dose per day**	*Dose per week**
	3-6 ml of 1:1 liquid extract	20-40 ml of 1:1 liquid extract

Tablets providing 50 to 120 mg per day of anthocyanins (equivalent to about 20 to 50 g of fresh fruit) have been typically used in clinical trials.

SUPPORTING INFORMATION

Traditional Prescribing

Traditional Western herbal medicine uses include:
- Digestive disorders (diarrhea, dyspepsia, gastrointestinal infections, and inflammations), hemorrhoids[1]
- Scurvy, urinary complaints[1]
- Vaginal discharges, to dry up breast milk[1]

Pharmacologic Research

Bilberry fruit contains a range of anthocyanins, some of which are blue pigments responsible for the color of the ripe berries.
- Bilberry extract has demonstrated vasoprotective and antiedema effects *in vivo*.
- *In vitro* studies have demonstrated the antioxidant activity of bilberry and its anthocyanins.
- Antiplatelet activity has been demonstrated *in vitro*, *in vivo*, and *ex vivo*. The mechanism of action may depend on an increase in the concentration of cAMP, a decrease in the concentration of platelet thromboxane, or both.
- Anthocyanins from bilberry protected collagen against nonenzymatic proteolytic activity *in vitro* and therefore may protect collagen from degradation during inflammatory processes.
- Bilberry extract demonstrated significant dose-dependent antiulcer activity *in vivo*.

Clinical Studies

All clinical studies have been conducted using bilberry preparations that were standardized for anthocyanin content. The oral doses used in the following clinical studies ranged from 54 to 288 mg per day of anthocyanins, with doses of 115 mg/day and 173 mg/day of anthocyanins most commonly administered.
- A review of uncontrolled trials from 1979 to 1985 concluded that bilberry extract caused rapid disappearance of symptoms and improvements in venous microcirculation and lymph drainage for patients with venous insufficiency.
- In a double-blind, placebo-controlled trial, patients with peripheral vascular disorders of various causes experienced a reduction in subjective symptoms, including paresthesia, pain, heaviness, and edema, after treatment with bilberry for 30 days. Mobilization of finger joints was improved in patients with Raynaud's syndrome.

Bilberry continued on page 95

*This dose range is extrapolated from traditional herbal texts[1] and pharmacologic and clinical trial data.

- Bilberry extract provided relief for patients with venous disorders, including hemorrhoids during pregnancy in an open trial lasting 2 to 3 months.
- In a double-blind, placebo-controlled trial, bilberry significantly reduced symptoms of dysmenorrhea, such as pelvic and lumbosacral pain, mammary tension, headache, nausea, and heaviness of the lower limbs.
- In uncontrolled trials, bilberry extract improved symptoms caused by decreased capillary resistance and reduced the microcirculatory changes induced by cortisone therapy in patients with asthma and chronic bronchitis after 6 months' treatment and improved diabetic retinopathy with a marked reduction or even disappearance of retinic hemorrhages. Other controlled studies support the use of bilberry for the treatment of both diabetic and hypertensive retinopathy.
- In a placebo-controlled trial, bilberry extract reduced nosebleed caused by abnormal capillary fragility of the mucous membranes.
- Studies have also shown the benefits of bilberry in patients with visual disorders, such as myopia, defective vision in bright light, simple glaucoma (in combination with retinol), and poor darkness adaptation. Bilberry also improved night vision in healthy volunteers, although a small double-blind, placebo-controlled trial published in 2000 cast doubt on this aspect of its efficacy.[2]
- Postoperative complications from surgery of the nose were reduced in patients who received bilberry extract administered for 7 days before and 10 days after surgery.
- In Germany, the Commission E supports the use of bilberry dried fruit and preparations to treat nonspecific acute diarrhea and externally for local therapy of mild inflammation of the mucous membranes of the mouth and throat.[3]

REFERENCES

Except when specifically referenced, the following book was referred to in the compilation of the pharmacologic and clinical information: Mills S, Bone K: *Principles and Practice of Phytotherapy: Modern Herbal Medicine*, Edinburgh, 2000, Churchill Livingstone.

1 Grieve M: *A modern herbal*, New York, 1971, Dover Publications.
2 Muth ER, Laurent JM, Jasper P: *Altern Med Rev* 5(2):164-173, 2000.
3 Blumenthal M et al, editors: *The complete German Commission E monographs: therapeutic guide to herbal medicines*, Austin, 1998, American Botanical Council.

BLACK COHOSH

Botanical Names: *Cimicifuga racemosa, Actaea racemosa*[#^]
Family: Ranunculaceae
Plant Part Used: Root and rhizome

PRESCRIBING INFORMATION

Actions	Antirheumatic, spasmolytic, estrogen modulating, uterine tonic
Potential Indications	Based on appropriate evaluation of the patient, practitioners should consider prescribing black cohosh in formulations in the context of: • Symptoms associated with menopause *(2,4)* • Dysmenorrhea *(4,5)* • Premenstrual syndrome *(4)* • Ovarian dysfunction and ovarian insufficiency *(4)* • Amenorrhea, ovarian pain, female infertility; arthritis, rheumatism, neuralgia, myalgia, sciatica; whooping cough, tinnitus *(5)*
Contraindications	Black cohosh should not be taken during pregnancy or lactation[2] except during the last month to assist with birth.[3] Until more information is available, women with estrogen-dependent tumors such as breast cancer should avoid using black cohosh.
Warnings and Precautions	Traditional sources note that overdose has caused nausea and vomiting and may produce vertigo, as well as visual and nervous disturbance.
Interactions	The antiproliferative effect of black cohosh extract in combination with tamoxifen was assessed *in vitro* on 17β-estradiol–stimulated MCF-7 human breast cancer cells. Black cohosh augmented the antiproliferative action of tamoxifen. Whether this interaction also applies *in vivo* has not been established.
Use in Pregnancy and Lactation	Contraindicated in pregnancy and lactation, except for assisting birth during the last month.
Side Effects	High doses cause frontal headache. Stomach complaints have been observed with a low frequency in clinical trials.

Dosage	***Dose per day*** *	***Dose per week*** *
	1.5-3.0 ml of 1:2 liquid extract	10-20 ml of 1:2 liquid extract

Black cohosh may be taken long term within the recommended dose, although the Commission E recommends not more than 6 months, perhaps because controlled studies over longer periods are lacking.

Black Cohosh *continued on page 97*

[#]Alternative name.
[^]Adopted by the American Herbal Products Association as the new botanical name.[1]
*This dose range is extrapolated from the British Pharmaceutical Codex 1934, the British Herbal Pharmacopoeia 1983, clinical trial information, and the author's education and experience.

Traditional Prescribing

Traditional Western herbal medicine uses include:
- Myalgia, chorea, arthritis, rheumatism, neuralgia, sciatica[3,4]
- Female reproductive disorders, dysmenorrhea, amenorrhea, ovarian pain, female infertility, partus preparator, leukorrhea[4,5]
- Whooping cough, tinnitus[4]

Pharmacologic Research

- Experimental studies have shown the luteinizing hormone (LH) suppressive effect of black cohosh when the extract was given both orally and via injection (the latter route produced greater activity). At least three compounds were found to be involved. Black cohosh extract has also increased LH secretion *in vivo* (oral route).[6]
- Although estrogenic compounds are present in black cohosh, no estrogenic activity was found *in vivo* after oral or subcutaneous administration. Black cohosh extracts reduced the number of skin flushes in an experimental menopausal model, which was considered to be indicative of an estrogenic effect.[7] Research presented in 2000 highlights the debate concerning the nature of any estrogenic activity of black cohosh.[8]
- Black cohosh is not overtly estrogenic, but the compounds within it act as phyto-SERMs (plant substances that act as selective estrogen-receptor modulators) that interact with certain types of estrogen receptors such as Erβ, which is present in many tissues.
- Black cohosh had no effect on uterine weight *in vivo* or on any of the estrogen-regulated genes in the uterus, whereas it mimicked many of the effects of estradiol in bone, liver, and the aorta.
- Oral administration of black cohosh extract did not promote estrogen-dependent mammary gland tumors *in vivo*.[9]
- Black cohosh extract inhibited monoamine oxidase in the striatum after long-term pretreatment *in vivo*.[10]

Clinical Studies

The clinical studies outlined here were conducted using a German proprietary medicine and reflect lower doses compared with those used traditionally. The tablets are quoted as containing 1 mg of a marker triterpene glycoside (27-deoxyactein). Current regulatory information indicates that these tablets now contain 24.8 to 42.7 mg dried herb equivalent and 0.8 to 1.2 mg triterpene glycosides.
- A review of clinical data indicates that black cohosh appears to have therapeutic efficacy for moderate to severe neurovegetative symptoms of menopause. Good tolerability and a low risk of side effects have been confirmed.[11] The data reviewed includes case reports dating back to the 1950s, a drug-monitoring study of over 700 individuals and clinical trials. Three of the trials were randomized and controlled and administered a dose containing 4 mg/day of marker triterpene glycoside. In the randomized, double-blind, placebo-controlled trial, black cohosh was superior in efficacy to that of conjugated estrogens (0.625 mg/day) after 3 months. In this trial, the black cohosh

Black Cohosh continued on page 98

treatment group also showed significant improvement in the proliferation status of vaginal epithelium. However, the administered dose of estrogens was considered too low. A pharmacologic study involving menopausal women observed that black cohosh (4 tablets/day) significantly reduced the mean serum LH level compared with a placebo group. This statistical reduction of LH was not observed in an earlier randomized, controlled trial using the same dose.

- Treatment with a high dose of black cohosh extract was not associated with changes in endometrial thickness, vaginal cell status, or hormone levels in a drug-monitoring study involving 28 menopausal women. Hormones measured included LH, follicle-stimulating hormone (FSH), prolactin, and estradiol. Approximately 80% of patients demonstrated good or very good efficacy in relation to the menopausal symptoms measured. The dosage of extract (similar to that discussed here) was 136 mg/day. The mean duration of treatment was 98 days.[12]

- Treatment with black cohosh (2 tablets/day) was not significantly better than was placebo for most menopausal symptoms in a randomized, double-blind trial involving women with a history of breast cancer. Of the seven menopausal symptoms assessed, sweating was the only symptom for which the improvement reported by the treatment group was statistically significant from placebo.[13] The dose administered was lower than that used in other clinical trials.

- In an open, multicenter, postmarketing surveillance study, a combination of St. John's wort and black cohosh demonstrated improvement in 90% of patients for the psychologic complaints experienced in menopause, with improved concentration and a reduction in hot flashes.[14] The same St. John's wort and black cohosh combination significantly reduced menopausal symptoms compared with placebo in a randomized, double-blind trial involving 179 women. The daily dose contained 0.5 mg of total hypericin and 2 mg of 27-deoxyactein (the active compound in black cohosh).[15]

- In Germany, the Commission E supports using black cohosh to treat premenstrual discomfort, dysmenorrhea, and menopausal symptoms.[16]

REFERENCES

Except when specifically referenced, the following book was referred to in the compilation of the pharmacologic and clinical information: Mills S, Bone K: *Principles and Practice of Phytotherapy: Modern Herbal Medicine*, Edinburgh, 2000, Churchill Livingstone.

1 McGuffin M, editor: *Herbs of Commerce*, ed 2, [draft 3.3], Bethesda, Md, 1998, American Herbal Products Association.

2 British Herbal Medicine Association: *British herbal compendium*, Bournemouth, 1992, BHMA.

3 Felter HW: *The eclectic materia medica, pharmacology and therapeutics*, Portland, 1922, reprinted 1983, Eclectic Medical Publications.

4 British Herbal Medicine Association's Scientific Committee: *British herbal pharmacopoeia*, Bournemouth, 1983, BHMA.

5 Felter HW, Lloyd JU: *King's American dispensatory*, ed 18, rev 3, Portland, 1905, reprinted 1983, Eclectic Medical Publications.

6 Knuvener E, Korte B, Winterhoff H: *Phytomed* 7(supp 2):12, 2000.

7 Lohning A, Verspohl EJ, Winterhoff H: *International Conference: 2000 Years of Natural Product Research – Past, Present and Future*, Amsterdam, July 26-30, 1999; Abstract 327.

Black Cohosh *continued on page 99*

8 *Third International Congress on Phytomedicine,* Munich, October 11-13, 2000. *Phytomed* 7(supp 2):11-12, 2000.

9 Freundenstein J, Dasenbrock C, Nisslein T: *Phytomed* 7(supp 2):13, 2000.

10 Lohning A, Winterhoff H: *Phytomed* 7(supp 2):13, 2000.

11 Liske E: *Adv Ther* 15(1):45-53, 1998.

12 Nesselhut T, Liske E: *10th Annual Meeting of the North American Menopause Society,* New York, September 23-25, 1999; Poster 8.

13 Jacobson JS et al: *J Clin Oncol* 19(10):2739-2745, 2001.

14 Gerhard I, Liske E, Wustenberg P: *Z Phytother Abstractband* 21-22, 1995.

15 Boblitz N et al: *Focus Alternat Complement Ther* 5(1):85-86, 1995.

16 Blumenthal M et al, editors: *The complete German Commission E monographs: therapeutic guide to herbal medicines,* Austin, 1998, American Botanical Council.

BLACK HAW

Botanical Name: *Viburnum prunifolium*
Family: Caprifoliaceae
Plant Part Used: Bark

Actions

Uterine sedative, bronchospasmolytic, antiasthmatic, hypotensive, astringent

Potential Indications

Based on appropriate evaluation of the patient, practitioners should consider prescribing black haw in formulations in the context of:
• Dysmenorrhea (5)
• False labor pains, threatened miscarriage, postpartum hemorrhage (5)
• Asthma, hiccup, leg cramps (5)

Contraindications

None known.

Warnings and Precautions

According to the American Herbal Products Association,[1] individuals with a history of kidney stones are cautioned against using black haw because of the presence of oxalate or oxalic acid in the dried bark. Oxalate, as the potassium or calcium salt, is present in the cell sap of many plants and vegetables. Calcium oxalate is practically insoluble in water[2] and is unlikely to be present in aqueous ethanolic liquid extracts of black haw in sufficient quantities to justify this precaution.

Interactions

Black haw contains scopoletin (a coumarin), and suggestions are that it may potentiate the effects of anticoagulant medications or cause hemorrhagic problems.[3] However, no evidence has been found to suggest that anticoagulant activity *in vivo*[4] and simple plant coumarins do not necessarily increase the risk of bleeding.

Use in Pregnancy and Lactation

No adverse effects expected.

Side Effects

None expected if taken within the recommended dose range. A traditional text reports that nausea and vomiting may occur with large doses.[5]

Dose per day*	Dose per week*
1.5-4.5 ml of 1:2 liquid extract	10-30 ml of 1:2 liquid extract

Traditional Prescribing

Traditional Western herbal medicine uses include:
• As a uterine tonic, for uterine irritation and inflammation[5,6]
• Dysmenorrhea, severe lumbar and bearing-down pains; cramplike, expulsive menstrual pains[5,6]

Black Haw *continued on page 101*

*This dose range is extrapolated from the British Pharmaceutical Codex 1949, the British Herbal Pharmacopoeia 1983, and the author's education and experience.

- Threatened miscarriage,[5,6] especially with a rise in blood pressure[6]
- False labor pains,[5,6] postpartum hemorrhage; menorrhagia, uterine hemorrhage in menopause, amenorrhea[5]
- Nervous disorders associated with menses, including epilepsy[5]
- Leg cramps, especially at night[5]
- Asthma,[6] hiccup, heart palpitations[5]
- Diarrhea, dysentery, jaundice[5]
- Sterility, spermatorrhea[5]
- Alcoholic hangover[5]
- Topically for indolent ulcers and ophthalmic disorders[5]

Native Americans used black haw for stomach troubles, dysentery, female reproductive problems, before and during parturition, and as an antispasmodic, diaphoretic, and tonic. Black haw was official in the USP from 1882 to 1926 and NF from 1926 to 1960.[3,7]

Pharmacologic Research

Black haw bark contains flavonoids (including the biflavone amentoflavone), iridoid glycosides, triterpenes and triterpenic acids, and coumarins (including scopoletin).[3]

The value of published research conducted before 1940 on *Viburnum* spp. must be questioned because of possible improper identification of the various species and possible adulteration with other species.[8]
- Early studies investigating the uterine spasmolytic effect for black haw had varying results.[9-15] Two reviews of these studies concluded that the findings were scientifically invalid because of significant design limitations.[16,17] More recent studies have confirmed the uterine spasmolytic activity of black haw ethanolic extracts *in vitro*.[18-21]
- Black haw has also demonstrated spasmolytic activity in isolated intestinal tissues.[21]
- Hypotensive and hypertensive effects have been reported for black haw. An indirect, dose-dependent, vasoconstricting effect was observed in isolated aortic tissue.[22] Intravenous administration of the total extract induced a slow but prolonged increase in mean blood pressure *in vivo*.[22] Conversely, early *in vivo* studies demonstrated a hypotensive effect for black haw (intravenous route).[15,23] Theories suggest that the hypotensive effect was a result of the absence of iridoid compounds in the extracts used in the early studies.[21] Moreover, because the herb was administered by injection in all these studies, their relevance is questionable.
- In an early study, dietary black haw root bark did not have a significant appetite-enhancing effect in an experimental model, suggesting a lack of bitter action.[24] (This finding is not surprising because modern herbal clinicians do not regard black haw as a bitter tonic.)

Clinical Studies

No clinical studies using black haw have been found.

Black Haw *continued on page 102*

REFERENCES

1 McGuffin M et al, editors: *American Herbal Products Association's botanical safety handbook*, Boca Raton, Fla, 1997, CRC Press.

2 Budavari S et al, editors: *The Merck index: an encyclopedia of chemicals, drugs and biologicals*, ed 12, Whitehouse Station, N.J., 1996, Merck and Co.

3 American Herbal Pharmacopoeia: *Black haw bark – Viburnum prunifolium: analytical, quality control, and therapeutic monograph*, Santa Cruz, Calif, June 2000, American Herbal Pharmacopoeia.

4 Patterson DSP, Roberts BA, O'Neill PA: *Vet Rec* 89(20):544-545, 1971.

5 Felter HW, Lloyd JU: *King's American dispensatory*, ed 18, rev 3, Portland, 1905, reprinted 1983, Eclectic Medical Publications.

6 British Herbal Medicine Association's Scientific Committee: *British herbal pharmacopoeia*, Bournemouth, 1983, BHMA.

7 Vogel VJ: *American Indian medicine*, Norman, Okla, 1970, University of Oklahoma Press.

8 American Herbal Pharmacopoeia: *Cramp bark–Viburnum opulus: analytical, quality control, and therapeutic monograph*, Santa Cruz, Calif, February 2000, American Herbal Pharmacopoeia.

9 Pilcher JD, Delzell WR, Burman GE: *Arch Intern Med* 18(5):557-583, 1916.

10 Pilcher JD, Delzell WR, Burman GE: *J Am Med Assoc* 67(7):490-492, 1916.

11 Pilcher JD: *Arch Int Med* 19(9):53-55, 1917.

12 Pilcher JD, Mauer RT: *Surgery Gynecol Obstet* 27:97-99, 1918.

13 Hager BH, Becht FC: *J Pharmacol ExpTher* 13(1):61-70, 1919.

14 Munch JC: *J Am Pharm Assoc* 28(11):886-887, 1939.

15 Munch JC, Pratt HJ: *Pharm Arch* 12:88-91, 1941.

16 Woodbury RA: *Drug Stand* 19(7-9):143-151, 1951.

17 Baldini L, Brambilla G, Parodi S: *Arch Ital Sci Farmacolog* 3(14):55-63, 1963.

18 Balansard G et al: *Med Plants Phytother* 17(3):123-132, 1983.

19 Jarboe CH et al: *Nature* 212(64):837, 1966.

20 Jarboe CH et al: *J Med Chem* 10:488-489, 1967.

21 Tomassini L et al: *Proceedings of the Societa Italiana di Fitochimica 9th National Congress*, Societa Italiana di Fitochimica, Florence, May 27-30, 1988.

22 Cometa MF, Tomassini L, Palmery M: *Fitoterapia* 69(5):23, 1998.

23 Evans Jr WE, Harne WG, Krantz Jr JC: *J Pharmacol* 75:174-177, 1942.

24 Garb S, Cattell M: *Drug Stand* 24(3):94-99, 1956.

BLADDERWRACK

Other Common Name:	Kelp (this common name is applied to several seaweed species, including bladderwrack)
Botanical Name:	*Fucus vesiculosus*
Family:	Fucaceae
Plant Part Used:	Thallus (plant body)

PRESCRIBING INFORMATION

Actions

Weight reducing, thyroid stimulant, demulcent

Potential Indications

Based on appropriate evaluation of the patient, practitioners should consider prescribing bladderwrack in formulations in the context of:
- Obesity associated with iodine deficiency *(3,5)*
- Thyroid conditions resulting from iodine deficiency *(5,7)*
- Rheumatic conditions, including arthritis *(5)*

Contraindications

Hyperthyroidism, pregnancy, lactation, and cardiac problems associated with hyperthyroidism[1]

Warnings and Precautions

None required.

Interactions

Bladderwrack may interact with thyroid replacement therapies (thyroxine).

Use in Pregnancy and Lactation

Contraindicated in pregnancy and lactation.

Side Effects

Kelp (species undefined) has caused transient hyperthyroidism (estimated iodine intake of 2.8 to 4.2 mg/day)[2,3] and raised levels of thyroid stimulating hormone (dose undefined).[4]

When consumed as a food, kelp (probably not bladderwrack) has caused subclinical hypothyroidism[5] and Hashimoto's thyroiditis.[6] Rare extrathyroidal effects may also occur in susceptible individuals as a result of iodine intake, such as the allergic reactions of edema (doses up to 25 mg/day iodine), iodine fever (50 to 500 mg/day iodine), and eosinophilia (dose not defined). However, iodine intake from iodine-rich foods and supplements are unlikely to reach these high levels.[7]

Other cases of side effects from bladderwrack or kelp ingestion have been recorded (including kidney damage) and were attributed to high levels of heavy metals, particularly arsenic. In one case, the ingested kelp tablets contained 20 µg of arsenic per tablet (27.8 µg/g). The dose taken was not indicated. Physicians linked a case of severe dyserythropoiesis and autoimmune thrombocytopenia to ingestion of a kelp tablet (probably not bladderwrack). Analysis of the tablets showed that they contained 1.3 µg/g of arsenic. The patient had been ingesting 2.2 µg of arsenic daily from this source.[8-10] The reader should note that marine organisms, including bladderwrack, naturally accumulate arsenic.

Bladderwrack *continued on page 104*

However, the arsenic is mainly organically bound and rapidly excreted. For this reason, the World Health Organization has established a tolerable weekly intake for inorganic arsenic only, which is present in bladderwrack at considerably lower levels.[11]

Dosage

Dose per day*	Dose per week*
4.5-8.5 ml of 1:1 liquid extract	30-60 ml of 1:1 liquid extract

SUPPORTING INFORMATION

Traditional Prescribing

Traditional Western herbal medicine uses include:
- Obesity, particularly associated with hypothyroidism.[12] (Eclectic texts note that bladderwrack may be beneficial for treating obesity but only in cases when the diet is deficient, presumably of the iodine that bladderwrack contains.[13])
- Myxedema (a condition resulting from advanced hypothyroidism), lymphadenoid goiter (most likely of the simple type resulting from iodine deficiency, rather than the exophthalmic type, which is indicative of hyperthyroidism)[12]
- Rheumatism and rheumatoid arthritis (internally and topically)[12]

Bladderwrack was thought by the Eclectics to tone muscular fibers, to act powerfully on the glandular system as a depurative, and to reduce renal congestion and bladder inflammation.[13]

Pharmacologic Research

Bladderwrack thallus contains trace minerals (particularly free and protein-bound iodide) and polysaccharides of several types (including alginic acid and fucans such as fucoidan). Other constituents include polyphenols, lipids, and sterols.[1]
- Experimental studies conducted and reported in 1910 found oral doses of bladderwrack have a stimulatory activity on the thyroid gland.[14]
- When administered by injection, a polysaccharide fraction of bladderwrack demonstrated hypoglycemic activity in a normoglycemic model and lowered serum lipid levels in hyperlipidemia.[15,16]
- Bladderwrack extract promoted collagen gel contraction by increasing the expression of integrin molecules on the surface of fibroblasts in an *in vitro* model of dermal tissue.[17] Polysaccharides from bladderwrack demonstrated strong adhesion to epithelial tissue *in vitro*.[18]
- Low molecular weight fucoidan fraction from bladderwrack demonstrated potent anticoagulant and fibrinolytic properties *in vitro*, with only minor platelet-activating effects.[19]
- Fractions of bladderwrack extract demonstrated anti-HIV activity *in vitro*.[20]

Bladderwrack *continued on page 105*

*This dose range is extrapolated from the British Herbal Pharmacopoeia 1983, the British Herbal Compendium 1992, and the author's education and experience.

Clinical Studies

- A clinical trial investigating several weight-reducing treatments in moderately overweight Swedish women was conducted over a 2-year period. Most of the treatments, including the kelp-lecithin-vitamin combination, produced poor results.[21] (The species used was probably not bladderwrack.)
- A hypocaloric diet combined with spirulina, bladderwrack, and gelatin did not change any of the measured parameters in hypertensive obese patients.[22]
- In a controlled clinical trial, obese volunteers taking bladderwrack extract in addition to a controlled diet achieved a significantly greater average weight loss than did those on diet alone.[23]

REFERENCES

1 British Herbal Medicine Association: *British herbal compendium,* Bournemouth, 1992, BHMA.
2 Eliason BC: *J Am Board Fam Pract* 11(6):478-480, 1998.
3 Shilo S, Hirsch HJ: *Postgrad Med J* 62:661-662, 1986.
4 Key TJA et al: *J Hum Nutr Diet* 5:323-326, 1992.
5 Konno N et al: *J Clin Endocrinol Metab* 78(2):393-397, 1994.
6 Okamura K, Inoue K, Omae T: *Acta Endocrinol* 88:703-712, 1978.
7 de Smet PAGM et al, editors: *Adverse effects of herbal drugs,* Berlin, 1997, Springer-Verlag.
8 Conz PA et al: *Nephrol Dial Transplant* 13:526-527, 1998.
9 Walkiw O, Douglas DE: *Clin Toxicol* 8(3):325-331, 1975.
10 Pye KG et al: *Lancet* 339(8808):1540, 1992.
11 de Smet PAGM et al, editors: *Adverse effects of herbal drugs,* Berlin, 1992, Springer-Verlag.
12 British Herbal Medicine Association's Scientific Committee: *British herbal pharmacopoeia,* Bournemouth, 1983, BHMA.
13 Felter HW, Lloyd JU: *King's American dispensatory,* ed 18, rev 3, Portland, 1905, reprinted 1983, Eclectic Medical Publications.
14 Hunt R, Seidell A: *J Pharmacol* 2:15-47, 1910.
15 Vazquez-Freire MJ, Lamela M, Calleja JM: *Phytother Res* 10(supp 1):S184-S185, 1996.
16 Lamela M, Vazquez-Freire MJ, Calleja JM: *Phytother Res* 10(supp 1):S175-S176, 1996.
17 Fujimura T et al: *Biol Pharm Bull* 23(3):291-297, 2000.
18 Schmidgall J, Schnetz E, Hensel A: *Planta Med* 66(1):48-53, 2000.
19 Durig J et al: *Thromb Res* 85(6):479-491, 1997.
20 Beress A et al: *J Nat Prod* 56(4):478-485, 1993.
21 Bjorvell H, Rossner S: *Int J Obes* 11(1):67-71, 1987.
22 Monego ET et al: *Arq Bras Cardiol* 66(6):343-347, 1996.
23 Curro F, Amadeo A: *Arch Med Interna* 28:1343-1349, 1976.

BLUE COHOSH

Botanical Name: *Caulophyllum thalictroides*
Family: Berberidaceae
Plant Part Used: Root

PRESCRIBING INFORMATION

Actions

Spasmolytic, uterine and ovarian tonic, emmenagogue, oxytocic

Potential Indications

Based on appropriate evaluation of the patient, practitioners should consider prescribing blue cohosh in formulations in the context of:
- Disorders of the female reproductive tract including amenorrhea, dysmenorrhea, menorrhagia, ovarian or uterine pain or inflammation, uterine prolapse or atony (5)
- Spasmodic conditions of smooth muscle, including abdominal cramping (5)
- Rheumatic conditions, muscular weakness, nervous debility (5)

Contraindications

Because of possible teratogenic effects, blue cohosh is contraindicated in early pregnancy and lactation. Traditional texts such as the *British Herbal Pharmacopoeia* 1983 support this contraindication by recommending that only small doses are advisable during the first trimester of pregnancy. Use in late pregnancy has been linked to adverse events and should be undertaken only by clinicians experienced with blue cohosh for this application.

Warnings and Precautions

None required.

Interactions

None known.

Use in Pregnancy and Lactation

Contraindicated in pregnancy and lactation.

Side Effects

High levels of the isolated alkaloid anagyrine in goat's milk have been associated with teratogenic effects in animals and in one human.[1] The relevance of this finding to use of blue cohosh is unclear.

Several adverse events have been associated with maternal ingestion of blue cohosh. A midwife attempted the induction of labor using a combination of blue cohosh and black cohosh given orally (dose undefined) at around 42 weeks of gestation.[2] After normal labor, the female baby was unable to breathe spontaneously and sustained central nervous system hypoxic-ischemic damage.[3] Profound neonatal congestive heart failure was linked to maternal consumption of blue cohosh tablets about 1 month before delivery. The dosage and content of the tablets was undefined. The woman had been advised to take 1 tablet per day, but she took three times that dose (3 tablets/day) for 3 weeks before delivery.[4] The infant exhibited signs of severe cardiac injury and was hospitalized. Follow-up at 2 years of age indicated that cardiomegaly and mildly reduced left ventricular function were evident.

Blue Cohosh *continued on page 107*

The U.S. Food and Drug Administration's (FDA) Special Nutritionals Adverse Event Monitoring System database (which lists adverse events but is not subject to preconditions, analysis, or peer review) also contains two cases possibly associated with blue cohosh, including stroke in an infant.

Toxic effects have occurred from overdose of blue cohosh tincture (cited as 10 to 20 doses/day in relation to attempted abortion). Symptoms included hyperthermia, hypertension, tachycardia, hyperventilation, diaphoresis, and weakness.[5]

The presence of oxytocic quinolizidine alkaloids such as sparteine or N-methylcytisine in blue cohosh might explain both its oxytocic activity and its occasional toxicity. Adverse effects may be the result of an inability by some people to metabolize sparteine and alkaloids of related structure. About 5% of male and female subjects studied in a trial were unable to metabolize sparteine by N-oxidation,[6] and this defect appears to have a genetic basis.[7]

Dosage

Dose per day*	Dose per week*
1.5-3.0 ml of 1:2 liquid extract	10-20 ml of 1:2 liquid extract

SUPPORTING INFORMATION

Traditional Prescribing

Traditional Western herbal medicine uses include:
- Uterine pain, amenorrhea, dysmenorrhea, irregular menstruation; threatened miscarriage, false labor pains, as a partus preparator; uterine atony[8,9]
- Rheumatic pain, muscular weakness, debility of the nervous system, epilepsy[9]
- Abdominal cramping, indigestion; dull frontal headache[9]

Blue cohosh was used by Native Americans to expedite parturition and menstruation, for lingering parturition, and for suppressing profuse menstruation, genitourinary complaints in both sexes, colic, sore throat, rheumatism, and dropsy. However, the modern understanding argues against using blue cohosh to facilitate labor except perhaps in practitioners already experienced with its use in this context. Blue cohosh was considered an effective fever remedy. Blue cohosh was official in the USP from 1882 to 1905 and the NF from 1916 to 1950 and was used for antispasmodic, emmenagogue, and diuretic purposes.[10]

Pharmacologic Research

Blue cohosh root contains quinolizidine alkaloids, including sparteine, methylcytisine, and anagyrine.[11] Blue cohosh also contains saponins such as caulosaponin.[12]

Blue Cohosh *continued on page 108*

*This dose range is extrapolated from the *British Herbal Pharmacopoeia* 1983 and the author's education and experience.

- Uterine stimulant effects were observed for the liquid extract, hot water extract and saponin fraction, and isolated caulosaponin *in vitro*.[12-14]
- Methylcytisine has demonstrated hypertensive activity when administered by injection. Caulosaponin demonstrated vasoconstrictive activity on isolated arteries and a cardiotoxic effect on cardiac muscle.[12]
- Nicotinic activity was observed after oral ingestion of methylcytisine by a human subject.[5]

Clinical Studies

- A survey published in 2000 reported that herbal therapy was recommended by 73.2% of 82 North Carolina–certified midwives for pregnant and postpartum patients. Blue cohosh was among the herbs commonly prescribed for women past their due dates.[15] Similar findings were obtained in a survey conducted a year earlier in which 64% of 90 midwives reported using blue cohosh. This survey recorded the following dosages: 5 drops of tincture every 4 hours for induction of labor or 10 drops of tincture every 2 hours in hot water.[16]

REFERENCES

1 Ortega JA, Lazerson J: *J Pediatr* 111(1):87-89, 1987.
2 Gunn TR, Wright IM: *N Z Med J* 109(1032):410-411, 1996.
3 Wright IMR: *J Pediatr* 134(3):384-385, 1999.
4 Jones TK, Lawson BM: *J Pediatr* 132:550-552, 1998.
5 Rao RB et al: *J Toxicol Clin Toxicol* 36(5):455, 1998.
6 Eichelbaum M et al: *Eur J Clin Pharmacol* 16:183-187, 1979.
7 Vinks A et al: *Clin Pharmacol Ther* 31(1):23-29, 1982.
8 British Herbal Medicine Association's Scientific Committee: *British herbal pharmacopoeia,* Bournemouth, 1983, BHMA.
9 Felter HW, Lloyd JU: *King's American dispensatory,* ed 18, rev 3, Portland, 1905, reprinted 1983, Eclectic Medical Publications.
10 Vogel VJ: *American Indian medicine,* Norman, Okla, 1970, University of Oklahoma Press.
11 Kennelly EJ et al: *J Nat Prod* 62(10):1385-1389, 1999.
12 Chandler F, editor: *Herbs: everyday reference for health professionals,* Ottawa, 2000, Canadian Pharmacists Association.
13 Pilcher JD, Delzell WR, Burman GE: *JAMA* 67:490-492, 1916.
14 Ferguson HC, Edwards LD: *J Am Pharm Assoc* 43(1):16-21, 1954.
15 Allaire AD, Moos MK, Wells SR: *Obstet Gynecol* 95(1):19-23, 2000.
16 McFarlin BL et al: *J Nurse Midwifery* 44(3):205-216, 1999.

BLUE FLAG

Botanical Names: *Iris versicolor, Iris caroliniana*[+]
Family: Iridaceae
Plant Part Used: Rhizome

PRESCRIBING INFORMATION

Actions	Depurative, laxative, cholagogue, lymphatic, diuretic
Potential Indications	Based on appropriate evaluation of the patient, practitioners should consider prescribing blue flag in formulations in the context of:

- Skin, liver, and gallbladder disorders, particularly when chronic in nature *(5)*
- Constipation, headache, or digestive problems related to poor liver function *(5)*
- Enlarged lymph nodes, enlarged thyroid, enlarged spleen, enlarged ovaries *(5)*
- Obesity *(7)*

Contraindications	None known.
Warnings and Precautions	None required.
Interactions	None known.
Use in Pregnancy and Lactation	No adverse effects expected.
Side Effects	None expected if taken within the recommended dose range.

Dosage

Dose per day*	Dose per week*
3-6 ml of 1:2 liquid extract	20-40 ml of 1:2 liquid extract

SUPPORTING INFORMATION

Traditional Prescribing

Traditional Western herbal medicine uses include:

- Skin diseases[1,2]
- Biliousness with constipation and liver dysfunction,[1] jaundice, poor gallbladder function, chronic liver disorders, including hepatitis; constipation; nausea, vomiting, headache, or digestive problems related to poor liver function[2]
- Reflex muscular pains resulting from gastric irritation[2]
- Enlarged lymph nodes, enlarged thyroid, enlarged spleen; chronic pancreatic, splenic, or renal disorders[2]
- Syphilis, scrofula (tuberculous infection of the cervical lymph nodes)[2]

Blue Flag *continued on page 110*

[+]Medicinally interchangeable species.
*This dose range is extrapolated from the British Herbal Pharmacopoeia 1983, the British Herbal Compendium 1992, and the author's education and experience.

- Enlarged uterus or ovary; leukorrhea, dysmenorrhea; prostatic discharges, nocturnal emissions[2]
- Vomiting with pregnancy; regarded as an emetic, but with antiemetic activity in small doses[3]

Blue flag was held in high regard by Native Americans and was one of the most widely used native medicines. Blue flag was used as a powerful cathartic and employed internally to treat the common cold and lung problems. Externally, blue flag was used as a poultice and wash for sores, bruises, and burns. The steamed root was taken internally to keep disease away because of its importance as a physic and panacea. The steeped root was a specific for cholera. Blue flag was official in the USP from 1820 to 1895 and in the NF from 1916 to 1942, with uses listed as cathartic, emetic, and diuretic.[4]

Pharmacologic Research

Blue flag root significantly increased plasma levels of free fatty acids and glycerol after oral administration (20 mg/kg) in an experimental model, demonstrating mobilization of fat tissue.[5]

Clinical Studies

No clinical studies using blue flag have been found.

REFERENCES

1 British Herbal Medicine Association's Scientific Committee: *British herbal pharmacopoeia*, Bournemouth, 1983, BHMA.

2 Felter HW, Lloyd JU: *King's American dispensatory*, ed 18, rev 3, Portland, 1905, reprinted 1983, Eclectic Medical Publications.

3 British Herbal Medicine Association: *British herbal compendium*, Bournemouth, 1992, BHMA.

4 Vogel VJ: *American Indian medicine*, Norman, Okla, 1970, University of Oklahoma Press.

5 Bambhole VD: *Ancient Sci Life* 8:117, 1988.

BUCHU

Botanical Names: *Agathosma betulina, Barosma betulina[#]*
Family: Rutaceae
Plant Part Used: Leaf

PRESCRIBING INFORMATION

Actions	Urinary antiseptic, mild diuretic
Potential Indications	Based on appropriate evaluation of the patient, practitioners should consider prescribing buchu in formulations in the context of urinary tract infection, dysuria, cystitis, urethritis, and prostatitis. *(5)*
Contraindications	None known.
Warnings and Precautions	None required.
Interactions	None known.
Use in Pregnancy and Lactation	Some writers suggest that buchu is contraindicated in pregnancy. However, this precaution would only be the case for buchu substitutions (e.g., *Agathosma crenulata*), which contain much higher levels of pulegone in their essential oil.
Side Effects	Occasional gastrointestinal irritation may occur if taken on an empty stomach.

Dosage

Dose per day[*]	*Dose per week*[*]
2.0-4.5 ml of 1:2 liquid extract	15-30 ml of 1:2 liquid extract

SUPPORTING INFORMATION

Traditional Prescribing

Traditional Western herbal medicine uses include:
- Diseases of the genitourinary tract, especially inflammation of the mucous membranes of the lower urinary system and prostate (e.g., cystitis, urethritis, prostatitis); urinary discharges, urinary gravel[1,2]
- Incontinence associated with a diseased prostate, desire to urinate with little relief from micturition[2]
- Improving appetite, relieving nausea and flatulence[2]

Traditional South African medicinal uses include stomach complaints, kidney and urinary tract diseases, and rheumatism.[3]

Buchu *continued on page 112*

[#]Alternative name.
[*]This dose is extrapolated from the British Herbal Pharmacopoeia 1983, the British Herbal Compendium 1992, and the author's education and experience.

Pharmacologic Research

An alcoholic extract of buchu demonstrated activity against microflora typical of urinary tract infections *in vitro*. Only the essential oil showed considerable activity against all the test organisms.

Clinical Studies

No clinical studies using buchu have been found.

REFERENCES

The following book was referred to in the compilation of the pharmacologic and clinical information that has not been referenced here: Mills S, Bone K: *Principles and Practice of Phytotherapy: Modern Herbal Medicine,* Edinburgh, 2000, Churchill Livingstone.

1 British Herbal Medicine Association's Scientific Committee: *British herbal pharmacopoeia,* Bournemouth, 1983, BHMA.
2 Felter HW, Lloyd JU: *King's American dispensatory,* ed 18, rev 3, Portland, 1905, reprinted 1983, Eclectic Medical Publications.
3 van Wyk B-E, van Oudtshoorn B, Gericke N: *Medicinal plants of South Africa,* Arcadia, South Africa, 1997, Briza Publications.

BUGLEWEED

Botanical Names: *Lycopus virginicus, Lycopus europaeus*[+]
Family: Labiatae
Plant Part Used: Aerial parts

PRESCRIBING INFORMATION

Actions
Thyroid-stimulating hormone (TSH) antagonist, antithyroid, reduces heart rate, mild sedative

Potential Indications
Based on appropriate evaluation of the patient, practitioners should consider prescribing bugleweed in formulations in the context of hyperthyroidism, especially Graves' disease and associated symptoms, such as tachycardia, rapid pulse, and exophthalmia. *(4,5)*

Contraindications
Thyroid hypofunction, enlargement of the thyroid without functional disorder;[1] pregnancy and lactation.[2]

Warnings and Precautions
None required.

Interactions
Bugleweed should not be administered concurrently with preparations containing thyroid hormone and may interfere with administration of thyroid diagnostic procedures that use radioactive isotopes.[1]

Use in Pregnancy and Lactation
Contraindicated in pregnancy and lactation because of potential antigonadotropic activity.

Side Effects
In rare cases, extended therapy and high (undefined) doses of bugleweed preparations have resulted in an enlargement of the thyroid. Sudden discontinuation of bugleweed preparations can cause increased symptoms of the disease.[1] The following side effects have been reported in the literature from clinical use of bugleweed preparations published between 1941 to 1968: headache, increase in size of thyroid, and occasionally an increase in hyperthyroid symptoms, including nervousness, tachycardia, and loss of weight. The increase in thyroid size was observed in patients with goiter not linked to thyroid malfunction.[2]

Dosage

Dose per day*	Dose per week*
2-6 ml of 1:2 liquid extract	15-40 ml of 1:2 liquid extract

SUPPORTING INFORMATION

Traditional Prescribing
Traditional Western herbal medicine uses include:
- Nervous tachycardia, Graves' disease with cardiac involvement; thyrotoxicosis with difficult breathing, tachycardia, and tremor;[3] exophthalmic goiter[4]

Bugleweed *continued on page 114*

[+]Medicinally interchangeable species.
*This dose range is extrapolated from the British Herbal Pharmacopoeia 1983 and the author's education and experience.

- Organic and functional cardiac disease; abnormally active circulation, rapid pulse with high temperature[4]
- Chronic cough, irritating and wet cough, pneumonia, bronchitis[3,4]
- Restlessness, insomnia, anxiety[4]

Bugleweed is considered in European herbal medicine as having antithyroid activity. Being less powerful than orthodox drugs, bugleweed is recommended for mild thyroid hyperfunction and can be used as a long-term treatment.[5]

Pharmacologic Research

- *Lycopus europaeus* aqueous ethanolic extract has demonstrated antithyrotropic and antigonadotropic activity in experimental models *in vivo* (both after injection and oral administration).[6] The following activities have been observed:
  - Decreased triiodothyronine (T_3) levels, possibly resulting from reduced peripheral thyroxin (T_4) deiodination
  - Decreased T_4 and TSH levels
  - Decreased LH levels
- In this series of experiments, testosterone levels were reduced, but prolactin remained unchanged after oral administration of bugleweed extracts.[6] In an earlier study, *L. virginicus* aqueous ethanolic extract strongly lowered prolactin levels after intravenous injection.[7] This activity was demonstrated at a dose much higher than was the dose that produced the previously noted antithyrotropic activity.[8] *L. virginicus* extract reduced the weight of the testes, but LH-dependent testosterone synthesis was not significantly changed (route unknown).[9]
- Injection of bugleweed extract reduced serum TSH and pituitary TSH levels under normal thyroid conditions but caused an increase in pituitary TSH levels under hypothyroid conditions (also with decreased serum TSH).[8]
- An antigonadotropic activity has been demonstrated for *L. virginicus* and *L. europaeus* extracts and for some of their constituents.[7,10] The antithyrotropic activity is probably exerted by the ability of phytochemicals in bugleweed to form adducts with TSH and inhibit its ability to bind to the TSH receptor. This inhibitory interaction has also been demonstrated for the Graves' autoantibody *in vitro*.[10,11] An intracellular mechanism of inhibition may also be present.[12]
- *L. europaeus* extract demonstrated antioxidant activity *in vitro*.[13]

Clinical Studies

- *Lycopus europaeus* inhibited iodine metabolism and thyroid T_4 output in human volunteers.[14]
- *Lycopus europaeus* extract has been beneficial for treating hyperthyroidism in uncontrolled trials conducted in the 1940s and 1950s.[15–18]
- In Germany, the Commission E supports using bugleweed to treat mild thyroid hyperfunction with disturbances of the autonomic nervous system and mastodynia (breast pain or tenderness).[1]

Bugleweed *continued on page 115*

REFERENCES

1 Blumenthal M et al, editors: *The complete German Commission E monographs: therapeutic guide to herbal medicines,* Austin, 1998, American Botanical Council.

2 de Smet PAGM et al, editors: *Adverse effects of herbal drugs,* Berlin, 1993, Springer-Verlag.

3 British Herbal Medicine Association's Scientific Committee: *British herbal pharmacopoeia,* Bournemouth, 1983, BHMA.

4 Felter HW, Lloyd JU: *King's American dispensatory,* ed 18, rev 3, Portland, 1905, reprinted 1983, Eclectic Medical Publications.

5 Weiss RF: *Herbal medicine,* translated by Meuss AR: *Lehrbuch der phytotherapie,* ed 6, Beaconsfield, U.K., 1988, Beaconsfield Publishers.

6 Winterhoff H et al: *Arzneim Forsch* 44(1):41-45, 1994.

7 Sourgens H et al: *Int J Crude Drug Res* 24(2):53-63, 1986.

8 Sourgens H et al: *Planta Med* 45:78-86, 1982.

9 Sourgens H et al: *Acta Endocrinol Suppl* 234:49, 1980.

10 Auf'mkolk M et al: *Endocrinology* 116(5):1687-1693, 1985.

11 Auf'mkolk M et al: *Endocrinology* 115(2):527-534, 1984.

12 Kleeman S, Winterhoff H: *Planta Med* 56:683P, 1990.

13 Lamaison JL, Petitjean-Freytet C, Carnat A: *Pharm Acta Helv* 66(7):185-188, 1991.

14 Hiller E, Deglmann H: *Arzneim Forsch* 5:465-470, 1955.

15 Mattausch F: *Hippokrates* 14:168-171, 1943.

16 Leppert H: *Therapiewoche* 952; 2:571-572, 1951.

17 Frank J: *Munch Med Wschr* 101:203-204, 1959.

18 Fiegel G: *Med Klin* 49:1221, 1954.

BUPLEURUM

Botanical Names: *Bupleurum falcatum, Bupleurum scorzonerifolium*[+]
Family: Umbelliferae
Plant Part Used: Root

Actions

Antiinflammatory, hepatoprotective, diaphoretic, antitussive

Potential Indications

Based on appropriate evaluation of the patient, practitioners should consider prescribing Bupleurum in formulations in the context of:
- Chronic inflammatory disorders (7)
- Poor liver function (5)
- Feverish conditions, influenza, the common cold (4,5)
- Prolapse of uterus and rectum, irregular menstruation (5)

Contraindications

According to TCM, Bupleurum is contraindicated in *deficient yin* cough (cough with debility) or *liver fire* ascending to the head, such as some cases of headache and hypertension. Bupleurum can occasionally cause nausea or vomiting, in which case the smallest dose possible is used.

Warnings and Precautions

Bupleurum has a sedative effect in some patients.

Interactions

None known.

Use in Pregnancy and Lactation

No adverse effects expected.

Side Effects

Large doses may cause a sedative effect in some patients, increase bowel movements, and flatulence. Bupleurum can occasionally cause nausea and reflux in sensitive patients, a property common to most saponin-rich herbs.

A traditional Chinese herbal formula, which included Bupleurum, has induced pneumonitis in some patients and liver damage in rare cases. Whether this condition was a result of Bupleurum or one of the other herbs present is unclear.

Dosage

Dose per day*	Dose per week*
3.5-8.5 ml of 1:2 liquid extract	25-60 ml of 1:2 liquid extract

Traditional Prescribing

Uses and properties from TCM include:
- Bitter and *cold*, acting as a diaphoretic (in fever management), to regulate and restore gastrointestinal and liver function[2]

Bupleurum *continued on page 117*

[+]Medicinally interchangeable species.
*This dose range is adapted from dried plant doses administered by decoction in TCM.[1] The author's experience and the fact that ethanol-water is a more effective solvent than water for many phytochemicals are taken into account.

• Alternating chills and fever (e.g., malaria), liver enlargement, prolapse of the uterus and rectum, menstrual problems, epigastric pain, nausea, indigestion[1-3]

Pharmacologic Research

Bupleurum root contains triterpenoid saponins, including the saikosaponins.

• The antiinflammatory activity of the saikosaponins appears to be related, at least partially, to their ability to both induce secretion of endogenous corticosterone and potentiate its antiinflammatory activity. Orally, saikosaponins may be used to reduce the dose of glucocorticoid drugs and to prevent glucocorticoid-induced adrenal suppression.

• The ability of saikosaponins to raise blood glucose levels was demonstrated in several pharmacologic studies following both oral and injected doses. This result may be a direct consequence of the ability of saikosaponins to increase the levels of endogenous glucocorticoids. Because saikosaponins also increase liver glycogen stores, Bupleurum may prove to be useful in treating reactive hypoglycemia.

• In experimental models, injection of saikosaponins stimulated immune function.

• Saikosaponins have increased hepatic protein synthesis *in vitro* and *in vivo*.

• Saikosaponins (by injection) have demonstrated nephroprotective activity. This activity was partly the result of antiplatelet and corticosterone-releasing activities, as well as an inhibition of the decrease in free-radical scavengers such as glutathione peroxidase.

• Saikosaponins have reduced gastric ulcer development, lowered cholesterol, and exerted antipyretic activity.

• Injection of saikosaponins demonstrated a potent antitussive effect in an experimental model.

Clinical Studies

• In an uncontrolled clinical study of 143 patients treated with Bupleurum, fever subsided within 24 hours in 98% of influenza cases and in 88% of patients with the common cold.

• In another study involving 40 patients with pathological fever, Bupleurum produced an antipyretic effect in 97.5% of patients and achieved a reduction of 1° to 2°C (1.8° to 3.6°F) in body temperature in 77.5% of all patients.

• Intravenous injection of Bupleurum gave positive results in treating infectious hepatitis.

REFERENCES

The following book was referred to in the compilation of the pharmacologic and clinical information that has not been referenced here: Mills S, Bone K: *Principles and Practice of Phytotherapy: Modern Herbal Medicine,* Edinburgh, 2000, Churchill Livingstone.

1 Pharmacopoeia Commission of the People's Republic of China: *Pharmacopoeia of the People's Republic of China* (English ed), Beijing, 1997, Chemical Industry Press.

2 Chang HM, But PP: *Pharmacology and applications of Chinese materia medica,* Singapore, 1987, World Scientific.

3 Bensky D, Gambel A: *Chinese herbal medicine materia medica,* Seattle, 1986, Eastland Press.

BURDOCK

Botanical Name: *Arctium lappa*
Family: Compositae
Plant Part Used: Root

Actions

Depurative, mild diuretic, mild laxative

Potential Indications

Based on appropriate evaluation of the patient, practitioners should consider prescribing burdock in formulations in the context of:
- Skin disorders, particularly eczema, psoriasis and other chronic skin disorders; boils *(5)*
- Disorders requiring increased elimination from the body, such as gout and rheumatism *(5)*

Contraindications

None known.

Warnings and Precautions

None required.

Interactions

None known.

Use in Pregnancy and Lactation

No adverse effects expected.

Side Effects

None expected when taken within the recommended dose range.

Dosage

*Dose per day**	*Dose per week**
1.5-3.5 ml of 1:2 liquid extract	10-25 ml of 1:2 liquid extract

SUPPORTING INFORMATION

Traditional Prescribing

Traditional Western herbal medicine uses include:
- Skin eruptions, particularly when weak circulation and impaired nutrition exist; eczema, venereal, and leprous disorders, long term use for psoriasis; boils, styes[1,2]
- Rheumatism, cystitis, gout[1,2]
- Anorexia nervosa, dyspepsia[1,2]
- Considered one of the best depuratives[3]

Native Americans used burdock for a wide variety of applications, including as a general tonic and blood purifier and as an ingredient in treatments for stomach pain and during labor. Burdock was official in the USP from 1831 to 1842 and 1851 to 1916 and in the NF from 1916 to 1947 and was listed as a diuretic and diaphoretic.[4]

Burdock *continued on page 119*

*This dose range is extrapolated from British Herbal Pharmacopoeia 1983, the British Herbal Compendium 1992, and the author's education and experience.

Pharmacologic Research

- Burdock extract antagonized platelet-activating factor *in vitro*.[5]
- Burdock extract has demonstrated free-radical scavenging activity *in vitro* and inhibited carrageenan-induced edema and carbon tetrachloride–induced hepatotoxicity *in vivo* after injection.[6] Isolated caffeoylquinic acid derivatives from burdock have been verified as antioxidants.[7]
- Methanol extract of burdock administered by injection demonstrated antitumor activity.[8]

Clinical Studies

No clinical studies using burdock have been found.

REFERENCES

1 British Herbal Medicine Association's Scientific Committee: *British herbal pharmacopoeia,* Bournemouth, 1983, BHMA.

2 Felter HW, Lloyd JU: *King's American dispensatory,* ed 18, rev 3, Portland, 1905, reprinted 1983, Eclectic Medical Publications.

3 Grieve M: *A modern herbal,* New York, 1971, Dover Publications.

4 Vogel VJ: *American Indian medicine,* Norman, Okla, 1970, University of Oklahoma Press.

5 Iwakami S et al: *Chem Pharm Bull* 40(5):1196-1198, 1992.

6 Lin CC et al: *Am J Chin Med* 24(2):127-137, 1996.

7 Maruta Y, Kawabata J, Niki R: *J Agric Food Chem* 43:2592-2595, 1995.

8 Dombradi CA, Foldeak S: *Tumori* 52(3):173-175, 1966.

CALENDULA

Other Common Name: Marigold
Botanical Name: *Calendula officinalis*
Family: Compositae
Plant Part Used: Flower

PRESCRIBING INFORMATION

Actions	Vulnerary, antiinflammatory, lymphatic, styptic (hemostatic), antimicrobial, antiviral (topically), antifungal (topically)
Potential Indications	Based on appropriate evaluation of the patient, practitioners should consider prescribing Calendula in formulations in the context of: • Internal and topical treatment for inflammation of the oral and pharyngeal mucosa *(4)* • Internal treatment for gastric and duodenal ulcers; enlarged or inflamed lymph nodes, acne, sebaceous cysts *(5)* • Internal treatment for spasmodic conditions, including dysmenorrhea *(5)* • Topical treatment for burns *(2)* • Topical treatment for inflammation of the skin and mucosa, wounds, especially poorly healing wounds *(4,5)* • Topical treatment for leg ulcers, venous circulatory problems, scalds; to help control bleeding *(4)* • Topical treatment for eczema, varicose veins, hemorrhoids, acne, vaginal discharges *(5)*
Contraindications	Known allergy.[1]
Warnings and Precautions	The likelihood of Calendula preparations causing a contact allergy is low. However, people with known sensitivity to other members of the Compositae family (e.g., ragweed, daisies, chrysanthemums) should avoid topical application of Calendula or Calendula products.[1] Sensitization to Calendula and allergic contact reactions have been reported.[2,3] Anaphylactic shock after gargling with an infusion of Calendula has also been reported.[4]
Interactions	None known.
Use in Pregnancy and Lactation	No adverse effects expected.
Side Effects	Allergic reaction occurs rarely following topical application.[1]

Dosage	Dose per day*	Dose per week*
	1.5-4.5 ml of 1:2 liquid extract	10-30 ml of 1:2 liquid extract

Calendula *continued on page 121*

*This dose range is extrapolated from the British Pharmaceutical Codex 1934, the British Herbal Pharmacopoeia 1983, and the author's education and experience.

SUPPORTING INFORMATION

Traditional Prescribing

Traditional Western herbal medicine uses include:

- Enlarged or inflamed lymph nodes, sebaceous cysts, gastric or duodenal ulcer, acute or chronic inflammatory skin lesions[5]
- Amenorrhea, dysmenorrhea; nosebleed[5]
- Spasmodic conditions, fever, chronic suppuration, capillary enlargement, varicose veins, chronic ulcers, stubborn acne, splenic and hepatic enlargement[6]
- Topically for wounds, acne, chaffed skin in infants, cracked nipples, eczema, leg ulcers, varicose veins, hemorrhoids, anal eczema and inflammation, vaginal discharges, lymphadenoma, inflamed skin lesions, conjunctivitis[5,6]

Pharmacologic Research

- Various Calendula extracts and Calendula essential oil have demonstrated antibacterial, antifungal, and trichomonacidal activity *in vitro*.[7]
- Calendula extract enhanced the proliferation of lymphocytes *in vitro*.[8] Polysaccharides from Calendula stimulated phagocytosis of human granulocytes *in vitro*.[9] This finding may be relevant to topical application.
- Calendula flavonoids inhibited the activity of lipoxygenase *in vitro*.[10] Calendula extract suppressed the inflammatory process and leukocyte infiltration caused by carrageenan and prostaglandin E_1 (route unknown).[11] Oral dose of aqueous ethanolic extract of Calendula produced antiinflammatory activity in carrageenan-induced rat paw edema. The activity was much milder than that with indomethacin.[12]
- Using the croton oil dermatitis mouse ear model, both the total extract of Calendula and the extract obtained after supercritical carbon dioxide extraction (which contains the lipophilic phytochemicals) demonstrated antiinflammatory activity after topical application. Fractionation and testing revealed that the triterpene alcohols caused the antiinflammatory activity, with the carotenoids and sterols almost inactive.[13] The most active topical antiinflammatory constituent is the triterpenoid compound faradiol monoester.[14]
- Calendula extract has demonstrated angiogenic activity (formation of new blood vessels, such as within a wound) in an *in vitro* assay. Calendula-treated tissue was positive for hyaluronan, a tissue glycan associated with neovascularization, unlike the control tissue, which lacked the presence of hyaluronan.[15] This finding is possibly relevant to topical use of Calendula.
- Topical application of an ointment containing Calendula fractions and allantoin stimulated physiological regeneration and epithelialization in experimentally induced wounds.[16] A Calendula ointment improved wound healing in experimentally induced wounds.[17] Calendula facilitated the collagen maturation phase of wound healing and influenced epithelial cell proliferation and migration.[18] Topical application of a Calendula glycetract had a vasoprotective activity on normal animal skin by decreasing capillary activity.[19]

Calendula *continued on page 122*

- Antiulcer activity was demonstrated in three experimental models after administrating an isolated saponin from Calendula. Antiinflammatory and sedative activities were also observed.[20,21] Fractions isolated from Calendula also showed activity (route unknown).[22]
- Calendula demonstrated antipyretic and analgesic activities in experimental models (route unknown).[23]
- The saponin fraction of Calendula normalized experimentally induced hyperlipidemia after oral administration over a 12-week period[7] but was without effect in normolipemia.[24]
- Oral administration of Calendula extract exhibited antitumor activity in experimentally induced carcinoma.[25]

Clinical Studies

- An herbal preparation containing Calendula, dandelion, St. John's wort, lemon balm, and fennel reduced intestinal pain in an uncontrolled trial in patients with chronic colitis. Defecation was normalized in these patients with diarrhea syndrome.[26]
- Calendula extract accelerated the healing time of an artificially induced skin abrasion in volunteers (most likely by topical application).[27] An evaluation of aerosol formulations designed to provide a protective film over wounds in human volunteers found that addition of Calendula tincture was satisfactory at controlling bleeding.[28]
- In a small, uncontrolled trial, Calendula was successful in treating periodontal inflammation.[29]
- Calendula ointment has been positively used in uncontrolled trials for treating bedsores, venous circulatory problems, and skin conditions such as leg ulcers and thrombophlebitis.[7] Calendula demonstrated benefit as an adjuvant therapy for rendering scar tissue more supple in patients with cleft lip and palate who were undergoing dermatography.[30]
- Calendula gel applied for 13 to 14 days provided good results for the healing of burns and scalds in 30 patients.[31] The effects of three ointments on managing burns were investigated in a randomized, controlled, multicenter clinical study involving 156 patients. Calendula and the proteolytic ointment showed similar efficacy, both superior to Vaseline. However, the Calendula ointment was better tolerated than the proteolytic ointment.[32]
- Improved outcomes and faster healing of ulceration were obtained when acyclovir treatment was combined with an herbal formula containing Calendula, burdock, and *Geranium robertianum* in patients with herpetic keratitis (most likely by topical application).[33]
- In Germany, the Commission E supports using Calendula to treat inflammation of the oral and pharyngeal mucosa internally and topically. Externally, Calendula is recommended for poorly healing wounds and leg ulcers.[34]
- ESCOP recommends Calendula for treating inflammations of the skin and mucosa and as an aid to wound healing.[1]

Calendula *continued on page 123*

REFERENCES

1 Scientific Committee of the European Scientific Cooperative on Phytotherapy (ESCOP): *ESCOP monographs: Calendulae flos,* European Scientific Cooperative on Phytotherapy, ESCOP Secretariat, Argyle House, Gandy Street, Exeter, Devon, EX4 3LS, United Kingdom, March 1996.

2 Wrangsjo K, Ros AM, Wahlberg JE: *Contact Dermatitis* 22(3):148-154, 1990.

3 Hausen BM, Oestmann G: *Derm Beruf Umwelt* 36(4):117-124, 1988.

4 Goldman II: *Klin Med* 52(4):142-143, 1974.

5 British Herbal Medicine Association's Scientific Committee: *British herbal pharmacopoeia,* Bournemouth, 1983, BHMA.

6 Felter HW, Lloyd JU: *King's American dispensatory,* ed 18, rev 3, Portland, 1905, reprinted 1983, Eclectic Medical Publications.

7 Isaac I: *Die Ringelblume: Botanik, Chemie, Pharmakologie, Toxikologie, Pharmazie und therapeutische Verwendung; Handbuch für Ärzte, Apotheker und andere Naturwissenschaftler,* Stuttgart, 1992, Wissenschaftliche Verlagsgesellschaft.

8 Amirghofran Z, Azadbakht M, Karimi MH: *J Ethnopharmacol* 72(1-2):167-172, 2000.

9 Varljen J, Liptak A, Wagner H: *Phytochem* 28(9):2379-2383, 1989.

10 Bezakova L et al: *Pharmazie* 51:126-127, 1996.

11 Shipochliev T, Dimitrov A, Aleksandrova E: *Vet Med Nauki* 18(6):87-94, 1981.

12 Mascolo N et al: *Phytother Res* 1:28-31, 1987.

13 Della Loggia R: *Z Phytother* 21:149-150, 2000.

14 Della Loggia R et al: *Planta Med* 60(6):516-520, 1994.

15 Patrick KFM et al: *Phytomed* 3(1):11-18, 1996.

16 Klouchek-Popova E et al: *Acta Physiol Pharmacol Bulg* 8(4):63-67, 1982.

17 Ansari MA et al: *Indian Vet J* 74(7):594-597, 1997.

18 Rao SG et al: *Fitoterapia* 62(6):508-510, 1991.

19 Russo M: *Riv Ital EPPOS* 54:730, 1972.

20 Yatsuno AI, Belova LF, Lipkina GS: *Pharmacol Toxicol SSSR* 41:193-198, 1978.

21 Iatsyno AI et al: *Farmakol Toksikol* 41(5):556-560, 1978.

22 Manolov P et al: *Probl Vatr Med* 11:70-74, 1983.

23 Ahmad S et al: *Pak J Sci Ind Res* 43(1):50-54, 2000.

24 Wojcicki J, Samochowiec L: *Herba Pol* 26:233-237, 1980.

25 Boucaud-Maitre Y, Algernon O, Raynaud J: *Pharmazie* 43:220-221, 1988.

26 Chakurski I et al: *Vutr Boles* 20(6):51-54, 1981.

27 Fleischner AM: *Cosmet Toiletries* 100:54-55, 1985.

28 Garg S, Sharma SN: *Pharmazie* 47(12):924-926, 1992.

29 Gasiorowska I et al: *Czas Stomatol* 36(4):307-311, 1983.

30 van der Velden EM, van der Dussen MFN: *J Oral Maxillofac Surg* 53(1):9-12, 1995.

31 Baranov AP: *Dtsch Apoth Ztg* 139:61-66, 1999.

32 Lievre M et al: *Clin Trials Meta-Analys* 28:9-12, 1992.

33 Corina P et al: *Oftalmologia* 46(1):55-57, 1999.

34 Blumenthal M et al, editors: *The complete German Commission E monographs: therapeutic guide to herbal medicines,* Austin, 1998, American Botanical Council.

CALIFORNIA POPPY

Other Common Name: Californian poppy
Botanical Names: *Eschscholzia californica, Eschscholtzia californica*[#]
Family: Papaveraceae
Plant Part Used: Aerial parts

PRESCRIBING INFORMATION

Actions	Anxiolytic, mild sedative, analgesic, hypnotic
Potential Indications	Based on appropriate evaluation of the patient, practitioners should consider prescribing California poppy in formulations in the context of: • Painful conditions involving the irritation or stimulation of pain fibers (similar to when morphine or codeine might be used) *(5)* • Disturbed sleep, in combination with *Corydalis cava (3)* • Disturbed sleep *(5)* • Anxiety and conditions in which anxiety plays a major role *(6,7)*
Contraindications	None known.
Warnings and Precautions	None required.
Interactions	None known.
Use in Pregnancy and Lactation	No adverse effects expected.
Side Effects	None expected if taken within the recommended dose range. Whether California poppy will interfere with standard drug tests for opiate alkaloids is unclear. However, this interference is unlikely.

Dosage	*Dose per day**	*Dose per week**
	3-6 ml of 1:2 liquid extract	20-40 ml of 1:2 liquid extract

SUPPORTING INFORMATION

Traditional Prescribing	Traditional Western herbal medicine uses include: • Reducing pain and producing calm sleep without the dangers of opiates[2] • Enhancing sleep, particularly for children with whooping cough[3] • Relieving pain of colic in children[4] • Migraine, nervous bowel, neuralgia, anxiety, depression, stress[1] • Topically for treating sores and ulcers[4] Native Americans and native Hispanics used the aerial parts, leaves, or flowers of California poppy for sedative and analgesic activity, to promote sleep, and for relief of toothache, particularly in children.[4]

California Poppy *continued on page 125*

[#]Alternative name.
*This dose range is extrapolated from traditional Western herbal medicine and the author's education and experience.[1]

California poppy was of interest to medical practitioners of the United States in the late nineteenth century, with the liquid extract entered into the Park-Davis catalog in 1890. California poppy was referred to in 1892 as an "excellent soporific (sleep inducing) and analgesic, above all harmless" and in 1893, reporting that, "...the effect produced by *Eschscholtzia californica* upon patients is the same as that of morphine, without the inconveniences of the latter drug."[5]

Pharmacologic Research

The aerial parts of California poppy contain isoquinoline alkaloids (mainly eschscholtzine and californidine, with smaller amounts of sanguinarine and chelerythrine)[6] and flavonol glycosides.[7]

- California poppy extract inhibits the enzymatic degradation of catecholamines and the synthesis of epinephrine (adrenaline) *in vitro*. Preserving high levels of catecholamines may explain the sedative and antidepressant activity of California poppy.[8] An extract formula containing 80% California poppy and 20% *Corydalis cava* has demonstrated the ability to interact with opiate receptors *in vitro*,[9] which indicates potential analgesic activity.
- Alkaloids from California poppy enhanced gamma-aminobutyric acid (GABA) binding to rat brain synaptic membrane receptors. This finding may indicate a benzodiazepine-like activity.[10] Constituents of California poppy exhibited dose-dependent binding to benzodiazepine receptors and displaced the benzodiazepine flurazepam from the receptor.[11]
- A sedative effect was observed for California poppy extract after injection in experimental models in terms of both behavioral effects and promotion of sleep.[12,13] At lower doses, an anxiolytic effect was observed.[12] Sedative effects have also been observed after treatment with high oral doses.[14] The sedative and anxiolytic effects of California poppy are most likely linked to benzodiazepine-receptor activation because they were antagonized by the benzodiazepine-receptor antagonist flumazenil *in vivo* (by injection).[15]
- Isoquinoline alkaloids are known to possess *in vivo* sedative activity.[9]
- Muscle relaxant and analgesic activities have been reported *in vivo*,[11] although no muscle relaxant activity was observed *in vivo* in a later study. Dose-dependent peripheral analgesic activity was demonstrated for California poppy *in vivo* (by injection), but central analgesic activity was not recorded.[15]
- California poppy tincture inhibited experimentally induced contractions of isolated smooth muscle.[13]
- Two alkaloids isolated from California poppy, chelerythrine and sanguinarine, exhibited affinity for vasopressin receptors and demonstrated competitive inhibition of vasopressin binding *in vitro*.[16] Substances that have this activity have been used pharmacologicly as renal agents, vasoconstricting agents, and hemostatics.

Clinical Studies

- Single administration of a California poppy extract (equivalent to 6.7 g of herb) to volunteers resulted in a quantitative electroencephalographic (EEG) recording that was distinguishable from that obtained

California Poppy *continued on page 126*

from placebo. Results from the self-rating assessment of alertness, however, did not differ from placebo.[17] An acute sedative effect was not demonstrated, but analysis after ongoing administration may demonstrate a sedative effect.

- In two controlled clinical trials, the combination of California poppy and *Corydalis cava* normalized disturbed sleeping behavior without evidence of carry-over effects or addiction. This preparation consisted of alcoholic extracts of California poppy (standardized for protopine) and Corydalis (standardized for bulbocapnine) in the ratio of 4:1. The dosage was not defined.[14]

REFERENCES

1 Bartram T: *Encyclopedia of herbal medicine,* ed 1, Dorset, England, 1995, Grace Publishers.

2 Felter HW, Lloyd JU: *King's American dispensatory,* ed 18, rev 3, Portland, 1905, reprinted 1983, Eclectic Medical Publications.

3 Cheney RH: *Quart J Crude Drugs* 3:413-416, 1963.

4 Brinker FJ: *Eclectic dispensatory of botanical therapeutics,* vol 2, Sandy, Oregon, 1995, Eclectic Medical Publications.

5 Davis GS: *The pharmacology of the newer materia medica,* Detroit, 1892, Davis. Cited in Bender GA: *Pharm Hist* 22(2):49-59, 1980.

6 Tome F, Colombo ML, Caldiroli L: *Phytochem Anal* 10:264-267, 1999.

7 Beck MA, Haberlein H: *Phytochem* 50(2):329-332, 1999.

8 Kleber E et al: *Arzneim Forsch* 45(2):127-131, 1995.

9 Reimeier C et al: *Arzneim Forsch* 45(2):132-136, 1995.

10 Kardos J, Blasko G, Simonyi M: *Arzneim Forsch* 36(6):939-940, 1986.

11 Rolland A: Doctoral thesis, University of Metz, France, 1988. Cited in Schafer HL et al: *Arzneim Forsch* 45(2):124-126, 1995.

12 Rolland A et al: *Planta Med* 57(3):212-216, 1991.

13 Vincieri FF et al: *Pharmacol Res Commun* 20(suppl 5):41-44, 1988.

14 Schafer HL et al: *Arzneim Forsch* 45(2):124-126, 1995.

15 Rolland A et al: *Phytother Res* 15:377-381, 2001.

16 Granger I et al: *Planta Med* 58(1):35-38, 1992.

17 Schulz H, Jobert M, Hubner WD: *Phytomed* 5(6):449-458, 1998.

CASCARA

Other Common Name:	Cascara sagrada
Botanical Names:	*Rhamnus purshiana, Rhamnus purshianus,#* *Frangula purshiana#*
Family:	Rhamnaceae
Plant Part Used:	Bark

PRESCRIBING INFORMATION

Actions	Laxative
Potential Indications	Based on appropriate evaluation of the patient, practitioners should consider prescribing cascara in formulations in the context of:
	• Constipation,* flatulence, abdominal fullness, in combination with boldo *(3)*
	• Dyspepsia,* stimulating gastric secretion, loss of appetite, asthenia, postprandial bloating, coated tongue, itching of skin, in combination with gentian, rhubarb, and boldo *(3)*
	• Headache resulting from constipation or intestinal weakness *(5)*
	• Conditions other than constipation in which easy defecation with a soft stool is desirable, such as with hemorrhoids and anal fissure *(5)*
	• Gastrointestinal conditions with hepatic involvement *(5)*
Contraindications	Intestinal obstruction,[1] intestinal inflammation, such as Crohn's disease, ulcerative colitis, and appendicitis; abdominal pain of unknown origin. Children under 12 years of age should not be prescribed cascara.[2]
Warnings and Precautions	Although short-term use of anthraquinone glycoside–containing laxatives is generally regarded as safe, long-term use is not recommended.[3] Stimulating laxatives should not be used over an extended period (more than 2 weeks) without medical advice. Using stimulating laxatives longer than is recommended can lead to intestinal sluggishness, although concurrent intake of fiber in sufficient quantities of water can counteract this condition. Cascara should be used only if no benefit can be obtained through change of diet or use of bulk-forming products.[2] As with all laxatives, cascara should not be prescribed when any undiagnosed acute or persistent abdominal symptoms are present.[4] Fresh or inadequately prepared cascara bark should not be used because severe vomiting and intestinal spasm can result.[2]
Interactions	Anthraquinone glycoside–containing laxatives may potentially decrease the transit time of concomitantly administered oral drugs and thereby decrease their absorption.[5]
	Excessive use of cascara can cause disturbance of fluid and electrolyte balance (especially potassium deficiency). Potassium deficiency

Cascara continued on page 128

#Alternative name.
*Cascara has also been used in traditional herbal medicine for treating constipation and dyspepsia and is recommended by both the Commission E and ESCOP for the short-term treatment of constipation. (4,5)

127

potentiates the action of cardiac glycosides[5] and interferes with antiarrhythmic drugs.[2] Simultaneous application of thiazide diuretics, corticosteroids, or licorice will increase potassium loss.[2,4] Speculations suggest that abuse of laxatives such as senna (*Cassia* spp.) may potentiate the development of analgesic nephropathy (resulting from dehydration).[5]

Use in Pregnancy and Lactation

According to the *British Herbal Compendium*, cascara is contraindicated in pregnancy and lactation.[1] However, this caution seems excessive provided that the dosage recommendations here are observed. Doses that cause an excessively loose stool should not be used during pregnancy.

Side Effects

Cramplike discomfort of the gastrointestinal tract may occur at normal therapeutic doses. These cases require a dose reduction.[2] Diarrhea resulting from abuse of cascara has been reported.[6]

Long-term use or abuse may cause disturbances of electrolyte balance, including potassium deficiency, which can lead to disorders of heart function and muscular weakness. A harmless pigmentation of the intestinal mucosa (pseudomelanosis coli) may occur with chronic use and usually reverses after discontinuing cascara.[2] Chronic intake of anthraquinone laxatives has been associated with an increased risk of colorectal cancer,[3] although this connection has been debated.[7,8]

A case of cascara-induced intrahepatic cholestasis causing portal hypertension has been reported. The dosage was one capsule three times per day for 3 days. Each capsule contained 425 mg of aged cascara bark, standardized to 5% cascarosides (1.3 g bark containing 64 mg cascarosides per day).[9]

Dosage

Dose per day**	Dose per week**
3-8 ml of 1:2 liquid extract	20-55 ml of 1:2 liquid extract

SUPPORTING INFORMATION

Traditional Prescribing

Traditional Western herbal medicine uses include:
- Constipation,[10] particularly when habitual or chronic in nature and when a tonic for the intestines is required[11]
- Dyspeptic conditions related to constipation and caused by intestinal weakness; headache resulting from similar causes[11]
- Loss of tone in the rectum[11]
- Conditions in which a soft stool is desirable, such as anal fissure or hemorrhoids[1]
- Rheumatism; gastric, duodenal, or biliary catarrh with jaundice; chronic diseases of the liver[11,12]

Cascara continued on page 129

**This dose range is extrapolated from the British *Pharmaceutical Codex* 1934, the British *Pharmacopoeia* 1932, and the author's education and experience.

Native Americans used cascara as a cathartic. Native South Americans also used cascara.[13]

Pharmacologic Research

Key constituents of cascara bark include hydroxyanthracene derivatives in a complex mixture (approximately 8%) consisting mainly of anthrone glycosides, especially cascarosides. Other constituents include aloins, deoxyaloins, and O-glycosides of the anthraquinones aloe-emodin, emodin, and chrysophanol.[1,14]

- The hydroxyanthracene derivatives are carried unabsorbed to the large bowel, where metabolism via glycosidases from intestinal flora results in the formation of the active aglycones.[3,15] (Because of this metabolism, defecation occurs several hours after ingestion.) These aglycones exert their laxative effect by local activity in the intestine by the following mechanisms: modification of intestinal motility (by stimulating intestinal muscle) and accumulation of fluid.[8] The increase in motility is a faster response than is the effect resulting from the increase in fecal water. A number of chemical mediators are implicated in producing these effects, including release of prostaglandins,[16] inhibition of intestinal tone and segmentation,[8] and production of high concentrations of nitric oxide synthase (which evokes net intestinal fluid secretion).[17]

- After absorption, the anthraquinones are transformed mainly to their corresponding glucuronide and sulfate derivatives, which finally appear in urine and bile. Therapy with anthraquinone glycosides such as those found in cascara and senna is regarded as preferable to therapy with free anthraquinones because the glycosides are less readily absorbed from the gastrointestinal tract and are active at much lower doses.[15] Anthraquinone glycosides hence have lower potential toxicity.

- The addition of a preparation containing *Curcuma aromatica* rhizome, whole roots of *Curcuma amara*, and cascara to a high-cholesterol diet was found to lower both serum and liver cholesterol in rats.[18]

Clinical Studies

- A preparation containing cascara, gentian, rhubarb, and boldo was tested in 24 healthy volunteers and in 80 patients with mild gastrointestinal disturbances. The herbal preparation induced a significant increase in salivary secretion from 1 to 30 minutes after oral administration, similar to the active control (citric acid) and unlike placebo or placebo plus alcohol. In this double-blind study, the herbal preparation was significantly better than placebo for the following symptoms: asthenia, loss of appetite, coated tongue, postprandial bloating, difficult digestion, constipation, flatulence, abdominal fullness, and itching of skin. The test preparation was more efficacious than the two pairs of its components (cascara and boldo; gentian and rhubarb).[19] The following herb equivalents were probably administered for the paired preparations: cascara (200 mg/day) and boldo (100 mg/day); gentian (40 mg/day) and rhubarb (200 mg/day).

Cascara continued on page 130

- A survey of 3257 elderly patients admitted to 58 hospitals in Italy in 1991 recorded that plant anthranoid laxatives were the second most frequently prescribed laxative (1.9% in hospital, 3.3% prehospital).[20]
- In Germany, the Commission E supports using cascara to treat constipation.[2]
- ESCOP recommends cascara for short-term use in cases of occasional constipation.[4]
- Cascara has remained official in the USP since the first entry in early 1890 and is currently official in the USP24-NF19.

REFERENCES

1 British Herbal Medicine Association: *British herbal compendium,* Bournemouth, 1992, BHMA.

2 Blumenthal M et al, editors: *The complete German Commission E monographs: therapeutic guide to herbal medicines,* Austin, 1998, American Botanical Council.

3 van Gorkom BA et al: *Aliment Pharmacol Ther* 13(4):443-452, 1999.

4 Scientific Committee of the European Scientific Cooperative on Phytotherapy [ESCOP]: *ESCOP monographs: Rhamni purshiani cortex,* European Scientific Cooperative on Phytotherapy, ESCOP Secretariat, Argyle House, Gandy Street, Exeter, Devon, EX4 3LS, United Kingdom, June 1997.

5 de Smet PAGM et al, editors: *Adverse effects of herbal drugs,* Berlin, 1993, Springer-Verlag.

6 Cummings JH et al: *Br Med J* 1:537-541, 1974.

7 Nusko G et al: *Gut* 46(5):651-655, 2000.

8 Mascolo N et al: *Phytother Res* 12(supp 1):S143-S145, 1998.

9 Nadir A, Reddy D, Van Thiel DH: *Am J Gastroenterol* 95(12):3634-3637, 2000.

10 British Herbal Medicine Association's Scientific Committee: *British herbal pharmacopoeia,* Bournemouth, 1983, BHMA.

11 Felter HW, Lloyd JU: *King's American dispensatory,* ed 18, rev 3, Portland, 1905, reprinted 1983, Eclectic Medical Publications.

12 Ellingwood F, Lloyd JU: *American materia medicam, therapeutics and pharmacognosy,* ed 11, Portland, 1983, Eclectic Medical Publications.

13 Vogel VJ: *American Indian medicine,* Norman, Okla, 1970, University of Oklahoma Press.

14 Wagner H, Bladt S: *Plant drug analysis: a thin layer chromatography atlas,* ed 2, Berlin, 1996, Springer-Verlag.

15 de Witte P, Lemli L: *Hepatogastroenterol* 37(6):601-605, 1990.

16 Geboes K: *Verh K Acad Geneeskd Belg* 57(1):51-74, 1995.

17 Izzo AA, Mascolo N, Capasso F: *Dig Dis Sci* 43(8):1605-1620, 1998.

18 Beynen AC: *Artery* 14(4):190-197, 1987.

19 Borgia M et al: *Curr Ther Res* 29(3):525-536, 1981.

20 Pahor M et al: *Aging (Milano)* 7(2):128-135, 1995.

CAT'S CLAW

Other Common Name: Uña de gato
Botanical Name: *Uncaria tomentosa*
Family: Rubiaceae
Plant Part Used: Stem bark

PRESCRIBING INFORMATION

Actions
Immune enhancing, antiinflammatory, antioxidant

Potential Indications
Based on appropriate evaluation of the patient, practitioners should consider prescribing cat's claw in formulations in the context of:
- Poor immunity, tendency to infections (7)
- Inflammatory conditions such as arthritis, gastritis, cystitis (6)
- Convalescence, debility (6)
- Adjuvant therapy for cancer (3,6)
- HIV infection, AIDS (4)

As cat's claw has been traditionally used as a tonic (6) and may also be used to treat other health issues requiring this action, including chronic fatigue syndrome.

Contraindications
None known.

Warnings and Precautions
None required.

Interactions
None known.

Use in Pregnancy and Lactation
Cat's claw should be used with caution in pregnancy and lactation. (The root of *Uncaria tomentosa* has been used traditionally as a contraceptive; pharmacologic results have demonstrated an antifertility effect in one animal model.[1] Oral use of the bark decoction is traditionally prescribed in Bolivia for irregular menstruation.[2])

Side Effects
Diarrhea and indigestion have occurred in several patients taking cat's claw. In one case, a high (undefined) dose had been consumed.[3]

Acute renal failure caused by "cat's claw" was reported in a 35-year-old Peruvian female with systemic lupus erythematosus (SLE). The contents of the capsules were not analyzed, and the duration of treatment was not stated. One month after discontinuing the herbal preparation, her condition had improved. The patient in all likelihood experienced an idiosyncratic adverse reaction to the herbal preparation.[4]

Dosage

Dose per day*	Dose per week*
4.5-11.0 ml of 1:2 liquid extract	30-75 ml of 1:2 liquid extract

Cat's Claw *continued on page 132*

*This dose range is extrapolated from traditional use of decoction of the bark.[3]

It is recommended that only the pentacyclic oxindole alkaloid-predominant type of cat's claw be used in therapy.

SUPPORTING INFORMATION

Traditional Prescribing

Traditional Peruvian medicinal uses include degenerative processes (e.g., cancer), inflammatory conditions (e.g., arthritis, gastritis, inflammation of the genitourinary tract and skin), gastric ulcers, diabetes, asthma, convalescence, and debility.[3,5]

Cat's claw is also regarded in traditional Peruvian medicine as a tonic or restorative.[3]

Cat's claw is one of the powerful plants that the Asháninka priests exclusively used to eliminate disturbance in the communication between body and spirit.[6]

Pharmacologic Research

Cat's claw stem bark contains a number of oxindole alkaloids.[7] Two different chemotypes of *U. tomentosa* that have been identified are likely to have distinctly different pharmacologic properties. One chemotype contains only, or predominantly, pentacyclic oxindole alkaloids (POA); the other contains POA and significant quantities of tetracyclic oxindole alkaloids (TOA). Intriguingly, indigenous priests are said to be able to identify the correct chemotype and harvest exclusively the chemotype containing POA, even though the two chemotypes are botanically identical.[6,7]

- Cat's claw extract has exhibited antioxidant activity *in vitro*[8] and antiinflammatory activity in experimental models after oral administration.[9–11] Results of an *in vitro* study suggested that the antiinflammatory action may be a result of immunomodulation via suppression of tumor necrosis factor-alpha synthesis.[12]
- Cat's claw extract has significantly stimulated interleukin-1 and interleukin-6 production *in vitro*.[13] Cat's claw extracts and POA stimulated phagocytosis *in vitro* and by injection.[14–16] POA were found to induce endothelial cells to release a factor that influences the proliferation of lymphocytes.[6,17] The TOA antagonized the effects of the POA.[6] These studies indicate immune enhancement for the POA chemotypes.
- POA demonstrated antitumor activity *in vitro*.[18]
- Cat's claw was shown to exhibit antiestrogenic effects *in vitro*.[19]

Clinical Studies

- A double-blind, randomized study assessed the effects of a freeze-dried aqueous extract of *U. tomentosa* on the mutagenic activity of urine collected from 12 smokers and 12 nonsmokers. A progressive decrease in mutagenic activity in the smokers' urine was observed with increasing dose.[20]

Cat's Claw *continued on page 133*

- In an uncontrolled trial, 13 patients with HIV took 20 mg/day of an aqueous hydrochloric acid extract of *U. tomentosa* root (containing 12 mg total POA/g) for 2.2 to 5.0 months. Although the total white blood cell count remained unchanged within the group, results indicated that low values were raised and high values were lowered. The lymphocyte count increased significantly to an average of approximately 35%. However, no significant changes in T4/T8 cell ratios were observed.[6]
- Standardized *U. tomentosa* root extract was used in a long-term, open study involving 44 patients with AIDS.[1] The daily dose varied from 20 to 60 mg per day (the dried herb equivalent would be much higher), with some patients also taking azidothymidine (AZT). Patients who had CD4 lymphocyte counts of 200 to 500 × 10^6/L demonstrated the best results for immunologic parameters:
  - CD4 cells increased significantly for the first year of therapy, and the increase persisted for the first 3 years. Patients continued to show stable counts for as long as 4 and 5 years after beginning treatment.
  - p24 antigen levels decreased.
  - B lymphocyte counts increased.

REFERENCES

1 Jones K: *Cat's claw: healing vine of Peru,* Seattle, 1995, Sylvan Press.
2 Bourdy G et al: *J Ethnopharmacol* 70(2):87, 2000.
3 Obregón Vilches, Lida E: *Cat's claw: Uncaria genus. Botanical, chemical, and pharmacological studies of Uncaria tomentosa and Uncaria guianensis,* Lima, 1995, Instituto de Fitoterapia Americano.
4 Hilepo JN, Bellucci AG, Mossey RT: *Nephron* 77(3):361, 1997.
5 Maxwell N: *Witch doctor's apprentice,* ed 3, New York, 1990, Citadel Press.
6 Keplinger K et al: *J Ethnopharmacol* 64:23, 1999.
7 Laus G, Brossner D, Keplinger K: *Phytochemistry* 45(4):855, 1997.
8 Desmarchelier C et al: *Phytother Res* 11(3):254, 1997.
9 Sandoval M et al: *Ailment Pharmacol Ther* 12(12):1279-1289, 1998.
10 Miller MJS et al: *Peditr Res* 45:114A, 1999.
11 Aquino R et al: *J Nat Prod* 54(2):453-459, 1991.
12 Sandoval M et al: *Free Radic Biol Med* 29(1):71-78, 2000.
13 LeMaire I et al: *J Ethnopharmacol* 64(2):109-115, 1999.
14 Wagner H et al: *Planta Med* 51(2):139, 1985.
15 Wagner H, Kreutzkamp B, Jurcic K: *Planta Med* 51(5):419, 1985.
16 United States Patent 5302611, April 12, 1994.
17 Wurm M et al: *Planta Med* 64(8):701-704, 1998.
18 Stuppner H et al: *Planta Med* 59(Suppl):A583, 1993.
19 Salazar EL, Jayme V: *Proc West Pharmacol Soc* 41:123-124, 1998.
20 Reinhard KH: *J Altern Complement Med* 5(2):143-151, 1999.

CELERY SEED

Botanical Name: *Apium graveolens*
Family: Umbelliferae
Plant Part Used: Fruit (sometimes referred to as seed)

Actions

Diuretic, antiinflammatory, antirheumatic

Potential Indications

Based on appropriate evaluation of the patient, practitioners should consider prescribing celery seed in formulations in the context of:
- Relief of osteoarthritis and rheumatism *(4,5)*
- Prevention of gout *(5)*

Contraindications

No evidence has been found that celery seed is contraindicated in pregnancy. This attribution comes from the mistaken assumption that the essential oil contains significant levels of apiol.

Warnings and Precautions

Caution is advised in kidney disorders, in particular inflammation of the kidneys, because the essential oil may increase the inflammation by causing epithelial irritation.[1,2]

Interactions

None known.

Use in Pregnancy and Lactation

No adverse effects expected.

Side Effects

Allergic reaction is possible but rare.[1] The furanocoumarins in combination with ultraviolet light may cause photodermatitis.[2]

Dosage

Dose per day*	Dose per week*
4.5-8.5 ml of 1:2 liquid extract	30-60 ml of 1:2 liquid extract

SUPPORTING INFORMATION

Traditional Prescribing

Traditional Western herbal medicine uses include:
- Rheumatism, arthritis, gout[3]
- Inflammation of the urinary tract, retention of urine, dropsy[3,4]
- Restlessness, nervous disorders, insomnia[5]

The Eclectics considered celery seed as a nervine tonic.[4]

Pharmacologic Research

Apium graveolens seeds contain an essential oil consisting of terpenes and phthalides (especially 3-n-butyl phthalide).[1]

Celery Seed continued on page 135

*This dose range is extrapolated from the British Pharmaceutical Codex 1934, the British Herbal Pharmacopoeia 1983, the British Herbal Compendium 1992, and the author's education and experience.

- Oral celery seed oil significantly elevated glutathione S-transferase activity *in vivo* compared with controls.[6,7] Two groups of components within celery seed oil (limonene-type monoterpenes and butyl phthalides) appeared to be responsible for this activity. Further testing showed that the phthalide compounds were more active than the limonene-type monoterpenes.[8]
- Celery seed oil administered orally increased liver tissue regeneration.[9] Methanolic extract of celery seed demonstrated significant hepatoprotective activity after oral administration in acetominophen (paracetamol)-induced and thioacetamide-induced hepatotoxicity.[10]
- Compared with controls, aqueous celery extract demonstrated a significant reduction in serum total cholesterol, LDL cholesterol, and triglycerides in a model of hyperlipidemia.[11]
- Ethanolic extract of celery seed demonstrated analgesic activity in two experimental models (by oral and injected routes). Antiinflammatory activity was also demonstrated in chronic inflammation (when given orally).[12]
- The essential oil has shown tranquilizing[13] and anticonvulsant effects on the central nervous system.[13–15] Phthalides are reported to possess antispasmodic, sedative, and diuretic actions.[16]
- In experimentally induced tumorigenesis, essential oil of celery seed markedly reduced tumor incidence and tumor multiplicity.[7]
- 3-n-butyl phthalide inhibited platelet aggregation *in vitro*[17] and demonstrated antispasmodic activity on isolated tissue.[18]
- 3-n-butyl phthalide demonstrated hypotensive activity after intraperitoneal injection.[19] Oral administration of 3-n-butyl phthalide resulted in a selective antianginal effect, without changing blood pressure or heart rate.[18] Oral administration of 3-n-butyl phthalide (80 to 240 mg/kg) prevented experimentally induced brain edema *in vivo*.[20]

Clinical Studies

In an uncontrolled, preclinical trial in Australia, 15 patients with long-running rheumatic pain received celery seed extract over 12 weeks. The parameters measured were usual pain, current pain, and usual and current body areas experiencing pain. Patients reported significant reduction in pain intensity for usual pain after weeks 3 and 6 and for current pain after weeks 3 and 12. The number of joints at which pain was experienced was significantly decreased over each 3-week period.[21]

REFERENCES

1 British Herbal Medicine Association: *British herbal compendium,* Bournemouth, 1992, BHMA.

2 Bisset NG, editor: *Herbal drugs and phytopharmaceuticals,* Stuttgart, 1994, Medpharm Scientific Publishers.

3 British Herbal Medicine Association's Scientific Committee: *British herbal pharmacopoeia,* Bournemouth, 1983, BHMA.

4 Felter HW, Lloyd JU: *King's American dispensatory,* ed 18, rev 3, Portland, 1905, reprinted 1983, Eclectic Medical Publications.

5 Grieve M: *A modern herbal,* New York, 1971, Dover Publications.

6 Banerjee S et al: *Nutr Cancer* 21(3):263-269, 1994.

7 Zheng GQ et al: *Nutr Cancer* 19(1):77-86, 1993.

Celery Seed *continued on page 136*

8 Ren S, Lien EJ: *Prog Drug Res* 48:147-171, 1997.

9 Gershebin LL: *Food Cosmet Toxicol* 15(3):173-181, 1977.

10 Singh A, Handa SS: *J Ethnopharmacol* 49(3):119-126, 1995.

11 Tsi D, Das NP, Tan KH: *Planta Med* 61(1):18-21, 1995.

12 Atta AH, Alkofahi A: *J Ethnopharmacol* 60:117-124, 1998.

13 Kohli RP et al: *Indian J Med Res* 55(10):1099-1102, 1967.

14 Yu S, You S: *Yao Hsueh Hsueh Pao* 19(8):566-570, 1984.

15 Yang J, Chen Y: *Yaoxue Tongbao* 19:670-671, 1984.

16 Gijbels MJM et al: *Riv Ital EPPOS* 61:335-341, 1979.

17 Teng CM et al: *Biochim Biophys Acta* 924(3):375-382, 1987.

18 Ko WC et al: *Planta Med* 64(3):229-232, 1998.

19 Tsi D, Tan BKH: *Phytother Res* 11(8):576-582, 1997.

20 Deng W, Feng Y: *Chin Med Sci J* 12(2):102, 1997.

21 Australian Patent 9946991O-A, January 1995.

CHAMOMILE

Other Common Name:	German chamomile
Botanical Names:	*Matricaria recutita, Matricaria chamomilla,*# *Chamomilla recutita*#
Family:	Compositae
Plant Part Used:	Flower

PRESCRIBING INFORMATION

Actions

Antiinflammatory, spasmolytic, carminative, mild sedative, antiulcer, vulnerary, diaphoretic

Potential Indications

Based on appropriate evaluation of the patient, practitioners should consider prescribing chamomile in formulations in the context of:
- Gastrointestinal spasm, inflammatory diseases of the gastrointestinal tract, irritable bowel syndrome, flatulence, bloating *(4,5)*
- Acute, uncomplicated diarrhea, in combination with pectin* *(2)*
- Infantile colic,** in combination with lemon balm, vervain, licorice, and fennel *(3)*
- Anxiety *(4)*
- Travel sickness, nervous diarrhea *(5)*
- Dysmenorrhea, amenorrhea *(5)*
- Restlessness, anxiety *(5)*
- Teething problems in children *(5)*
- Topical treatment for eczema and wound healing *(2,5)*
- Topical treatment for leg ulcers *(3,5)*
- Topical treatment for skin inflammation *(3,5)*
- Topical treatment for mucous membrane inflammations, including those of the oral cavity and gums; anogenita inflammation *(4,5)*
- Topical treatment for bacterial skin diseases *(4)*

Contraindications

Known allergy.

Warnings and Precautions

Despite reports of skin reactions and dermatitis from topical use of chamomile, the likelihood of chamomile preparations causing a contact allergy is low. However, people with known sensitivity to other members of the Compositae family (e.g., ragweed, daisies, chrysanthemums) should avoid oral and topical application of chamomile or chamomile products.

Interactions

Chamomile tea (compared with a water control) reduced the absorption of iron by 47% following a bread meal in adult volunteers. The inhibition was dose-dependent and related to its polyphenol content

Chamomile *continued on page 138*

#Alternative name.

*Apple may be added to the patient's diet to supply pectin.

**Chamomile has also been used in traditional herbal therapy for treating colic. (5)

137

(phenolic acids, monomeric flavonoids, and polymerized polyphenols). Inhibition of iron absorption by black tea was 79% to 94%.[1] This finding indicates a potential interaction for concomitant administration of chamomile during iron intake. In anemia and cases in which iron supplementation is required, chamomile should not be taken simultaneously with meals or iron supplements.

Use in Pregnancy and Lactation

No adverse effects expected.

Side Effects

Contact dermatitis and skin reactions have been reported from the topical use of chamomile preparations. One case of severe anaphylactic reaction after ingesting chamomile tea has been reported. Given the widespread consumption of chamomile tea and the few reported cases of anaphylaxis, this type of reaction is extremely rare. Additionally, using ethanolic extracts denatures the proteins and renders this type of reaction unlikely.

Eye washing with chamomile tea can induce allergic conjunctivitis; the pollen contained in these infusions appears to be responsible for the allergic reaction. Pollens and their proteins are unlikely to be present or active in aqueous alcohol extracts of chamomile.

Dosage

Dose per day***	Dose per week***
3-6 ml of 1:2 high-grade liquid extract	20-40 ml of 1:2 high-grade liquid extract

High-grade liquid extracts providing quantified levels of bisabolol are recommended. Ideally, aqueous ethanol extracts should contain not less than 0.4 mg/ml of bisabolol.

SUPPORTING INFORMATION

Traditional Prescribing

Traditional Western herbal medicine uses include:
- Flatulent or nervous dyspepsia, travel sickness, nervous diarrhea, nervous disorders of the stomach and bowel, flatulent colic with distention, catarrhal conditions of the bowel; dysmenorrhea, amenorrhea[2,3]
- Restlessness, nervous irritability in children, teething problems, infantile convulsions, rheumatic and neuralgic pain[2,3]
- Catarrhal conditions of the nose, ears, and eyes; for earache, as a diaphoretic[2,3]
- Topically for inflammations and irritations of the skin and mucosa, including hemorrhoids, mastitis, leukorrhea, and leg ulcers[2-4]

Chamomile *continued on page 139*

***This dose range is extrapolated from the British Herbal Compendium 1992 and the author's education and experience.

Pharmacologic Research

Active constituents of chamomile flowers include an essential oil (containing α-bisabolol and chamazulene) and flavonoids. Chamomile preparations used in research are often standardized for α-bisabolol and chamazulene content.

- *In vitro* studies showed chamomile extracts to have antiinflammatory and antioxidant effects. Experimental studies of both oral and topical application of chamomile extract also demonstrated this antiinflammatory action.
- Experimental models showed chamomile extract to have an antispasmodic action *in vitro*.
- Injection of the flavonoid apigenin demonstrated clear antianxiety activity and slight sedative activity without muscle relaxant effects.
- Chamomile extract and α-bisabolol demonstrated antiulcer activity in experimental models after oral administration.
- Chamomile extract, essential oil, and isolated constituents have demonstrated antimicrobial activity *in vitro*.
- The wound-healing activity of chamomile is closely linked to its antiinflammatory activity. Chamomile extract and its isolated constituents demonstrated wound-healing activity in several experimental models.

Clinical Studies

- Oral administration of chamomile tea during cardiac catheterization induced a deep sleep in 10 of 12 patients tested, despite the pain and anxiety experienced from the medical procedure. Two chamomile tea bags were used in a 6-oz (175-ml) cup of hot water. The patients drank the tea in less than 10 minutes.
- A combination of a chamomile extract and pectin showed superior results to placebo in treating acute, uncomplicated diarrhea in a double-blind, randomized trial. The preparation contained 2.5% of chamomile extract standardized to 0.0035% chamazulene and 0.05% α-bisabolol and 3.2% pectin.
- A double-blind study on babies approximately 3 weeks of age with infantile colic investigated the effect of an instant herb tea containing chamomile, lemon balm, vervain, licorice, and fennel. After 7 days, the improvement in colic scores was significantly better in the herbal tea group. More babies in the treatment group had their colic eliminated. The tea preparation was offered with every episode of colic, up to 150 ml per dose, but not more than three times per day. The exact composition of the preparation was not defined.
- Uncontrolled trials demonstrated that a standardized chamomile mouthwash was beneficial for treating chronic oral inflammations (except in the case of glossodynia) and oral mucositis caused by head and neck irradiation and systemic chemotherapy. The chamomile rinse accelerated the resolution of mucositis, and prophylactic use was also favorable. However, chamomile did not decrease the incidence of stomatitis in patients undergoing chemotherapy. The mouthwash contained 50 mg of α-bisabolol and 150 to 300 mg apigenin-7-glucoside per 100 g and was applied three times daily.

Chamomile *continued on page 140*

- Topical application of standardized chamomile preparations has shown benefit in treating eczema, varicose eczema, and varicose ulcers in uncontrolled trials, surveys, and controlled trials. Standardized chamomile cream showed mild superiority over 0.5% hydrocortisone cream and marginal improvement compared with placebo in medium-degree atopic eczema. This trial was a partially blinded, randomized trial carried out as a half-side comparison (one side of the body compared with the other).[5]
- Standardized chamomile cream was compared with steroidal and nonsteroidal dermal preparations in the maintenance therapy of eczema. Chamomile cream showed similar efficacy to 0.25% hydrocortisone and was superior to the nonsteroidal antiinflammatory agent (5% bufexamac) and a glucocorticoid preparation (0.75% fluocortin butyl ester).
- Standardized chamomile extract demonstrated a statistically significant benefit on wound healing following tattoo dermabrasion in a randomized, double-blind, placebo-controlled clinical trial involving 14 patients. In a randomized, controlled trial, standardized chamomile cream was preferred over almond cream by patients for treating the erythema and moist desquamation acquired after receiving radiotherapy.
- Standardized chamomile ointment had similar efficacy as 5% dexpanthenol cream in healing episiotomy wounds in an open, randomized trial.[6] An open, randomized trial that compared several procedures for second-degree hemorrhoid treatment found best results in the group receiving application of a standardized chamomile ointment in conjunction with the surgical procedures (ligature and anal dilation).[7]
- In Germany, the Commission E supports using chamomile internally to treat gastrointestinal spasm and inflammatory diseases of the gastrointestinal tract. Chamomile is recommended externally to treat skin and mucous membrane inflammations, bacterial skin diseases, including those of the oral cavity and gums, inflammation and irritation of the respiratory tract (by inhalation), and anogenital inflammation (by bath or enema).[8] ESCOP also recommends chamomile for these indications, specifically indicating internal use for the following gastrointestinal complaints: minor spasm, epigastric distension, flatulence, and belching.[9]
- Chamomile has been reinstated to the USP and is official in the USP24-NF19.

REFERENCES

Except when specifically referenced, the following book was referred to in the compilation of the pharmacologic and clinical information: Mills S, Bone K: *Principles and Practice of Phytotherapy: Modern Herbal Medicine*, Edinburgh, 2000, Churchill Livingstone.

1 Hurrell RF, Reddy M, Cook JD: *Br J Nutr* 81(4):289-295, 1999.
2 British Herbal Medicine Association's Scientific Committee: *British herbal pharmacopoeia*, Bournemouth, 1983, BHMA.
3 Felter HW, Lloyd JU: *King's American dispensatory*, ed 18, rev 3, Portland, 1905, reprinted 1983, Eclectic Medical Publications.

Chamomile *continued on page 141*

4 British Herbal Medicine Association: *British herbal compendium,* Bournemouth, 1992, BHMA.

5 Patzelt-Wenczler R, Ponce-Poschl E: *Eur J Med Res* 5(4):171-175, 2000.

6 Kaltenbach FJ. Cited in Nasemann Th, Patzelt-Wenczler R, editors: *Kamillosan im Spiegel der Literatur,* Frankfurt, 1991, PMI Verlag.

7 Forster CF, Sussmann HE, Patzelt-Wenczler R: *Schweiz Rundsch Med Prax* 85(46):1476-1481, 1996.

8 Blumenthal M et al, editors: *The complete German Commission E monographs: therapeutic guide to herbal medicines,* Austin, 1998, American Botanical Council.

9 Scientific Committee of the European Scientific Cooperative on Phytotherapy [ESCOP]: *ESCOP monographs: Matricariae flos.* European Scientific Cooperative on Phytotherapy, ESCOP Secretariat, Argyle House, Gandy Street, Exeter, Devon, EX4 3LS, United Kingdom, October 1999.

CHASTE TREE

Botanical Name: *Vitex agnus-castus*
Family: Labiatae
Plant Part Used: Fruit

PRESCRIBING INFORMATION

Actions	Prolactin inhibitor, dopaminergic agonist, indirectly progesterogenic, galactagogue
Potential Indications	Based on appropriate evaluation of the patient, practitioners should consider prescribing chaste tree in formulations in the context of:

- Premenstrual syndrome, especially with mastalgia and fluid retention *(2,4,5)*
- Progesterone deficiency, corpus luteal insufficiency, latent hyperprolactinemia *(3)*
- Cystic hyperplasia of the endometrium, infertility resulting from decreased progesterone levels or hyperprolactinemia *(4)*
- Acne *(3)*
- Secondary amenorrhea *(4,5)*
- Metrorrhagia (from functional causes), menorrhagia, polymenorrhea, oligomenorrhea *(4,6)*
- Insufficient lactation *(3,5)*
- Possible benefit in menopausal symptoms, withdrawal from hormone replacement therapy, and conditions in which unopposed estrogen plays a role (e.g., fibroids, endometriosis, follicular ovarian cysts) because of its supposed progesterone-favoring effect *(7)*
- Possible benefit in conditions in which raised prolactin secretion is implicated (e.g., breast cysts, fibrocystic breast disease, benign prostatic hyperplasia) *(7)*

Contraindications	None required.
Warnings and Precautions	In general, chaste tree is best not taken in conjunction with progesterone drugs, contraceptive pill, or hormone-replacement therapy (HRT). Chaste tree may aggravate pure spasmodic dysmenorrhea not associated with premenstrual syndrome (PMS).
Interactions	Chaste tree may interact antagonistically with dopamine receptor antagonists.
Use in Pregnancy and Lactation	Chaste tree should be used cautiously during pregnancy and only in the early stages for treating insufficient corpus luteal function.
	Although the dopaminergic activity might suggest that chaste tree is best avoided during lactation, clinical trials have demonstrated its positive activity on milk production, albeit at low doses.

Chaste Tree *continued on page 143*

Side Effects

Rare occurrences of generalized itching and urticaria have been reported. Herbalists have reported that chaste tree can rarely cause headache.

In several trials, side effects were noted in 1% to 13% of participants. These side effects centered on the gastrointestinal tract and were not considered significant.

A 45-year-old woman who had been taking herbal preparations containing black cohosh, chaste tree, and evening primrose oil for 4 months had three seizures within a 3-month period. The herbal preparations were stopped, and the patient was treated with anticonvulsants.

Dosage

Dose per day*	Dose per week*
1.0-2.5 ml of 1:2 liquid extract	6 to 18 ml of 1:2 liquid extract

SUPPORTING INFORMATION

Traditional Prescribing

Traditional Western herbal medicine uses include:
- As a galactagogue and emmenagogue by the Eclectics; said to "repress the sexual passions"; for impotence, sexual melancholia, sexual irritability with nervousness, melancholia, or mild dementia[2]
- Gynecologic problems and insufficient lactation (European use)[3,4]

Pharmacologic Research

Constituents of chaste tree berries include essential oil, diterpenes of the labdane- and clerodane-type, including rotundifuran, 6ß,7ß-diacetoxy-13-hydroxy-labda-8, and 14-diene, flavonoids (e.g., casticin), and iridoid glycosides, including aucubin and agnuside.
- *In vitro* studies indicate that chaste tree has a dopaminergic effect, inhibiting prolactin release from the anterior pituitary.
- Labdane diterpenes inhibited spiperone[5] and sulpiride[6] binding at dopamine D_2 receptors *in vitro*. Chaste tree extract produced similar inhibition of binding as the isolated diterpenes. Agnuside, aucubin, casticin, and other flavonoids did not show an inhibitory effect in this assay.[5]
- Rotundifuran dose-dependently inhibited prolactin secretion from cultured pituitary cells. Both rotundifuran and dopamine inhibited forskolin-induced prolactin secretion and cAMP formation in pituitary cells *in vitro*.[6]
- An early experimental model found that low oral doses of chaste tree produced a decrease of estrogen effects and a promotion of progesterone effects, which was presumably mediated through the pituitary gland. At high doses (up to 20 times the low dose), an inhibition of all gonadotropic hormones and growth hormone resulted.

Chaste Tree *continued on page 144*

*This dose range is extrapolated from a published survey of United Kingdom herbalists conducted in 1997.[1]

Clinical Research

The doses used in most of the German clinical trials summarized here (around 40 mg/day) are much lower than those that Western herbalists typically use. Recent trials with chaste tree have used higher doses (around 200 mg/day).

- In an open, placebo-controlled, crossover trial, 20 male volunteers received special extract of chaste tree (equivalent to 120, 240, or 480 mg/day dried extract) or placebo for 14 days. The results suggested that the activity of chaste tree on prolactin secretion was dependent on dosage and the initial level of the prolactin concentration. Men were used in this trial because their hormones are under less cyclical influence compared with women. Chaste tree caused an increase in prolactin secretion at the lowest dose and a decrease at the highest dose. Chaste tree did not alter the serum concentrations of LH, FSH, or testosterone.
- Chaste tree extract (equivalent to 40 mg/day of dried fruit for 1 month) reduced prolactin levels in women with hyperprolactinemia in an uncontrolled study.[7]
- Early uncontrolled clinical studies on chaste tree observed improvement in patients with a variety of menstrual disorders. Results were particularly marked for patients suffering from cystic hyperplasia of the endometrium (which is caused by a relative progesterone deficiency). Chaste tree was particularly indicated in patients with deficient corpus luteum function. The dosage most often used was equivalent to 36 mg/day of dried fruit.
- Observation by 153 gynecologists of 551 patients with symptoms of corpus luteal insufficiency, cyclic disorders, or PMS over several menstrual cycles revealed that chaste tree treatment was beneficial in 68.8% of cases. The average dose of chaste tree was equivalent to 36 mg/day of dried fruit. Over 80% of patients were relieved of complaints or stated that their condition had improved.
- Thirty-seven women with luteal phase defects caused by latent hyperprolactinemia completed a double-blind, placebo-controlled trial testing the efficacy of a chaste tree preparation (equivalent to 20 mg/day of dried fruit for 3 months). With chaste tree treatment, prolactin release following administration of thyroxin-releasing hormone was significantly reduced. Shortened luteal phases were normalized, and luteal phase progesterone deficiencies were corrected. Two women receiving chaste tree became pregnant, and PMS symptoms were significantly reduced in the chaste tree group.
- Chaste tree extract (equivalent to 180 mg/day of dried fruit for three cycles) improved PMS symptoms (irritability, mood alteration, anger, headache, breast fullness, and bloating) and clinical global impression scores in a randomized, double-blind, placebo-controlled trial.[8]
- In a controlled clinical trial, significant benefit was observed for all types of PMS except type PMS-C (characterized by symptoms such as headache, craving for sweets, palpitations, and dizziness).

Chaste Tree *continued on page 145*

- In contrast, 93% of 1634 patients with PMS reported a decrease in, or cessation of, symptoms in all four PMS symptom complexes, including PMS-C, after treatment with chaste tree extract (equivalent to 40 mg/day of dried fruit for three cycles) in a recent postmarketing study. Eighty-five percent of physicians rated chaste tree as good or very good.[9]

- In a multicenter, randomized, double-blind, comparative trial, 175 women with PMS received either chaste tree or vitamin B_6 (100 mg pyridoxine) over three cycles. Patients received chaste tree extract (equivalent to 40 mg dried fruit) each day or one capsule of placebo twice daily on days 1 to 15, and one capsule of pyridoxine (100 mg) twice daily on days 16 to 35 of the menstrual cycle. PMS scores decreased for both treatments, however, chaste tree treatment was superior to pyridoxine overall. Compared with pyridoxine, chaste tree showed a significant improvement in reducing characteristic symptoms such as breast tenderness, edemas, abdominal tension, headaches, constipation, and depressed mood.

- In a prospective, multicenter trial on PMS, chaste tree extract (equivalent to 180 mg/day of dried fruit for three cycles) reduced patient's symptom scores. Global efficacy was rated as moderate to excellent by 88% of patients. Improvement was maintained for up to three cycles after medication. No differences were seen between patients taking oral contraceptives and those who were not. No effect was observed on resting levels of blood prolactin.[10]

- In two uncontrolled studies, the influence of chaste tree on corpus luteal function was investigated. The women were considered to be capable of reproduction, had normal prolactinemia, but showed pathologically low serum progesterone levels at day 20 of the menstrual cycle. After 3 months, chaste tree treatment (equivalent to 36 mg/day dried fruit) was considered to be successful in 39 of 45 cases. Seven women became pregnant, 25 women had normal serum progesterone levels at day 20, and another seven women tended towards normal levels.

- In a randomized, double-blind, clinical trial, 160 patients with premenstrual mastalgia received a homeopathic formula also containing chaste tree tincture, gestagen therapy (lynestrenol), or placebo. Treatment with the chaste tree–homeopathic combination gave good relief of symptoms in 74.5% of patients and a lower incidence of side effects. Improvements were 82.1% for lynestrenol and 36.8% for placebo. Chaste tree solution or chaste tree tablets (both equivalent to 32 mg/day dried fruit) for three cycles reduced mastalgia and prolactin levels in a randomized, double-blind, placebo-controlled trial.[11] In an earlier trial involving 20 patients that used the same design but included crossover, a statistically significant reduction of symptoms was observed for chaste tree treatment (equivalent to 32 mg/day dried fruit). Short-lived nausea was reported in some cases.

Chaste Tree *continued on page 146*

- A favorable effect was observed on milk production for participants treated with chaste tree in a case observation study. In a controlled trial, average milk production was approximately three times that of controls after 20 days of treatment (equivalent to 40 mg/day dried fruit). This finding suggests, consistent with the study in men cited previously, that low doses might increase prolactin and promote milk production.
- In a controlled trial of 161 male and female patients with acne, a minimum of 3 months' treatment with chaste tree resulted in an improvement for 70% of patients, which was significantly better than placebo. Patients were treated with chaste tree (equivalent to 36 mg/day of dried fruit) for 4 to 6 weeks, followed by a lower dose for 1 to 2 years. The mechanism for the beneficial effect of chaste tree on acne is not known but may be a result of a mild antiandrogenic effect.
- In Germany, the Commission E supports using chaste tree to treat irregularities of the menstrual cycle, premenstrual complaints, and mastodynia.[12]

REFERENCES

Except when specifically referenced, the following book was referred to in the compilation of the pharmacologic and clinical information: Mills S, Bone K: *Principles and Practice of Phytotherapy: Modern Herbal Medicine,* Edinburgh, 2000, Churchill Livingstone.

1 Christie S, Walker AF: *Eur J Herb Med* 3(3):29-45, 1997-1998.
2 Felter HW, Lloyd JU: *King's American dispensatory,* ed 18, rev 3, Portland, 1905, reprinted 1983, Eclectic Medical Publications.
3 Mills SY: *Out of the earth: the essential book of herbal medicine,* London, 1991, Viking Arkana (Penguin).
4 Mills SY: *Women's medicine: Vitex agnus castus, the herb,* Christchurch, UK, 1992, Amberwood.
5 Meier B et al: *Phytomed* 7(5):373-381, 2000.
6 Christoffel V et al. Cited in Loew D, Blume H, Dingermann TH, editors: *Phytopharmaka v, Forschung und Klinische Anwendung,* Darmstadt, 1999, Steinkopff.
7 Gorkow C: *Z Phytother* 20:159-168, 1999.
8 Schellenberg R: *BMJ* 322:134-137, 2001.
9 Loch EG, Selle H, Boblitz N: *J Womens Health Gend Based Med* 9(3):315-320, 2000.
10 Berger D et al: *Arch Gynecol Obstet* 264(3):150-153, 2000.
11 Wuttke W et al: *Geb Fra* 57(10):569-574, 1997.
12 Blumenthal M et al, editors: *The complete German Commission E monographs: therapeutic guide to herbal medicines,* Austin, 1998, American Botanical Council.

CHICKWEED

Botanical Name: Stellaria media
Family: Caryophyllaceae
Plant Part Used: Aerial parts

PRESCRIBING INFORMATION

Actions
Demulcent, astringent, refrigerant, antiulcer (peptic)

Potential Indications
Based on appropriate evaluation of the patient, practitioners should consider prescribing chickweed in formulations in the context of:
- Rheumatic and gouty conditions, gastrointestinal ulceration *(5)*
- Topical treatment for skin disorders, especially eczema and psoriasis, itchy skin, rashes, burns, ulceration, and boils; inflammation of the eye *(5)*
- Topical treatment for hemorrhoids *(6)*

Contraindications
Known allergy.

Warnings and Precautions
None required.

Interactions
None known.

Use in Pregnancy and Lactation
No adverse effects expected.

Side Effects
Allergic rashes may rarely result from topical use.

Dosage

*Dose per day**	*Dose per week**
3-6 ml of fresh plant succus	20-40 ml of fresh plant succus

SUPPORTING INFORMATION

Traditional Prescribing
Traditional Western herbal medicine uses include:
- Rheumatism[1,2]
- Constipation, cough, hoarseness[3]
- Topically for eczema, psoriasis, skin inflammation, poorly healing ulcers, carbuncle, abscess[1,2]
- Hemorrhoids[3]

Pharmacologic Research
The aerial parts of chickweed contain flavonoids, phenolic acids, triterpenoid saponins, phytosterols, and carotenoids.[4]

No pharmacologic information has been found for chickweed.

Clinical Studies
No clinical studies using chickweed have been found.

Chickweed *continued on page 148*

*This dose range is extrapolated from the dried herb tincture dosages listed in the British Herbal Pharmacopoeia 1983 and the author's education and experience.

REFERENCES

1 British Herbal Medicine Association's Scientific Committee: *British herbal pharmacopoeia*, Bournemouth, 1983, BHMA.

2 Felter HW, Lloyd JU: *King's American dispensatory*, ed 18, rev 3, Portland, 1905, reprinted 1983, Eclectic Medical Publications.

3 Grieve M: *A modern herbal*, New York, 1971, Dover Publications.

4 Kitanov GM: *Pharmazie* 47:470-471, 1992.

CINNAMON

Botanical Names: *Cinnamomum zeylanicum, Cinnamomum verum*[#]
Family: Lauraceae
Plant Part Used: Bark

PRESCRIBING INFORMATION

Actions
Carminative, aromatic digestive, astringent

Potential Indications
Based on appropriate evaluation of the patient, practitioners should consider prescribing cinnamon in formulations in the context of:
- Loss of appetite, dyspeptic complaints, bloating, flatulence, mild, spastic conditions of the gastrointestinal tract *(4,5)*
- The common cold and influenza *(5)*
- Nausea, vomiting, diarrhea *(5)*
- Conditions requiring warmth and circulatory stimulation, such as cold hands and feet *(5)*
- Uterine hemorrhage, menorrhagia *(5)*

Contraindications
Known allergy to cinnamon and Peruvian balsam.[1] Cross-reactions with Peruvian balsam have been observed for people who are sensitive to cinnamic aldehyde.[2]

Warnings and Precautions
None required.

Interactions
None known.

Use in Pregnancy and Lactation
The German Commission E recommends that cinnamon is contraindicated in pregnancy. However, a review of the safety literature suggests that cinnamon does not present any special risk in pregnancy.[3]

Side Effects
Allergic reactions of the skin and mucosa have been reported.[1] This finding is most likely a result of cinnamic aldehyde, which is a potent contact sensitizer.[3]

Dosage

Dose per day*	Dose per week*
3-6 ml of 1:2 liquid extract	20-40 ml of 1:2 liquid extract

SUPPORTING INFORMATION

Traditional Prescribing
Traditional Western herbal medicine uses include:
- Flatulent dyspepsia, anorexia, intestinal colic, infantile diarrhea, nausea and vomiting[4,5]
- The common cold, influenza,[4] cold extremities[5]

Cinnamon *continued on page 150*

[#]Alternative name.
*This dose range is extrapolated from the British Pharmaceutical Codex 1949, the British Herbal Pharmacopoeia 1983, and the author's education and experience.

- Uterine hemorrhage, menorrhagia[5]
- Correcting the effects of certain remedies (e.g., the nausea caused by Cinchona) and improving the flavor of other herbs[5]

Pharmacologic Research

Cinnamon bark contains an essential oil, with the major constituent being cinnamic aldehyde (cinnamaldehyde).[6]

- The oral pungency of cinnamic aldehyde was found to be a result of burning, tingling, and numbing, with quick onset and rapid decay.[7]
- Cinnamon oil has demonstrated antibacterial and antifungal activities *in vitro*,[8] including activity against a range of dermatophytes.[9] Cinnamic aldehyde has been identified as an active fungitoxic constituent.[10]
- Cinnamon oil has demonstrated antispasmodic activity on isolated smooth muscle tissue,[11] decreased stomach and intestinal motility, and reduced stress-induced gastric ulcers *in vivo*.[8] The *in vivo* studies used relatively large doses of oil administered by injection.
- Cinnamon extract demonstrated analgesic activity in two experimental models testing central and peripheral effects (400 mg/kg pretreatment by injection; 200 mg/kg oral pretreatment, respectively).[12]
- Cinnamon has demonstrated antioxidant activity *in vitro*[13] and exerted antioxidant activity in rats fed a high-fat diet. The antioxidant protection occurred through its ability to activate antioxidant enzymes.[14] Cinnamon did not lower cholesterol in induced hypercholesterolemia.[15]
- *In vitro* studies indicate that cinnamon and a compound extracted from it potentiate insulin activity.[16,17] Similar to insulin, the compound affects protein phosphorylation in the intact fat cell.[17] The insulin-potentiating activity of cinnamon was not correlated with its total chromium content.[16]

Clinical Studies

- Administration of a cinnamon treatment for 1 week improved oral candidiasis in five patients with HIV infection.[18]
- In Germany, the Commission E supports using cinnamon to treat loss of appetite, dyspeptic complaints (e.g., mild, spastic conditions of the gastrointestinal tract), bloating, and flatulence.[1]

REFERENCES

1 Blumenthal M et al, editors: *The Complete German Commission E monographs: therapeutic guide to herbal medicines,* Austin, 1998, American Botanical Council.

2 Collins FW, Mitchell JC: *Contact Dermatitis* 1(1):43-47, 1975.

3 de Smet PAGM et al, editors: *Adverse effects of herbal drugs,* Berlin, 1992, Springer-Verlag.

4 British Herbal Medicine Association's Scientific Committee: *British herbal pharmacopoeia,* Bournemouth, 1983, BHMA.

5 Felter HW, Lloyd JU: *King's American dispensatory,* ed 18, rev 3, Portland, 1905, reprinted 1983, Eclectic Medical Publications.

6 Wagner H, Bladt S: *Plant drug analysis: a thin layer chromatography atlas,* ed 2, Berlin, 1996, Springer-Verlag.

7 Cliff M, Heymann H: *J Sensory Stud* 7(4):2792-290, 1992.

8 World Health Organization: *WHO monographs on selected medicinal plants,* Geneva, 1999, WHO.

Cinnamon *continued on page 151*

9 Lima EO et al: *Mycoses* 36(9-10):333-336, 1993.

10 Singh HB et al: *Allergy* 50(12):995-999, 1995.

11 Reiter M, Brandt W: *Arzneim Forsch* 35(1A):408-414, 1985.

12 Atta AH, Alkofahi A: *J Ethnopharmacol* 60(2):117-124, 1998.

13 Hirayama T et al: *Shokuhin Eiseigaku Zasshi* 27(6):615-618, 1986.

14 Dhuley JN: *Indian J Exp Biol* 37(3):238-242, 1999.

15 Sambaiah K, Srinivasan K: *Nahrung* 35(1):47-51, 1991.

16 Khan A et al: *Biol Trace Elem Res* 24(3):183-188, 1990.

17 Imparl-Radosevich J et al: *Hormone Res* 50(3):177-182, 1998.

18 Quale JM et al: *Am J Chin Med* 24(2):103-109, 1996.

CLEAVERS

Other Common Names: Clivers, Galium
Botanical Name: *Galium aparine*
Family: Rubiaceae
Plant Part Used: Aerial parts

PRESCRIBING INFORMATION

Actions	Diuretic, depurative
Potential Indications	Based on appropriate evaluation of the patient, practitioners should consider prescribing cleavers in formulations in the context of:
	• Skin diseases, including psoriasis and eczema (5)
	• Enlarged or inflamed lymph nodes (5)
	• Painful or difficult urination, cystitis (5)
	• Kidney stones (6)
Contraindications	None known.
Warnings and Precautions	None required.
Interactions	None known.
Use in Pregnancy and Lactation	No adverse effects expected.
Side Effects	None expected if taken within the recommended dose range.

Dosage

Dose per day*	Dose per week*
3.5-7.0 ml of 1:2 liquid extract	25-50 ml of 1:2 liquid extract

SUPPORTING INFORMATION

Traditional Prescribing	Traditional Western herbal medicine uses include:
	• Painful or difficult urination, inflammation of kidneys and bladder, lymphadenitis, enlarged lymph nodes, scrofula (tuberculous infection of the cervical lymph nodes)[1,2]
	• Skin diseases and eruptions, especially psoriasis and eczema[2]
	• Cancer[2]
	• Kidney stones[3]
Pharmacologic Research	The iridoid glycosides of the aerial parts of cleavers have shown mild laxative activity *in vivo*.[4]
Clinical Studies	No clinical studies using cleavers have been found.

Cleavers *continued on page 153*

*This dose range is extrapolated from the British Herbal Pharmacopoeia 1983, the British Herbal Compendium 1992, and the author's education and experience.

REFERENCES

1 British Herbal Medicine Association's Scientific Committee: *British herbal pharmacopoeia,* Bournemouth, 1983, BHMA.

2 Felter HW, Lloyd JU: *King's American dispensatory,* ed 18, rev 3, Portland, 1905, reprinted 1983, Eclectic Medical Publications.

3 Grieve M: *A modern herbal,* New York, 1971, Dover Publications.

4 Steinegger E, Hansel R: *Lehrbuch der pharmakognosie und phytopharmazie,* Berlin, 1988, Springer-Verlag.

CODONOPSIS

Botanical Name: *Codonopsis pilosula*
Family: Campanulaceae
Plant Part Used: Root

PRESCRIBING INFORMATION

Actions

Tonic

Potential Indications

Based on appropriate evaluation of the patient, practitioners should consider prescribing Codonopsis in formulations in the context of:
- Fatigue, loss of appetite, shortness of breath associated with chronic cough or palpitation (5)
- Coronary heart disease (4)
- Improving red blood cell production and hemoglobin concentration (7)
- Adjuvant therapy for cancer (3)

Contraindications

None known.

Warnings and Precautions

None required.

Interactions

None known.

Use in Pregnancy and Lactation

No adverse effects expected.

Side Effects

None expected if taken within the recommended dose range.

Dosage

Dose per day*	**Dose per week***
4.5-8.5 ml of 1:2 liquid extract	30-60 ml of 1:2 liquid extract

SUPPORTING INFORMATION

Traditional Prescribing

Uses and properties from TCM include:
- Reinforcing *qi* and invigorating the functions of the *spleen* and *lung*[1,2]
- Lack of appetite, fatigue, tired limbs, diarrhea, vomiting[2]
- Chronic cough and shortness of breath, shortness of breath with palpitation[2,3]
- Symptoms of prolapse of the uterus, stomach, and anus[2]

Codonopsis is regarded in TCM as having similar functions to those of Korean ginseng root, although not as strong.[2] Codonopsis contains different constituents to Korean ginseng and does not contain triterpenoid saponins.[4]

Codonopsis *continued on page 155*

*This dose range is adapted from dried plant doses administered by decoction in TCM.[1] The author's experience and the fact that ethanol-water is a more effective solvent than water for many phytochemicals are taken into account.

Pharmacologic Research

- Codonopsis extract weakly stimulated human lymphocytes *in vitro*.[5]
- Codonopsis demonstrated the following effects in experimental models:[3]
- Promoted phagocytic activity of peritoneal macrophages (*in vitro*, *in vivo*)
- Increased red blood cell production and hemoglobin concentration (oral)
- Elevated blood glucose (oral)
- Codonopsis extract demonstrated protective activity in experimentally induced gastric ulcers, including the stress-induced model. Pepsin secretion was also reduced.[6] In another model, oral decoction of Codonopsis increased serum gastrin levels with no change in gastric acidity or plasma somatostatin.[7]
- Codonopsis prolonged life span in an experimental model of SLE. Production of anti-double-stranded deoxyribonucleic acid (DNA) antibodies was also inhibited.[8]

Clinical Studies

- Preliminary studies indicate that Codonopsis can improve the defective *in vitro* interleukin-2 production in patients with SLE.[8]
- Codonopsis liquor significantly decreased platelet aggregation in patients with coronary heart disease with blood stasis after 4 weeks of treatment. The inhibition of platelet aggregation did not occur via elevation of fibrinolytic activity.[9]
- Some benefit was observed for patients with cancer who were treated with Codonopsis as an adjuvant during radiotherapy. Compared with controls, Codonopsis reduced the immunosuppressive effect of radiotherapy but had no effect on most humoral immune parameters. A slight increase in immunoglobulin M (IgM) was observed in the treated patients.[10]

REFERENCES

1 Pharmacopoeia Commission of the People's Republic of China: *Pharmacopoeia of the People's Republic of China*, English ed, Beijing, 1997, Chemical Industry Press.
2 Bensky D, Gamble A: *Chinese herbal medicine materia medica*, Seattle, 1986, Eastland Press.
3 Chang HM, But PP: *Pharmacology and applications of Chinese materia medica*, Singapore, 1987, World Scientific.
4 Wong MP, Chiang TC, Chang HM: *Planta Med* 49(1):60, 1983.
5 Shan BE et al: *Int J Immunopharmacol* 21(3):149-159, 1999.
6 Wang ZT et al: *Gen Pharmacol* 28(3):469-473, 1997.
7 Chen SF et al: *Zhongguo Zhongyao Zazhi* 23(5):299-301, 1998.
8 Chen JR et al: *Am J Chin Med* 21(3-4):257-262, 1993.
9 Xu X, Wang SR, Lin Q: *Chung Kuo Chung Hsi I Chieh Ho Tsa Chih* 15(7):398-400, 1995.
10 Zeng XL, Li XA, Zhang BY: *Chung Kuo Chung Hsi I Chieh Ho Tsa Chih* 12(10):607, 581, 1992.

COLEUS

Botanical Names: *Coleus forskohlii, Plectranthus forskohlii#*
Family: Labiatae
Plant Part Used: Root

PRESCRIBING INFORMATION

Actions	Hypotensive, antiplatelet, bronchospasmolytic, spasmolytic, cardiotonic, digestive stimulant, aromatic digestive
Potential Indications	Based on appropriate evaluation of the patient, practitioners should consider prescribing Coleus in formulations in the context of: • Congestive heart disease *(4a)* • Asthma, psoriasis *(4a)* • Topical treatment for glaucoma* *(4a)* • Hypertension, ischemic heart disease, thrombosis (resulting from antiplatelet activity) *(7)*
Contraindications	Given its hypotensive effect, Coleus is contraindicated in patients with hypotension.
Warnings and Precautions	Coleus should be used cautiously in patients taking prescribed medication and those with peptic ulcer.
Interactions	Because of its unique pharmacologic activity, forskolin, the active constituent of Coleus, has the ability to potentiate many drugs. Coleus should therefore be used cautiously in patients taking prescribed medication, especially hypotensive and antiplatelet drugs.
Use in Pregnancy and Lactation	No adverse effects expected.
Side Effects	None expected if taken within the recommended dose range.

Dosage

Dose per day**	Dose per week**
6-13 ml of 1:1 liquid extract	40-90 ml of 1:1 liquid extract

Extracts providing quantified levels of forskolin are recommended. Ideally, aqueous ethanol extracts should contain not less than 2.5 mg/ml of forskolin.

For glaucoma, a solution of approximately 4 to 6 drops of a 1:1 extract is prepared in an eye bath of recently boiled water or saline. Liquid should be allowed to cool before applying to the eye. (Allowing the alcohol to evaporate before putting near the eye is important.)**

Coleus *continued on page 157*

#Alternative name.
*The alcohol must be evaporated before putting the liquid extract near the eye. (See "Dosage" section in this monograph.)
**This dose range is extrapolated from scientific and clinical investigations of forskolin.[1]

SUPPORTING INFORMATION

Traditional Prescribing

Although closely related species of Coleus are used in traditional Ayurvedic medicine, *Coleus forskohlii* has been used only as a condiment in India, with the roots prepared as a pickle.[2]

Pharmacologic Research

Coleus root contains the diterpene forskolin.[3]

Forskolin has demonstrated extensive pharmacologic activity (usually *in vitro* or *in vivo* by injection). Forskolin is known to activate adenylate cyclase, which catalyzes the production of cAMP.[3] Most of the pharmacologic properties described here are a consequence of this property. Forskolin:

- Lowered normal or elevated blood pressure *in vivo* (injection, oral) by relaxing arteriolar smooth muscle[4]
- Demonstrated positive inotropic action (increased force of contraction) on isolated heart muscle[4] and *in vivo* (by injection)[5]
- Inhibited platelet aggregation *in vitro*[4] and *in vivo*[6] (Oral administration of *Coleus forskohlii* extract [standardized for forskolin] demonstrated antithrombotic activity *in vivo*.)[6]
- Increased cerebral blood flow *in vivo* (by injection), having a direct vasodilator effect[7]
- Relaxed isolated bronchial smooth muscle[8] and prevented experimentally induced bronchospasm *in vivo* (by intravenous and intraduodenal injection)[9]
- Stimulated lipolysis *in vitro*[10] and inhibited glucose uptake *in vitro*[11]
- Potentiated the secretagogue effects of glucose *in vitro*[12] and stimulated the release of somatostatin and glucagon from isolated pancreatic islet cells[13]
- Stimulated thyroid function with increased thyroid hormone production in the isolated organ[14] (However, low concentrations of forskolin inhibited thyroid function *in vitro* [thyroid cells].)[15]
- Enhanced secretion of acid and pepsinogen from the gastric mucosa of isolated tissue[16]
- Stimulated amylase secretion from parotid gland tissue[17] and acted synergistically with cholecystokinin in stimulating amylase release from exocrine pancreatic tissue[18]
- Acted synergistically with FSH and LH on estrogen and progesterone production and with adrenocorticotropin hormone (ACTH) on corticosteroid production *in vitro*[19]
- Inhibited melanoma cell–induced platelet aggregation and reduced pulmonary tumor colonization *in vivo* (by injection)[20]
- Lowered intraocular pressure[19]
- Inhibited the release of inflammatory mediators *in vitro*[21] and partially inhibited B-lymphocyte activation *in vitro*[22]

Coleus continued on page 158

Clinical Studies

No clinical studies have been conducted using Coleus. The following studies have been conducted using forskolin or a water-soluble derivative.

- Human studies confirmed that topical application of forskolin (50 µl of a 1% solution) lowers intraocular pressure[23,24] by reducing the flow of aqueous humor. In India, the clinical value by topical application of forskolin for glaucoma has been confirmed.[25]

- Forskolin improved symptoms in a small number of patients with psoriasis.[26]

- Initial studies on patients with congestive cardiomyopathy and coronary artery disease confirmed that forskolin improved cardiac function and myocardial contractility.[25] In another trial (open, controlled design), no increase in myocardial contractility at the tested intravenous dose of forskolin was observed, but left ventricular function was improved. Although higher doses of forskolin did increase myocardial contractility, the accompanying large reduction in blood pressure may preclude such doses in congestive heart failure.[27] Although these trials used forskolin by injection, clinical trials have successfully used oral doses of a water-soluble forskolin derivative to treat acute heart failure.[28]

- Clinical studies demonstrated a bronchodilating effect in patients with asthma, as well as those with and without chemically induced bronchoconstriction. Forskolin was inhaled at a dose of 1 to 10 mg per puff and, by this route, caused no side effects, although its action was short-lived.[29,30] Forskolin also countered chemically induced bronchoconstriction in a double-blind, placebo-controlled, crossover, comparative trial involving healthy volunteers. The administered doses were 2 mg and 10 mg of forskolin by inhalation.[31]

REFERENCES

1 Wagner H, Hikino H, Farnsworth NR, editors: *Economic and medicinal plant research*, London, 1988, Academic Press.

2 Valdes LJ, Mislankar SG, Paul AG: *Econ Bot* 41(4):474-483, 1987.

3 Seamon KB, Daly JW: *J Cyclic Nucleotide Res* 7(4):201-224, 1981.

4 de Souza NJ, Dohadwalla AN, Reden J: *Med Res Rev* 3(2):201-219, 1983.

5 Dubey MP et al: *J Ethnopharmacol* 3(1):1-13, 1981.

6 de Souza NJ: *J Ethnopharmacol* 38(2-3):177-180, 1993.

7 Wysham DG, Brotherton AF, Heistad DD: *Stroke* 17(6):1299-1303, 1986.

8 Burka JF: *J Pharmacol Exp Ther* 225(2):427-435, 1983.

9 Chang J et al: *Eur J Pharmacol* 101(3-4):271-274, 1984.

10 Ho R, Shi QH: *Biochem Biophys Res Commun* 107(1):157-164, 1982.

11 Laurenza A, Sutkowski EM, Seamon KB: *Trends Pharmacol Sci* 10(11):442-447, 1989.

12 Henquin JC, Meissner HP: *Endocrinology* 115(3):1125-1134, 1984.

13 Hermansen K: *Endocrinology* 116(6):2251-2258, 1985.

14 Laurberg P: *FEBS Lett* 170(2):273-276, 1984.

15 Brandi ML et al: *Acta Endocrinol* 107(2):225-229, 1984.

16 Hersey SJ, Owirodu A, Miller M: *Biochim Biophys Acta* 755(2):293-299, 1983.

17 Watson EL, Dowd FJ: *Biochem Biophys Res Commun* 111(1):21-27, 1983.

18 Willems PH et al: *Biochim Biophys Acta* 802(2):209-214, 1984.

Coleus *continued on page 159*

19 Season KB, Daly JW: Cited in Greengard P, Robison GA, editors: *Advances in cyclic nucleotide and protein phosphorylation research,* vol 20, New York, 1986, Raven Press.

20 Agarwal KC, Parks RE Jr: *Int J Cancer* 32(6):801-804, 1983.

21 Marone G et al: *Biochem Pharmacol* 36(1):13-20, 1987.

22 Holte H et al: *Eur J Immunol* 18(9):1359-1366, 1988.

23 Burstein NL, Sears ML, Mead A: *Exp Eye Res* 39(6):745-749, 1984.

24 Caprioli J, Sears M: *Lancet* 1(8331):958-960, 1983.

25 Rupp RH, de Souza NJ, Dohadwalla AN, editors: From the proceedings of the International Symposium on Forskolin: Its Chemical, Biologic and Medical Potential, Bombay, January 28-29, 1985, Bombay, 1986, Alfredo Borges Associates.

26 Bonczkowitz H, Methner GF: *Akt Dermatol* 10:12, 1984.

27 Kramer W et al: *Arzneim Forsch* 37(3):364-367, 1987.

28 Hosono M: *Nippon Yakurigaku Zasshi* 114(2):83-88, 1999.

29 Lichey I et al: *Lancet* 2(8395):167, 1984.

30 Bauer K et al: *Clin Pharmacol Ther* 3(1):76-83, 1993.

31 Kaik G, Witte PU: *Wien Med Wochenschr* 136(23-24):637-641, 1986.

CORN SILK

Botanical Name: *Zea mays*
Family: Gramineae
Plant Part Used: Style and stigma

PRESCRIBING INFORMATION

Actions

Diuretic, antilithic, urinary demulcent

Potential Indications

Based on appropriate evaluation of the patient, practitioners should consider prescribing corn silk in formulations in the context of:
- Cystitis, urethritis, bedwetting, bladder disorders of children, urinary calculi, prostatitis (5)
- Stimulating diuresis, improving renal function (4,5)

Contraindications

None known.

Warnings and Precautions

None required.

Interactions

None known.

Use in Pregnancy and Lactation

No adverse effects expected.

Side Effects

None expected if taken within the recommended dose range.

Dosage

Dose per day*	Dose per week*
2-6 ml of 1:1 liquid extract	15-40 ml of 1:1 liquid extract

SUPPORTING INFORMATION

Traditional Prescribing

Traditional Western herbal medicine uses include:
- Cystitis, urethritis, pyelitis, nocturnal enuresis, urinary calculi or gravel, strangury, prostatitis, gonorrhea[1,2]
- Bladder disorders of children[2]

Uses and properties from TCM include edema, hepatitis, nephritis, cholelithiasis, jaundice, and hypertension.[3,4]

Corn silk has also been used traditionally as a diuretic and for treating dropsy in Indonesia[5] and urinary retention in Fiji.[6]

Corn silk was official in the USP from 1894 to 1906 and NF from 1916 to 1946 and was used as a diuretic. From as far back as the sixteenth century, Native Americans used corn products for medicinal purposes.[7]

Corn Silk *continued on page 161*

*This dose range is extrapolated from British Herbal Pharmacopoeia 1983, the British Herbal Compendium 1992, and the author's education and experience.

Pharmacologic Research

- Diuretic activity has been confirmed *in vivo*.[8]
- Corn silk extract inhibited tumor necrosis factor-alpha–induced and bacterial lipopolysaccharide–induced epithelial cell adhesion *in vitro*.[9]

Clinical Studies

- Eight to 10 grams of corn silk decoction produced a mild diuretic effect in normal volunteers.[2]
- In uncontrolled trials in China, corn silk decoction produced diuretic effects in renal edema, ascites, and nutritional edema and improved renal function and albuminuria in patients with chronic nephritis and nephrotic syndrome. Decoction of 50 g of fresh herb was recommended, with the dose not exceeding the daily urine output.[2]

REFERENCES

1 British Herbal Medicine Association's Scientific Committee: *British herbal pharmacopoeia,* Bournemouth, 1983, BHMA.

2 Felter HW, Lloyd JU: *King's American dispensatory,* ed 18, rev 3, Portland, 1905, reprinted 1983, Eclectic Medical Publications.

3 Chang HM, But PP: *Pharmacology and applications of Chinese materia medica,* Singapore, 1987, World Scientific.

4 Bensky D, Gamble A: *Chinese herbal medicine materia medica,* Seattle, 1986, Eastland Press.

5 Dharma AP: *Indonesian medicinal plants,* Jakarta, 1987, Balai Pustaka.

6 Cambie RC, Ash J: *Fijian medicinal plants,* Melbourne, Australia, 1994, CSIRO Publishing.

7 Vogel VJ: *American Indian medicine,* Norman, Okla, 1970, University of Oklahoma Press.

8 Rebuelta M et al: *Plantes Med Phytother* 21:2672-275, 1987.

9 Habtemariam S: *Plant Med* 64(4):314-318, 1998.

COUCH GRASS

Botanical Names: *Agropyron repens, Elymus repens,*[#^] *Elytrigia repens*[#]
Family: Gramineae
Plant Part Used: Rhizome

PRESCRIBING INFORMATION

Actions

Soothing diuretic, urinary demulcent

Potential Indications

Based on appropriate evaluation of the patient, practitioners should consider prescribing couch grass in formulations in the context of:
- Inflammation and infection of the urinary tract, preventing kidney gravel *(4,5)*
- Prostatitis, benign prostatic hyperplasia *(5)*
- Gout, rheumatism, jaundice *(5)*

Contraindications

The Commission E recommends copious fluid intake to assist in reducing microorganisms in the urinary tract, but this should not be undertaken if edema resulting from impaired cardiac or renal function is present.[2]

Warnings and Precautions

None required.

Interactions

None known.

Use in Pregnancy and Lactation

No adverse effects expected.

Side Effects

None expected if taken within the recommended dose range.

Dosage

Dose per day*	Dose per week*
3-6 ml of 1:1 liquid extract	20-40 ml of 1:1 liquid extract

SUPPORTING INFORMATION

Traditional Prescribing

Traditional Western herbal medicine uses include:
- Irritation or inflammation of the urinary tract, including cystitis, urethritis, prostatitis, benign prostatic hyperplasia, and urinary calculi[3,4]
- Gout, rheumatism, jaundice[2]

Pharmacologic Research

Oral administration of couch grass infusion demonstrated the following results in a calcium oxalate urolithiasis model: a decrease in citraturia when combined with a high carbohydrate diet and an increase in calciuria and decrease in magnesiuria when combined with a standard diet.[5]

Couch Grass *continued on page 163*

[#]Alternative name.
[^]Adopted by the American Herbal Products Association as the new botanical name.[1]
*This dose range is extrapolated from the *British Herbal Pharmacopoeia* 1983 and the author's education and experience.

Clinical Studies

No clinical studies using couch grass have been found.

In Germany, the Commission E supports using couch grass with copious fluid intake to treat inflammatory diseases of the urinary tract and for preventing kidney gravel.[2]

REFERENCES

1 McGuffin M, editor: *Herbs of commerce*, ed 2 [draft 3.3], Bethesda, Md, 1998, American Herbal Products Association.
2 Blumenthal M et al, editors: *The complete German Commission E monographs: therapeutic guide to herbal medicines*, Austin, 1998, American Botanical Council.
3 British Herbal Medicine Association's Scientific Committee: *British herbal pharmacopoeia*, Bournemouth, 1983, BHMA.
4 Felter HW, Lloyd JU: *King's American dispensatory*, ed 18, rev 3, Portland, 1905, reprinted 1983, Eclectic Medical Publications.
5 Grases F et al: *J Ethnopharmacol* 45(3):211-214, 1995.

CRAMP BARK

Botanical Names: *Viburnum opulus, Viburnum opulus* var. *americanum*[+]
Family: Caprifoliaceae
Plant Part Used: Bark

PRESCRIBING INFORMATION

Actions

Spasmolytic, mild sedative, astringent, hypotensive, peripheral vasodilator

Potential Indications

Based on appropriate evaluation of the patient, practitioners should consider prescribing cramp bark in formulations in the context of:
- Uterine pain, dysmenorrhea (5)
- Cramps of both skeletal and smooth muscle (5)
- Threatened miscarriage, preparation for parturition (5)
- Hypertension (6)

Contraindications

None known.

Warnings and Precautions

None required.

Interactions

None known.

Use in Pregnancy and Lactation

No adverse effects expected.

Side Effects

None expected if taken within the recommended dose range.

Dosage

*Dose per day**	*Dose per week**
2.0-4.5 ml of 1:2 liquid extract	15-30 ml of 1:2 liquid extract

SUPPORTING INFORMATION

Traditional Prescribing

Traditional Western herbal medicine uses include:
- Cramps and spasms of all kinds; cramps in the legs[1,2]
- Uterine dysfunction, uterine pain, with spasmodic action; ovarian pain[1,2]
- Dysmenorrhea, bearing-down, expulsive pains; menopausal metrorrhagia, pain in thighs and back[1,2]
- Convulsions during pregnancy or labor; threatened miscarriage; as a partus preparator[1,2]
- Spasmodic contraction of the bladder, infantile enuresis; asthma[1,2]
- Angina, palpitations,[3] hypertension[4]

Native Americans used cramp bark as a treatment for stomach cramps, other cramps, "pain over the whole body," and uterine prolapse.

Cramp Bark *continued on page 165*

[+]Medicinally interchangeable species.
*This dose range is extrapolated from the *American Herbal Pharmacopoeia* and the author's education and experience.

Cramp bark was also used as a febrifuge, emetic, and tonic. Cramp bark was official in the USP from 1894 to 1916 and NF from 1916 to 1960 and was listed as a sedative and antispasmodic.[4,5]

Pharmacologic Research

The constituents of cramp bark are not well defined, but the presence of catechin and epicatechin and the absence of amentoflavone is considered characteristic (for differentiation from *Viburnum prunifolium* [black haw]). The coumarins scopoletin and scopolin are also present, although apparently only in trace amounts.[4]

- Laboratory studies conducted subsequent to 1940 have shown cramp bark extract and its constituents to have relaxing effects on isolated uterine tissue and organ.[6-8] An *in vitro* study found the methanol extract of cramp bark to be the most active uterine spasmolytic compared with other *Viburnum* species, including black haw.[7] (Pharmacologic studies conducted before 1940 cannot be trusted for the correct identification of plant material.[4])

- Intravenous injection of a sesquiterpene dialdehyde fraction of cramp bark lowered heart rate and blood pressure *in vivo*. The authors suggested that cramp bark had a direct musculotrophic action in addition to weakly potentiating the action of acetylcholinesterase.[9]

- Alcoholic extracts of cramp bark increased blood coaguability and demonstrated hemostatic activity in experimental models (route unknown).[10]

- Aqueous extracts of cramp bark exhibited a digitalis-type cardiotonic effect in the isolated heart, but cramp bark does not contain cardiac glycosides.[11]

- Crude aqueous-alcoholic extracts of cramp bark were found to have inhibitory effects on the enzymes elastase, trypsin, α-chymotrypsin, and angiotensin I *in vitro*. This activity was attributed to the polyphenolic component (stannins) such as catechin.[12]

Clinical Studies

No clinical trials have been conducted, although case reports from the mid-1800s in the United States indicate that cramp bark was effective as a uterine sedative.[13]

REFERENCES

1 Felter HW, Lloyd JU: *King's American dispensatory*, ed 18, rev 3, Portland, 1905, reprinted 1983, Eclectic Medical Publications.

2 British Herbal Medicine Association's Scientific Committee: *British herbal pharmacopoeia*, Bournemouth, 1983, BHMA.

3 Bartram T: *Encyclopedia of herbal medicine*, ed 1, Dorset, UK, 1995, Grace Publishers.

4 *American Herbal Pharmacopoeia: Cramp bark—Viburnum opulus: analytical, quality control, and therapeutic monograph*, Santa Cruz, February 2000, American Herbal Pharmacopoeia.

5 Vogel VJ: *American Indian medicine*, Norman, Okla, 1970, University of Oklahoma Press.

6 Costello CH, Lynn EV: *J Am Pharm Assoc* 32:20-22, 1943.

7 Jarboe CH et al: *Nature* 212(64):837, 1966.

8 Jarboe CH et al: *J Med Chem* 10:488-489, 1967.

9 Nicholson JA, Darby TD, Jarboe CH: *Proc Soc Exp Biol Med* 140(2):457-461, 1972.

10 Smirnova AS, Yadrova VM: *Farmatsiya* 17(4):42-45, 1968.

11 Vlad L, Munta A, Crisan IG: *Planta Med* 31:228-231, 1977.

12 Jonadet M et al: *Pharm Acta Helv* 64(3):94-96, 1989.

13 Munch JC: *Pharm Arch* 11(3):33-37, 1940.

CRANESBILL

Botanical Name: *Geranium maculatum*
Family: Geraniaceae
Plant Part Used: Root

PRESCRIBING INFORMATION

Actions

Astringent, antidiarrheal, antihemorrhagic

Potential Indications

Based on appropriate evaluation of the patient, practitioners should consider prescribing cranesbill root in formulations in the context of:
- Diarrhea, dysentery, gastrointestinal ulceration or bleeding *(5)*
- Menorrhagia, metrorrhagia *(5)*
- Topical treatment for leukorrhea, indolent ulcers *(5)*

Contraindications

None known.

Warnings and Precautions

Because of the tannin content of this herb, long-term use should be avoided. Cranesbill should be used cautiously in highly inflamed or ulcerated conditions of the gastrointestinal tract.

Interactions

None known.

Use in Pregnancy and Lactation

No adverse effects expected.

Side Effects

None expected if taken within the recommended dose range.

Dosage

Dose per day*	Dose per week*
2-5 ml of 1:2 liquid extract	15-35 ml of 1:2 liquid extract

SUPPORTING INFORMATION

Traditional Prescribing

Traditional Western herbal medicine uses include:
- Diarrhea, dysentery, hemorrhoids, peptic and duodenal ulceration, hematemesis, melena, chronic mucous discharges[1,2]
- Menorrhagia, metrorrhagia[1]
- Topically for leukorrhea, indolent ulcers[1]

Native Americans used cranesbill root for hemoptysis and venereal disease. Externally, cranesbill root was used for bleeding wounds, burns, leukorrhea, intestinal ailments, diarrhea, sore gums, gum disease, toothache, neuralgia, and hemorrhoids. Cranesbill root was official in the USP from 1820 to 1916, the NF from 1916 to 1936, and was used as a tonic and astringent.[3]

Cranesbill *continued on page 167*

*This dose range is extrapolated from the British Herbal Pharmacopoeia 1983.

Pharmacologic Research

No pharmacologic information relevant to the current use of cranesbill root has been found.

Clinical Studies

No clinical studies using cranesbill root have been found.

REFERENCES

1 British Herbal Medicine Association's Scientific Committee: *British herbal pharmacopoeia,* Bournemouth, 1983, BHMA.
2 Felter HW, Lloyd JU: *King's American dispensatory,* ed 18, rev 3, Portland, 1905, reprinted 1983, Eclectic Medical Publications.
3 Vogel VJ: *American Indian medicine,* Norman, Okla, 1970, University of Oklahoma Press.

CRATAEVA

Botanical Names: *Crataeva nurvala, Crateva nurvala*[#]
Family: Capparidaceae (=Capparaceae)
Plant Part Used: Bark

PRESCRIBING INFORMATION

Actions

Antilithic, bladder tonic, antiinflammatory

Potential Indications

Based on appropriate evaluation of the patient, practitioners should consider prescribing Crataeva in formulations in the context of:
- Chronic and acute urinary tract infections *(4)*
- Hypotonic, atonic or neurogenic bladder *(4)*
- Incontinence and possibly enuresis *(4)*
- Prevention and treatment of kidney, ureter, and bladder stones *(4,5)*
- Other urinary system disorders *(5)*

Contraindications

None known.

Warnings and Precautions

None required.

Interactions

None known.

Use in Pregnancy and Lactation

No adverse effects expected.

Side Effects

None expected if taken within the recommended dose range.

Dosage

Dose per day[*]	*Dose per week*[*]
6-14 ml of 1:2 liquid extract	40-100 ml of 1:2 liquid extract

Crataeva may also be administered as a decoction of the dried bark.

SUPPORTING INFORMATION

Traditional Prescribing

Traditional Ayurvedic uses include:
- Disorders of urinary system, especially kidney and bladder stones[1]
- Deep-seated suppurative inflammation, small joint diseases, osteomyelitis[2]
- Intestinal and hepatic infestation[2]
- Snakebite; also used as an antiperiodic (to treat a periodic illness such as malaria)[1]

Pharmacologic Research

Key constituents of Crataeva bark include sterols (especially lupeol, a pentacyclic triterpene) and flavonoids. The Capparidaceae family is also characterized by the presence of glucosinolates.[3]

Crataeva *continued on page 169*

[#]Alternative name.
[*]This dose range is extrapolated from traditional Ayurvedic medicine[1] and the author's education and experience.

- Crataeva increased the tone of smooth and skeletal muscle *in vitro*.[4]
- The petroleum ether extract of Crataeva was shown to inhibit both acute and chronic inflammation *in vivo* (route unknown).[5] Oral lupeol exerted significant dose-dependent antiinflammatory activity in several models of acute and chronic inflammation. Analgesic or antipyretic properties were not displayed.[6]
- Lupeol reduced foot pad thickness (a measure of inflammation) and complement activity in an experimental model of arthritis (route unknown).[7] Lupeol reduced paw swelling, loss of body weight, and cellular infiltration into the synovial cavity of proximal interphalangeal joints in a model of adjuvant-induced arthritis (oral administration).[8]
- Crataeva significantly decreased bladder stone formation and reduced bladder edema, ulceration, and cellular infiltration compared with controls in an experimental model (route unknown).[9] Oral treatment increased bladder tone[9] and decreased the tendency to form calcium oxalate kidney stones.[10]
- Oral doses of an alcoholic extract of Crataeva demonstrated significant dose-dependent protective activity against experimental urinary stone formation and reversed the biochemical parameters associated with urolith formation toward normal levels.[11]
- Crataeva decoction lowered the induced levels of small intestinal sodium and potassium-adenosinetriphosphatase (Na^+,K^+-ATPase) compared with controls in animals fed a calculi-producing diet. Changes in Na^+,K^+-ATPase levels may regulate the uptake of minerals.[12]
- Changes in the activities of Na^+,K^+-ATPase, aspartate aminotransferase, and glychollate oxidase (the major oxalate-synthesizing enzyme) were reduced by treatment with Crataeva decoction in an experimental model of calcium oxalate urolithiasis.[13]
- Oral administration of lupeol inhibited stone formation, exhibited stone-dissolving activity, and facilitated the passage of very small calculi from the bladder. Altered levels of urea and creatinine, indicative of kidney dysfunction, were restored to normal.[14] Oral lupeol also dose-dependently reduced the weight of urinary stones, prevented formation of vesical calculi by reducing calcium phosphate and oxalate levels in the urine, normalized serum and urine biochemical parameters, and reduced inflammation and other damage in the bladder and kidneys in an experimental model of urolithiasis.[15]
- Lupeol reduced markers of crystal deposition in the kidneys and minimized renal tubular damage in experimental models of calcium oxalate stone formation.[16,17] Oral lupeol administration reduced kidney oxalate levels and counteracted free-radical toxicity (indicating cytoprotective and antioxidant actions) in experimental urolithiasis.[18] Lupeol also restored renal thiol status and restored antioxidant enzymes in the kidney and bladder of stone-forming animals. The mechanism behind the protective activity may involve inhibiting calcium oxalate crystal aggregation and enhancing defense systems.[19]

Crataeva *continued on page 170*

- Lupeol produced improvement in renal antioxidant status when coadministered (route unknown) with cadmium (a nephrotoxin) in a chronic toxicity model.[20]

Clinical Studies

- Crataeva decoction relieved frequency, incontinence, pain, and urine retention, increased bladder tone, and increased the force of urination in patients with hypotonic bladder resulting from benign prostatic hyperplasia. Bladder tone, residual volume, and symptoms also improved in cases of persistent hypotonia, atony, and neurogenic bladder after Crataeva treatment.[9]
- The urine of patients became less lithogenic (urinary calcium was reduced, and urinary sodium and magnesium significantly increased) after treatment with Crataeva decoction.[9]
- Twenty six of forty six patients with kidney, ureter, or bladder stones not requiring surgery passed the stones within 10 weeks' treatment with Crataeva decoction. The majority of the remaining patients experienced symptom relief.[9]
- Eighty five percent of patients with proven chronic urinary tract infections were symptom-free after 4 weeks' treatment with Crataeva decoction.[9]

REFERENCES

1 Chopra RN et al: *Chopra's indigenous drugs of India,* ed 2, Calcutta, 1958, reprinted 1982, Academic Publishers.
2 Bharatiya Vidya Bhavan's Swami Prakashananda Ayurveda Research Centre: *Selected medicinal plants of India,* Bombay, 1992, Chemexcil.
3 Prabhakar YS, Suresh Kumar D: *Fitoterapia* 61(2):99-111, 1990.
4 Prasad DN, Das PK, Singh RS: *J Res Ind Med* 1:120, 1966.
5 Das PK et al: *J Res Ind Med* 9:49, 1974.
6 Singh S et al: *Fitoterapia* 68(1):9-16, 1997.
7 Geetha T, Varalakshmi P: *Gen Pharmacol* 32(4):495-497, 1999.
8 Geetha T, Varalakshmi P: *Fitoterapia* 69(1):13-19, 1998.
9 Deshpande PJ, Sahu M, Kamur P: *Indian J Med Res* 76(suppl):46-53, 1982.
10 Varalakshmi P, Shamila Y, Latha E: *J Ethnopharmacol* 28(3):313-321, 1990.
11 Anand R et al: *Fitoterapia* 64:345, 1993.
12 Varalakshmi P et al: *J Ethnopharmacol* 31(1):67-73, 1991.
13 Baskar R, Saravanan N, Varalakshmi P: *Indian J Clin Biochem* 10(2):98-102, 1995.
14 Anand R et al: From the proceedings of the 24th Indian Pharmacologic Society Conference, Ahmedabad, Gujarat, India, December 29-31, 1991, abstract A10.
15 Anand R et al: *Phytother Res* 8(7):417-421, 1994.
16 Malini MM, Baskar R, Varalakshmi P: *Jpn J Med Sci Biol* 48(5-6):211-220, 1995.
17 Vidya L, Varalakshmi P: *Fitoterapia* 71(5):535-543, 2000.
18 Baskar R et al: *Fitoterapia* 67(2):121-125, 1996.
19 Malini MM, Lenin M, Varalakshmi P: *Pharmacol Res* 41(4):413-418, 2000.
20 Nagaraj M, Sunitha S, Varalakshmi P: *J Appl Toxicol* 20(5):413-417, 2000.

DAMIANA

Botanical Names: *Turnera diffusa, Turnera aphrodisiaca*[#]
Family: Turneraceae
Plant Part Used: Leaf

PRESCRIBING INFORMATION

Actions	Nervine tonic, tonic, mild laxative

Potential Indications

Based on appropriate evaluation of the patient, practitioners should consider prescribing damiana in formulations in the context of:
- Nervousness, anxiety, depression *(5)*
- Sexual inadequacy: impotence, frigidity *(5,7)*
- Nervous dyspepsia, constipation *(5)*

Contraindications

None known.

Warnings and Precautions

None required.

Interactions

None known.

Use in Pregnancy and Lactation

No adverse effects expected.

Side Effects

None expected if taken within the recommended dose range.

Dosage

Dose per day*	*Dose per week**
3-6 ml of 1:2 liquid extract	20-40 ml of 1:2 liquid extract

SUPPORTING INFORMATION

Traditional Prescribing

Traditional Western herbal medicine uses include:
- Anxiety, depression, nervous dyspepsia, constipation[1]
- Impotence and frigidity in both sexes,[1,2] irritation of the urinary mucous membranes, renal catarrh[2]

Native Brazilians and Mexicans used damiana, with early documented use by the Mayan people. Uses by native northern Mexicans included muscular and nervous debility, as an aphrodisiac and emmenagogue, for menstrual disorders, to aid in childbirth, and for spermatorrhea, orchitis, nephritis, and irritable bladder. In addition to the aphrodisiac uses, Hispanic herbalists of Mexico used damiana for sterility, nervous disorders, and diabetes.[3-5] Damiana was also consumed in Mexico as a pleasant, stimulating, tonic beverage without the side effects of tea or coffee and was employed therapeutically as a hot drink for suppressed menstruation.[6]

Damiana *continued on page 172*

[#]Alternative name.
*This dose range is extrapolated from the British Pharmaceutical Codex 1934, the British Herbal Pharmacopoeia 1983, the British Herbal Compendium 1992, and the author's education and experience.

Damiana was official in the NF from 1916 to 1942 and was referred to as a stimulant and laxative, with a reputation as an aphrodisiac.[7]

Pharmacologic Research

- A postulated explanation for the aphrodisiac effect of damiana is that its volatile oil might irritate the urethral mucous membranes.[4]
- A methanol extract of damiana induced relaxation of isolated smooth muscle from the corpus cavernosum.[8] Oral administration of damiana extract (0.25 to 1.0 ml/kg) demonstrated a stimulating effect on the sexual behavior of male rats. Copulatory performance was improved in sexually sluggish or impotent animals, but not in potent animals.[9]
- Oral administration of damiana infusion resulted in hypoglycemic activity in an experimental model.[10] Aqueous alcohol (70%) and 100% alcohol extracts of damiana inhibited the formation of gastric lesions in several experimental models after oral or intragastric administration.[11]
- Damiana extract decreased psychomotor activity in an experimental model (administered by injection).[12]

Clinical Studies

No clinical studies using damiana have been found.

REFERENCES

1 British Herbal Medicine Association's Scientific Committee: *British herbal pharmacopoeia,* Bournemouth, 1983, BHMA.

2 Felter HW, Lloyd JU: *King's American dispensatory,* ed 18, rev 3, Portland, 1905, reprinted 1983, Eclectic Medical Publications.

3 Grieve M: *A modern herbal,* New York, 1971, Dover Publications.

4 Tyler VE: *Pharm Hist* 25(2):55-60, 1983.

5 Brinker FJ: *Eclectic dispensatory of botanical therapeutics,* vol 2, Sandy, Oregon, 1995, Eclectic Medical Publications.

6 Lloyd JU: *Pharm Rev* 22:126, 1904.

7 Vogel VJ: *American Indian medicine,* Norman, Okla, 1970, University of Oklahoma Press.

8 Hnatyszyn O et al: From the International Congress and 48th Annual Meeting of the Society for Medicinal Plant Research and the 6th International Congress on Ethnopharmacology of the International Society for Ethnopharmacology, Zurich, September 3-7, 2000, abstract P2A/39.

9 Arletti R et al: *Psychopharmacology* 143(1):15-19, 1999.

10 Perez RM et al: *J Ethnopharmacol* 12(3):253-262, 1984.

11 Gracioso JS et al: *Phytomed* 7(supp 2):92-93, 2000.

12 Jui J: *Lloydia* 29(3):250-259, 1966.

DANDELION

Botanical Name: *Taraxacum officinale*
Family: Compositae
Plant Parts Used: Leaf, root

PRESCRIBING INFORMATION

Actions

Dandelion leaf and root are considered to have similar actions: bitter tonic, choleretic, diuretic (especially leaf), mild laxative, and antirheumatic.

Potential Indications

Based on appropriate evaluation of the patient, practitioners should consider prescribing dandelion leaf or dandelion root in formulations in the context of:
- Cystitis, in combination with uva ursi *(2)*
- Restoration of hepatic and biliary function, dyspepsia *(4,5)*
- Loss of appetite, flatulence, intestinal bloating, to stimulate diuresis *(4)*
- Edema *(5,7)*
- Oliguria, jaundice, gallstones, constipation, muscular rheumatism, chronic skin diseases *(5)*

Both the traditional prescribing information and the information obtained from pharmacologic research suggest that dandelion leaf has the stronger diuretic activity and dandelion root has the stronger choleretic and cholagogue activities. This data should be reflected in the preferred use of the specific plant parts.

Contraindications

Dandelion leaf and root are contraindicated in closure of the bile ducts, cholecystitis, intestinal obstruction,[1] and known allergy. (A sesquiterpene lactone found in both leaf and root is responsible for causing allergic dermatitis. Other constituents within dandelion may also be allergenic.[2])

Warnings and Precautions

Dandelion leaf: despite reports of skin reactions and dermatitis from topical use of dandelion aerial parts, the likelihood of dandelion leaf preparations causing a contact allergy is low. However, people with known sensitivity to other members of the Compositae family (e.g., ragweed, daisies, chrysanthemums) should avoid topical application of dandelion leaf or dandelion leaf products.

Dandelion root: caution is required if gallstones are present.[3]

Interactions

None known.

Use in Pregnancy and Lactation

No adverse effects expected.

Side Effects

None expected if taken within the recommended dose range.

Dandelion *continued on page 174*

Dosage

Dandelion leaf:

*Dose per day**	*Dose per week**
6.0-11.5 ml of 1:1 liquid extract	40-80 ml of 1:1 liquid extract

Dandelion root:

*Dose per day**	*Dose per week**
3 to 6 ml of 1:2 liquid extract	20 to 40 ml of 1:2 liquid extract

SUPPORTING INFORMATION

Traditional Prescribing

Traditional Western herbal medicine uses of dandelion root include:
- Cholecystitis, gallstones, jaundice; atonic dyspepsia with constipation, muscular rheumatism, oliguria[4]
- Sluggishness and enlargement of the liver or spleen; impaired digestion, constipation[5]
- Dropsy, uterine obstruction, chronic skin diseases[5]

In traditional Western herbal medicine, the uses of dandelion leaf are similar to those of dandelion root, but the leaf was considered to be weaker in activity than the root (except for diuretic activity).[4]

Native Americans used dandelion root for heartburn and as a bitter tonic. Dandelion root was official in the USP from 1831 to 1926 and remained official in the NF until 1965. Dandelion root was used as a diuretic, tonic, and mild laxative.[6]

Native Americans also used dandelion leaf as a tonic.[6]

Pharmacologic Research

Dandelion leaf:
- In an early experimental study, a decoction of dandelion leaf administered by injection was shown to increase bile secretion.[7]
- Oral administration of dandelion leaf extract had a strong diuretic effect (even compared with frusemide) in an experimental model. Using high doses, long-term weight loss resulting from diuresis was observed. Because dandelion leaf contains potassium, depletion of this mineral is not a problem. In fact, the diuretic activity may be the result of the potassium content (see later discussion). Dandelion leaf demonstrated stronger activity than did dandelion root.[8]

Dandelion root:
- Dandelion root decoction increased bile secretion *in vivo* when administered by injection. The activity was stronger than that observed for dandelion leaf.[7]

Dandelion *continued on page 175*

*This dose range is extrapolated from the British Herbal Pharmacopoeia 1983, the British Herbal Compendium 1992, and the author's education and experience.

- As previously mentioned, dandelion root extract also demonstrated a mild diuretic effect in an experimental model.[8] Diuretic activity was, however, not observed in another study after either oral or intraperitoneal administration during a 2-hour observation period.[9]
- From the results of their experimental study, the authors concluded that no organic secondary metabolites showing major diuretic activity were present in dandelion root. The high potassium content of dandelion was considered to be the agent responsible for any diuretic activity.[10]
- Ethanol extract of dandelion root demonstrated analgesic and antiinflammatory activity when administered by injection.[9]
- Oral preadministration of an aqueous-ethanolic extract of dandelion root inhibited experimentally induced edema.[11] In another experiment, intraperitoneal treatment also demonstrated partial inhibition.[9]
- An ethanolic extract of dandelion root caused a dose-dependent inhibition of adenosine diphosphate (ADP)–induced aggregation in a preparation of human platelet-rich plasma. Arachidonic acid– and collagen-induced platelet aggregation were not influenced.[12]

Dandelion (part undefined or combined):
- In an *in vitro* study, extracts of dandelion reduced enzymatically induced lipid peroxidation and cytochrome c (with and without the reduced form of nicotinamide-adenine dinnucleotide phosphate [NADPH]) in a dose-dependent manner.[13]
- Dandelion inhibited the production of tumor necrosis factor-alpha (TNF-α) from primary cultures of astrocytes by inhibiting interleukin-1 production.[14] In an earlier *in vitro* study, aqueous solution of dandelion restored the nitric oxide production from γ-interferon-primed peritoneal macrophages as a result of TNF-α secretion.[15]
- Dandelion extracts were shown to increase bile secretion in experimental models. A choleretic effect was described after administering the dose of dandelion by cannula.[16,17]
- Oral administration of dandelion root and leaf did not significantly affect glucose homeostasis in either nondiabetic animals or streptozotocin-induced diabetes.[18] In another study, oral doses of whole dandelion produced a hypoglycemic effect in normal animals, without a significant response in alloxan-induced diabetes.[19]
- Dandelion extract increased the activity of cytostatic and surgical treatments in a transplantable tumor model. An independent inhibitory action on the tumor and metastases was also shown. The toxic effect of cyclophosphamide on red blood cells was lessened.[20] A hot water extract from dandelion also showed antitumor activity following intraperitoneal administration.[21]

Clinical Studies

- An herbal preparation containing Calendula, dandelion, St. John's wort, lemon balm, and fennel reduced intestinal pain in an uncontrolled trial involving patients with chronic colitis. Defecation was normalized in patients with diarrhea syndrome.[22]

Dandelion *continued on page 176*

- In a randomized, prospective study, treatment of ureteric calculi with either spasmoanalgesic therapy or an herbal preparation was compared. The preparation contained dandelion root and leaf, golden rod, *Rubia tinctorum*, *Ammi visnaga*, and a small amount of escin (a constituent of horsechestnut seed). No significant difference was observed with regard to the transit times of the stones between the two groups, but side effects and treatment costs were less in the herbal therapy group. The strength of the herbal extracts in these capsules was not defined.[23]
- In a double-blind, placebo-controlled, randomized, clinical trial, 57 women with recurrent cystitis received either herbal treatment (standardized uva ursi extract and dandelion leaf and root extract) or placebo. Treatment for 1 month significantly reduced the recurrence of cystitis during the 1-year follow-up period, with no incidence of cystitis in the herbal group and a 23% occurrence in the placebo group. No side effects were reported. The dose of the individual herbs was not specified.[24]
- In Germany, the Commission E supports using dandelion leaf to treat loss of appetite, dyspepsia, bloating, and flatulence. Dandelion root with leaf is recommended to treat disturbed bile flow, loss of appetite, and dyspepsia. This combination is also used to stimulate diuresis.[3]
- ESCOP recommends dandelion leaf as adjuvant therapy for treatments when enhanced urinary output is desirable, for example, in cases of rheumatism and for preventing renal gravel.[25]
- ESCOP recommends dandelion root for restoring hepatic and biliary function, dyspepsia, and loss of appetite.[25]

REFERENCES

1 British Herbal Medicine Association: *British herbal compendium,* Bournemouth, 1992, BHMA.
2 de Smet PAGM et al, editors: *Adverse effects of herbal drugs,* Berlin, 1993, Springer-Verlag.
3 Blumenthal M et al, editors: *The complete German Commission E monographs: therapeutic guide to herbal medicines,* Austin, 1998, American Botanical Council.
4 British Herbal Medicine Association's Scientific Committee: *British herbal pharmacopoeia,* Bournemouth, 1983, BHMA.
5 Felter HW, Lloyd JU: *King's American dispensatory,* ed 18, rev 3, Portland, 1905, reprinted 1983, Eclectic Medical Publications.
6 Vogel VJ: *American Indian medicine,* Norman, Okla, 1970, University of Oklahoma Press.
7 Chabrol E et al: *CR Soc Biol* 108:1100-1102, 1931.
8 Racz-Kotilla E, Racz G, Solomon A: *Planta Med* 26:212-217, 1974.
9 Tita B et al: *Pharmacology Research* 27(suppl 1):23-24, 1993.
10 Hook I, McGee A, Henman A: *Int J Pharmacog* 31(1):29-34, 1993.
11 Mascolo N et al: *Phytother Res* 1:28-31, 1987.
12 Neef H et al: *Phytother Res* 10:S138-S140, 1996.
13 Hagymasi K et al: *Phytother Res* 14(1):43-44, 2000.
14 Kim HM et al: *Immunopharmacol Immunotoxicol* 22(3):519-530, 2000.
15 Kim HM et al: *Immunopharmacol Immunotoxicol* 20(2):283-297, 1998.
16 Bussemaker J: *Naunyn-Schmied Arch Exper Pathol Pharm* 181:512-513, 1936.
17 Bohm K: *Arzneim Forsch* 9:376-378, 1959.
18 Swanston-Flatt SK et al: *Diabetes Res* 10(2):69-73, 1989.
19 Akhtar MS, Khan QM, Khaliq T: *JPMA J Pak Med Assoc* 35(7):207-210, 1985.
20 Razina TG et al: *Rastitel'nye Resursy* 34(1):64-68, 1998.

Dandelion *continued on page 177*

21 Baba K, Abe S, Mizuno D: *Yakugaku Zasshi* 101:538-543, 1981.

22 Chakurski I et al: *Vutr Boles* 20(6):51-54, 1981.

23 Bach D et al: *Forschr Med* 101(8):337-342, 1983.

24 Larsson B, Jonasson A, Fianu S: *Curr Ther Res Clin Exp* 53(4):441-443, 1993.

25 Scientific Committee of the European Scientific Cooperative on Phytotherapy [ESCOP]: *ESCOP monographs: Taraxaci folium/radix*. European Scientific Cooperative on Phytotherapy, ESCOP Secretariat, Argyle House, Gandy Street, Exeter, Devon, EX4 3LS, United Kingdom, March 1996.

DEVIL'S CLAW

Other Common Names: Harpagophytum, grapple plant
Botanical Name: *Harpagophytum procumbens*
Family: Pedaliaceae
Plant Part Used: Root

PRESCRIBING INFORMATION

Actions	Antiinflammatory, antirheumatic, analgesic, bitter tonic
Potential Indications	Based on appropriate evaluation of the patient, practitioners should consider prescribing devil's claw in formulations in the context of: • Rheumatic and arthritic conditions *(2,4,5)* • Osteoarthritis *(2,4)* • Chronic back pain *(2,5)* • Tendinitis *(4)* • Loss of appetite, dyspepsia *(4,6)* • Topical treatment for skin lesions, such as wounds and ulcers *(6)*
Contraindications	The Commission E advises the following contraindications: gastric and duodenal ulcers and gallstones. However, any health risks are theoretical in nature, being projected from the bitter tonic activity.
Warnings and Precautions	None required.
Interactions	A case of purpurea was reported in a patient taking warfarin and devil's claw.[1] However, key details of this case, including the patient's medical condition, other medications, and the doses and duration of the warfarin and devil's claw ingestion were not reported.
Use in Pregnancy and Lactation	No adverse effects expected.
Side Effects	Mild gastrointestinal disturbances may occur in sensitive individuals, especially at the higher dose levels.

Dosage

Dose per day	*Dose per week*
6.0-11.5 ml of 1:2 liquid extract for analgesic and antirheumatic activity*	40-80 ml of 1:2 liquid extract for analgesic and antirheumatic activity*
3 ml of 1:2 liquid extract for gastrointestinal complaints**	20 ml of 1:2 liquid extract for gastrointestinal complaints**

Pharmacologic studies have indicated that stomach acidity might decrease the analgesic and antiinflammatory activity. However, a recent study has established that this indication is not the case.[2]

Devil's Claw *continued on page 179*

*This dose range is extrapolated from clinical studies.
**This dosage is extrapolated from the German Commission E.

Traditional Prescribing

Traditional Western herbal medicine uses include:
- Rheumatism, arthritis, gout, myalgia, fibrositis, lumbago, pleurodynia[3]
- As a general tonic, loss of appetite, digestive disorders[4]

Traditional South African medicinal uses include:
- As a purgative and bitter tonic[5]
- As an analgesic, especially during and after childbirth[5]
- Febrile diseases, allergic reactions[5]
- Topically for ulcers, wounds, cutaneous lesions, and after childbirth[5]

Pharmacologic Research

Key constituents of devil's claw root include iridoid glycosides (0.5% to 3.0%), primarily harpagoside, which has a bitter taste.
- Devil's claw extract reduced subacute inflammation in an *in vivo* model of arthritis after oral and intraperitoneal administration. Results were comparable to phenylbutazone. Another study using different but similar models found that devil's claw did not produce significant effects on either primary or secondary inflammatory reactions.
- Oral doses of devil's claw aqueous extract and harpagoside demonstrated little or no activity in acute models of inflammation, such as carrageenan-induced edema. However, intraperitoneal pretreatment with devil's claw extract produced significant, dose-dependent, antiinflammatory effects in this model. Devil's claw root treated with acid at levels similar to that in the stomach lost all activity (when administered by intraperitoneal injection). However, more recent experiments with simulated stomach conditions found that harpagoside was stable.[2]
- The iridoids from devil's claw may possibly be transformed into alkaloids in the gastrointestinal tract. *In vitro* tests indicate that several of the devil's claw iridoids, including harpagoside, undergo microbial transformation to form the alkaloid aucubinine B.[6]
- Both *in vitro* and *in vivo* studies have demonstrated that devil's claw has minimal effect on prostaglandin biosynthesis. These studies indicate that devil's claw is unlikely to act by a similar mechanism to NSAIDs. Hence the herb will not have the same irritant effects on the stomach.
- Injections of devil's claw extract and harpagoside exhibited dose-dependent peripheral analgesic effects comparable to aspirin. Intraperitoneal administration of harpagoside produced an analgesic effect comparable to phenylbutazone. However, the aglycone of harpagoside was inactive. No consistent analgesic effects were found in an experimental model after oral doses of devil's claw extract.
- Devil's claw extract inhibited the synthesis of prostaglandins by inhibiting cyclooxygenase-2 and inhibited the release of TNF-α from primary human monocytes (an *in vitro* model of peripheral inflammation).[7]

Devil's Claw *continued on page 180*

- After oral administration, devil's claw extract lowered arterial blood pressure dose-dependently, with a concomitant decrease in heart rate, in an experimental model.[8] Devil's claw extract protected against experimentally induced arrhythmia *in vitro* and *in vivo* after oral and intraperitoneal administration.[8,9]

Clinical Studies

- In a randomized, double-blind, controlled, multicenter study, devil's claw powder taken over a period of 4 months significantly reduced both spontaneous pain and functional disability, and it was as efficacious as was diacerhein (an anthrone analgesic) in patients with osteoarthritis of the knee and hip. The number of patients using NSAIDs and other analgesic drugs at the completion of the study, and the frequency of adverse events, was significantly lower in the devil's claw group. The daily dose was 2.6 g of freeze-dried powder containing 87 mg of total iridoid and 57 mg of harpagoside.[10,11]
- In patients with arthrosis and articular pain, devil's claw extract decreased the severity of pain when compared with placebo in two randomized, double-blind studies. Improvements were more frequent in moderate cases of arthrosis than they were in severe cases. Spinal mobility was also increased compared with placebo in the articular pain trial. The arthrosis patients received 2.4 g per day of an extract (containing 36 mg/day of iridoid glycosides) for 3 to 9 weeks and those with articular pain received 2.0 g per day of an extract (containing 60 mg/day of iridoid glycosides) for 8 weeks.
- In another randomized study in patients with chronic back pain, treatment with devil's claw extract (equivalent to 6 g/day of root and containing 50 mg/day of harpagoside) for 4 weeks demonstrated a greater reduction in a back pain index than did placebo. The reduction in pain, however, was confined almost exclusively to the subgroup of patients whose pain did not radiate to one or both legs. More patients in the treatment group were pain-free compared with the placebo group at the end of the treatment. A subsequent study of similar design confirmed that more patients receiving devil's claw extract (equivalent to 4.5 g/day or 9 g/day of root and containing 50 mg/day or 100 mg/day of harpagoside, respectively) for 4 weeks were pain-free compared with placebo.[12]
- In a large, uncontrolled study of patients with various rheumatic illnesses, 42% to 85% of patients showed significant improvement after 6 months' treatment with devil's claw extract (75 to 225 mg/day of iridoid glycosides). However, one open study of 13 patients with rheumatoid arthritis and psoriatic arthropathy found no benefit from devil's claw treatment.
- In Germany, the Commission E supports using devil's claw to treat loss of appetite and dyspepsia and as supportive therapy for degenerative disorders of the musculoskeletal system.[13]
- ESCOP recommends devil's claw for treating painful arthrosis, tendinitis, loss of appetite, and dyspepsia.[14]

Devil's Claw *continued on page 181*

REFERENCES

Except when specifically referenced, the following book was referred to in the compilation of the pharmacologic and clinical information: Mills S, Bone K: *Principles and Practice of Phytotherapy: Modern Herbal Medicine,* Edinburgh, 2000, Churchill Livingstone.

1 Heck AM, Dewitt BA, Lukes AL: *Am J Health-Syst Pharm* 57(13):1221-1227, 2000.

2 Loew D, Puttkammer S. Cited in Chrubasik S, Roufogalis BD, editors: *Herbal medicinal products for the treatment of pain,* Lismore, NSW, Australia, 2000, Southern Cross University Press.

3 British Herbal Medicine Association's Scientific Committee: *British herbal pharmacopoeia,* Bournemouth, 1983, BHMA.

4 van Wyk B-E, van Oudtshoorn B, Gericke N: *Medicinal plants of South Africa,* Arcadia, South Africa, 1997, Briza Publications.

5 Ragusa S et al: *J Ethnopharmacol* 11(3):245-257, 1984.

6 Fleurentin F. Cited in Chrubasik S, Roufogalis BD, editors: *Herbal medicinal products for the treatment of pain,* Lismore, NSW, Australia, 2000, Southern Cross University Press.

7 Kammerer N, Fiebich B. Cited in Chrubasik S, Roufogalis BD, editors: *Herbal medicinal products for the treatment of pain,* Lismore, NSW, Australia, 2000, Southern Cross University Press.

8 Circosta C et al: *J Ethnopharmacol* 11(3):259-274, 1984.

9 Costa de Pasquale R et al: *J Ethnopharmacol* 13(2):193-194, 1985.

10 Chantre P et al: *Phytomed* 7(3):177-183, 2000.

11 Leblan D, Chantre P, Fournie B: *Joint Bone Spine* 67(5):462-467, 2000.

12 Chrubasik S et al: *Eur J Anaesthesiol* 16(2):118-129, 1999.

13 Blumenthal M et al, editors: *The complete German Commission E monographs: therapeutic guide to herbal medicines,* Austin, 1998, American Botanical Council.

14 Scientific Committee of the European Scientific Cooperative on Phytotherapy [ESCOP]: *ESCOP monographs: Harpagophyti radix.* European Scientific Cooperative on Phytotherapy, ESCOP Secretariat, Argyle House, Gandy Street, Exeter, Devon, EX4 3LS, United Kingdom, March 1996.

DONG QUAI

Botanical Names: *Angelica sinensis, Angelica polymorpha* var. *sinensis#*
Family: Umbelliferae
Plant Part Used: Root

PRESCRIBING INFORMATION

Actions	Antiinflammatory, antianemic, antiplatelet, female tonic, mild laxative, antiarrhythmic
Potential Indications	Based on appropriate evaluation of the patient, practitioners should consider prescribing dong quai in formulations in the context of: • Dysmenorrhea,* in combination with Corydalis, white peony, and Ligusticum *(4)* • Female reproductive disorders, irregular menstruation, amenorrhea *(5)* • Chronic hepatitis and cirrhosis *(4)* • Constipation, abdominal pain, swellings, bruising *(5)* • Tinnitus, blurred vision, palpitations *(5)* • A douche for infertility *(4)*
Contraindications	The following contraindications apply from TCM: diarrhea caused by weak digestion, hemorrhagic disease, bleeding tendency or very heavy periods, first trimester of pregnancy, tendency to spontaneous abortion, and acute viral infections such as the common cold and influenza.
Warnings and Precautions	None required.
Interactions	Caution is advised for patients receiving chronic treatment with warfarin.
Use in Pregnancy and Lactation	Contraindicated in the first trimester of pregnancy, especially in higher doses.
Side Effects	A case of a man who developed gynecomastia (mammary glandular hyperplasia) after ingestion of dong quai capsules has been reported. The label indicated "100% dong quai *(Angelica sinensis)* root powder. No fillers or additives."[1]

Dosage	*Dose per day***	*Dose per week***
	4.5-8.5 ml of 1:2 liquid extract	30-60 ml of 1:2 liquid extract

Dong Quai *continued on page 183*

#Alternative name.
*Dong quai has also been used in TCM for treating dysmenorrhea. (5)
**This dose range is adapted from dried plant doses administered by decoction in TCM.[2] The author's experience and the fact that ethanol-water is a more effective solvent than water for many phytochemicals are taken into account.

Traditional Prescribing

Uses and properties from TCM include:
- Strengthening the *heart, lung,* and *liver* meridians, lubricating the bowel, invigorating and *harmonizing* the *blood,* treating congealed blood conditions[1]
- Irregular menstruation, amenorrhea, dysmenorrhea resulting from blood stasis or anemia[2-4]
- Constipation, abdominal pain; tissue trauma, swellings, bruising, boils, rheumatism; headache, tinnitus, blurred vision, palpitations.[2-4]

Pharmacologic Research

- The whole root has shown a stimulant effect *in vivo.* Other studies have shown that dong quai can relax or coordinate uterine contractions, depending on uterine tone. The root is devoid of estrogenic action.
- Dong quai can prolong the refractory period and correct experimental atrial fibrillation. Both the aqueous extract of dong quai and ferulic acid inhibited platelet aggregation and serotonin release *in vitro.*
- In experimental models, dong quai was shown to prevent coronary atherosclerosis, lower blood pressure, dilate the coronary vessels, increase coronary flow, reduce blood cholesterol, and reduce respiratory rate.
- Dong quai exerted a stimulating effect on hematopoiesis in bone marrow.
- Dong quai might somewhat counter the immunosuppressive effects of hydrocortisone *in vivo* but is not as effective as is Astragalus.
- Dong quai had a proliferative effect on muscle cells *in vitro.*
- Dong quai has demonstrated hepatoprotective effects, a stimulating effect on the liver, an antiinflammatory effect, and muscle relaxant properties, all *in vivo.*

Clinical Studies

- A combination of dong quai, Corydalis, white peony, and *Ligusticum wallichii* showed a 93% improvement rate for treating dysmenorrhea in an uncontrolled trial.
- Infertility resulting from tubal occlusion was treated for up to 9 months with uterine irrigation of dong quai extract in an uncontrolled trial. Nearly 80% of patients regained tubal patency, and 53% became pregnant.
- In an uncontrolled trial, dong quai improved abnormal protein metabolism, improved abnormal thymol turbidity test results, and increased plasma protein levels in 60% of patients with chronic hepatitis or hepatic cirrhosis.
- In China, an injection containing dong quai has been successfully used to treat Buerger's disease and constrictive aortitis.

Dong Quai *continued on page 184*

REFERENCES

The following book was referred to in the compilation of the pharmacologic and clinical information: Mills S, Bone K: *Principles and Practice of Phytotherapy: Modern Herbal Medicine,* Edinburgh, 2000, Churchill Livingstone.

1 Goh SY, Loh KC: *Singapore Med J* 42(3):115-116, 2001.
2 Pharmacopoeia Commission of the People's Republic of China: *Pharmacopoeia of the People's Republic of China,* English ed, Beijing, 1997, Chemical Industry Press.
3 Bensky D, Gamble A: *Chinese herbal medicine materia medica,* Seattle, 1986, Eastland Press.
4 Chang HM, But PP: *Pharmacology and applications of Chinese materia medica,* Singapore, 1987, World Scientific.

ECHINACEA

Other Common Name:	Purple coneflower
Botanical Names:	*Echinacea angustifolia, Echinacea purpurea*
Family:	Compositae
Plant Parts Used:	Root, aerial parts

PRESCRIBING INFORMATION

Actions

Immune modulating, immune enhancing, depurative, antiinflammatory, vulnerary, lymphatic, sialagogue

Potential Indications

Based on appropriate evaluation of the patient, practitioners should consider prescribing Echinacea root in formulations in the context of:
- Treating and preventing upper respiratory tract infections *(1,4,5)*
- Treating and preventing infections in general *(5)*
- Enhancing immune response in healthy individuals *(4)*
- Nasopharyngeal catarrh, respiratory catarrh, chronic bronchitis *(5)*
- Sinusitis, in combination with Thuja and Baptisia *(3)*
- Adjuvant therapy for cancer *(5)*
- Abscess, boils, poorly healing wounds, furunculosis, eczema, psoriasis, mouth ulcers, venomous bites, skin and glandular inflammations *(5)*

Contraindications

No conclusive evidence has been found that using Echinacea for long periods is detrimental or that it is contraindicated in disorders such as autoimmune disease, allergies, and asthma. The risk of allergic reaction to Echinacea itself is very small, especially if preparations of the root are used, given that these are free of pollens.

Warnings and Precautions

Caution is advised for transplant patients taking immunosuppressive drugs; short-term therapy only is suggested. Misinformation exists that Echinacea is potentially hepatotoxic because of the presence of pyrrolizidine alkaloids (PAs). However, the PAs found in Echinacea possess chemical structures that are known to be nontoxic.

Allergic reactions, mainly contact dermatitis, may occur rarely in susceptible patients sensitized to Echinacea aerial parts and plants from the Compositae family. The likelihood of Echinacea root preparations causing allergy is very low.

Interactions

See the "Warnings and Precautions" section in this monograph.

Use in Pregnancy and Lactation

No adverse effects expected.

A prospective, controlled study published in 2000 concluded that gestational use of Echinacea (generally for 5 to 7 days) during organogenesis was not associated with an increased risk of major malformations. No significant differences were found in pregnancy outcome between the study group, including 206 women who had used Echinacea during pregnancy (112 women in the first trimester) and their matched controls.[1]

Echinacea *continued on page 186*

Side Effects

Side effects are generally not expected for oral or topical administration.

Dosage

Flowering tops, aerial parts, root, and whole plant of Echinacea are used medicinally. In traditional herbal medicine, the root was the preferred plant part that Native Americans and the Eclectic physicians used. Only doses for the use of the root of the preferred Echinacea species are provided here.

Echinacea purpurea root:

Dose per day*	**Dose per week***
3-6 ml of 1:2 liquid extract	20-40 ml of 1:2 liquid extract
4.5-8.5 ml of 1:3 glycetract	30-60 ml of 1:3 glycetract

Echinacea angustifolia root:

Dose per day*	**Dose per week***
3-6 ml of 1:2 liquid extract	20-40 ml of 1:2 liquid extract

Preparations containing a blend of *Echinacea purpurea* root and *Echinacea angustifolia* root:

Dose per day*	**Dose per week***
3-6 ml of blended 1:2 liquid extracts	20-40 ml of blended 1:2 liquid extracts

SUPPORTING INFORMATION

Traditional Prescribing

The Eclectic physicians use *Echinacea angustifolia* root internally and topically for:
- Boils, carbuncles, abscesses, septicemia, snakebite, insect bite, wounds, ulcerated and fetid mucous surfaces, gangrene, eczema, psoriasis[2]
- Tonsillitis, nasopharyngeal catarrh, respiratory catarrh, chronic bronchitis[2]
- Fermentative dyspepsia, indigestion, ulcerative stomatitis, diarrhea, dysentery[2]
- Fevers, influenza, measles, chickenpox, scarlet fever, smallpox, tuberculosis, typhoid pneumonia, diphtheria, malaria, meningitis[2]
- Mastitis, salpingitis, leucorrhea, vulvitis, gonorrhea, syphilis, impotence[2]
- Glandular inflammations, cancer pain[2]

Echinacea purpurea root was used to treat syphilis[2] and was often used by the Eclectics for the same purposes as those for which *E. angustifolia* was used but was considered to have weaker activity.[3] Echinacea was listed primarily as a depurative with antiseptic properties.[2,3]

Echinacea *continued on page 187*

*This dose range is extrapolated from the British Herbal Compendium 1992 and the author's education and experience.

Native Americans used *Echinacea angustifolia* root as a "remedy for more ailments than any other plant," a universal antidote for snakebite, and other venomous bites, stings, and poisonous conditions. Other native uses included enlarged glands, sore throat, septic conditions, rabies, and toothache (topically as well). *Echinacea angustifolia* root was official in the NF from 1916 to 1950 and used to induce saliva and as a depurative and diaphoretic.[4]

Medicinal use of the fresh flowering plant of *Echinacea purpurea* originated in Germany in the late 1930s where it was popularized by Dr. Gerhard Madaus. The homeopathic use of fresh plant tinctures influenced Madaus.

Pharmacologic Research

Many potentially active constituents are in Echinacea, including alkylamides, cichoric acid, polysaccharides, and glycoproteins. Many herbalists regard the alkylamides as the most important active constituents.[5]

The roots of both species contain alkylamides and caffeic acid esters (especially cichoric acid in *E. purpurea* and echinacoside in *E. angustifolia*). When tasted, the alkylamides cause a characteristic tingling in the mouth. Polysaccharides are present in Echinacea roots, but the quantity of polysaccharides present in extract preparations containing 50% ethanol or more will be negligible.

- Experimental findings support well the nonspecific enhancement of phagocytic activity for oral doses of Echinacea. Extracts of the aerial parts of the three species demonstrated lower activity than that of the roots. Lipophilic fractions from root extracts (containing mainly alkylamides and polyacetylenes) were more active than hydrophilic fractions (containing caffeic acid derivatives). Alkylamide fractions from the root of both species and cichoric acid also demonstrated activity.
- *E. angustifolia* root extract accelerated the IgG immune response after initial antigen exposure and retained the improved immune response after booster injection of antigen in experimental models *in vivo* (oral route).[6]
- Caffeic acid esters obtained from *E. angustifolia* root demonstrated antihyaluronidase activity *in vitro*. Antihyaluronidase activity may help enhance tissue resistance to the spread of infection and facilitate connective tissue regeneration.
- Purified root extract from the three Echinacea species demonstrated antiviral activity toward herpes simplex virus *in vitro*. An indirect effect via stimulation of α- and β-interferon production was also observed. Cichoric acid produced an antiviral effect against vesicular stomatitis virus *in vitro*.
- Polyacetylenes from *E. angustifolia* and *E. purpurea* roots had bacteriostatic and fungistatic activity against *Escherichia coli* and *Pseudomonas aeruginosa*. Echinacoside had only weak antimicrobial activity against *Staphylococcus aureus in vitro*. The basis of the use of Echinacea in infections is not the result of direct antimicrobial activity.

Echinacea *continued on page 188*

• *Echinacea angustifolia* root extract inhibited edema and the crude polysaccharide fraction had an antiinflammatory effect in the croton oil mouse ear test when applied topically. Echinacea was more potent than was the topical NSAID benzydamine in its antiedematous effect. Alkylamides from Echinacea inhibit cyclooxygenase and 5-lipoxygenase *in vitro*, thus they may possibly be antiinflammatory agents.

Clinical Studies

Although three species of Echinacea are used therapeutically (*Echinacea angustifolia, E. purpurea,* and *E. pallida*), *Echinacea pallida* is considered by many herbalists to be the least effective of the three species.

• Nine treatment trials and four prevention trials, which were randomized, double-blind, and placebo-controlled, investigating the efficacy of Echinacea on upper respiratory tract infections (URTIs) have been reviewed.[7] Eight of the nine treatment trials support the ability of Echinacea to decrease the severity and duration of acute URTIs. One unpublished trial reported a negative result. All of the prevention trials trended toward statistical significance for Echinacea treatments. Methodological quality of the majority of the trials was modest. The Echinacea treatment used in these trials is defined here. A subgroup analysis of infection-prone participants in one of the prevention trials using an herbal formulation of *E. angustifolia* aerial parts and root, *Eupatorium perfoliatum, Baptisia tinctoria,* and homeopathic *Arnica montana* showed a statistically significant relative risk reduction for the treated group compared with placebo. One of the prevention trials used a relatively low dose of Echinacea root (200 mg/day). The review concluded that Echinacea may be beneficial for the early treatment of acute URTIs but little evidence exists from the trials reviewed for prolonged use of Echinacea for preventing URTIs. However, the clinical experience of many herbalists would support the latter application.

Treatment Trials		Prevention Trials	
Herbal Formulation	**No. of Trials**	**Herbal Formulation**	**No. of Trials**
E. purpurea root, 1800 mg/day	1	E. angustifolia root or E. purpurea root (200 mg/day of either for 5 days/wk for 12 wks)	1
E. pallida root, 900 mg/day	1	E. purpurea aerial parts	1
E. purpurea aerial parts	1	Herbal formulation containing E. angustifolia aerial parts and root, Eupatorium perfoliatum, Baptisia tinctoria, and homeopathic Arnica montana[†]	1

Echinacea *continued on page 189*

E. purpurea aerial parts 95%, E. purpurea root 5% (equivalent to 1.6 g/day fresh aerial parts and root for 8 days) — 1	Herbal formulation containing E. angustifolia and E. pallida roots, Baptisia tinctoria, Thuja occidentalis, and homeopathics§ — 1

E. purpurea aerial parts 95%, E. purpurea root 5% (equivalent to 1.6 g/day fresh aerial parts and root for 8 days)   1

Herbal formulation containing E. angustifolia aerial parts and root, Eupatorium perfoliatum, Baptisia tinctoria, and homeopathic Arnica montana*   2

E. angustifolia part undefined, 750 mg/day dried preparation   1

Herbal formulation containing E. angustifolia and E. pallida roots, Baptisia tinctoria, and Thuja occidentalis‡   1

Herbal formulation containing E. angustifolia and E. pallida roots, Baptisia tinctoria, Thuja occidentalis, and homeopathics§   1

Herbal formulation containing E. angustifolia and E. pallida roots, Baptisia tinctoria, Thuja occidentalis, and homeopathics§   1

- Trials investigating the use of Echinacea root preparations for URTIs, published or presented at conferences since this review, include the following:
  - A randomized, double-blind, placebo-controlled trial investigated the efficacy of two herbal formulas in preventing the common cold in highly stressed medical students over a period of 15 weeks. Both the immunomodulatory formula (E. angustifolia root and E. purpurea root) and the adaptogenic formula (ashwaganda, Korean ginseng, and Astragalus) significantly reduced the incidence of infection by the end of the tenth week when given in adequate doses as prophylactic agents for acute URTIs. The daily dose of both formulas was

Echinacea continued on page 190

---

*The daily dose in these trials ranged from 1.5 to 3.0 g of the total formulation (dry weight equivalent), including the homeopathic Arnica. In one trial, the higher dose (3 g) was administered for the first 2 days followed by the lower dose (1.5 g) from the third to sixth days.

†Dosage was equivalent to 1.2 g/day of the total formulation, including the homeopathic Arnica for 8 weeks.

‡On the basis of the current formulation, the daily dose of herbs was well below the normal therapeutic limit (more similar to a homeopathic protocol).

§The tablets used in these trials contained herbs in quantities well below the normal therapeutic levels: 5 mg Thuja, 7.5 mg Echinacea, and 10 mg Baptisia per tablet. The number of tablets prescribed in these trials ranged from three to six per day.

equivalent to 3.5 g dry weight of total herb as the starting dose, decreasing to one half that amount.[8]

- Treatment with an Echinacea tea at early onset of cold or influenza relieved symptoms in a shorter period than did placebo. The trial was of randomized, double-blind design. The tea contained *Echinacea purpurea* root, *E. purpurea*, and *E. angustifolia* aerial parts, lemongrass, and spearmint. The tea bag delivered 1.3 g of Echinacea and the dosage began at 5 to 6 cups per day at early symptoms, tapering down to 1 cup per day over a period of 5 days.[9]
- No significant difference compared with placebo in the incidence of infection or the total daily symptom score was observed after treatment with an Echinacea preparation in volunteers challenged with rhinovirus in a randomized, double-blind trial. The Echinacea preparation was a combination of the extracts of *E. purpurea* and *E. angustifolia* (parts undefined) given at a dosage of 900 mg/day and appeared to be of poor quality, containing cichoric acid (0.16%) with almost no alkylamides or echinacoside present.[10]
- The prospective, controlled trial previously listed that investigated the use of Echinacea during pregnancy also found that 81% of participants reported that Echinacea improved the symptoms of their URTI.[1] (See the "Use in Pregnancy and Lactation" section.)
- Patients with acute sinusitis taking tablets containing extracts of *E. angustifolia* and *E. pallida* roots, *Thuja occidentalis*, and *Baptisia tinctoria* with the antibiotic doxycycline had much better x-ray and global assessment results than those taking doxycycline alone.
- Standardized alcoholic extract of *E. purpurea* root given orally over 5 days (containing 1 mg each of chicoric acid and alkylamides per day) maximally stimulated granulocyte phagocytosis on the fifth day (120% of the starting value) in healthy men.
- ESCOP recommends *E. purpurea* root for adjuvant therapy and prophylaxis of recurrent infections of the upper respiratory tract.[11]

REFERENCES

Except when specifically referenced, the following book was referred to in the compilation of the pharmacologic and clinical information: Mills S, Bone K: *Principles and Practice of Phytotherapy: Modern Herbal Medicine,* Edinburgh, 2000, Churchill Livingstone.

1 Gallo M et al: *Arch Intern Med* 160(20):3141-3143, 2000.
2 Felter HW, Lloyd JU: *King's American dispensatory,* ed 18, rev 3, Portland, 1905, reprinted 1983, Eclectic Medical Publications.
3 Ellingwood F, Lloyd JU: *American materia medica, therapeutics and pharmacognosy,* ed 11, Portland, 1983, Eclectic Medical Publications.
4 Vogel VJ: *American Indian medicine,* Norman, Okla, 1970, University of Oklahoma Press.
5 Awang DVC: *Altern Ther Women's Health* July:57-59, 1999.
6 Rehman J et al: *Immun Lett* 68(2-3):391-395, 1999.
7 Barrett B, Vohman M, Calabrese C: *J Fam Prac* 48(8):628-635, 1999.
8 MacIntosh A et al: Publication in press.
9 Lindenmuth GF, Lindenmuth EB: *J Altern Complement Med* 6(4):327-334, 2000.
10 Turner RB, Riker DK, Gangemi JD: *Antimicrob Agents Chemother* 44(6):1708-1709, 2000.
11 Scientific Committee of the European Scientific Cooperative on Phytotherapy [ESCOP]: *ESCOP monographs: Echinaceae purpureae radix.* European Scientific Cooperative on Phytotherapy, ESCOP Secretariat, Argyle House, Gandy Street, Exeter, Devon, EX4 3LS, United Kingdom, October 1999.

ELDER FLOWER

Botanical Name: *Sambucus nigra*
Family: Caprifoliaceae
Plant Part Used: Flower

PRESCRIBING INFORMATION

Actions	Diaphoretic, anticatarrhal
Potential Indications	Based on appropriate evaluation of the patient, practitioners should consider prescribing elder flower in formulations in the context of: • The common cold *(4,5)* • Conditions requiring diaphoresis, such as fevers and influenza *(5)* • Acute and chronic sinusitis, hay fever *(5)* • Pleurisy, bronchitis, sore throat, measles *(6)*
Contraindications	None known.
Warnings and Precautions	None required.
Interactions	None known.
Use in Pregnancy and Lactation	No adverse effects expected.
Side Effects	None expected if taken within the recommended dose range.

Dosage

Dose per day*	Dose per week*
2-6 ml of 1:2 liquid extract	15-40 ml of 1:2 liquid extract

SUPPORTING INFORMATION

Traditional Prescribing	Traditional Western herbal medicine uses include: • As a diaphoretic in any condition requiring fever management, including the common cold and influenza (particularly in the early stages); sinusitis, chronic nasal catarrh with deafness,[1] pleurisy, bronchitis, sore throat, measles, fevers, scarlet fever[2] • Topically for inflammation of the eyes, skin disorders, wounds,[2] and burns[3] Eclectic physicians regarded warm infusions of *Sambucus canadensis*, a similar herb, as diaphoretic and warming and cold infusions as diuretic and depurative. Therefore *Sambucus canadensis* was also used to treat skin infections and liver disorders.[3]
Pharmacologic Research	• Aqueous extract of elder (part undefined) demonstrated an insulin-releasing and insulinlike activity *in vivo* (route unknown). The following isolated constituents did not stimulate insulin secretion: lectin, rutin,

Elder Flower *continued on page 192*

*This dose range is extrapolated from the British Herbal Pharmacopoeia 1983 and the author's education and experience.

lupeol, and β-sitosterol.[4] In an earlier trial, oral administration of aqueous extract of elder (part unknown) did not affect glucose homeostasis under either normal or induced diabetic conditions.[5]

- Aqueous extract of elder (part unknown) increased urine flow and urinary sodium excretion *in vivo* (route unknown).[6] A diuretic effect was observed after intragastric administration of elder flower infusion and an extract high in potassium and flavonoids.[7]
- A methanolic extract of elder flower inhibited the biosynthesis of the following cytokines *in vitro*: interleukin-1α, interleukin-1β, and TNF-α.[8] Mild antiinflammatory activity was demonstrated after intragastric administration of elder flower extract in an experimental model.[9]
- Intraperitoneal administration of an unsaponifiable fraction of elder flower moderately enhanced phagocytosis *in vivo*.[10]
- Early studies reported that elder flower increased the response of the sweat glands to heat stimuli.[11,12]

Clinical Studies

- An increase in diaphoresis in healthy volunteers has been reported,[12] although theories suggested that the effect was caused by the large amount of hot fluid consumed.[13]
- In Germany, the Commission E supports using elder flower to treat the common cold.[14]

REFERENCES

1 British Herbal Medicine Association's Scientific Committee: *British herbal pharmacopoeia,* Bournemouth, 1983, BHMA.
2 Grieve M: *A modern herbal,* New York, 1971, Dover Publications.
3 Felter HW, Lloyd JU: *King's American dispensatory,* ed 18, rev 3, Portland, 1905, reprinted 1983, Eclectic Medical Publications.
4 Gray AM, Abdel-Wahab YH, Flatt PR: *J Nutr* 130(1):15-20, 2000.
5 Swanston-Flatt SK et al: *Diabetes Res* 10(2):69-73, 1989.
6 Beaux D, Fleurentin J, Mortier F: *Phytother Res* 13(3):222-225, 1999.
7 Rebuelta M et al: *Plantes Med Phytother* 17:173-181, 1983.
8 Yesilada E et al: *J Ethnopharmacol* 58(1):59-73, 1997.
9 Mascolo N et al: *Phytother Res* 1:28-31, 1987.
10 Delaveau P, Lallouette P, Tessier AM: *Planta Med* 40(1):49-54, 1980.
11 Schmersahl KJ: *Naturwissenschaften* 51:361, 1964.
12 Wiechowski W: *Med Klin* 23:590-592, 1927.
13 Bisset NG, editor: *Herbal drugs and phytopharmaceuticals,* Stuttgart, 1994, Medpharm Scientific Publishers.
14 Blumenthal M et al, editors: *The complete German Commission E monographs: therapeutic guide to herbal medicines,* Austin, 1998, American Botanical Council.

ELECAMPANE

Botanical Name: *Inula helenium*
Family: Compositae
Plant Part Used: Root

PRESCRIBING INFORMATION

Actions	Expectorant, diaphoretic, antibacterial, spasmolytic, bronchospasmolytic
Potential Indications	Based on appropriate evaluation of the patient, practitioners should consider prescribing elecampane in formulations in the context of: • Respiratory catarrh and infections *(5)* • The common cold, influenza, bronchitis, asthma *(5)* • Possible treatment for peptic ulcer disease and intestinal worms *(4a)*
Contraindications	See the "Use in Pregnancy and Lactation" section in this monograph.
Warnings and Precautions	Caution is advised in people with known sensitivity to elecampane or to other members of the Compositae family.
Interactions	None known.
Use in Pregnancy and Lactation	According to the British Herbal Compendium, elecampane is contraindicated in pregnancy and lactation.[1] However, no substantial basis has been found for this concern.
Side Effects	Occasional allergic reactions may occur because of sensitivity caused by the sesquiterpene lactones present in elecampane.[2,3]

Dosage

Dose per day*	Dose per week*
3-6 ml of 1:2 liquid extract	20-40 ml of 1:2 liquid extract

SUPPORTING INFORMATION

Traditional Prescribing

Traditional Western herbal medicine uses include:
• Catarrhal conditions of the respiratory tract, especially bronchitis, irritating cough in children, tuberculosis, and asthma[1,4,5]
• Sustaining the strength of the patient in chronic disorders of the respiratory tract[5]
• Dyspepsia, night sweats[4]
• Internally and externally for skin conditions[4]

Eclectic physicians regarded elecampane as an important remedy for irritation of the trachea and bronchi, thus elecampane was used in cases with free and abundant expectoration, teasing cough, and substernal pain, such as severe forms of the common cold and influenza.[5]

Elecampane *continued on page 194*

*This dose range is extrapolated from the *British Herbal Compendium* 1992 and the author's education and experience.

Pharmacologic Research

Elecampane root contains sesquiterpene lactones of the eudesmanolide-type: alantolactone, isoalantolactone, and their derivatives.[1]

- Elecampane extract demonstrated activity against *Mycobacterium tuberculosis in vitro*. The eudesmanolides were the active constituents.[6] Antibacterial activity was demonstrated against organisms that cause brucellosis and anthrax for an elecampane extract (0.5% to 1.0%). Activity against staphylococci and hemolytic streptococci were weakly displayed. No significant results were obtained *in vivo* for brucellosis or anthrax.[7]
- Elecampane essential oil demonstrated antibacterial activity *in vitro* against *Staphylococcus aureus* and *Streptococcus pyogenes* in concentrations as low as 1.2%.[8]
- Elecampane essential oil demonstrated a relaxant effect on isolated tracheal and ileal smooth muscle.[9]
- Oral or intragastric administration of eudesmanolides increased intragastric temperature in an experimental model, which was indicative of increased blood supply and blood flow in the gastric mucosa.[10]
- Japanese scientists demonstrated the *in vivo* anthelmintic properties of the eudesmanolides from elecampane, particularly alantolactone, in the 1940s.[11,12]

Clinical Studies

- A preparation of isolated eudesmanolides demonstrated ulcer healing properties, relieved symptoms, and improved gastric mucosal circulation in an uncontrolled trial involving 102 patients with peptic ulcer disease.[13]
- Oral administration of alantolactone (9 to 200 mg) to children from 7 to 14 years of age produced a safe, favorable anthelmintic effect for Ascaris infestation.[14]

REFERENCES

1 British Herbal Medicine Association: *British herbal compendium,* Bournemouth, 1992, BHMA.

2 Lamminpaa A et al: *Contact Dermatitis* 34(5):330-335, 1996.

3 Alonso Blasi N et al: *Arch Dermatol Res* 284(5):297-302, 1992.

4 British Herbal Medicine Association's Scientific Committee: *British herbal pharmacopoeia,* Bournemouth, 1983, BHMA.

5 Felter HW, Lloyd JU: *King's American dispensatory,* ed 18, rev 3, Portland, 1905, reprinted 1983, Eclectic Medical Publications.

6 Cantrell CL et al: *Planta Med* 65(4):351-355, 1999.

7 Bulanov PA: *Izvest Akad Nauk Kazakh SSR Ser Microbiol* 1:40-46, 1949.

8 Boatto G, Pintore G, Palomba M: *Fitoterapia* 65(3):279-280, 1994.

9 Reiter M, Brandt W: *Arzneim Forsch* 35(1A):408-414, 1985.

10 Luchkova MM: *Fiziolohichnyi Zh* 23(5):685-687, 1977.

11 Anon: *Japan J Med Sci IV Pharmacol* 13(3):75-93, 1941.

12 Anon: *Japan J Med Sci IV Pharmacol* 11(2-3):110-112, 1941.

13 Luchkova MM: *Vrachebnoe Delo* 6:69-71, 1978.

14 Ozeki S, Kotake M, Hayashi K: *Proc Imp Acad* 12:233-234, 1936.

ELEUTHEROCOCCUS

Other Common Name:	Eleuthero, Siberian ginseng
Botanical Names:	*Eleutherococcus senticosus, Acanthopanax senticosus*[#]
Family:	Araliaceae
Plant Part Used:	Root

PRESCRIBING INFORMATION

Actions

Adaptogenic, immune modulating, tonic

Potential Indications

Based on appropriate evaluation of the patient, practitioners should consider prescribing Eleutherococcus in formulations in the context of:
- Enhancing immune function in healthy individuals *(2)*
- Improving mental performance *(4)*
- Improving physical performance *(4,5)*
- Environmental and occupational stress *(3,4)*
- Minimizing the effects of stress in patients subject to chronic illness *(4)*
- Convalescence, including after antibiotic therapy; adjuvant therapy for dysentery *(4)*
- Adjuvant therapy for cancer, to improve immune function and decrease side effects from orthodox therapy *(4)*
- Exhaustion, insomnia, mild depression *(4,5)*

Contraindications

Eleutherococcus is best not used during the acute phase of infections. Although some medical scientists and regulatory bodies consider Eleutherococcus to be contraindicated in hypertension, it also has been used to treat hypertension.

Warnings and Precautions

None required.

Interactions

A case of apparent elevated serum digoxin levels attributed to consumption of an unauthenticated "Eleutherococcus" product has been reported. As to whether Eleutherococcus caused a real increase in serum digoxin levels rather than an interference was inconclusive with the test method used.

Use in Pregnancy and Lactation

No adverse effects expected.

Side Effects

Russian studies on Eleutherococcus have noted a general absence of side effects. However, care should be exercised in patients with cardiovascular disorders because insomnia, palpitations, tachycardia, and hypertension have been reported in a few cases. Side effects are more likely if normal doses are exceeded. "Ginseng abuse syndrome" with insomnia, diarrhea, and hypertension has been described, but the study did not differentiate between Korean ginseng *(Panax ginseng)* and Eleutherococcus.

Eleutherococcus *continued on page 196*

[#]Alternative name.

Dosage

*Dose per day**	*Dose per week**
2-8 ml of 1:2 liquid extract	15-55 ml of 1:2 liquid extract

Extracts providing standardized levels of eleutheroside E are recommended. Ideally, aqueous ethanol extracts should contain at least 0.5 mg/ml of eleutheroside E.

Maintenance doses for healthy individuals should be toward the lower end of the dose range, but higher doses should be used for treating illness and for high stress situations, including athletic training.

The recommended regime for healthy people is a course of 6 weeks followed by a 2-week break. This regime can be repeated for as long as is necessary. For treating specific illnesses, continuous use is preferable.

SUPPORTING INFORMATION

Traditional Prescribing

Uses and properties from TCM include:
- To reinforce *qi*, to *invigorate* the function of the *spleen* and *kidney*, to calm the nerves[1]
- Poor functioning of the *spleen* and *kidney* marked by general weakness, fatigue, anorexia, and aching of the lower back and knees[1]
- Insomnia and dream-disturbed sleep[1]

Traditional Western herbal medicine uses include temporary fatigue, general debility, and chronic inflammatory conditions[2]

Pharmacologic Research

Key constituents of Eleutherococcus root include the eleutherosides (a chemically diverse group of compounds), triterpenoid saponins, and glycans.
- Experimental studies have shown that Eleutherococcus, its components, or both increased stamina and resistance to stressors (heat, cold, immobilization, trauma, surgery, blood loss, increased or decreased barometric pressure, narcotics, toxins, and bacteria), protected against the physical, behavioral, functional, and biochemical effects of stress (oral route), improved learning and memory (oral route), and exerted an immune-enhancing effect in immuno-compromised mice.
- Eleutherococcus increased survival and promoted the self-repair mechanism in experimental irradiation studies after intraperitoneal or oral administration.
- Eleutherococcus inhibited spontaneous malignant tumors and tumors induced by a number of carcinogens *in vivo.* Eleutherococcus potentiated the effect of some cytotoxic drugs *in vitro,* thus reducing the amount of drug needed.

Eleutherococcus *continued on page 197*

*This dose range is based on those used in clinical trials.

- Resistance to bacterial infection was increased in experimental models by prior dosing with Eleutherococcus. However, simultaneous administration with the infecting organism increased the severity of the disease. Antiviral immunity was also stimulated *in vivo* and *in vitro* by prior administration of Eleutherococcus.
- Eleutherococcus impeded both hypertrophy and atrophy of the adrenal and thyroid glands, reduced blood sugar in hyperglycemia and increased it in hypoglycemia (*in vivo* by oral route), and normalized both leukopenia and leukocytosis.
- Eleutherococcus enhanced the protective effect of the anticoagulant system against coagulant drugs *in vivo* by oral administration, increased repair in damaged heart muscle, increased the number of mitochondria in cardiac muscle, increased the conversion of fat into glycogen for energy, and countered the effects of cerebral ischemia in experimental models.
- Eleutherococcus demonstrated an anabolic effect by stimulating weight gain *in vivo* when given orally and, in other models, improved egg weight and yield and increased reproductive capacity.
- An antitoxic effect has been demonstrated *in vivo* by the simultaneous administration of drugs or toxins with Eleutherococcus.

Clinical Studies

- A placebo-controlled, double-blind study demonstrated that Eleutherococcus extract improved maximal work capacity by 23.3% in male athletes compared with a 7.5% increase in the placebo group. The dose used was equivalent to 300 mg/day of dried root and contained 2.12 mg of eleutheroside B and 0.48 mg of eleutheroside E. The dose was administered for 8 days. However, Eleutherococcus extract did not increase work capacity in highly trained distance runners in a randomized, double-blind, placebo-controlled trial.
- A randomized, double-blind, placebo-controlled, crossover trial involving nine athletes concluded that Eleutherococcus supplementation at 1.2 g/day for 7 days before each of the two trial periods did not alter steady-state substrate utilization or 10-km cycling performance time.[3]
- A 40% reduction in lost work days and a 50% reduction in general illness over a 1-year period was observed in a controlled study of 1000 workers in a Siberian factory who received Eleutherococcus. The mean daily temperature of the region was $-5°$ C ($23°$ F).
- The following results (compared with baseline values) were obtained in healthy volunteers treated with Eleutherococcus extract for 1 month in a randomized, comparative trial: increased cellular immunity, increased oxygen consumption during maximal physical exercise, increased aerobic metabolism of tissues, and decreased blood levels of total cholesterol, LDL-cholesterol, and triglyceride. (The comparison was with administration of *Echinacea purpurea* aerial parts, which did not produce significant results.)[4]
- Eleutherococcus extract (equivalent to approximately 6 g/day of dried root) significantly increased T-helper cell and natural killer cell numbers in healthy volunteers in a double-blind, placebo-controlled trial.

Eleutherococcus *continued on page 198*

- In uncontrolled trials, Eleutherococcus extract:
  - Improved the performance and stamina of explorers, sailors, deep sea divers, mine and mountain rescue workers, truck drivers, pilots, factory workers, laborers, and cosmonauts
  - Increased endurance and concentration in track and field athletes, gymnasts, and weight lifters
  - Improved running times by an average of 9% in long-distance runners
  - Improved the strength of larger muscles in athletes
  - Caused faster activation and greater intensity of perspiration in healthy participants exposed to heat stress
  - Accelerated reading time and decreased errors in proofreaders
  - Enhanced nonspecific immunity, minimized the side effects from radiation, chemotherapy and surgery, and improved healing and well being in patients with cancer
  - Alleviated the effects of protracted disease and lengthened survival time in patients with terminal disease
  - Improved well being and lung capacity in patients with chronic bronchitis, pneumoconiosis, and pneumonia
  - Improved cardiovascular function and general well being in patients with atherosclerotic conditions and patients with rheumatic heart lesions
  - Lowered blood pressure in patients with hypertension and raised it in those with low blood pressure
  - Significantly raised blood pressure and peripheral resistance in children with hypotension
  - Caused a faster response to medical treatment in children with dysentery
  - Alleviated exhaustion, irritability, insomnia, and mild depression
  - Assisted resettled people to adapt to their new and harsh environment in the mountainous, desert area of Mongolia, as measured by normalization in the parameters measured, including work capacity[5]
- Patients with antibiotic-induced diarrhea benefited from Eleutherococcus in a postmarketing surveillance study.
- In Germany, the Commission E supports using Eleutherococcus as a tonic for invigoration and fortification in times of fatigue and debility, reduced capacity for work and concentration, and during convalescence.[6]

REFERENCES

Except when specifically referenced, the following book was referred to in the compilation of the pharmacologic and clinical information: Mills S, Bone K: *Principles and Practice of Phytotherapy: Modern Herbal Medicine,* Edinburgh, 2000, Churchill Livingstone.

1 Pharmacopoeia Commission of the People's Republic of China: *Pharmacopoeia of the People's Republic of China,* English ed, Beijing, 1997, Chemical Industry Press.

2 British Herbal Medicine Association: *British herbal compendium,* Bournemouth, 1992, BHMA.

3 Eschbach LF et al: *Int J Sport Nutr Exerc Metab* 10(4):444-451, 2000.

4 Szolomicki J et al: *Phytother Res* 14(1):30-35, 2000.

5 Zhekalov AN: *Rastit Resur* 31(4):87-91, 1995.

6 Blumenthal M et al, editors: *The complete German Commission E monographs: therapeutic guide to herbal medicines,* Austin, 1998, American Botanical Council.

EUPHORBIA

Botanical Names: *Euphorbia hirta, Euphorbia pilulifera*[#]
Family: Euphorbiaceae
Plant Part Used: Aerial parts

PRESCRIBING INFORMATION

Actions	Expectorant, antiasthmatic, spasmolytic, antiprotozoal
Potential Indications	Based on appropriate evaluation of the patient, practitioners should consider prescribing Euphorbia in formulations in the context of:

• Congestion and spasm of the respiratory tract, especially chronic bronchitis, laryngitis, asthma, emphysema, and whooping cough *(5)*
• Amebic dysentery and possibly other gastrointestinal protozoal infections *(4,6)*
• Intestinal worms, bowel disorders *(6)*

Contraindications	None known.
Warnings and Precautions	None required.
Interactions	None known.
Use in Pregnancy and Lactation	No adverse effects expected.
Side Effects	None expected if taken within the recommended dose range. Based on traditional literature, large (undefined) doses of Euphorbia may cause nausea and vomiting,[1] and it may occasionally cause epigastric distress with nausea.[2]

Dosage

Dose per day*	Dose per week*
0.7-2.0 ml of 1:2 liquid extract	5-12 ml of 1:2 liquid extract

Clinical studies show that Euphorbia can remove intestinal protozoal parasites.[3,4] In chronic cases, 15 to 20 ml of 1:2 extract can be used for up to 7 days' continuous treatment at a time.

SUPPORTING INFORMATION

Traditional Prescribing

Traditional Western herbal medicine uses include:
• Asthma, bronchitis, laryngeal spasm, difficult breathing of cardiac disease, tuberculosis, emphysema,[2,5] the common cold[1]
• Intestinal amebiasis,[5] intestinal worms, bowel disorders, colic, dysentery, warts[6]

Euphorbia *continued on page 200*

[#]Alternative name.
*This dose range is extrapolated from the British Pharmaceutical Codex 1949, the British Herbal Pharmacopoeia 1983, and the author's education and experience.

Aboriginal Australians used Euphorbia for asthma, bronchitis, and emphysema and as a sedative in respiratory conditions, although findings suggest that it was not always effective for asthma.[6] A decoction of the whole plant was taken as a treatment for debility.[7]

Euphorbia was official in the NF from 1916 to 1947 and had "some reputation as antiasthmatic."[8] Eclectic physicians regarded Euphorbia as a reliable antiasthmatic.[2]

Pharmacologic Research

Some of the pharmacologic research listed here used "whole plant" extracts, which probably included the root. The roots of Euphorbia species have been traditionally used for their emetic and cathartic properties. This research may not be relevant to Euphorbia extract manufactured from aerial parts.

- A polyphenolic-rich extract of Euphorbia whole plant demonstrated antiamebic and spasmolytic activity *in vitro*.[9] Aqueous extract of Euphorbia whole plant demonstrated antibacterial, antiamebic, and spasmolytic activity *in vitro*. These activities support the traditional Congolese use of Euphorbia as an antidiarrheal agent.[10] Freeze-dried decoction of Euphorbia whole plant demonstrated antidiarrheal activity in three experimental models of diarrhea. The flavonoid quercitrin, isolated from Euphorbia, has displayed antidiarrheal activity.[11]
- A study using an *in vitro* model verified inhibitory activity against *Amoeba proteus* for Euphorbia. Aqueous extract of fresh aerial parts demonstrated greater cytotoxic activity than did extracts of dried plant material.[12]
- Oral administration of Euphorbia whole plant extract demonstrated significant suppression of parasitemia in a malaria model.[13]
- Water and ethanol extracts of Euphorbia leaf administered by intraperitoneal injection demonstrated a diuretic effect by increasing the rate of urine output and increasing electrolyte excretion.[14] Freeze-dried aqueous extract of Euphorbia aerial parts strongly inhibited the activity of angiotensin converting enzyme (ACE) *in vitro* and decreased water intake when administered by injection, which is also indicative of ACE inhibition.[15]
- Euphorbia extract reduced the release of prostaglandins and inhibited platelet aggregation *in vitro*. The extract also decreased the formation of carrageenan-induced paw edema (route unknown).[16] Freeze-dried aqueous extract of Euphorbia had analgesic, antipyretic, and antiinflammatory activity experimentally (most likely by injection). Euphorbia also exerted central analgesic activity. The antiinflammatory activity was stronger in acute models compared with chronic models.[17] Sedative and anxiolytic effects have also been demonstrated.[17,18] The extract did not protect against induced convulsions, did not cause muscle relaxant effects, and did not have affinity for benzodiazepine receptors. No hypnotic, neuroleptic, or significant antidepressant activity was observed. However, the extract intensified the activity of barbiturates.[19]

Euphorbia *continued on page 201*

Clinical Studies

The clinical antiprotozoal activity of Euphorbia has been documented. Initial observations of 53 cases of amebic dysentery demonstrated that a 1:2 extract of Euphorbia quickly and effectively controlled acute symptoms.[3] The dosage protocol for adults was 20 ml (equivalent to 10 g of herb) with soup over 3 hours, then 15 ml (7.5 g of herb) with soup over 3 hours, followed by 10 ml (5 g of herb) with soup over 3 hours. Chronic cases also showed benefit, the dose being 20 ml per day. A subsequent trial using a tabletted concentrate of Euphorbia demonstrated a successful outcome in 83% of 150 patients with amebic dysentery. Disappearance of the parasite and pain improvement were rapidly established, and follow-up showed no recurrence after 5 to 12 months.[4]

REFERENCES

1 Grieve M: *A modern herbal,* New York, 1971, Dover Publications.
2 Felter HW, Lloyd JU: *King's American dispensatory,* ed 18, rev 3, Portland, 1905, reprinted 1983, Eclectic Medical Publications.
3 Ridet J, Chartol A: *Med Trop* 24:119-143, 1964.
4 Martin M et al: *Med Trop* 24:250-261, 1964.
5 British Herbal Medicine Association's Scientific Committee: *British herbal pharmacopoeia,* Bournemouth, 1983, BHMA.
6 Lassak EV, McCarthy T: *Australian medicinal plants,* North Ryde, NSW, Australia, 1983, Methuen Australia.
7 Aboriginal Communities of the Northern Territory of Australia, Conservation Commission of the Northern Territory: *Traditional aboriginal medicines in the Northern Territory of Australia,* Darwin, NT, Australia, 1993, Conservation Commission of the Northern Territory of Australia.
8 Vogel VJ: *American Indian medicine,* Norman, Okla, 1970, University of Oklahoma Press.
9 Tona L et al: *Phytomed* 7(1):31-38, 2000.
10 Tona L et al: *Phytomed* 6(1):59-66, 1999.
11 Galvez J et al: *Planta Med* 59(4):333-336, 1995.
12 Duez P et al: *J Ethnopharmacol* 34(2-3):235-246, 1991.
13 Tona L et al: *J Ethnopharmacol* 68(1-3):193-203, 1999.
14 Johnson PB et al: *J Ethanopharmacol* 65(1):63-69, 1999.
15 Williams LAD et al: *Phytother Res* 11(5):401-402, 1997.
16 Hiermann A, Bucar F: *J Ethnopharmacol* 42(2):111-116, 1994.
17 Lanhers MC et al: *Planta Med* 57(3):225-231, 1991.
18 Lanhers MC et al: *J Ethnopharmacol* 29(2):189-198, 1990.
19 Lanhers MC et al: *Phytother Res* 10(8):670-676, 1996.

EYEBRIGHT

Botanical Names: *Euphrasia officinalis, Euphrasia rostkoviana,*[#/+^] *Euphrasia stricta*[#^]
Family: Scrophulariaceae
Plant Part Used: Aerial parts

PRESCRIBING INFORMATION

Actions

Astringent, anticatarrhal, mucous membrane tonic, antiinflammatory

Potential Indications

Based on appropriate evaluation of the patient, practitioners should consider prescribing eyebright in formulations in the context of:
- Catarrhal conditions of the upper respiratory tract, sinusitis, chronic sneezing, hay fever, middle ear problems, sore throat, catarrhal phase of measles, the common cold (5)
- Inflammation or infection of the eyes, including conjunctivitis (5)

Contraindications

None known.

Warnings and Precautions

None required.

Interactions

None known.

Use in Pregnancy and Lactation

No adverse effects expected.

Side Effects

None expected if taken within the recommended dose range.

Dosage

Dose per day*	Dose per week*
2.0-4.5 ml of 1:2 liquid extract	15-30 ml of 1:2 liquid extract

For topical use of eyebright (such as for treatment of conjunctivitis), a solution of approximately 5 to 6 drops of a 1:2 extract is prepared in an eye bath of recently boiled water or saline. The liquid should be allowed to cool before applying to the eye. (Allowing the alcohol to evaporate before applying to the eye is important.)

SUPPORTING INFORMATION

Traditional Prescribing

Traditional Western herbal medicine uses include:
- Catarrhal conditions of the eyes, nose and ears; sinusitis, conjunctivitis (internally and locally); the common cold with copious discharge; the catarrhal phase during and following measles[2,3]
- Weakness of the eyes and eyesight disorders[4]
- Catarrhal conditions of the intestinal tract; epilepsy[3]

Eyebright *continued on page 203*

[#]Alternative name.
[+]Medicinally interchangeable species.
[^]Adopted by the American Herbal Products Association as the new botanical name.[1]
*This dose range is extrapolated from the *British Herbal Pharmacopoeia* 1983 and the author's education and experience.

Pharmacologic Research

The aerial parts of eyebright contain iridoid glycosides, including aucubin.

- Aucubigenin, the aglycone of aucubin, demonstrated antibacterial and antifungal activity *in vitro*.
- Aucubin alone had no antiviral activity *in vitro*. However, when mixed with β-glucosidase (an enzyme that releases the aglycone from the glycoside), aucubin displayed significant antiviral activity against hepatitis B.
- Aucubigenin by injection showed antitumor activity in experimental models, but aucubin did not.
- Aucubin demonstrated antispasmodic activity on isolated tissue. Both oral and topical administration resulted in an antiinflammatory effect in models of edema.

Clinical Studies

No clinical studies of internal use of eyebright have been found.

REFERENCES

The following book was referred to in the compilation of the pharmacologic and clinical information: Mills S, Bone K: *Principles and Practice of Phytotherapy: Modern Herbal Medicine,* Edinburgh, 2000, Churchill Livingstone.

1 McGuffin M, editor: *Herbs of commerce,* ed 2 [draft 3.3], Bethesda, Md, 1998, American Herbal Products Association.
2 British Herbal Medicine Association's Scientific Committee: *British herbal pharmacopoeia,* Bournemouth, 1983, BHMA.
3 Felter HW, Lloyd JU: *King's American dispensatory,* ed 18, rev 3, Portland, 1905, reprinted 1983, Eclectic Medical Publications.
4 Grieve M: *A modern herbal,* New York, 1971, Dover Publications.

FALSE UNICORN

Other Common Name:	Helonias root
Botanical Names:	*Chamaelirium luteum, Helonias luteum*[#]
Family:	Melanthiaceae
Plant Part Used:	Root

PRESCRIBING INFORMATION

Actions

Uterine tonic, ovarian tonic, estrogen modulating

Potential Indications

Based on appropriate evaluation of the patient, practitioners should consider prescribing false unicorn root in formulations in the context of:
- Disorders of the female reproductive tract, including amenorrhea, dysmenorrhea, ovarian pain, leukorrhea, prolapse, atony of the reproductive organs, threatened miscarriage, and morning sickness (5)
- Menopausal symptoms, especially hot flashes (5)
- Infertility, sexual lassitude (5)

Contraindications

None known.

Warnings and Precautions

None required.

Interactions

None known.

Use in Pregnancy and Lactation

No adverse effects expected.

Side Effects

None expected if taken within the recommended dose range. Very large (undefined) doses are said to cause nausea and vomiting.[1,2]

Dosage

Dose per day*	Dose per week*
2-6 ml of 1:2 liquid extract	15-40 ml of 1:2 liquid extract

SUPPORTING INFORMATION

Traditional Prescribing

Traditional Western herbal medicine uses include:
- Disorders of the female reproductive tract, especially amenorrhea, dysmenorrhea (particularly of a congestive nature), anemia associated with reproductive problems, ovarian pain, leukorrhea, prolapse, atony of the reproductive organs, threatened miscarriage, and morning sickness[1,3,4]
- Menopausal complaints[2]
- Infertility and sexual lassitude in both sexes[3]

The Eclectic physicians regarded false unicorn root as a valuable uterine tonic, imparting tone and vigor to the female reproductive organs, and used it to promote normal activity of the glandular organs.[3,5]

False Unicorn *continued on page 205*

[#]Alternative name.

*This dose range is extrapolated from the British Herbal Pharmacopoeia 1983, the British Herbal Compendium 1992, and the author's education and experience.

Native Americans used false unicorn root. False unicorn was official in the NF from 1916 to 1947 and was used as a diuretic and uterine tonic.[6]

Pharmacologic Research

False unicorn root contains steroidal saponins that may exert estrogenic effects by binding with estrogen receptors of the hypothalamus.[2] In the premenopausal woman, this action may provide an estrogenic effect, and in the low-estrogen environment of menopause, these saponins may relieve menopausal symptoms, especially hot flashes.
- In an early study, false unicorn root extract did not demonstrate any activity on isolated uterine tissue.[7] A later study confirmed a lack of stimulatory activity on the uterus *in vivo* after injection.[8]

Clinical Studies

No clinical studies using false unicorn root have been found.

REFERENCES

1 British Herbal Medicine Association's Scientific Committee: *British herbal pharmacopoeia,* Bournemouth, 1983, BHMA.
2 British Herbal Medicine Association: *British herbal compendium,* Bournemouth, 1992, BHMA.
3 Felter HW, Lloyd JU: *King's American dispensatory,* ed 18, rev 3, Portland, 1905, reprinted 1983, Eclectic Medical Publications.
4 Felter HW: *The eclectic materia medica, pharmacology and therapeutics,* Portland, 1922, reprinted 1983, Eclectic Medical Publications.
5 Ellingwood F, Lloyd JU: *American materia medica, therapeutics and pharmacognosy,* ed 11, Portland, 1983, Eclectic Medical Publications.
6 Vogel VJ: *American Indian medicine,* Norman, Okla, 1970, University of Oklahoma Press.
7 Pilcher JD: *J Pharmacol Exp Therapeut* 8:110-111, 1916.
8 Pilcher JD, Mauer RT: *Surg Gynecol Obstet* 27:97-99, 1918.

FENNEL

Botanical Name: *Foeniculum vulgare*
Family: Umbelliferae
Plant Part Used: Fruit (sometimes referred to as seed)

PRESCRIBING INFORMATION

Actions	Carminative, appetite stimulating, spasmolytic, galactagogue, estrogen modulating, antimicrobial, expectorant
Potential Indications	Based on appropriate evaluation of the patient, practitioners should consider prescribing fennel in formulations in the context of: • Dyspepsia,* in combination with wormwood, caraway, and peppermint (2) • Chronic digestive problems, bloating, flatulence,** in combination with caraway, peppermint, and gentian (2) • Infantile colic,** in combination with lemon balm, chamomile, vervain, and licorice (3) • Mild spasmodic gastrointestinal complaints, bloating, flatulence (4) • Chronic nonspecific colitis, in combination with dandelion root, St. John's wort, lemon balm, and Calendula (4) • Upper respiratory tract catarrh (4) • Abdominal pain with anorexia, vomiting, and diarrhea (5) • Wheeze, shortness of breath, chronic cough, as a gargle for pharyngitis (5) • Suppressed lactation (5) • Irritable bowel syndrome (6) • Possible benefit for obesity (6)
Contraindications	Contraindicated in patients who suffer from "celery-carrot-mugwort-spice" syndrome.
Warnings and Precautions	Allergic reactions to fennel are rare and seem to be limited to occupational exposure. A percentage of patients who are allergic to celery also display allergic reactions to fennel. Individuals sensitized to carrot, for example, may also have allergic reactions to other vegetables or spices of the Umbelliferae family (celery-carrot-mugwort-spice syndrome). Allergic reactions in the skin and respiratory tract have been reported.
Interactions	None known.
Use in Pregnancy and Lactation	No adverse effects expected, especially when administered as infusions that contain a lower essential oil content than do extracts. Fennel has a long history of use as a galactagogue.

Fennel *continued on page 207*

*ESCOP recommends fennel for treating dyspepsia. (4,5)
**Fennel has been used in traditional herbal medicine for treating the following conditions: infantile colic, chronic digestive problems, and flatulence. (5)

Side Effects   Allergic reaction occurs rarely, as previously indicated.

Dosage

Dose per day***	*Dose per week****
3-6 ml of 1:2 liquid extract	20-40 ml of 1:2 liquid extract

SUPPORTING INFORMATION

Traditional Prescribing

Traditional Western herbal medicine uses include:
- Flatulent colic, especially in infants; flatulent dyspepsia,[1,2] irritable bowel syndrome[3]
- Increasing reduced appetite[1] and suppression of food cravings[4]
- Wheezing, shortness of breath, chronic cough[1]
- Amenorrhea, suppressed lactation[2]
- Topically to treat conjunctivitis and blepharitis, as a gargle for pharyngitis[1]
- Improving the taste of unpleasant medicines[2]

Uses and properties from TCM include:
- To dispel *cold* and relieve pain, to regulate stomach function[5]
- Abdominal pain with anorexia, vomiting, and diarrhea; dysmenorrhea with cold sensation[5]

Pharmacologic Research

Fennel fruit contains an essential oil, the quantity and composition of which depends on the subspecies: *F. vulgare* subsp. *vulgare* var. *vulgare* (bitter fennel) contains more than 4% essential oil; *F. vulgare* subsp. *vulgare* var. *dulce* (sweet fennel) contains more than 2%.[6]
- Fennel oil and alcohol extracts of fennel demonstrated antispasmodic activity in several *in vitro* models using isolated smooth muscle. This activity was confirmed in an *in vivo* model following injection.
- Fennel water was used to decrease the tone and amplitude of peristalsis in the stomach, small intestine, and colon in an experimental model. Another study found that fennel appeared to relax smooth muscle by a direct local activity and to stimulate it via the sympathetic nervous system.
- In experimental models, acetone extracts of fennel (route unknown) induced estrus (changes in the uterine mucosa related to the mating period) and caused growth of mammary glands, oviducts, the cervix, and vagina. An antiandrogenic effect was also observed.
- In an experimental model, oral administration of fennel fruit extract caused a significant increase in collected bile when compared with controls.
- An ethanolic extract of fennel fruit showed significant diuretic activity compared with controls. The diuresis was not associated with changes in sodium or potassium excretion.

Fennel *continued on page 208*

***This dose range is extrapolated from the British Herbal Pharmacopoeia 1983 and the author's education and experience. The dosage listed in the British Pharmaceutical Codex 1934 indicates that the essential oil is an integral aspect of the dosage.

- Fennel oil administered by inhalation was shown to have a mild antitussive or cough suppressant effect.
- Several studies have demonstrated the *in vitro* antibacterial activity of fennel oil.
- Fennel oil displayed a favorable influence on the total quantity of milk (and its fat content) produced by goats.

Clinical Studies

- A liquid herbal formula containing fennel, wormwood, caraway *(Carum carvi)*, and peppermint was found to be superior to the spasmolytic drug metoclopramide in relieving pain, nausea, belching, and heartburn in a randomized, double-blind, clinical trial assessing treating dyspepsia.
- In another randomized, double-blind, placebo-controlled, clinical trial, patients with marked chronic digestive problems such as flatulence or bloating were treated with either an herbal formula containing caraway, fennel, peppermint, and gentian in tablet form or a placebo over a 14-day period. Significant improvement was achieved in the herbal group compared with placebo.
- Patients with chronic nonspecific colitis were treated with a combination containing dandelion root, St. John's wort, lemon balm, Calendula, and fennel. By the fifteenth day of treatment, spontaneous and palpable pains along the large intestine had disappeared in 96% of the patients. Defecation was normalized in patients with diarrhea syndrome.
- The effect of an instant herbal tea preparation containing chamomile, vervain, licorice, fennel, and lemon balm on infantile colic was assessed in a prospective, randomized, double-blind study involving babies approximately 3 weeks of age. After 7 days, colic scores were significantly lower in the herbal tea group compared with the placebo group. The tea preparation was offered with every episode of colic, up to 150 ml per dose, but not more than three times per day. The exact composition of the preparation was not defined.
- In Germany, the Commission E supports using fennel to treat mild, spasmodic gastrointestinal complaints, bloating, flatulence, and upper respiratory tract catarrh.[7]
- ESCOP recommends fennel for treating dyspepsia and upper respiratory catarrh.[8]

REFERENCES

The following book was referred to in the compilation of the pharmacologic and clinical information: Mills S, Bone K: *Principles and Practice of Phytotherapy: Modern Herbal Medicine*, Edinburgh, 2000, Churchill Livingstone.

1 British Herbal Medicine Association's Scientific Committee: *British herbal pharmacopoeia*, Bournemouth, 1983, BHMA.
2 Felter HW, Lloyd JU: *King's American dispensatory*, ed 18, rev 3, Portland, 1905, reprinted 1983, Eclectic Medical Publications.
3 Bartram T: *Encyclopedia of herbal medicine*, ed 1, Dorset, UK, 1995, Grace Publishers.
4 Grieve M: *A modern herbal*, New York, 1971, Dover Publications.

Fennel *continued on page 209*

5 Pharmacopoeia Commission of the People's Republic of China: *Pharmacopoeia of the People's Republic of China*, English ed, Beijing, 1997, Chemical Industry Press.

6 European Pharmacopoeia Commission: *European pharmacopoeia*, ed 3, Strasbourg, France, 1996, European Department for the Quality of Medicines within the Council of Europe.

7 Blumenthal M et al, editors: *The complete German Commission E monographs: therapeutic guide to herbal medicines*, Austin, 1998, American Botanical Council.

8 Scientific Committee of the European Scientific Cooperative on Phytotherapy [ESCOP]: *ESCOP monographs: Foeniculi fructus*. European Scientific Cooperative on Phytotherapy, ESCOP Secretariat, Argyle House, Gandy Street, Exeter, Devon, EX4 3LS, United Kingdom, March 1996.

FENUGREEK

Botanical Name: *Trigonella foenum-graecum*
Family: Leguminosae
Plant Part Used: Seed

PRESCRIBING INFORMATION

Actions	Appetite stimulating, galactagogue, antiinflammatory, demulcent, hypoglycemic, hypocholesterolemic
Potential Indications	Based on appropriate evaluation of the patient, practitioners should consider prescribing fenugreek in formulations in the context of:

- Managing diabetes mellitus (both insulin-dependent and non-insulin–dependent) *(3,5)*
- Loss of appetite *(4,5)*
- Dyspepsia, gastritis, debility, gastrointestinal inflammation *(5)*
- Preventing atherosclerosis *(5,7)*
- Promoting lactation *(5)*

Contraindications	None known.
Warnings and Precautions	Based on a recent pharmacologic study (see later discussion), high doses of fenugreek are not recommended in patients with low thyroid activity.
Interactions	A medical source cites fenugreek as having the potential to interact with warfarin and potentially increase the risk of bleeding.[1] Another source indicates this caution is based on the fact that fenugreek contains coumarin.[2] One scientific reference does cite the presence of coumarin in fenugreek seed.[3] Coumarin does not, however, increase the risk of bleeding. Dicoumarol, a compound formed from coumarin by bacterial action in spoiled sweet clover hay, has powerful anticoagulant activity. The requirement for powerful anticoagulant activity is hydroxylation of the coumarin molecule in the 4 position. Common plant coumarins are not substituted at this position and therefore lack significant clinical anticoagulant activity, although some do possess measurable activity when given to animals in high doses.[4]

A clinical trial has found that administration of fenugreek seed (5 g/day for 3 months) did not affect platelet aggregation, fibrinolytic activity, and fibrinogen levels.[5] A case has been reported suggesting a probable interaction between warfarin and fenugreek, boldo *(Peumus boldus)*, or any combination. A patient being treated with warfarin developed an increase in international normalized ratio (indicating decreased coagulation), which returned to normal after cessation of the herbs. This herb-drug interaction was observed a second time after both herbs were reintroduced a few days later.[6]

Large or frequent dose of fenugreek may inhibit iron absorption.[7]

Fenugreek *continued on page 211*

Use in Pregnancy and Lactation

No adverse effects expected. Fenugreek is traditionally used to promote lactation.

Side Effects

None expected for internal use if fenugreek is taken within the recommended dose range. Mild gastrointestinal upset has been recorded in a small percentage of patients during a clinical trial using high doses of fenugreek seed (25 g/day).[8]

Excessive consumption of fenugreek can lead to a currylike body odor and may be responsible for the incorrect diagnosis of maple syrup urine disease.[9] (The substance responsible for the characteristic odor of maple syrup urine disease is 4,5-dimethyl-3-hydroxy-2[5H]-furanone [sotolone], which is also present in both fenugreek and maple syrup.[10])

Frequent consumption of (dietary) fenugreek has been associated with anemia in Ethiopian children resulting from the inhibition of iron absorption.[7]

According to the Commission E, repeated external use can result in undesirable skin reactions.[11] Two cases of severe allergic reaction have been reported after internal and topical use of fenugreek seed.[12]

Dosage

Dose per day*	Dose per week*
2.0-4.5 ml of 1:2 liquid extract	15-30 ml of 1:2 liquid extract

SUPPORTING INFORMATION

Traditional Prescribing

Traditional Western herbal medicine uses include:
- Dyspepsia, anorexia, gastritis[13,14]
- Debility and anorexia of convalescence[1]
- To increase milk flow in nursing mothers[15]
- Uterine irritation; lower respiratory tract irritation[2]
- Topically for sore throat, boils, myalgia, lymphadenitis, gout, wounds, and leg ulcers; vaginal or rectal irritation or inflammation; chronic disorders of the stomach, bowel, and liver[1,2]

Traditional Ayurvedic uses include:
- As a carminative, tonic, and aphrodisiac[16]
- Dyspepsia, diarrhea, dysentery, colic, flatulence, rheumatism, enlarged liver or spleen, chronic cough[17]
- As a cooling drink for patients with smallpox (by infusion)[16]
- In a gruel with milk and sugar as a galactagogue[17]
- Lowering serum cholesterol, triglyceride, and glucose; for antiatherosclerotic action[18]

Fenugreek *continued on page 212*

*This dosage is extrapolated from the British Herbal Pharmacopoeia 1983.

Uses and properties from TCM include:
- *Cold* syndrome of the *kidney* resulting from *yang* deficiency marked by pain and coldness in the lower abdomen[19]
- Hernia; weakness and edema of the legs caused by *cold damp*[19]

Fenugreek is also used in the traditional herbal medicine of Southeast Asia for treating female disorders such as reduced menstrual flow, dysmenorrhea, leucorrhea, and postpartum pain and fever.[20] In the Middle East and northern Africa, fenugreek seed has traditionally been added to the diet of patients with diabetes.[3,21,22]

Pharmacologic Research

Constituents of fenugreek seeds include steroidal saponins of the furanostanolic type, alkaloids (including trigonelline), flavonoids, sterols, protein, amino acids, proteinase inhibitors, and carbohydrates.[23] Coumarin is also listed as present in fenugreek seed.[3] The furanostanol glycosides are bitter in taste.[23] Alcoholic extracts of fenugreek will not contain as much carbohydrate (including the mucilaginous galactomannans) as will a decoction of seed. Defatted fenugreek contains similar levels of amino acids, minerals, and vitamins but less fat and saponin than does fenugreek seed.

The whole seeds and defatted seeds, being rich in mucilage (soluble fiber), lower blood cholesterol levels. Whether alcoholic liquid extracts of fenugreek seed will have this effect is uncertain, although saponins will be present (which are known to lower cholesterol and lipids; see later discussion).

Both fenugreek seed and fenugreek leaf have shown hypoglycemic activity. In the studies outlined in this monograph, only information on the seed (or part undefined) is listed. (The seed might possibly contain the same hypoglycemic components as does the leaf.)
- Various results have been obtained for hypoglycemic activity *in vivo* using different types of fenugreek preparations. A summary of results for these preparations follows:
- Seed powder: hypoglycemic activity in diabetic and normal models[24]
- Suspension: no effect on oral glucose tolerance test in a normal model, hypoglycemic effect in a diabetic model[24]
- Decoction: hypoglycemic activity in both diabetic and normal models[24] and in transient hyperglycemia[25]
- Defatted seed: hypoglycemic activity in a diabetic model but no activity in normal models[24]
- Defatted seed subfractions: hypoglycemic activity in a diabetic model for the subfraction containing fiber; no activity for the subfractions containing protein plus saponin, protein, or saponin[24]
- Ethanol extract: hypoglycemic activity in both diabetic and normal models[24]
- Saponins: high doses given with food increased food intake and motivation to eat in normal animals and stabilized food consumption in a diabetic model[26]

Fenugreek *continued on page 213*

- The mechanism behind the hypoglycemic activity and the components responsible for this activity are not certain. The following results have been obtained:
  - 4-Hydroxyisoleucine, a free amino acid isolated from fenugreek, stimulated glucose-induced insulin secretion from pancreatic islet cells and demonstrated hypoglycemic activity *in vivo* following intravenous injection in normal and diabetic models.[27,28]
  - Trigonelline displayed hypoglycemic activity in early research[29] but in more recent human trials has been discounted as an active component.[24]
  - Although the fiber subfraction has demonstrated activity, excluding the coexistence of active compounds other than fiber is not possible. Fiber and other fenugreek components acting at the gastrointestinal level may be responsible for improved glucose and starch tolerance.[24]
  - Fenugreek improves peripheral glucose utilization and may exert antidiabetic activity at the insulin receptor, as well as at the gastrointestinal level.[24]
  - High doses of an ethanol extract (which were rich in saponins) increased food intake, increased the motivation to eat, and increased insulin levels in normal animals. This activity is a result of either a direct stimulatory effect on the beta cells or an indirect effect related to the palatability and the flavor-enhancing property of the fenugreek extract. However, the extract was inactive against chemically induced anorexia.[24] In normal rats or mice, the isolated saponins also increased food intake and the motivation to eat, while modifying the circadian rhythm of feeding behavior.[26]
- Fenugreek seed has been shown in various animal models to have beneficial effects on serum lipid profiles.[24] Hypocholesterolemic activity has been associated mainly with reduced intestinal reabsorption of cholesterol and bile acids, which has been attributed to the saponins-sapogenins and the galactomannan gum fiber (mucilage). Hypolipidemic activity has only been associated with the saponins-sapogenins and not with the fiber.[24] Fenugreek also lowered lipid peroxidation and increased the level of antioxidants in blood in a diabetic model, compared with controls.[30] Fenugreek extract reduced the deposition of cholesterol on aorta walls and reduced the number of aortic lesions in an experimental model of early atherosclerotic progression.[31]
- Fenugreek (2% of the diet) enhanced pancreatic lipase activity[32] and decreased the levels of intestinal phosphatases and sucrase[33] *in vivo*.
- Pretreatment with aqueous fenugreek extract did not protect against drug-induced gastric ulceration but promoted healing when administered to animals with ulcers, possibly because of its mild anticholinergic and demulcent properties.[34]
- Dietary fenugreek had no adverse effect on fertility or birth outcome *in vivo*.[35] This finding is in contrast to earlier research published in 1969 indicating that aqueous and alcoholic fenugreek extracts had a stimulating effect on isolated uterus (and highlights the issue that herbal research on isolated organs often has little relevance to

Fenugreek *continued on page 214*

213

effects after oral intake).[36] The addition of fenugreek to the mother's diet during pregnancy and lactation, or only during lactation, did not increase the weight gain of young rat pups compared with controls.[37]

- Administration of a dried, aqueous ethanol extract of fenugreek seed (0.1 g/kg) to both mice and rats significantly decreased serum T_3 concentration and T_3/T_4 ratio, but increased T_4 levels. The inhibition in T_4 to T_3 conversion was not peroxidation-mediated. A significant decrease in superoxide dismutase activity was also observed.[38]
- Fenugreek decreased the quantity of renal calcium oxalate deposited in an experimental model of kidney stone formation.[39]
- Dietary levels of fenugreek stimulated cytochrome P-450, cytochrome b5, and cytochrome P-450–dependent aryl hydroxylase *in vivo*.[40]
- Oral administration of an aqueous suspension of fenugreek seed (powder dissolved in water) promoted wound healing in three wound models.[41]
- Antiinflammatory and antineoplastic activity has been demonstrated in an experimental model for alcoholic extract of fenugreek seed administered by intraperitoneal injection.[42]

Clinical Studies

Dietary fiber from fenugreek has been shown in open, controlled trials to alleviate the imbalances associated with lipid metabolism disorders and non-insulin–dependent diabetes mellitus.[43] The bitter taste of fenugreek has been suggested as a limitation for its use in the daily diets of patients with diabetes,[44] which may explain the common use of defatted (debitterized) extracts of seed in trials. Many clinical trials evaluating fenugreek have used whole seed or defatted seed, and in some cases, high doses were administered. Defatted seed contains mainly fiber and protein, with the lipids and saponins removed, and is odorless and tasteless. Whole seed contains mainly fiber and protein but with lipids and saponins intact.

- A weak and transient hypoglycemic effect was observed in 50% of patients with diabetes treated orally with 500 mg of trigonelline during fasting. Administration of trigonelline at doses of 500 mg up to three times per day for 5 days did not decrease diurnal blood sugar levels.[29]
- Fenugreek (5 g/day) administered to healthy volunteers for 3 months did not affect blood sugar levels compared with baseline values either after fasting or after meals.[5] In healthy volunteers, a single dose of whole fenugreek seed (25 g) prevented the increase in blood glucose following glucose intake and decreased blood insulin levels. Response was greatest in volunteers treated with whole seed, followed by the gum isolate, defatted seed, and cooked seed. Degummed seeds and cooked leaves showed no activity. Whole seed, defatted seed, and gum isolate were rich in galactomannan.[45]
- Clinical trials investigating the hypoglycemic activity of fenugreek in diabetes are summarized in Table 1. In many of these trials, patients continued to take their orthodox medications.

Fenugreek *continued on page 215*

TABLE I

Clinical Trials Investigating the Hypoglycemic Activity of Fenugreek

Dosage and Duration of Trial	Trial Design	Condition	Results
Seed (5 g/day; 3 mos)	Open, placebo-controlled	NIDDM (40 patients)	Significantly reduced both postprandial and fasting blood sugar levels compared with baseline values in mild cases; no significant activity in severe cases. Blood sugar levels were unchanged in the placebo group.[5]
Defatted seed (100 g/day; 2 × 10-day periods)	Open, controlled	IDDM (10 patients); NIDDM (15 patients)	Reduced fasting blood sugar, improved glucose tolerance, and reduced urinary glucose excretion compared with a controlled diet (patients with IDDM).[46] Similar results were obtained with patients with NIDDM.[47]
Seed (25 g/day; 25 wks including 1 wk controlled diet alone)	Open, controlled	NIDDM (60 patients)	Decreased fasting blood glucose and insulin, improved glucose tolerance, decreased 24-hour urinary glucose excretion, and reduced glycosylated hemoglobin concentration compared with a controlled diet.[48] Blood urea levels decreased after 12 weeks. Renal or hepatic toxicity was not observed in these patients.[49]
Defatted seed (25 g/day; 5 wks including 2 wks controlled diet alone)	Open, controlled	NIDDM (5 patients)	Improved plasma glucose and insulin responses and 24-hr urinary glucose output compared with a controlled diet.[45]
Seed (20 g, single dose)	Open, controlled	NIDDM (10 patients/group)	Elevation in glucose response was significantly lower compared with those consuming glucose alone.[50] Comparing the different plant parts of fenugreek, the hypoglycemic activity of seed or root was greater than that of leaf or stalk.
Seed (15 g, single dose)	Open, controlled	NIDDM (21 patients)	Decreased blood glucose in 80% of patients compared with the control meal alone; plasma insulin was nonsignificantly lower.[51]
Seed (25 g/day; 15 days)	Open, controlled	NIDDM	Improved glucose tolerance compared with a controlled diet alone. Fenugreek also increased molar insulin-binding sites on erythrocytes. These results suggest an improvement in peripheral glucose utilization.[52]

NIDDM, Non-insulin–dependent diabetes mellitus; IDDM, insulin-dependent diabetes mellitus.

Fenugreek *continued on page 216*

- Fenugreek (5 g/day) administered to 30 healthy volunteers for 3 months did not affect blood lipid levels compared with baseline values.[5] Clinical trials investigating the hypolipidemic activity of fenugreek in patients with diabetes are summarized in Table 2. Hypocholesterolemic activity has also been

TABLE 2

Clinical Studies Investigating the Hypolipidemic Activity of Fenugreek

Dosage	Trial Design	Condition	Result
Seed (5 g/day; 1 mo)	Open, placebo-controlled	Coronary artery disease with NIDDM (60 patients)	Significantly decreased total cholesterol and triglycerides compared with baseline values after 3 months' treatment. HDL-cholesterol was unchanged. Lipid levels were unchanged in the placebo group.[5]
Defatted seed (100 g/day; 2 × 10-day periods)	Open, controlled	IDDM (10 patients); NIDDM (15 patients)	Improved serum lipid levels (excluding HDL-cholesterol) compared with a controlled diet alone.[46] Similar results were obtained with NIDDM patients.[47]
Defatted seed (100 g/day; 2 × 20-day periods)	Open, controlled	Hypercholesterolemia (10 patients)	Significant reduction in serum total cholesterol, LDL- and VLDL-cholesterol, and triglyceride levels compared with a controlled diet alone. HDL-cholesterol levels were unchanged.[53]
Defatted seed (25 g/day; 5 wks including 2 wks controlled diet alone)	Open, controlled	NIDDM (5 patients)	Reduced serum cholesterol levels compared with a controlled diet alone.[45]
Seed (15 g, single dose)	Open, controlled	NIDDM (21 patients)	No effect on lipid levels compared with the control meal alone.[51]
Seed (25 g/day; 25 wks including 1 wk controlled diet alone)	Open, controlled	NIDDM (60 patients)	Significantly reduced total cholesterol, LDL- and VLDL-cholesterol, and triglycerides compared with a controlled diet. HDL-cholesterol showed a slight, nonsignificant rise.[8]
Defatted seed (25-50 g/day, 20 days)	Open, placebo-controlled	Hypercholesterolemia (18 patients)	Significant decreases in serum total cholesterol, VLDL-cholesterol, and triglycerides compared with the placebo group.[54]

NIDDM, Non-insulin–dependent diabetes mellitus; HDL, high-density lipoproteins; IDDM, insulin-dependent diabetes mellitus; LDL, low-density lipoproteins; VLDL, very low-density lipoproteins.

Fenugreek *continued on page 217*

demonstrated clinically for sprouted fenugreek, suggesting an activity for the saponins, other components, or both, but this information is not covered in the table.

- In Germany, the Commission E supports using fenugreek to treat loss of appetite. Externally, a decoction of fenugreek seed can be used for local inflammation.[11]

REFERENCES

1 Heck AM, Dewitt BA, Lukes AL: *Am J Health Syst Pharm* 57(13):1221-1227, 2000.
2 Newall CA, Anderson LA, Phillipson JD: *Herbal medicines, a guide for health-care professionals,* London, 1996, Pharmaceutical Press.
3 Shani J et al: *Arch Int Pharmacodyn* 210:27-37, 1974.
4 Arora RB, Mathur CN: *Br J Pharmacol* 20:29-35, 1963.
5 Bordia A, Verma SK, Srivastava KC: *Prostaglandins Leukot Essent Fatty Acids* 56(5):379-384, 1997.
6 Lambert JP, Cormier A: *Pharmacother* 21(4):509-512, 2001.
7 Adish AA et al: *Public Health Nutr* 2(3):243-252, 1999.
8 Sharma RD et al: *Phytother Res* 10(4):332-334, 1996.
9 Sewell AC, Mosandi A, Bohles H: *N Engl J Med* 341(10):769, 1999.
10 Podebrad F et al: *J Inherit Metab Dis* 22(2):107-114, 1999.
11 Blumenthal M et al, editors: *The complete German Commission E monographs: therapeutic guide to herbal medicines,* Austin, 1998, American Botanical Council.
12 Patil SP, Niphadkar PV, Bapat MM: *Ann Allergy Asthma Immunol* 78(3):297-300, 1997.
13 British Herbal Medicine Association's Scientific Committee: *British herbal pharmacopoeia,* Bournemouth, 1983, BHMA.
14 Felter HW, Lloyd JU: *King's American dispensatory,* ed 18, rev 3, Portland, 1905, reprinted 1983, Eclectic Medical Publications.
15 Bartram T: *Encyclopedia of herbal medicine,* ed 1, Dorset, UK, 1995, Grace Publishers.
16 Chopra RN et al: *Chopra's indigenous drugs of India,* ed 2, Calcutta, 1958, reprinted 1982, Academic Publishers.
17 Kapoor LD: *CRC handbook of Ayurvedic medicinal plants,* Boca Raton, Fla, 1990, CRC Press.
18 Puri D, Baral N, Upadhyaya BP: *J Nepal Med Assoc* 36(123):334-337, 1997.
19 Pharmacopoeia Commission of the People's Republic of China: *Pharmacopoeia of the People's Republic of China,* English ed, Beijing, 1997, Chemical Industry Press.
20 World Health Organization: *The use of traditional medicine in primary health care: a manual for health workers in Southeast Asia,* New Delhi, 1990, WHO Regional Office for Southeast Asia.
21 Merzouki A, Ed-derfoufi F, Molero Mesa J: *Fitoterapia* 71:278-307, 2000.
22 Iwu MM: *Handbook of African medicinal plants,* Boca Raton, Fla, 1993, CRC Press.
23 Bisset NG, editor: *Herbal drugs and phytopharmaceuticals,* Stuttgart, 1994, Medpharm Scientific Publishers.
24 Al-Habori M, Raman A: *Phytother Res* 12:233-242, 1998.
25 Alarcon-Aguilara FJ et al: *J Ethnopharmacol* 61:101-110, 1998.
26 Petit PR et al: *Steroids* 60(10):674-680, 1995.
27 Sauvaire Y et al. From the 2nd International Congress on Phytomedicine, Munich, September 11-14, 1996, abstract P-92.
28 Broca C et al: *Am J Physiol* 277(4, pt 1):E617-623, 1999.
29 Mishkinsky J, Joseph B, Sulman FG: *Lancet* 2(7529):1311-1312, 1967.
30 Ravikumar P, Anuradha CV: *Phytother Res* 13(3):197-201, 1999.
31 Bhandari U, Grover JK, Sharma JN: *Hamdard Med* 41(4):56-59, 1998.
32 Platel K, Srinivasan K: *Nahrung* 44(1):42-46, 2000.
33 Platel K, Srinivasan K: *Int J Food Sci Nutr* 47(1):55-59, 1996.
34 Al-Meshal IA et al: *Fitoterapia* 56(4):232-235, 1985.
35 Mital N, Gopaldas T: *Nutr Rep Int* 33(2):363-369, 1986.
36 Abdo MS, Al-Kafawi AA: *Planta Med* 17(1):14-18, 1969.
37 Mital N, Gopaldas T: *Nutr Rep Int* 33(3):477-484, 1986.
38 Panda S, Tahiliani P, Kar A: *Pharmacol Res* 40(5):405-409, 1999.
39 Ahsan SK et al: *J Ethnopharmacol* 26(3):249-254, 1989.
40 Sambaiah K, Srinivasan K: *Indian J Biochem Biophys* 26(4):254-258, 1989.

Fenugreek *continued on page 218*

41 Taranalli AD, Kuppast IJ: *Indian J Pharm Sci* 58(3):117-119, 1996.

42 Sur P et al: *Phytother Res* 15(3):257-259, 2001.

43 Madar Z. From the proceedings of the Joint CEC-NCRD Workshop held in Israel (Ginozar Kibbutz) in January 1989 on lupin production and bio-processing for feed, food, and other by-products, EUR-Publication No. 12641, Luxembourg, 1990.

44 Pathak P, Srivastava S, Grover S: *Int J Food Sci Nutr* 51(5):409-414, 2000.

45 Sharma RD: *Nutr Res* 6(12):1353-1364, 1986.

46 Sharma RD, Raghuram TC, Rao NS: *Eur J Clin Nutr* 44(4):301-306, 1990.

47 Sharma RD, Raghuram TC: *Nutr Res* 10(7):731-739, 1990.

48 Sharma RD et al: *Nutr Res* 16(8):1331-1339, 1996.

49 Sharma RD et al: *Phytother Res* 10(6):519-520, 1996.

50 Nair LD, Kapoor R: *Indian J Nutr Diet* 37(3):76-84, 2000.

51 Madar Z et al: *Eur J Clin Nutr* 42(1):51-54, 1988.

52 Raghuram TC et al: *Phytother Res* 8:83-86, 1994.

53 Sharma RD, Raghuram TC: *Phytother Res* 5:145-147, 1991.

54 Prasanna M: *Indian J Pharmacol* 32(1):34-36, 2000.

FEVERFEW

Botanical Names: *Tanacetum parthenium, Chrysanthemum parthenium*[#]
Family: Compositae
Plant Part Used: Leaf

PRESCRIBING INFORMATION

Actions	Antiinflammatory, antiallergic, bitter tonic, emmenagogue (in high doses), anthelmintic
Potential Indications	Based on appropriate evaluation of the patient, practitioners should consider prescribing feverfew in formulations in the context of: • Prophylaxis and treatment of migraine headaches and associated symptoms *(2,4,6)* • Prophylaxis and treatment of tension headache *(3,6)* • Possible benefit in inflammatory arthritis, such as rheumatoid arthritis *(4)*
Contraindications	Individuals with a known hypersensitivity to feverfew, parthenolide, or other members of the Compositae family should not take feverfew internally.
Warnings and Precautions	None required.
Interactions	None known.
Use in Pregnancy and Lactation	Doses during pregnancy should be kept to a minimum (no more than 1.5 ml of a 1:5 tincture/day). No adverse effects expected during lactation as long as the recommended dosage levels are observed.
Side Effects	Allergic contact dermatitis has been noted in many cases after contact with fresh feverfew leaves. The side effects were considered mild and included mouth ulcers, sore tongue, abdominal pain, indigestion, unpleasant taste, tingling sensation, urinary problems, headache, swollen lips or mouth, and diarrhea.

Dosage

Dose per day*	Dose per week*
1-3 ml of 1:5 dried plant tincture	7-20 ml of 1:5 dried plant tincture

Extracts providing quantified levels of parthenolide are recommended. Ideally, aqueous ethanol extracts should contain not less than 0.4 mg/ml of parthenolide.

Feverfew *continued on page 220*

[#]Alternative name.
*This dose range is extrapolated from the British Herbal Compendium 1992 and ESCOP but is somewhat higher than the recommendations from these sources. This higher dose level was given to establish the prophylactic effect at a faster rate.

Traditional Prescribing

Traditional Western herbal medicine uses include:
- Headache[1]
- As a bitter tonic to increase appetite, improve digestion, and promote digestive secretions[2]
- As a warm infusion for cholera, the common cold, febrile diseases, cleansing the kidneys, bringing on menstruation, and expelling worms[3]
- As a honey or sugar sweetened decoction for coughs, wheezing, and difficult breathing[4]
- As a cold infusion, as a tonic, and to relieve facial and ear pain in dyspeptic or rheumatic patients[4]
- Topically as a poultice for pain, bowel swelling, flatulence, and colic[3]

Pharmacologic Research

Key constituents of feverfew leaf include sesquiterpene lactones containing an α-methylene-γ-lactone group, including parthenolide.
- A likely mechanism for the action of feverfew is the inhibition of granule secretion from platelets (antimigraine effect) and polymorphs (antiarthritic effect). Several *in vitro* studies support this mechanism.
- Although the platelets of patients taking feverfew aggregated normally to adenosine diphosphate and thrombin, aggregation in response to serotonin was greatly reduced. This finding implies that although normal clotting mechanisms are still intact, the biochemical chain of events leading to a migraine might be broken.
- Feverfew extracts markedly inhibited phagocytosis of *Candida guilliermondii in vitro*. However, intracellular killing was not affected. The fact that feverfew can inhibit phagocytosis, as well as degranulation, gives it potential as an antiinflammatory agent.
- *In vitro* studies have demonstrated an inhibitory effect of feverfew on eicosanoid production. The relevance of these studies to normal oral use of the herb is uncertain.
- Extracts of fresh feverfew caused a dose- and time-dependent inhibition of the contractile activity of isolated smooth tissue in response to receptor-acting agonists such as serotonin and phenylephrine.
- Compounds containing the α-methylene-γ-lactone group have inhibited tumor growth, respiration, and nucleic acid synthesis *in vitro* and *ex vivo*; demonstrated antihyperlipidemic activity; inhibited carrageenan-induced edema and chronic adjuvant-induced arthritis; and delayed hypersensitivity reactions in experimental models.
- Adding feverfew extract to isolated tissue samples protected against endothelial cell perfusion–induced injury, indicating that feverfew may have a vasoprotective effect in addition to its effects on platelets.
- Extracts of feverfew, as well as the essential oil, have demonstrated antimicrobial activity *in vitro*.

Clinical Studies

- A survey of people with headache using feverfew leaf revealed that the frequency and severity of migraines and tension headaches were reduced. Associated nausea and vomiting decreased or disappeared.

Feverfew continued on page 221

The effectiveness of conventional painkillers increased with concurrent feverfew use. Relief of arthritis symptoms was also experienced. The dosage was low (2. 5 fresh leaves/day, 3.8 cm × 3.1 cm, weight not defined), and the onset of any effect often took several months.

- Following the previous survey, a double-blind, placebo-controlled trial in patients who had been self-medicating with raw feverfew every day for 3 months prior found no change in the frequency or severity of symptoms when the treatment was switched to feverfew capsules (50 mg/day). Patients who switched to a placebo group experienced a significant increase in the frequency and severity of headaches, nausea, and vomiting.
- In a randomized, double-blind, placebo-controlled, crossover study, treatment with powdered feverfew (82 mg/day for 4 months standardized to 2.2 µmol/day parthenolide) was associated with a reduction in the number and severity of attacks and a significant reduction in the degree of vomiting in migraine sufferers.
- These results were not observed in another randomized, double-blind, placebo-controlled, crossover trial. Feverfew did not exert any significant preventative effect on the frequency of migraine attacks, although patients seemed to have a tendency to use fewer analgesic drugs while they were using feverfew. Active treatment occurred for only 4 months, which might be insufficient time to establish the prophylactic effect at the dosage tested. The daily dose was 143 mg of a granulated ethanolic extract corresponding to approximately 170 mg of original dried herb and standardized to 0.5 mg of parthenolide.
- A double-blind, placebo-controlled, crossover study involving people with chronic migraine observed that capsules of powdered feverfew (100 mg/day for 2 months standardized to 0.2 mg/day parthenolide) produced a highly significant decrease in pain intensity. In the second phase of this trial, the group who remained on feverfew continued to experience a decrease in pain intensity and a highly significant reduction in vomiting, nausea, and sensitivity to noise and light during attacks. Participants who switched to placebo experienced an increase in pain sensitivity. The difference between the two groups was significant. In phase 3, transferring the feverfew-treated group to placebo resulted in an increase in pain intensity and other symptoms, and shifting the placebo group to feverfew therapy resulted in an improvement in pain and other symptoms.
- ESCOP recommends feverfew for treating migraine.[5]
- Feverfew is official in the USP24-NF19.

REFERENCES

The following book was referred to in the compilation of the pharmacologic and clinical information: Mills S, Bone K: *Principles and Practice of Phytotherapy: Modern Herbal Medicine,* Edinburgh, 2000, Churchill Livingstone.

1 Johnson ES: *Feverfew,* London, 1984, Sheldon Press.

2 Felter HW, Lloyd JU: *King's American dispensatory,* ed 18, rev 3, Portland, 1905, reprinted 1983, Eclectic Medical Publications.

3 le Strange R: *A history of herbal plants,* London, 1977, Angus & Robertson.

4 Grieve M: *A modern herbal,* New York, 1971, Dover Publications.

5 Scientific Committee of the European Scientific Cooperative on Phytotherapy [ESCOP]: *ESCOP monographs: Tanaceti partheni herba/folium.* European Scientific Cooperative on Phytotherapy, ESCOP Secretariat, Argyle House, Gandy Street, Exeter, Devon, EX4 3LS, United Kingdom, March 1996.

FRINGE TREE

Botanical Name: Chionanthus virginicus
Family: Oleaceae
Plant Part Used: Root bark

PRESCRIBING INFORMATION

Actions

Cholagogue, choleretic, mild laxative, antiemetic, depurative

Potential Indications

Based on appropriate evaluation of the patient, practitioners should consider prescribing fringe tree in formulations in the context of:
- Liver and gallbladder disorders, particularly jaundice, cholecystitis, hepatitis, and gallstones (5)
- Skin and gastrointestinal disorders associated with reduced or disordered liver function (5)
- Other gastrointestinal disorders, such as colic, gastritis, duodenitis, gastric ulcer or pancreatitis (5)
- Splenic enlargement, portal hypertension (5)

Contraindications

None known.

Warnings and Precautions

None required.

Interactions

None known.

Use in Pregnancy and Lactation

No adverse effects expected.

Side Effects

None expected if taken within the recommended dose range.

Dosage

Dose per day*	Dose per week*
3-6 ml of 1:2 liquid extract	20-40 ml of 1:2 liquid extract

SUPPORTING INFORMATION

Traditional Prescribing

Traditional Western herbal medicine uses include:
- Jaundice, hepatic disease, hepatic inflammation, cholecystitis, gallstones, duodenitis, glycosuria of hepatic or alimentary origin, colic, irritation of the stomach, dyspepsia (including infantile), nausea, vomiting, pancreatic disease (including pancreatitis), splenic enlargement, portal hypertension[1,2]
- Skin and bowel disorders resulting from reduced or disordered liver function; syphilis, scrofula (tuberculous infection of the cervical lymph nodes)[2]

Fringe Tree *continued on page 223*

*This dose range is extrapolated from the British Herbal Pharmacopoeia 1983 and the author's education and experience.

Native Americans used fringe tree externally for cuts, bruises, wounds, toothache, and internal pains. Fringe tree was official in the NF from 1916 to 1947 and was used as a tonic.[3] The Eclectic physicians regarded fringe tree as an excellent tonic in convalescence from debilitating diseases.[2]

Pharmacologic Research

No pharmacologic information has been found for fringe tree.

Clinical Studies

No clinical studies using fringe tree have been found.

REFERENCES

1 British Herbal Medicine Association's Scientific Committee: *British herbal pharmacopoeia,* Bournemouth, 1983, BHMA.
2 Felter HW, Lloyd JU: *King's American dispensatory,* ed 18, rev 3, Portland, 1905, reprinted 1983, Eclectic Medical Publications.
3 Vogel VJ: *American Indian medicine,* Norman, Okla, 1970, University of Oklahoma Press.

GENTIAN

Botanical Name: Gentiana lutea
Family: Gentianaceae
Plant Part Used: Root

PRESCRIBING INFORMATION

Actions
Bitter tonic, gastric stimulant, sialagogue, cholagogue

Potential Indications
Based on appropriate evaluation of the patient, practitioners should consider prescribing gentian in formulations in the context of:
- Stimulating gastric secretion, bile release from the gallbladder, bile production by the liver (4)
- Loss of appetite,* dyspepsia,* asthenia, coated tongue, postprandial bloating, in combination with rhubarb (3)
- Stimulating gastric secretion, constipation, flatulence, abdominal fullness,* itching of skin, in combination with rhubarb, cascara, and boldo (3)
- Nausea, vomiting, heartburn, abdominal pain, constipation (4)
- Stimulating pancreatic enzyme secretion (7)

Contraindications
Gastric and duodenal ulcers,[1] hyperacidity,[2] gastric inflammation[3]

Warnings and Precautions
None required.

Interactions
None known.

Use in Pregnancy and Lactation
No adverse effects expected.

Side Effects
Very sensitive individuals may occasionally experience headaches.[1]
Doses at the higher end of the recommended range in liquid form may cause nausea in some people.

Dosage

Dose per day**	Dose per week**
0.7-2.0 ml of 1:2 liquid extract	5-15 ml of 1:2 liquid extract

SUPPORTING INFORMATION

Traditional Prescribing
Traditional Western herbal medicine uses include:
- Anorexia (loss of appetite), particularly after feverish conditions, to assist in assimilation of food[3]
- Atonic dyspepsia, gastrointestinal atony; debility, gout, amenorrhea[3,4]
- Diarrhea, intestinal worms[3]

Gentian *continued on page 225*

*Gentian has also been used in traditional herbal medicine. ESCOP recommends gentian for treating appetite loss and dyspepsia. The Commission E also recommends gentian for abdominal fullness and flatulence. (4,5)

**This dose range is extrapolated from the British Pharmaceutical Codex 1934, the British Pharmacopoeia 1932, and the author's education and experience.

Pharmacologic Research

- Isolated stomach cells exposed to different levels of an extract of gentian showed a concentration-dependent rise in gastric acid production.[5]
- In an experimental model, oral doses of gentian were shown to stimulate secretion of enzymes in the small intestine.[6]
- In another laboratory study, gentian extract increased gastric secretion in a dose-dependent fashion compared with controls. A dose of 0.5 ml/kg had no effect on gastric ulceration.[7]
- Gentian tincture given orally or directly into the stomach increased appetite in an experimental model of cachexia (weight loss in chronic diseases). A marked increase in gastric secretion and its acid and pepsin content was demonstrated only when gentian was given by mouth.[8]
- Gentian extract elevated bronchosecretion when compared with controls in a laboratory study.[9]

Clinical Studies

- In one uncontrolled study involving 18 volunteers using gentian tincture, gastric emptying was slightly increased in 16 of these cases. Gastric evacuation showed no significant change.[10]
- Nineteen patients with inflammatory conditions of the gastrointestinal tract associated with elevated IgA levels, and a healthy control group, were given 20 drops of a gentian tincture three times daily for 8 days. Secretory IgA levels were lowered in both groups; a correlation to clinical findings was reported, but statistical analysis was lacking.[11]
- In healthy volunteers, gentian induced a significant increase in salivary secretion from 1 to 30 minutes after oral administration, similar to the active control (citric acid) and unlike placebo or placebo plus alcohol. From 30 until 120 minutes, the volume per minute of saliva decreased but still remained higher than baseline values. In a double-blind study, an herbal preparation (containing gentian, rhubarb, cascara, and boldo) was significantly better than placebo for the following symptoms: asthenia, loss of appetite, coated tongue, postprandial bloating, difficult digestion, constipation, flatulence, abdominal fullness, and itching of skin. With regard to the other symptoms investigated, no significant difference was observed. The test preparation was more efficacious than the two pairs of its components (cascara and boldo; gentian and rhubarb).[12] The following herb equivalents were probably administered for the paired preparations: cascara (200 mg/day) and boldo (100 mg/day); gentian (40 mg/day) and rhubarb (200 mg/day).
- One oral dose of an alcoholic extract of gentian (containing 0.2 g root) given to volunteers 5 minutes before a meal stimulated gastric secretion, release of bile from the gallbladder and bile production by the liver.[13]
- In a multicenter, uncontrolled study, 205 patients were prescribed on average five gentian capsules per day (equivalent to 600 mg of root). Rapid relief of symptoms such as constipation, flatulence, appetite loss, vomiting, heartburn, abdominal pain, and nausea was achieved.[14]

Gentian continued on page 226

- In Germany, the Commission E supports using gentian to treat digestive disorders, such as loss of appetite, fullness, and flatulence.[1]
- ESCOP recommends gentian for treating appetite loss, particularly after illness, and dyspepsia.[2]

REFERENCES

1 Blumenthal M et al, editors: *The complete German Commission E monographs: therapeutic guide to herbal medicines*, Austin, 1998, American Botanical Council.

2 Scientific Committee of the European Scientific Cooperative on Phytotherapy [ESCOP]: *ESCOP monographs: Gentianae radix*. European Scientific Cooperative on Phytotherapy, ESCOP Secretariat, Argyle House, Gandy Street, Exeter, Devon, EX4 3LS, United Kingdom, July 1997.

3 Felter HW, Lloyd JU: *King's American dispensatory*, ed 18, rev 3, Portland, 1905, reprinted 1983, Eclectic Medical Publications.

4 British Herbal Medicine Association's Scientific Committee: *British herbal pharmacopoeia*, Bournemouth, 1983, BHMA.

5 Gebhardt R: *Pharm Pharmacol Lett* 7(2-3):106-108, 1997.

6 Kazakov BN. Cited in Scientific Committee of ESCOP: ESCOP monographs: Gentianae radix, European Scientific Cooperative on Phytotherapy, ESCOP Secretariat, Argyle House, Gandy Street, Exeter, Devon, EX4 3LS, United Kingdom, July 1997.

7 Leslie GB: *Medita* 8:31-47, 1978.

8 Moorhead LD: *J Pharmacol Exp Ther* 7:577-589, 1915.

9 Chibanguza G, Marz R, Sterner W: *Arzneim Forsch* 34(1):32-36, 1984.

10 Goetzl FR: *Drug Stand* 24:111, 1956.

11 Zimmerman W, Gaisbauer G, Gaisbauer M: *Z Phytother* 7:59-64, 1986.

12 Borgia M et al: *Curr Ther Res* 29(3):525-536, 1981.

13 Glatzel H, Hackenberg K: *Planta Med* 15(3):223-232, 1967.

14 Wegener T: *Z Phytother* 19:163-164, 1998.

GINGER

Botanical Name: *Zingiber officinale*
Family: Zingiberaceae
Plant Part Used: Rhizome

Actions	Carminative, antiemetic, peripheral circulatory stimulant, spasmolytic, antiinflammatory, antiplatelet, diaphoretic, digestive stimulant, pungent
Potential Indications	Based on appropriate evaluation of the patient, practitioners should consider prescribing ginger in formulations in the context of: • Prophylaxis and treatment of nausea and vomiting from motion sickness *(2,4)* • Prophylaxis and treatment of postoperative nausea *(2,4)* • Morning sickness *(2)* • Drug-induced nausea *(2)* • Osteoarthritis *(2)* • Dyspepsia *(4)* • Digestive problems, nausea, vomiting, colic, flatulent dyspepsia, cramping *(5)* • Fever, the common cold (especially the fresh rhizome), conditions requiring expectoration *(5)* • Dysmenorrhea *(5)*
Contraindications	According to the Commission E, using ginger is contraindicated in patients with gallstones, except under close supervision. In TCM, dried ginger is used cautiously during pregnancy. A daily dose of 2 g of dried ginger should not be exceeded in pregnancy.
Warnings and Precautions	The user should proceed with caution in cases of peptic ulceration, gastroesophageal reflux, or other gastric diseases.
Interactions	Ginger may increase the absorption of pharmaceutical drugs. Although no problems have been reported in humans, ginger may increase the chance of bleeding. Daily doses of (dried) ginger in excess of 4 g should be prescribed with caution in patients who are already taking blood-thinning drugs such as warfarin or aspirin or who have increased risk of hemorrhage.
Use in Pregnancy and Lactation	No adverse effects are expected within the recommended dose (0.7 to 2.0 ml of 1:2 liquid extract). A daily dose of 2 g of dried ginger should not be exceeded in pregnancy. Ginger has been successfully used in clinical trials to treat pregnant women with nausea.
Side Effects	At doses approaching or greater than the maximum recommended dose, a blood-thinning effect and an increase in gastric secretory activity leading to heartburn is possible. Topical application of ginger may

Ginger continued on page 228

cause contact dermatitis in sensitive patients. Occupational allergic contact dermatitis from spices, including ginger, has been reported.

Dosage

*Dose per day**	*Dose per week**
0.7-2.0 ml of 1:2 liquid extract	5-15 ml of 1:2 liquid extract

SUPPORTING INFORMATION

Traditional Prescribing

Traditional Western herbal medicine uses include:
- Nausea, anorexia, colic, flatulent dyspepsia[1,2]
- Amenorrhea,[3] dysmenorrhea;[2] to improve circulation[2]

Uses and properties from TCM include:
- For dried ginger: epigastric pain with cold feeling, vomiting and diarrhea with cold extremities, and faint pulse; dyspnea and cough with copious frothy expectoration[4]
- For fresh ginger: the common cold, vomiting caused by *cold* in the stomach, cough with thin white sputum[4]

Pharmacologic Research

Major constituents of ginger rhizome include an essential oil (1% to 3%, containing zingiberene and sesquiphellandrene) and pungent (hot) principles (1.0% to 2.5%, including gingerols and shogaols).
- Several studies have examined the antiemetic and antinausea effects of ginger. The mechanism of action responsible for the antiemetic effect is still controversial, however, possibilities include a central effect via gastrointestinal serotonin antagonism, central and peripheral anticholinergic and antihistaminic effects, and a dampening of induced vestibular impulses to the autonomic centers of the central nervous system.
- Oral administration of spray-dried ginger extract significantly prevented ethanol-induced gastric mucosal damage. Ginger and 6-gingerol inhibited experimental gastric ulcers *in vivo* after oral administration.
- Ginger and its pungent components exert an antiinflammatory effect by inhibiting both the cyclooxygenase and lipoxygenase enzymes belonging to the prostaglandin and leukotriene biosynthetic pathways, respectively. Oral intake of ginger extract inhibited carrageenan-induced paw swelling and was as active as aspirin in this model (although it was devoid of analgesic activity). Essential oil of ginger inhibited chronic adjuvant arthritis when given orally.
- Fever reduction in an experimental model after oral doses of ginger extract was comparable to aspirin.
- Several studies have demonstrated that ginger inhibits platelet aggregation *in vitro*. The inhibition of thromboxane formation appears to be the main cause of this antiplatelet action of ginger.

Ginger continued on page 229

*This dose range is extrapolated from the British Pharmaceutical Codex 1934, the British Herbal Pharmacopoeia 1983, the British Pharmacopoeia 1975, and the author's education and experience.

- Oral doses of ginger and its constituents have been shown to: increase saliva production, gastric secretions, and activity and intestinal transit; decrease pepsin activity; inhibit gastric contraction and serotonin-induced diarrhea; and reverse the cisplatin-induced delay in gastric emptying.
- Ginger and its components were thermogenic in perfused isolated tissues and significantly inhibited serotonin-induced hypothermia.
- Pungent principles of ginger had antihepatotoxic effects *in vitro,* inhibited histamine release from mast cells *in vitro,* and exhibited antiallergic activity *in vivo.* Ginger, ginger extract, and its pungent principles have demonstrated antioxidant activity *in vitro.*
- Ginger and its constituents have demonstrated antifungal activity, mild growth inhibition of gram-positive and gram-negative bacteria, antirhinoviral activity, and direct antiparasitic activity, all *in vitro.*
- Ginger as a thromboxane synthetase inhibitor and prostacyclin agonist was postulated to have therapeutic potential in alcohol withdrawal and the complications of liver damage, recovery from serious burns, peptic ulceration, Kawasaki disease, preventing aging penile vascular changes and impotence, as an antidepressant, and as an analgesic in dysmenorrhea.

Clinical Studies

- A systematic review of randomized controlled trials has evaluated the efficacy of ginger for nausea and vomiting. Six trials conducted before the year 2000 were evaluated. The pooled absolute risk reduction for the incidence of postoperative nausea calculated from three trials indicated a nonsignificant difference between the ginger and placebo groups. The dose was 1 g powdered ginger given preoperatively. Two of these trials suggested that ginger was superior to placebo and equally efficacious as metoclopramide. Three studies (investigating seasickness, morning sickness, and chemotherapy-induced nausea) collectively favored ginger over placebo.[5] The Cochrane Review of treatments for vomiting of pregnancy suggests ginger may be of benefit (based on two clinical trials) but that the evidence was weak to date (year 2000).[6]
- Many clinical studies have been published documenting the antinausea and antiemetic properties of ginger. However, several clinical studies have also been conducted that produced negative findings. The following summary indicates the trial design, effect on nausea and vomiting (positive-negative), and condition investigated in these trials (see Mills and Bone: *Principles and Practice of Phytotherapy*). Some of these trials were assessed in the previously listed reviews. Overall, the weight of evidence suggests that ginger may be beneficial for treating nausea and vomiting.
  - A positive effect was observed for ginger (0.25 to 1.5 g/day) in: two randomized, double-blind, placebo-controlled trials and one randomized, controlled trial[7] investigating seasickness; two randomized, double-blind, controlled trials investigating postoperative nausea; one randomized, double-blind, placebo-controlled,

Ginger continued on page 230

crossover trial in vomiting of pregnancy; one double-blind, controlled trial in hyperketonaemia patients; and one uncontrolled trial of psoralen-induced nausea.

- A negative effect was observed for ginger (0.5 to 1.0 g) in: two controlled trials and one double-blind, controlled trial investigating motion sickness; and one randomized, double-blind, placebo-controlled trial investigating postoperative nausea. A possible criticism of these motion sickness trials is that they were conducted in a laboratory setting that used rotating chairs and other machinery (although other such trials on ginger have been positive).

- A number of trials involving ginger for treating nausea and motion sickness have been conducted since the previously listed reviews.

  - A randomized, double-blind, placebo-controlled trial found that treatment with ginger (0.25 g four times/day) provided relief from pregnancy-induced nausea in 76% of women treated. In the placebo group, 46% reported relief. The reduction in nausea was maintained for the 4 days of the trial, and relief often started within 30 minutes of taking the ginger capsule.[8]

  - A study involving a small number of healthy volunteers confirmed the efficacy of ginger (1 g) in relieving symptoms of experimentally induced motion sickness. Volunteers who took ginger experienced a greater delay in developing nausea than did the placebo group.[9]

  - Symptoms of motion sickness were alleviated in a group of children (4 to 8 years of age) administered ginger before the start of a journey. In the children who were prescribed dimenhydrinate, symptoms were only improved. The ginger group experienced a reduction in symptoms within 30 minutes; for those taking dimenhydrinate the reduction occurred within 60 minutes. Test substances were administered 30 minutes before the start of the journey and every 4 hours thereafter as necessary: ginger powder 250 to 500 mg, dimenhydrinate 12.5 to 25.0 mg. The study was of randomized, double-blind design.[10]

- Seventy five percent of arthritis patients (rheumatoid and osteoarthritis) experienced relief in pain and swelling, and all of the patients with muscular discomfort experienced relief of pain, in an uncontrolled clinical study using dried ginger.

- Ginger extract was compared with ibuprofen and placebo in patients with osteoarthritis of the hip or knee in a double-blind, crossover trial. The effect of ginger was mild compared with placebo and was observed only in the first treatment period before crossover.[11]

- A combination of ginger and *Alpinia galanga* was tested against placebo in 261 patients with osteoarthritis of the knee. Although significant effects were observed from the herbal treatment, such as reduction in knee pain on standing, the overall benefit was mild. Mild gastrointestinal adverse events occurred more often in the ginger group compared with the placebo group.[12]

Ginger continued on page 231

- Oral ingestion of ginger improved gastroduodenal motility, both in the fasting state and after a standard test meal, in healthy volunteers who participated in a randomized, placebo-controlled, double-blind, crossover trial.[13]
- Powdered ginger (4 g/day) given to patients with coronary artery disease (CAD) did not affect platelet aggregation, fibrinolytic activity, and fibrinogen levels tested at 1½ and 3 months. No information was provided for controls. However, a single dose of ginger (10 g) produced a significant reduction in platelet aggregation after 4 hours in patients with CAD in a placebo-controlled trial.
- Adding ginger (5 g) to a fatty meal prevented the decrease in fibrinolytic activity caused by the fat intake in a randomized, placebo-controlled, crossover trial involving healthy volunteers. Placebo did not produce this preventative effect.[14]
- Treatment with ginger (approximately 2 g) plus soda water dropped the platelet count from 1.8 million to 240,000 in 1 day in a case study of thrombocytosis resulting from a myeloproliferative disorder in a 78-year-old man. The platelet count rose to over 1.5 million when ginger treatment was subsequently withdrawn. In a controlled trial, dried ginger (5 g/day) significantly inhibited platelet aggregation induced by dietary butter supplementation (100 g/day) in healthy males.
- In Germany, the Commission E supports using ginger to treat dyspepsia and prevent motion sickness.[15]
- ESCOP recommends ginger for the prophylaxis of the nausea and vomiting of motion sickness and as a postoperative antiemetic for minor day-case surgical procedures.[16]
- Ginger has been reinstated to the USP and is official in the USP24-NF19.

REFERENCES

Except when specifically referenced, the following book was referred to in the compilation of the pharmacologic and clinical information: Mills S, Bone K: *Principles and Practice of Phytotherapy: Modern Herbal Medicine,* Edinburgh, 2000, Churchill Livingstone.

1　British Herbal Medicine Association's Scientific Committee: *British herbal pharmacopoeia,* Bournemouth, 1983, BHMA.

2　Felter HW: *The eclectic materia medica, pharmacology and therapeutics,* Portland, 1922, reprinted 1983, Eclectic Medical Publications.

3　Grieve M: *A modern herbal,* New York, 1971, Dover Publications.

4　Pharmacopoeia Commission of the People's Republic of China: *Pharmacopoeia of the People's Republic of China,* English ed, Beijing, 1997, Chemical Industry Press.

5　Ernst E, Pittler MH: *Br J Anaesth* 84(3):367-371, 2000.

6　Jewell D, Young G: *Cochrane Database Syst Rev* (2):CD000145, 2000.

7　Ribenfeld D, Borzone L: *Healthnotes Rev Complement Integr Med* 6(2):98, 1999.

8　Eden J: *Medical Observer* July 21, 2000.

9　Lien HC, Sun WM: *Digestive Disease Week 2000,* San Diego, May 20-24, 2000.

10　Careddu P: *HealthNotes Rev* 6:102-107, 1999.

11　Bliddal H et al: *Osteoarthritis Cartilage* 8(1):9-12, 2000.

12　Altman RD, Marcussen KC: *Arthritis Rheum* 44(11):2531-2538, 2001.

13　Micklefield GH et al: *Int J Clin Pharmacol Ther* 37(7):341-346, 1999.

14　Verma SK, Bordia A: *Indian J Med Sci* 55(2):83-86, 2001.

15　Blumenthal M et al, editors: *The complete German Commission E monographs: therapeutic guide to herbal medicines,* Austin, 1998, American Botanical Council.

16　Scientific Committee of the European Scientific Cooperative on Phytotherapy [ESCOP]: *ESCOP monographs: Zingiberis rhizoma.* European Scientific Cooperative on Phytotherapy, ESCOP Secretariat, Argyle House, Gandy Street, Exeter, Devon, EX4 3LS, United Kingdom, March 1996.

GINKGO

Botanical Name: *Ginkgo biloba*
Family: Ginkgoaceae
Plant Part Used: Leaf

PRESCRIBING INFORMATION

Actions	Antioxidant, antiplatelet activating factor (anti-PAF) activity, tissue perfusion enhancing, circulatory stimulant, cognition enhancing, neuroprotective
Potential Indications	Based on appropriate evaluation of the patient, practitioners should consider prescribing Ginkgo in formulations in the context of:

- Cerebral insufficiency (restricted cerebral blood flow) and its related symptoms, such as memory and cognitive impairment, dizziness, tinnitus, acute cochlear deafness, headaches, anxiety and depression, and fatigue *(1,4)*
- Early stages of primary degenerative dementia (Alzheimer's-type) *(1,4)*
- Multiinfarct (vascular) dementia *(2,4)*
- Stroke of recent onset *(2)*
- A tonic for older adults *(2)*
- Vertigo or dizziness of vascular origin *(2)*
- Tinnitus of vascular and involutional origin *(4)*
- Peripheral arterial occlusive disease (Fontaine stage II [intermittent claudication] or stage III) *(1,4)*
- Idiopathic sudden hearing loss *(2)*
- Disorders resulting from reduced retinal blood flow, senile macular *degeneration (3)*
- Enhancing cognitive function, including working and long-term memory, abstract reasoning, and processing speed in healthy individuals and particularly in older adults *(2)*
- Improving attention in healthy young individuals *(3)*
- Improving memory and cognitive performance in healthy individuals *(2)*
- The effects of high altitude or hypoxia *(2)*
- Antioxidant activity *(3)*
- Congestive dysmenorrhea *(3)*
- Anti-PAF activity *(4a)*
- Asthma *(4)*

Contraindications	None known.
Warnings and Precautions	Ginkgo should be used with caution in patients on anticoagulant or antiplatelet medication.
Interactions	Based on some case reports of possible interaction, caution should be exercised when prescribing Ginkgo with warfarin and aspirin.
Use in Pregnancy and Lactation	No adverse effects expected.

Ginkgo *continued on page 233*

Side Effects

Analyses of clinical trials have shown that Ginkgo has a remarkably low incidence of side effects. Isolated episodes of spontaneous bleeding attributed to intake of Ginkgo have been reported. However, a clinical trial (see later discussion) found that treatment with Ginkgo limited oxidative stress in cardiovascular surgery because of a membrane-protective effect. Recovery of Ginkgo-treated patients was slightly improved compared with untreated patients.

A case of Stevens-Johnson syndrome that appeared to be associated with use of tablets containing standardized Ginkgo extract, choline, and B vitamins was reported. The authors advised that the reaction was unlikely to have been caused by the choline or B vitamins.[1] (Stevens-Johnson syndrome is an acute inflammatory skin disease that affects the skin and mucous membranes of the face and mouth.)

Dosage

*Dose per day**	*Dose per week**
3-4 ml of the standardized (2:1) liquid extract	21-28 ml of the standardized (2:1) liquid extract

Extracts providing standardized levels of ginkgo flavone glycosides are recommended. Ideally, aqueous ethanol extracts should contain 9.6 mg/ml of ginkgo flavone glycosides.

No restriction was found on the long-term use of Ginkgo. However, Ginkgo should be recommended for at least 6 weeks before any assessment of clinical benefit is made.

SUPPORTING INFORMATION

Traditional Prescribing

No information has been found for the traditional use of Ginkgo leaf. Ginkgo nuts were used in TCM.

Pharmacologic Research

Pharmacologic and clinical studies usually tested a special concentrated standardized extract of Ginkgo leaves, which is chemically complex, containing at least 26 identified components. The 50:1 concentrated extract is standardized to contain 22.5% to 25.0% flavonoid glycosides (ginkgo flavone glycosides) and 6% to 8% terpenoids (ginkgolides and bilobalide).

- The ginkgolides are potent and specific PAF antagonists; the effects are long-lived and are rapidly established after oral doses.
- Many experimental models have demonstrated the preventative and protective effects of standardized Ginkgo extract (high doses) and ginkgolides against hypoxia- or ischemia-induced damage of cerebral and cardiovascular tissues, both *in vitro* and *in vivo* after oral administration.

Ginkgo continued on page 234

*This dose range is based on those used in clinical trials.

- Standardized Ginkgo extracts have demonstrated potent antioxidant activity in many *in vitro* models.
- Prior oral dosing with standardized Ginkgo extract enhanced the performance of a tested task, indicating improved retrieval of the learned response, in a well-controlled animal study. Oral administration of standardized Ginkgo extract to young and old rats facilitated behavioral adaptation despite adverse environmental influences.
- Oral administration of standardized Ginkgo extract in conjunction with a high-fat diet reduced disturbances of lipid metabolism and the severity of plaque formation in an experimental model when compared with placebo and rutin. Ginkgo also affected metabolic processes in the liver and may modify lipid deposition in major arteries.
- Chronic administration of standardized Ginkgo extract inhibited stress-induced corticosterone hyposecretion through a reduction in the number of adrenal peripheral benzodiazepine receptors. Ginkgo extract and ginkgolide B were also found to act at the hypothalamic level and were able to reduce corticotropin-releasing hormone expression and secretion.
- Intragastric administration of a combined preparation of standardized extracts of Ginkgo and ginger demonstrated anxiolytic effects comparable to diazepam injection *in vivo*.
- Ginkgo extract fractions relaxed penile corpus cavernosal tissues *in vitro,* an effect that may help maintain erection.
- Topical application of standardized Ginkgo extract had antiinflammatory activity comparable to indomethacin in the croton oil test and promoted hair regrowth in shaved mice.

Clinical Studies

The following clinical trials were conducted using a standardized Ginkgo extract (50:1), with the majority of trials employing a daily dose range of 120 to 160 mg, which equates to 6 to 8 g of original dried herb (or 3 to 4 ml of a 2:1 standardized liquid extract).

- A critical review of 40 clinical trials conducted from 1975 to 1991 on the clinical use of standardized Ginkgo extracts in patients with cerebral insufficiency and related conditions (primary degenerative dementia; dizziness associated with labyrinth, vestibular disorders, or both; acute cochlear deafness; senile cognitive decline; and tinnitus) found that all except one of the 40 trials showed positive results, with significant results in 26. The inconclusive result was obtained for a trial on senile dementia of vascular origin. In most of the trials, the daily dose was 120 to 160 mg of standardized extract, given for at least 4 to 6 weeks. Meta-analysis of 11 randomized, double-blind, placebo-controlled trials confirmed the global effectiveness of Ginkgo in five studies and concluded that standardized Ginkgo extract provides a better therapeutic effect compared with placebo in treating cerebral insufficiency. In most cases, 150 mg/day was administered for 12 weeks. A more recent review confirmed these results and noted that no significant differences in the frequency or types of side effects were observed between Ginkgo and placebo groups.[2]

Ginkgo *continued on page 235*

- Improvements in cerebral blood flow, motor recovery, intellectual performance, memory, mood, and behavior were observed in recent stroke victims after treatment with standardized Ginkgo extract in uncontrolled and in randomized, double-blind, placebo-controlled, and comparative trials. Although the general dosage used was 120 mg/day of standardized extract for 1 to 2 months, in one of these trials, some patients received up to 360 mg/day.
- A meta-analysis of four randomized, double-blind, placebo-controlled trials found a small but significant effect after 3 to 6 months treatment with 120 to 240 mg/day of standardized Ginkgo extract on objective measures of cognitive function in patients with Alzheimer's disease. A subsequent randomized, double-blind, placebo-controlled, multicenter trial in patients with mild to severe Alzheimer's disease or multiinfarct dementia found that, compared with baseline values, treatment with standardized Ginkgo extract (120 mg/day for 26 weeks) slightly improved daily living and social behavior and cognitive assessment. The placebo group showed a statistically significant worsening in all domains of assessment. Regarding safety, no differences between Ginkgo and placebo were observed.[3] Two randomized, double-blind trials (included in the previously mentioned meta-analysis) demonstrated that standardized Ginkgo extract improved the cognitive performance and social function of patients with mild to severe Alzheimer's disease or multiinfarct dementia compared with placebo. No significant difference compared with placebo was observed in the number of patients reporting adverse events or in the incidence and severity of these events. The dosage administered in these trials was 240 mg/day for 24 weeks and 120 mg/day for 52 weeks. A recent meta-analysis found no major differences between standardized Ginkgo extract and four cholinesterase inhibitors (tacrine, donepezil, rivastigmine, and metrifonate) for delaying symptom progression in Alzheimer's disease or response rate compared with placebo. The authors suggested that all treatments compared were equally efficacious in treating mild to moderate Alzheimer dementia.[4]
- In contrast, results from a randomized, double-blind, placebo-controlled, parallel-group, multicenter trial published in 2000 suggest that Ginkgo is not efficacious as is a treatment for older people with age-associated memory impairment or mild to moderate Alzheimer's or vascular dementia. Patients were randomized to receive placebo or standardized Ginkgo extract in one of two doses: 160 mg/day or 240 mg/day for 12 or 24 weeks.[5] However, given the mixed nature of the participants in this trial, its significance can be questioned.
- Supplementation with standardized Ginkgo extract (120 mg/day for 4 months) improved mood, sleep, and coping ability for daily activities in a randomized, placebo-controlled study involving 5028 free-living elderly volunteers.[6]
- In a randomized, double-blind, placebo-controlled study involving healthy adults, standardized Ginkgo extract (100 mg/day for 30 days) produced a significant improvement in a wide range of cognitive

Ginkgo *continued on page 236*

abilities, including long-term memory and abstract reasoning, using the multidimensional aptitude battery. Standardized Ginkgo extract (180 mg/day for 6 weeks) significantly increased cognitive processing speed and subjective ratings of memory improvement, compared with placebo, in cognitively intact older adults (55 to 86 years of age) in a randomized, double-blind, placebo-controlled, parallel-group study.[7] The effects of acute doses of standardized Ginkgo extract on memory and psychomotor performance in asymptomatic volunteers aged 30 to 59 years was tested in a randomized, double-blind, placebo-controlled, five-way crossover design. The results confirm that the effects of Ginkgo on cognition are more pronounced for memory, particularly working memory. The most efficacious dose was a single dose of 120 mg and the cognitive enhancing effects were more likely to be apparent in individuals aged 50 to 59 years.[8] In a double-blind, controlled, crossover trial, acute administration of standardized Ginkgo extract (240 mg and 360 mg) to healthy young volunteers produced a sustained improvement in attention compared with placebo.[9,10] A randomized, double-blind, placebo-controlled trial demonstrated significant improvement in speed of information processing, working memory, and executive processing for healthy volunteers treated with standardized Ginkgo extract.[11] A combination containing standardized extracts of Ginkgo (120 mg/day) and Korean ginseng (200 mg/day standardized to 4% ginsenosides) demonstrated improvement in the working and long-term memories of healthy middle-aged volunteers after 14 weeks in a multicenter, double-blind, placebo-controlled trial.[12]

- In a meta-analysis that included five placebo-controlled trials, standardized Ginkgo extract (120 to 160 mg/day for 4 to 6 weeks) was found to have a highly significant therapeutic effect over placebo in peripheral arterial occlusive disease (Fontaine stage II or III). A review of randomized, double-blind, placebo-controlled trials of either standardized Ginkgo extract (120 to 160 mg/day) or the drug pentoxifylline in treating intermittent claudication found that the trials had similar clinical outcomes and were of the same methodological quality. Eight randomized, double-blind, placebo-controlled trials were included in a recent meta-analysis, concluding that standardized Ginkgo extract was superior to placebo in the symptomatic treatment of patients with intermittent claudication. The daily dose in these trials ranged from 120 mg to 160 mg for a period of 24 weeks in six of the trials and for a shorter duration in the other trials.[13]

- A review of randomized controlled trials found inconsistent results for Ginkgo in treating patients with tinnitus without accompanying symptoms of cerebral insufficiency.[14] A large, double-blind, placebo-controlled trial published in early 2001 found that standardized Ginkgo extract (150 mg/day) was no more beneficial than was placebo in treating tinnitus. The treatment did not significantly affect other symptoms of cerebral insufficiency. Given the positive results of previous trials, the authors suggested that Ginkgo appears

Ginkgo continued on page 237

ineffective in treating tinnitus alone, but it may be effective in treating tinnitus in patients who also have other symptoms of cerebral insufficiency.[15]

- A randomized trial comparing standardized Ginkgo extract (160 mg/day) and betahistine (a vasodilator, 32 mg/day) demonstrated the efficacy of both treatments on subjective and objective measurements of equilibrium in patients complaining of vertigo, dizziness, or both caused by vascular vestibular disorders. The results indicated that the sites of action of Ginkgo and betahistine for compensation of equilibrium are different and that Ginkgo improved oculomotor and visuovestibular function to a greater extent.[16]

- A significant borderline benefit for Ginkgo over naftidrofuryl (a vasodilator) in idiopathic sudden hearing loss (existing no longer than 10 days) was shown after 3 weeks' treatment in a randomized, comparative study. Ginkgo treatment was preferred because of the lack of side effects. Both treatment groups also received infusion therapy.

- A randomized, double-blind, placebo-controlled trial found standardized Ginkgo treatment (containing 48 mg/day flavone glycosides for 10 weeks) was unable to prevent the development of the symptoms of winter depression (the most prevalent type of seasonal affective disorder).[17] Standardized Ginkgo extract (240 mg/day) improved sleep in patients with major depression. In this open, pilot trial, patients taking the antidepressant trimipramine plus Ginkgo were compared with those taking the drug alone.[18]

- In a multicenter, double-blind, placebo-controlled study, Ginkgo significantly improved breast tenderness and markedly improved edema, anxiety, depression, and headaches in 165 women with congestive symptoms of PMS. Standardized Ginkgo extract was administered at 160 mg/day from day 16 to day 5 of the next menstrual cycle.

- In patients with blockage of veins in the retina, standardized Ginkgo extract improved blood vessels, visual acuity, field of vision, near and far vision, and color recognition in a randomized, double-blind, placebo-controlled trial. Marked improvements in vision in 86% of patients with poor blood supply to the retina (or the areas of the brain that interpret the signals from the eyes) were observed in an uncontrolled trial. The dosage of standardized extract was 120 mg/day for 3 months. A small, double-blind, placebo-controlled trial found standardized Ginkgo treatment (160 mg/day for 6 months) improved visual acuity (compared with placebo) in patients with senile macular degeneration. A recent placebo-controlled study found acute administration of Ginkgo significantly increased end-diastolic velocity in the ophthalmic artery in healthy volunteers, indicating possible benefit for optic neuropathy linked to glaucoma and other ischemic ocular diseases. The dosage of standardized Ginkgo extract was 120 mg/day for 2 days.[19]

- In a randomized, placebo-controlled trial, administering standardized Ginkgo extract (160 mg/day) for the duration of an expedition significantly prevented acute mountain sickness at moderate altitude

Ginkgo continued on page 238

(5400 meters, or over 17,700 feet) and decreased vasomotor disorders of the extremities.

- Ingestion of standardized Ginkgo extract (120 mg/day for 3 months) by healthy volunteers resulted in the inhibition of collagen-induced platelet aggregation and reduced urinary excretion of 11-dehydrothromboxane B_2 (a metabolite of thromboxane A_2).[20]
- A high dose of ginkgolide mixture (120 mg) inhibited PAF activity in healthy human volunteers in a small, double-blind, placebo-controlled study. The mixture contained 40% ginkgolide A, 40% ginkgolide B, and 20% ginkgolide C.
- Ginkgo limited free radical–induced oxidative stress generated throughout surgery in patients undergoing aortic valve replacement in a double-blind, placebo-controlled study. The dosage prescribed was 320 mg/day of standardized extract for 5 days before surgery.
- In small, uncontrolled trials standardized Ginkgo extract has:
  - Significantly reduced fibrinogen levels and blood viscosity in out-patients with a long history of elevated levels (240 mg/day for 12 weeks)
  - Increased hypoxia tolerance in healthy volunteers (200 mg/day for 1 week)
  - Decreased clastogenic (a form of mutagenic) activity of blood taken from salvage personnel working on the Chernobyl reactor accident (120 mg/day for 2 months)
  - Alleviated sexual dysfunction secondary to antidepressant drug use (average dose: 207 mg/day for 4 weeks)
  - Improved peak flow rates in asthmatic children
  - Caused significant clinical improvement in asthmatic adults
- In Germany, the Commission E supports using standardized Ginkgo leaf extract for:[21]
  - The symptomatic treatment of dementia syndromes, including primary degenerative dementia, vascular dementia, and mixed forms of both, characterized by the following symptoms: memory deficit, disturbances in concentration, depression, dizziness, tinnitus, and headache
  - Improvement in pain-free walking distance in intermittent claudication (peripheral arterial occlusive disease, Fontaine stage IIb) within a regimen of physical therapeutic measures
  - Vertigo and tinnitus of vascular and involutional origin
- Ginkgo is official in the USP24-NF19

REFERENCES

Except when specifically referenced, the following book was referred to in the compilation of the pharmacologic and clinical information: Mills S, Bone K: *Principles and Practice of Phytotherapy: Modern Herbal Medicine,* Edinburgh, 2000, Churchill Livingstone.

1 Davydov L, Stirling AL: *J Herbal Pharmacother* 1(3):65-69, 2001.
2 Soholm B: *Adv Ther* 15(1):54-65, 1998.
3 Le Bars PL, Kieser M, Itil KZ: *Dement Geriatr Cogn Discord* 11(4):230-237, 2000.

Ginkgo *continued on page 239*

4 Wettstein A: *Phytomed* 6(6):393-401, 2000.

5 van Dongen MC et al: *J Am Geriatr Soc* 48(10):1183-1194, 2000.

6 Cockle SM, Kimber S, Hindmarch I: *Phytomed* 7(supp 2):21, 2000.

7 Mix JA, Crews WD: *J Altern Complement Med* 6(3):219-229, 2000.

8 Rigney U, Kimber S, Hindmarch I: *Phytother Res* 13(5):408-415, 1999.

9 Kennedy DO, Scholey AB, Wesnes KA: *Psychopharmacology* 151(4):416-423, 2000.

10 Kennedy DO, Scholey AB, Wesnes KA: *Phytomed* 7(supp 2):21, 2000.

11 Stough C et al: *Int J Neuropsychopharmacol* 4(2):131-134, 2001.

12 Wesnes KA et al: *Psychopharmacology* 152(4):353-361, 2000.

13 Pittler MH, Ernst E: *Am J Med* 108(4):276-281, 2000.

14 Ernst E, Stevinson C: *Clin Otoloaryngol* 24(3):164-167, 1999.

15 Drew S, Davies E: *BMJ* 322(7278):73-75, 2001.

16 Cesarani A et al: *Adv Ther* 15(5):291-304, 1998.

17 Lingaerde O, Foreland AR, Magnusson A: *Acta Psychiatr Scand* 100(1):62-66, 1999.

18 Hemmeter U et al: *Pharmacopsychiatry* 34(2):50-59, 2001.

19 Chung HS et al: *J Ocul Pharmacol Ther* 15(3):233-240, 1999.

20 Kudolo G: *Altern Ther Health Med* 7(3):105, 2001.

21 Blumenthal M et al, editors: *The complete German Commission E monographs: therapeutic guide to herbal medicines*, Austin, 1998, American Botanical Council.

GLOBE ARTICHOKE

Botanical Name: *Cynara scolymus*
Family: Compositae
Plant Part Used: Leaf

PRESCRIBING INFORMATION

Actions	Hepatoprotective, hepatic trophorestorative, choleretic, cholagogue, bitter tonic, hypocholesterolemic, antiemetic, diuretic, depurative
Potential Indications	Based on appropriate evaluation of the patient, practitioners should consider prescribing globe artichoke in formulations in the context of:

- Hyperlipidemia (2,6)
- Conditions requiring an increase in bile flow (2)
- Dyspepsia and associated symptoms (e.g., constipation, abdominal pain, nausea, vomiting, flatulence, belching, fat intolerance) (4)
- Non-ulcer dyspepsia, in combination with boldo and greater celandine (2)
- Irritable bowel syndrome (4)
- Biliary fistula (4)
- Jaundice, gout (5)
- Conditions requiring a depurative action (such as itchy skin) (5)
- Long-term prevention and treatment of cardiovascular disease (7)

Contraindications	Closure of the gallbladder
Warnings and Precautions	Globe artichoke should be used only with professional supervision in cholelithiasis (gallstones). The Commission E advises caution for patients with known allergy to globe artichoke and to other plants of the Compositae family. The likelihood of globe artichoke preparations causing an allergy is very low.
Interactions	None known.
Use in Pregnancy and Lactation	No adverse effects expected.
Side Effects	Clinical trials indicate that the safety and tolerability of globe artichoke is good. Contact with the fresh plant can cause contact dermatitis. No cases of allergic reaction after oral intake have been reported.

Dosage

Dose per day*	Dose per week*
3-8 ml of 1:2 liquid extract	20-55 ml of 1:2 liquid extract

Globe Artichoke *continued on page 241*

*This dose range is extrapolated from clinical trials.

240

SUPPORTING INFORMATION

Traditional Prescribing

Traditional Western herbal medicine uses include:
- Jaundice,[1,2] hypercholesterolemia, anorexia; as a liver tonic and antitoxic[2]
- Clearing the complexion,[2] as a depurative for simple itch in children[3]
- Rheumatism, arthritis,[2] gout, dropsies[1]
- Nephrosclerosis, urinary stones, oliguria, uremia[3]

Pharmacologic Research

Key constituents of globe artichoke leaves include caffeic acid derivatives, especially cynarin.
- Studies from the 1930s indicate that globe artichoke increased bile flow from the liver, lowered cholesterol, and caused diuresis. More recently, globe artichoke extract demonstrated a marked choleretic effect in experimental models after intraperitoneal administration. Cynarin also increased bile secretion *in vitro* and *in vivo* after intraperitoneal administration.
- Studies have demonstrated the hepatoprotective and hepatorestorative activity of globe artichoke extracts against liver toxins *in vitro* and *in vivo* by the oral route.
- Globe artichoke extract exhibited strong antioxidant activity *in vitro*.
- Globe artichoke extract and cynarin inhibited cholesterol synthesis *in vitro* and countered an increase in serum lipids *in vivo* after intraperitoneal and oral administration.
- An antiatherosclerotic effect was demonstrated for globe artichoke extract *in vivo* after oral administration.
- Oral administration of globe artichoke extract stimulated the movement of gastrointestinal contents along the small intestine in an acute experimental model.

Clinical Studies

- A review of the clinical data from mostly uncontrolled trials conducted from 1936 to 1994 indicated that globe artichoke extract lowered lipid levels (cholesterol, triglycerides, or both) from between just below 5% to approximately 45%.
- In a trial of randomized, double-blind, placebo-controlled design, total cholesterol levels significantly decreased after globe artichoke administration to patients with baseline values above 220 mg/dl. High-density lipoprotein (HDL) cholesterol tended to increase. These results were confirmed in another trial of similar design in which a high dose of globe artichoke concentrated extract (equivalent to approximately 6 to 8 g/day of dried leaf for 6 weeks) decreased total cholesterol, LDL cholesterol, and the LDL/HDL ratio in adults with an initial total cholesterol of more than 280 mg/dl.[4]
- Oral doses of cynarin significantly reduced levels of total serum cholesterol in patients with elevated serum lipids in uncontrolled studies (750 to 1500 mg/day) and a double-blind, placebo-controlled trial (500 mg/day for 50 days). Average body weight was also significantly reduced in the controlled trial. Triglyceride levels in elderly patients

Globe Artichoke *continued on page 242*

with hypertriglyceridemia were significantly lowered in a double-blind, placebo-controlled study with cynarin (500 mg/day).
- Mean cholesterol and triglyceride values were significantly lowered in a postmarketing surveillance study involving 553 patients with dyspepsia. Substantial improvement was recorded for vomiting, nausea, abdominal pain, constipation, flatulence, belching, and fat intolerance. Physicians rated globe artichoke extract treatment (average dose of approximately 7 g/day of dried leaf for 6 weeks) as excellent or good in 87% of patients.
- Globe artichoke extract (average dose of approximately 7 g/day of dried leaf for 6 weeks) improved nausea, vomiting, abdominal pain, right-sided cramping pain, flatulence, and fat intolerance in patients with functional bowel disorders in a postmarketing surveillance study. Mean total cholesterol was also significantly reduced.
- Treatment with a standardized globe artichoke extract (equivalent to 8.6 g/day dried leaf) reduced the severity of symptoms of patients with irritable bowel syndrome in a postmarketing surveillance study. The overall effectiveness of globe artichoke rated favorably with both physicians and patients. Ninety-six percent of patients rated the herb as better than or at least equal to previous therapies.[5]
- Globe artichoke extract demonstrated choleretic and cholagogic effects and clinical improvement in an open study involving 198 patients with biliary fistula. Intraduodenal administration of globe artichoke extract (equivalent to 9.1 g of dried leaf, standardized to 1.2 mg cynarin) produced a significant increase in bile secretion at 120 and 150 minutes (compared with placebo) in healthy volunteers. The trial was of randomized, double-blind, crossover design.
- A randomized, placebo-controlled, double-blind study found an herbal formula containing globe artichoke extract (50%), boldo (*Peumus boldus*, 30%), and greater celandine (20%) significantly increased bile secretion and improved bloating, nausea, and heartburn in patients with non-ulcer dyspepsia.
- Prophylactic globe artichoke treatment significantly reduced platelet aggregation in workers chronically exposed to carbon disulfide.
- In Germany, the Commission E supports using globe artichoke to treat dyspeptic problems.[6]

REFERENCES

Except when specifically referenced, the following book was referred to in the compilation of the pharmacologic and clinical information: Mills S, Bone K: *Principles and Practice of Phytotherapy: Modern Herbal Medicine,* Edinburgh, 2000, Churchill Livingstone.

1 Felter HW: *The eclectic materia medica, pharmacology and therapeutics,* Portland, 1922, reprinted 1983, Eclectic Medical Publications.
2 Leclerc H: *Precis de phytotherapie,* ed 5, Paris, 1983, Masson.
3 Rocchietta S: *Minerva Med* 50:612-618, 1959.
4 Englisch W et al: *Arzneim Forsch* 50:260-265, 2000.
5 Walker AF, Middleton RW, Petrowicz O: *Phytother Res* 15(1):58-61, 2001.
6 Blumenthal M et al, editors: *The complete German Commission E monographs: therapeutic guide to herbal medicines,* Austin, 1998, American Botanical Council.

GOAT'S RUE

Botanical Name: *Galega officinalis*
Family: Leguminosae
Plant Part Used: Aerial parts

PRESCRIBING INFORMATION

Actions

Hypoglycemic, antidiabetic, galactagogue

Potential Indications

Based on appropriate evaluation of the patient, practitioners should consider prescribing goat's rue in formulations in the context of:
- Non-insulin–dependent diabetes mellitus *(4,5)*
- Improving lactation *(4,5)*
- Possibly assisting weight loss *(7)*

Contraindications

None known.

Warnings and Precautions

None required.

Interactions

None known.

Use in Pregnancy and Lactation

No adverse effects expected.

Side Effects

None expected if taken within the recommended dose range.

Consumption of goat's rue by sheep has caused poisoning.[1,2] (Toxic doses far exceeded those used therapeutically in humans.)

Dosage

*Dose per day**	*Dose per week**
4.5-8.5 ml of 1:2 liquid extract	30-60 ml of 1:2 liquid extract

SUPPORTING INFORMATION

Traditional Prescribing

Traditional Western herbal medicine uses include:
- Diabetes mellitus[3]
- As a galactagogue, vermifuge, nervous system stimulant, and diuretic[4]
- As a tonic in infectious diseases such as typhoid[4]

Pharmacologic Research

Key constituents of the aerial parts of goat's rue include the alkaloid galegine, which is a guanidine derivative.[5] In 1927, findings indicated that galegine possessed hypoglycemic properties, which led to the development of the related biguanide drugs. Biguanide drugs, such as metformin, increase the peripheral uptake of glucose by increasing the efficiency of available insulin; that is, they increase insulin sensitivity.[6]

Goat's Rue *continued on page 244*

*This dose range is extrapolated from the British Herbal Pharmacopoeia 1983 and the author's education and experience.

243

- Dietary goat's rue reduced serum glucose and body weight in both normal and genetically obese mice when compared with controls. Serum insulin was significantly reduced only in obese animals. Weight loss was associated with a persistent reduction in food intake by obese animals and an initial reduction in normal animals. However, weight loss in normal animals was then maintained, even with increased food intake above the control level.[7]
- Aqueous and ethanolic extracts of goat's rue improved glucose tolerance *in vivo* after oral administration. Hypoglycemic activity was demonstrated for the fractions containing galegine.[8]
- Oral doses of goat's rue extract and galegine both reduced blood glucose in an experimental model of diabetes.[9] Another study found no hypoglycemic effect for oral goat's rue extracts in normal or diabetic animals.[10]
- Goat's rue had a regenerative effect on the insulin-producing cells (β cells) of the pancreas *in vivo* (route unknown).[11]
- A purified galegine-containing extract of goat's rue dose-dependently inhibited the transport and uptake of glucose into human intestinal epithelial cells *in vitro*.[12]
- Aqueous extracts of goat's rue inhibited platelet aggregation *in vitro*[13-16] and *in vivo* by intravenous route.[17]

Clinical Studies

- Early clinical research demonstrated hypoglycemic activity for goat's rue.[18,19] Unlike the biguanide drugs, the herb did not have unpleasant side effects.[19]
- In an early controlled trial, nursing mothers receiving a preparation containing goat's rue extract and mineral salts (dose undefined) produced a larger increase in colostrum volume (125%) between the third and fifth days after delivery than did women not receiving the preparation (75% increase). Volume of milk, but not percentage of milk solids, had increased by the fifth day in the treated group.[20]

REFERENCES

1 Keeler RF et al: *Vet Hum Toxicol* 28(4):309-315, 1986.
2 Keeler RF, Baker DC, Evans JO: *Vet Hum Toxicol* 30(5):420-423, 1988.
3 British Herbal Medicine Association's Scientific Committee: *British herbal pharmacopoeia*, Bournemouth, 1983, BHMA.
4 Felter HW, Lloyd JU: *King's American dispensatory*, ed 18, rev 3, Portland, 1905, reprinted 1983, Eclectic Medical Publications.
5 Bisset NG, editor: *Herbal drugs and phytopharmaceuticals*, Stuttgart, 1994, Medpharm Scientific Publishers.
6 *E-MIMS*, version 4.00.0457, St. Leonard's, NSW, Australia, 2000, MIMS Australia.
7 Palit P, Furman BL, Gray AI: *J Pharm Pharmacol* 51(11):1313-1319, 1999.
8 Neef H, Declercq HN, Laekeman G: *Phytother Res* 9(1):45-48, 1995.
9 Petricic J, Kalodera Z: *Acta Pharm Jugosl* 32(3):219-223, 1982.
10 Pundarikakshudu K, Gray AI, Furman BL: *Fitoterapia* 65(5):423-426, 1994.
11 Sendrail M et al: *La semaine des Hopitaux* 37:389, 1961.
12 Neef H et al: *Pharm Pharmacol Lett* 6(2):86-89, 1996.
13 Atanasov AT, Spasov V: *J Ethnopharmacol* 69(3):235-240, 2000.
14 Atanasov AT, Spasov V: *Folia Med* 41(1):46-50, 1999.
15 Atanasov AT: *Phytother Res* 8(5):314-316, 1994.

Goat's Rue *continued on page 245*

16 Atanasov AT: *Bulgarian Med* 1:17-20, 1993.

17 Atanasov AT: *J Herbs Spices Med Plants* 3(3):71, 1995.

18 Leclerc H: *Presse Med* 36:1634, 1928.

19 Parturier G, Hugonot G: *Presse Med* 43:258, 1935.

20 Heiss H: *Wien Med Wochenschr* 24:546-549, 1968.

GOLDEN ROD

Botanical Name: *Solidago virgaurea*
Family: Compositae
Plant Part Used: Aerial parts

PRESCRIBING INFORMATION

Actions Antiinflammatory, diaphoretic, diuretic, anticatarrhal

Potential Indications Based on appropriate evaluation of the patient, practitioners should consider prescribing golden rod in formulations in the context of:
- Upper respiratory tract catarrh or inflammation, especially of a chronic nature; influenza (5)
- Rheumatoid arthritis and osteoarthritis, in combination with *Fraxinus excelsior* and *Populus tremula* (1)
- Promoting diuresis (3)
- Inflammation and infection of the urinary tract (4,5)
- Prophylaxis and treatment of kidney or bladder stones (4,5)

Contraindications Contraindicated in people with known allergy to golden rod. Golden rod is a medium level sensitizer[1] and has caused allergic reaction after systemic administration.[2]

The Commission E recommends copious fluid intake to assist in reducing microorganisms in the urinary tract, but this should not be undertaken if edema resulting from impaired cardiac or renal function exists.[3]

Warnings and Precautions Allergic reactions may occur in susceptible patients sensitized to plants from the Compositae family.

Interactions None known.

Use in Pregnancy and Lactation No adverse effects expected.

Side Effects None expected if taken within the recommended dose range.

Dosage

Dose per day*	Dose per week*
3-6 ml of 1:2 liquid extract	20-40 ml of 1:2 liquid extract

SUPPORTING INFORMATION

Traditional Prescribing Traditional Western herbal medicine uses include:
- Chronic upper respiratory tract catarrh or inflammation, influenza; flatulent dyspepsia;[4] cystitis, urinary disorders[4,5]
- As a spray or gargle for nose and throat infection[4]
- Topically as a powder for hemorrhage[5]

Golden Rod *continued on page 247*

*This dose range is extrapolated from the British Herbal Pharmacopoeia 1983 and the author's education and experience.

Native Americans used the flowers or leaves of several species of golden rod as a tea for fevers and pain in the chest.[6]

Pharmacologic Research

- A proprietary herbal formula containing golden rod, *Fraxinus excelsior* and *Populus tremula* (1:1:3), demonstrated antiinflammatory, antipyretic, and analgesic activities in experimental models, including carrageenan-induced edema and adjuvant-induced arthritis (route unknown).[7-9] In the case of the antiinflammatory models, each of the individual herbs also demonstrated activity.[9] The antiinflammatory activity is the result, at least in part, of the antioxidant properties of the individual herbal extracts that have been established in several *in vitro* models.[10] Similar to many NSAIDs, the combined extract and individual extracts inhibited dihydrofolate reductase *in vitro*.[8]
- Constituents of golden rod (3,5-O-caffeoylquinic acid and flavonoids) have inhibited leukocyte elastase (an enzyme involved in the progression of inflammation) *in vitro*. The ester saponins from golden rod induced the release of stored adrenocorticotropic hormone (ACTH) from pituitary corticotropic cells. The authors postulated that the release of ACTH might influence the release of glucocorticoids from the adrenal gland *in vivo*.[11]
- The flavonoid fraction of golden rod flowers demonstrated diuretic activity after oral administration in an experimental model.[12] A low oral dose of an aqueous extract of golden rod containing 0.3% flavonoids produced diuresis and an increase in electrolyte excretion in an experimental model.[13,14]
- Golden rod extract demonstrated spasmolytic activity in acetylcholine-pretreated isolated ileum.[15]
- An *in vitro* antifungal effect towards pathogenic species of Candida was demonstrated for triterpenoid saponins from golden rod.[16,17] The whole plant did not possess broad-spectrum activity toward *Candida* spp. and dermatophytes *in vitro*.[18] Essential oil of golden rod demonstrated antimicrobial activity against several bacteria, including *Streptococcus faecalis* and *Escherichia coli*, and exerted a strong fungicidal effect on dermatophyte strains *in vitro*.[19]
- Saponins from golden rod have displayed immunomodulatory and antitumoral effects *in vitro*.[20]

Clinical Studies

- A diuretic effect was observed in healthy volunteers after a single dose of golden rod tincture (100 drops, or approximately 4 ml) under double-blind, placebo-controlled conditions. In an uncontrolled trial, 70% of patients with urinary tract inflammation or symptomatic bacteriuria experienced complete disappearance of symptoms such as dysuria, frequency, and tenesmus when treated with the same preparation and dosage (duration of treatment not known). The fresh plant tincture (0.57 g/g) was made according to *German Homoeopathic Pharmacopoeia* (HAB).[21]

Golden Rod *continued on page 248*

- Two reviews assessing a formulation containing golden rod, *Fraxinus excelsior* and *Populus tremula,* for treating rheumatic conditions, including arthritis, have been published. One review assessed that the randomized, double-blind, controlled trials were of medium methodological quality.[22] The formulation demonstrated superior activity compared with placebo and was comparable to NSAID drugs but had a much lower incidence of adverse effects.[7,23] The formulation consists of 60% *Fraxinus excelsior,* 20% golden rod, and 20% *Populus tremula* and is standardized for salicylates, flavonoids, and coumarins.
- In a randomized, drug prospective study, treatment of ureteric calculi with either spasmoanalgesic drug therapy or an herbal preparation was compared. The preparation contained golden rod, dandelion root and leaf, *Rubia tinctorum, Ammi visnaga,* and a small amount of escin (a constituent of horsechestnut seed). Although no significant difference was observed with regard to transit times of the stones between the two groups, side effects and treatment costs were less in the herbal therapy group. The strength of the herbal extracts in these capsules was not defined.[23]
- In Germany, the Commission E supports using golden rod in conjunction with copious fluid intake to treat inflammatory diseases of the lower urinary tract, urinary calculi, and kidney gravel. Golden rod is also recommended as a prophylaxis for urinary calculi and kidney gravel.[3]
- ESCOP recommends golden rod for inflammatory conditions of the urinary tract, kidney gravel, and as an adjuvant therapy for bacterial infections of the urinary tract.[24]

REFERENCES

1 Zeller W, de Gols M, Hausen BM: *Arch Dermatol Res* 277(1):28-35, 1985.
2 Schatzle M, Agathos M, Breit R: *Contact Dermatitis* 39(5):271-272, 1998.
3 Blumenthal M et al, editors: *The complete German Commission E monographs: therapeutic guide to herbal medicines,* Austin 1998, American Botanical Council.
4 British Herbal Medicine Association's Scientific Committee: *British herbal pharmacopoeia,* Bournemouth, 1983, BHMA.
5 Felter HW, Lloyd JU: *King's American dispensatory,* ed 18, rev 3, Portland, 1905, reprinted 1983, Eclectic Medical Publications.
6 Vogel VJ: *American Indian medicine,* Norman, Okla, 1970, University of Oklahoma Press.
7 Klein-Galczinsky C: *Wien Med Wochenschr* 149(8-10):248-253, 1999.
8 Strehl E et al: *Arzneim Forsch* 45(2):174-176, 1995.
9 el-Ghazaly M et al: *Arzneim Forsch* 42(3):333-336, 1992.
10 Meyer B et al: *Arzneim Forsch* 45(2):174-176, 1995.
11 Melzig MF et al: *Z Phytother* 21(2):67-70, 2000.
12 Chodea A et al: *Acta Pol Pharm* 48(5-6):35-37, 1991.
13 Schilcher H: *Dtsch Apoth Ztg* 124:2429-2436, 1984.
14 Schilcher H, Rau H: *Urologe B* 28:274-280, 1988.
15 Westendorf J, Vahlensieck W: *Arzneim Forsch* 31(1):40-43, 1981.
16 Hiller K, Bader G: *4th International Congress on Phytotherapy,* Munich, Sept 10-13, 1992, Abstract SL 18.
17 Bader G et al: *Pharmazie* 55(1):72-74, 2000.
18 Pepeljnjak S et al: *Pharm Pharmacol Lett* 8(2):85-86, 1998.
19 Pepeljnjak S et al: *International Congress and 48th Annual Meeting of the Society for Medicinal Plant Research and the 6th International Congress on Ethnopharmacology of the International Society for Ethnopharmacology,* Zurich, September 3-7, 2000; Abstract P2A/74.

Golden Rod *continued on page 249*

20 Plohmann B et al: *Pharmazie* 52(12):953-957, 1997.

21 Bruhwiler K et al: *4th International Congress on Phytotherapy*, Munich, September 10-13, 1992; Abstract SL 20.

22 Ernst E, Chrubasik S: *Rheum Dis Clin North Am* 26(1):13-27, 2000.

23 Bach D et al: *Forsch Med* 101(8):337-342, 1983.

24 Scientific Committee of ESCOP (European Scientific Cooperative on Phytotherapy): *ESCOP Monographs: Solidaginis virgaureae herba*, ESCOP, Exter, UK, March 1996.

GOLDEN SEAL

Other Common Names: Hydrastis, goldenseal
Botanical Name: *Hydrastis canadensis*
Family: Ranunculaceae
Plant Part Used: Root and rhizome

PRESCRIBING INFORMATION

Actions	Antihemorrhagic, anticatarrhal, mucous membrane trophorestorative, antimicrobial, antibacterial, bitter tonic, antiinflammatory, depurative, vulnerary, choleretic, reputed oxytocic
Potential Indications	Based on appropriate evaluation of the patient, practitioners should consider prescribing golden seal in formulations in the context of: • Catarrhal states of the mucous membranes when unaccompanied by acute inflammation *(5)* • Acute infectious diarrhea *(4a,5)* • Giardiasis, hypertyraminemia *(4a)* • Gastritis, peptic ulcer *(4a,5)* • Adjuvant therapy for non-insulin–dependent diabetes mellitus *(4a)* • Hepatic symptoms, skin disorders *(5)* • Disorders of the ear, nose, mouth, throat *(5)* • Uterine and pelvic hemorrhagic conditions, genitourinary tract discharges *(5)* • A tonic during convalescence *(5)*
Contraindications	Berberine-containing plants are not recommended for use during pregnancy or for jaundiced neonates. Some reports suggest that golden seal is contraindicated in hypertensive conditions.
Warnings and Precautions	None required.
Interactions	Berberine may reinforce the effects of other drugs that displace the protein binding of bilirubin. Rather than possible uterine-contracting effects, this activity might explain the traditional contraindication for berberine-containing herbs in pregnancy.
Use in Pregnancy and Lactation	Contraindicated in pregnancy.
Side Effects	At daily doses higher than 0.5 g, berberine may cause dizziness, nose bleeds, dyspnea, skin and eye irritation, gastrointestinal irritation, nausea, diarrhea, nephritis, and urinary tract disorders. Such doses of berberine will not be reached using the recommended liquid doses outlined in this monograph.

Golden Seal *continued on page 251*

Dosage

*Dose per day**	*Dose per week**
2.0-4.5 ml of 1:3 tincture	15-30 ml of 1:3 tincture

Extracts providing quantified levels of hydrastine and berberine are recommended. Ideally, aqueous ethanol extracts should contain not less than 8 mg/ml of hydrastine and not less than 8 mg/ml of berberine.

SUPPORTING INFORMATION

Traditional Prescribing

Traditional Western herbal medicine uses include:
- Golden seal was specifically indicated by Eclectic physicians for subacute or chronic inflammation of the mucous membranes, particularly when accompanied by discharge or catarrh. In general, golden seal was contraindicated in acute inflammation of the mucous membranes. However, in the case of otitis media, golden seal was indicated for both acute and chronic inflammation, especially when copious discharge was present.[1]
- Digestive disorders, gastritis, peptic ulceration, colitis, anorexia, atonic dyspepsia with hepatic symptoms[2]
- Upper respiratory catarrh; skin diseases, especially when dependent on gastric difficulties; as a tonic during convalescence[1,2]
- Menorrhagia, postpartum hemorrhage, submucosal myoma (fibroids), hemorrhagic endometriosis, dysmenorrhea[1,2]
- Topically for affections of the nose and throat, eczema, pruritus, otorrhea, catarrhal deafness and tinnitus, conjunctivitis[1,2]

Native Americans used golden seal for dropsy, skin diseases, indolent ulcers, gonorrhea, liver and stomach disorders, and as a tonic. Externally, the infusion was used as a remedy for sore eyes, and the root was chewed for sore mouth. Golden seal was official in the USP from 1831 to 1842 and 1863 to 1936 and in the NF from 1936 to 1960. Golden seal was used as a bitter tonic and an astringent to treat inflammation of the mucous membranes.[3]

Pharmacologic Research

Key constituents of golden seal include alkaloids of the isoquinoline group, particularly berberine and hydrastine.
- *In vitro* and *in vivo* studies have demonstrated that berberine has antimicrobial activity against a wide variety of microorganisms, including bacteria, fungi, and parasites. Hydrastine has been found to produce 70% mortality in the tapeworm *Echinococcus granulosus,* both *in vitro* and *in vivo*.
- Berberine combined with Geranium leaf extract (oral doses) significantly inhibited diarrhea. Oral berberine, given with *Escherichia coli* enterotoxin, significantly reduced intestinal fluid accumulation *in vivo*.

Golden Seal *continued on page 252*

*This dose range is extrapolated from the British Pharmaceutical Codex 1934, the British Herbal Pharmacopoeia 1983, the British Herbal Compendium 1992, and the author's education and experience.

- Intravenous berberine blocked arrhythmias and decreased the amplitude of delayed after-depolarizations in isolated ventricular muscles *in vivo* and *in vitro*.
- Berberine increased thrombocytes, decreased factor XIII activity, inhibited platelet aggregation and adhesiveness, and inhibited clot retraction in experimental models (route unknown).
- Berberine has demonstrated cytotoxic activity in several *in vitro* models.
- Oral administration of berberine hydrochloride significantly increased bilirubin excretion in experimental hyperbilirubinemia without affecting the functional capacity of the liver.
- Lipogenesis was suppressed in isolated sebaceous glands by berberine.
- Berberine significantly decreased scopolamine-induced amnesia in an experimental model.
- Treatment with berberine in an experimental model of diabetes led to healthier pancreatic tissue compared with controls.
- Berberine had an immunosuppressive effect in an experimental model of renal autoimmune disease (route unknown).[4]
- Golden seal extract and its alkaloids demonstrated an antispasmodic action on isolated intestinal and uterine tissues.
- Although golden seal extract produced a vasoconstrictive effect, it also inhibited epinephrine- (adrenaline), serotonin-, and histamine-induced contraction of isolated aorta. However, although isolated berberine or hydrastine did not show this vasoconstrictive effect, berberine demonstrated some inhibitory activity on aortic contraction induced by epinephrine. Hydrastine was inactive. The observed vasoconstrictive effect of golden seal extract may result from the presence of hydrastinine, a decomposition product of hydrastine.

For more information on the pharmacology of berberine, the reader should review the barberry *(Berberis vulgaris)* and Indian barberry *(Berberis aristata)* monographs.

Clinical Studies

No clinical studies using golden seal have been found. Clinical trials using berberine are outlined here.
- Berberine (100 mg/day) demonstrated an antidiarrheal action and compared well against standard antidiarrheal drugs in an uncontrolled study involving children with gastroenteritis. In randomized, controlled trials, berberine has exhibited benefit in treating diarrhea caused by *Escherichia coli* infection but was of little value against *Vibrio cholerae* infectious diarrhea (cholera). The trials with positive outcomes for *E. coli* diarrhea were conducted with either untreated controls (400 mg of berberine sulfate as a single dose) or comparing rehydration therapy against rehydration therapy and berberine (200 mg). In another trial, neither berberine (400 mg/day) nor tetracycline exhibited any benefit over placebo in patients with noncholera diarrhea.

Golden Seal *continued on page 253*

- Berberine (900 mg/day) was more efficacious than ranitidine in clearing *Helicobacter pylori* and improving gastritis in *H. pylori*-associated duodenal ulcer in a randomized, comparative, clinical trial. Ranitidine was the more superior treatment for ulcer healing.
- In two controlled trials, berberine (5 to 10 mg/kg/day for 6 to 10 days) was superior to placebo and compared favorably with established drugs in treating giardiasis in children.
- In an uncontrolled trial, berberine (600 to 800 mg/day) corrected hypertyraminemia and prevented the elevation of serum tyramine after tyramine stimulation in patients with liver cirrhosis.
- In an uncontrolled trial, berberine (0.9 to 1.5 g/day for 1 to 3 months) in combination with a therapeutic diet improved the major symptoms of patients with non-insulin–dependent diabetes. Berberine improved patients' strength, normalized blood pressure, decreased blood lipids, and (in 60% of patients) normalized fasting glycemic levels.
- Berberine (15 mg/day for 15 days) increased platelet counts in patients with primary and secondary thrombocytopenia in an uncontrolled clinical trial.
- In a randomized, controlled trial, berberine chloride (1.5 g/day) was more efficacious than both tetracycline and a sulfamethoxazole-trimethoprim combination in clearing asexual parasitemia in patients with chloroquine-resistant malaria (when all agents were used in conjunction with pyrimethamine).
- Weekly intralesional injection of berberine salt solution (1%) healed cutaneous leishmaniasis after 4 to 8 weeks in a small, uncontrolled trial.

REFERENCES

Except when specifically referenced, the following book was referred to in the compilation of the pharmacologic and clinical information that has not been referenced in this monograph: Mills S, Bone K: *Principles and Practice of Phytotherapy: Modern Herbal Medicine,* Edinburgh, 2000, Churchill Livingstone.

1 Felter HW, Lloyd JU: *King's American dispensatory,* ed 18, rev 3, Portland, 1905, reprinted 1983, Eclectic Medical Publications.
2 British Herbal Medicine Association's Scientific Committee: *British herbal pharmacopoeia,* Bournemouth, 1983, BHMA.
3 Vogel VJ: *American Indian medicine,* Norman, Okla, 1970, University of Oklahoma Press.
4 Ekaterina KM et al: *Immunopharmacol* 48(1):9-16, 2000.

GOTU KOLA

Other Common Name:	Indian pennywort
Botanical Names:	*Centella asiatica, Hydrocotyle asiatica*[#]
Family:	Umbelliferae
Plant Part Used:	Aerial parts

PRESCRIBING INFORMATION

Actions

Vulnerary, antiinflammatory, depurative, adaptogenic, nervine tonic

Potential Indications

Based on appropriate evaluation of the patient, practitioners should consider prescribing gotu kola in formulations in the context of:

- Improving the healing response of the skin and subcutaneous tissue *(4a,5)*
- Diabetic microangiopathy *(4a)*
- Cellulitis; gastric or duodenal ulcer *(4a)*
- Leg ulcers *(4a,5)*
- Leprosy *(4,5)*
- Scleroderma *(4a)*
- Venous insufficiency of the lower limbs *(4a)*
- Varicose and postthrombotic syndromes *(4a)*
- Keloids and hypertrophic scars *(4a)*
- Hemorrhoids, in combination with bulking laxatives, if required *(4a)*
- Mouth ulcers *(6)*
- Chronic skin and rheumatic conditions *(5)*
- Improving mental function *(2,5)*
- Anxiety *(4)*
- Improving adaptation to stressors *(7)*
- Producing a rejuvenating tonic effect *(4,5)*
- Chronic hepatic disorders *(4a,6)*
- Topical treatment for postthrombotic syndrome and varicose veins *(4a)*
- Topical treatment for psoriasis, wounds *(4,5)*
- Topical treatment for burns, leg ulcers, cellulitis *(4)*
- Topical treatment for leprous ulcers, scar formation after surgery, eczema *(5)*
- Topical treatment for stretch marks, in combination with α-tocopherol and collagen-elastin hydrolysates *(4a)*

Contraindications

Known allergy.

Warnings and Precautions

None required.

Interactions

None known.

Use in Pregnancy and Lactation

No adverse effects expected.

Gotu Kola *continued on page 255*

[#]Alternative name.

Side Effects

Allergic contact dermatitis has been reported from using gotu kola, but it is a low risk treatment. Both the extract and the triterpene constituents are weak sensitizers.[1]

Dosage

Dose per day*	Dose per week*
3-6 ml of 1:2 liquid extract	20-40 ml of 1:2 liquid extract

Many of the successful clinical trials used a triterpene fraction of gotu kola at higher doses (approximately equivalent to 2.5 to 7.0 g of leaf per day) than the previously outlined liquid doses. Hence these liquid doses may possibly need to be exceeded to achieve similar results. However, on the other hand, an advantage might exist from using the whole extract rather than an isolated fraction.

SUPPORTING INFORMATION

Traditional Prescribing

Traditional Western herbal medicine uses include:
- Skin and rheumatic conditions, including chronic eczema, chronic rheumatism, leprosy, ulcers[2,3]
- Topically for poorly healing wounds, leprous ulcers, scar formation after surgery[2]

Traditional Ayurvedic uses include:
- As a depurative and tonic[4]
- As a *rasayana* (rejuvenating) remedy, hence it is used to improve memory and prolong life span[5]
- Topically for eczema, leprosy, secondary syphilitic ulcers, psoriasis[4,5]

Gotu kola has been traditionally used in many countries. In Thailand, the whole plant has been used as a depurative, particularly to treat skin diseases and as a diuretic and antidiarrheal remedy.[6] In Indonesia, gotu kola has been used for mouth ulcers and oral thrush.[7] In Fijian traditional herbal medicine, gotu kola was employed as a tonic for wasting diseases, such as tuberculosis, stomach problems, and rheumatic swelling and pain. Gotu kola was used both internally and topically to relieve pain.[8] In TCM, gotu kola is used for traumatic injuries, boils, urinary stones, and to counteract toxicity and reduce swelling.[9] In Hong Kong, gotu kola is also used for hepatitis, measles, the common cold, tonsillitis, bronchitis, and to treat poisoning. External uses include treatment of snakebite and bleeding wounds.[10] In South Africa, gotu kola has been employed to treat wounds, cancer, leprosy, fever, and syphilis.[11]

Pharmacologic Research

The aerial parts of gotu kola contain pentacyclic triterpene ester saponins,[12] the most abundant of which is asiaticoside. The triterpenoid

Gotu Kola continued on page 256

---

*This dose range is extrapolated from the British Herbal Pharmacopoeia 1983. Higher relative doses of the triterpene fraction have been used in most clinical trials.

content of good quality gotu kola dried herb is commonly 2% to 3% when analyzed by high-performance liquid chromatography (HPLC).[13]

- Gotu kola and asiaticoside demonstrated activity against herpes simplex virus-1 (HSV-1) and HSV-2 *in vitro*.[14]
- The triterpene fraction of gotu kola has demonstrated wound-healing activity in many experimental models (by injection, oral, and topical administration). The mechanism of action includes the stimulation of maturation of scar tissue by the increased production of type I collagen (and hence collagen synthesis) and a decrease in the inflammatory reaction and myofibroblast production.[15] The constituents also stimulated glycosaminoglycan synthesis[16] and acted specifically to shorten the immediate phase of healing.[17] Aqueous extract of gotu kola, particularly as a gel formulation, promoted healing in experimental open wounds.[18] Oral and topical administration of gotu kola extract produced faster epithelialization and a higher rate of wound contraction *in vivo* compared with controls.[19]
- Asiaticoside demonstrated activity in models of both normal and delayed wound healing after both topical and oral administration. Angiogenesis was promoted in isolated tissue.[20] Topical asiaticoside enhanced the induction of antioxidants at the initial stage of healing.[21]
- Oral administration of gotu kola extract inhibited gastric ulceration in cold- and restraint-induced stress models. Brain GABA levels were increased.[22] Complete mucosal cytoprotection was observed in an experimental model (by oral route).[23]
- The antiulcer activity may be related to a protective effect on stress. Gotu kola extract also prevented the experimental rise in plasma corticosterone levels following immobilization stress.[24] In other studies, oral gotu kola extract demonstrated normalizing effects against a variety of stressors.[25]
- The triterpene fraction of gotu kola reduced experimentally induced acute radiation dermatitis via its antiinflammatory activity (after topical application).[26]
- Oral administration of gotu kola and the partially purified triterpenoid fraction retarded the development of solid and ascites tumors and increased life span in an experimental model.[27]
- An antianxiety effect was demonstrated in several experimental models for an aqueous extract of gotu kola (by injection[28] and orally[29]). Sedative and antidepressant activity has also been demonstrated.[30] Oral administration of an aqueous extract of gotu kola caused a decrease in the turnover of central monoamines and improved learning and memory in experimental models.[31]

Clinical Studies

Most of the clinical trials listed here used the triterpene fraction of gotu kola (TFGK), with doses ranging from 60 to 180 mg per day (approximately 2.5 to 7.0 g of dried herb equivalent). The majority of these preparations contained 40% asiaticosides, 30% madecassic acid, and 30% asiatic acid.

Gotu Kola *continued on page 257*

- Oral administration of TFGK for 60 days demonstrated efficacy in a double-blind, placebo-controlled trial in patients with venous hypertensive microangiopathy.[32] In an uncontrolled trial[33] and in a randomized, single-blind, placebo-controlled trial,[34] TFGK improved symptoms, microcirculation, and capillary permeability in patients with venous hypertension. In another trial, symptoms and ankle edema were improved in patients with venous hypertension after TFGK treatment, with no significant change observed in the placebo group.[35] TFGK treatment (120 mg/day) for 6 months was beneficial for diabetic microangiopathy by improving microcirculation and decreasing capillary permeability. This trial was of prospective, randomized, placebo-controlled design.[36]
- TFGK treatment produced significant improvement in symptoms of heaviness in the lower limbs and edema in a randomized, double-blind, multicenter, placebo-controlled trial involving patients with venous insufficiency of the lower limbs. Two oral doses were trialled (60 mg/day or 120 mg/day) for 8 weeks.[37] Benefit was also demonstrated for TFGK treatment of patients with chronic venous insufficiency in an open study.[38] In a randomized, double-blind, comparative trial, TFGK demonstrated superior efficacy over hydroxyethylrutoside in treating venous insufficiency.[39] In an open trial, TFGK treatment provided an increase in venous return and improvement of symptoms in patients with varicose and postthrombotic syndromes.[40] In a controlled, crossover study involving patients with postphlebitic syndrome and venous insufficiency, oral treatment with TFGK provided better results in microcirculatory measurements than treatment with the flavonoids diosmin or hydroxyethylrutoside.[41]
- Oral treatment with TFGK produced a decrease in the elevated mucopolysaccharide turnover observed in patients with varicose veins.[42]
- Treatment with TFGK caused a significant reduction of circulating endothelial cells in patients with postphlebitic syndrome compared with baseline values.[43] Oral administration of TFGK and bulking laxatives (when required) produced a beneficial effect in patients with first- and second-degree hemorrhoids in an uncontrolled trial.[44]
- Positive results have been recorded in uncontrolled trials for treating gastric and duodenal ulcers (TFGK, oral),[45,46] gastritis (asiaticoside, oral),[47] and bladder lesions caused by bilharzial infection (TFGK, injection).[48] No benefit was observed for the healing of leg ulcers in patients treated with asiaticoside (by injection) compared with placebo.[49] However, positive results were obtained for oral use of TFGK taken for 3 to 8 weeks in 50 patients with leg ulcers.[50]
- Oral treatment with TFGK for an average of 55 days was successful in treating patients with cellulitis.[51] After 3 months' oral TFGK treatment, reduced tendency to sclerosis in cellulitic tissue was observed in a double-blind, placebo-controlled study.[52]
- Oral administration of TFGK has been successfully used to treat keloids and hypertrophic scars. In a study involving 227 patients, treatment with TFGK for a period of 2 to 18 months had therapeutic

Gotu Kola *continued on page 258*

value in both preventing (together with surgical revision) and reducing keloids. A subset of the patients involved in the curative study confirmed the activity of TFGK in a double-blind, placebo-controlled trial.[53]

- In a preliminary trial, TFGK taken for 3 to 24 months improved histology in 5 of 12 patients with chronic hepatic disorders, including alcoholic cirrhosis and cirrhosis of undetermined origin.[54]
- Gotu kola dried herb (0.5 g/day for 3 months) increased the intelligence quotient, general mental ability, and behavior in mentally disabled children in a randomized, placebo-controlled, clinical trial in India.[55]
- In an uncontrolled trial, gotu kola relieved the symptoms of patients with anxiety and improved mental functioning.[56]
- In a double-blind trial, gotu kola tended to increase the mean level of red blood cells, blood sugar, serum cholesterol, vital capacity, and total protein in normal volunteers. An increase in hemoglobin was statistically significant. This finding was thought to be indicative of a corticosteroid-like activity.[57,58]
- Gotu kola has been used to treat leprosy patients from very early times and in recent years in both uncontrolled trials[59-61] and a controlled trial (gotu kola powder or asiaticoside compared with diaminodiphenylsulfone over a period of 1 year).[62]
- Asiaticoside was not successful in treating scleroderma in children.[63] However, TFGK demonstrated symptomatic relief in a small group of patients with systemic scleroderma. The 13 patients received TFGK by intramuscular injection ranging from 1½ months to 1½ years. Two patients received TFGK orally for a portion of their treatment.[64] In another small, uncontrolled trial, oral doses of TFGK improved arthralgia and finger joint movement in scleroderma patients.[65]
- A systematic review published in 2000 concluded that, compared with placebo, treatment with a cream containing gotu kola extract, α-tocopherol, and collagen-elastin hydrolysates is associated with fewer women developing stretch marks. This result occurred only for women who had previously encountered stretch marks during pregnancy.[66]
- Topical application of gotu kola or TFGK has been successfully used to treat:
  - Postthrombotic syndrome and varicose veins (double-blind, placebo-controlled trial; TFGK)[67]
  - Chronic venous insufficiency (single-blind, controlled trial of TFGK against oral administration of the drug tribenoside)[68]
  - Psoriasis (uncontrolled trial; water and oil extract of gotu kola)[69]
  - Leg ulcers (uncontrolled trial;[70] placebo-controlled trial, TFGK by injection or topical[71])
  - Soiled wounds resistant to other treatments (standardized gotu kola extract combined with essential oils; uncontrolled trial)[72]
  - Burns (topical, injection, or both; uncontrolled trials with TFGK or gotu kola extract)[73,74]
  - Cellulitis (uncontrolled trial; standardized gotu kola extract)[75]

Gotu Kola *continued on page 259*

REFERENCES

1 Hausen BM: *Contact Dermatitis* 29(4):175-179, 1993.

2 British Herbal Medicine Association's Scientific Committee: *British herbal pharmacopoeia,* Bournemouth, 1983, BHMA.

3 Felter HW, Lloyd JU: *King's American dispensatory,* ed 18, rev 3, Portland, 1905, reprinted 1983, Eclectic Medical Publications.

4 Chopra RN et al: *Chopra's indigenous drugs of India,* ed 2, Calcutta, 1958, reprinted 1982, Academic Publishers.

5 Thakur RS, Puri HS, Husain A: *Major medicinal plants of India,* Lucknow, India, 1989, Central Institute of Medicinal and Aromatic Plants.

6 Farnsworth NR, Bunyapraphatsara N, editors: *Thai medicinal plants,* Bangkok, 1992, Medicinal Plant Information Center.

7 Dharma AP: *Indonesian medicinal plants,* Jakarta, 1987, Balai Pustaka.

8 Cambie RC, Ash J: *Fijian medicinal plants,* Melbourne, Australia, 1994, CSIRO Publishing.

9 Pharmacopoeia Commission of the People's Republic of China: *Pharmacopoeia of the People's Republic of China,* English ed, Beijing, 1997, Chemical Industry Press.

10 Chung CH, Li NH: *Chinese medicinal herbs of Hong Kong: Chinese-English,* Hong Kong, 1978, Shang wu yin shu kuan.

11 van Wyk B-E, van Oudtshoorn B, Gericke N: *Medicinal plants of South Africa,* Arcadia, South Africa, 1997, Briza Publications.

12 Wagner H, Bladt S: *Plant drug analysis: a thin layer chromatography atlas,* ed 2, Berlin, 1996, Springer-Verlag.

13 Gunther B, Wagner H: *Phytomed* 3(1):59-65, 1996.

14 Yoosook C et al: *Phytomed* 6(6):411-419, 2000.

15 Widgerow AD et al: *Aesthetic Plast Surg* 24(3):227-234, 2000.

16 Maquart FX et al: *Eur J Dermatol* 9(4):289-296, 1999.

17 Poizot A, Dumez D: *C R Acad Sci Hebd Seances Acad Sci D* 286(10):789-792, 1978.

18 Sunilkumar, Parameshwaraiah S, Shivakumar HG: *Indian J Exp Biol* 36(6):569-572, 1998.

19 Suguna L, Sivakumar P, Chandrakasan G: *Indian J Exp Biol* 34(12):1208-1211, 1996.

20 Shukla A et al: *J Ethnopharmacol* 65(1):1-11, 1999.

21 Shukla A, Rasik AM, Dhawan BN: *Phytother Res* 13(1):50-54, 1999.

22 Chatterjee TK et al: *Indian J Exp Biol* 30(10):889-891, 1992.

23 Tan PV, Njimi CK, Ayafor JF: *Phytother Res* 11:45-47, 1997.

24 Upadhyay SC et al: *Indian Drugs* 25(6):388-389, 1991.

25 Sarma DNK, Khosa RL: *Phytother Res* 10:181-183, 1996.

26 Chen YJ et al: *Biol Pharm Bull* 22(7):703-706, 1999.

27 Babu TD, Kuttan G, Padikkala J: *J Ethnopharmacol* 48(1):53-57, 1995.

28 Diwan PV, Karwande I, Singh AK: *Fitoterapia* 62(3):253-257, 1991.

29 de Lucia R, Sertie JAA: *Fitoterapia* 68(5):413-416, 1997.

30 Sakina MR, Dandiya PC: *Fitoterapia* 61(4):291-296, 1990.

31 Nalini K, Aroor AR: *Fitoterapia* 63(3):232-237, 1992.

32 Cesarone MR et al: *Minerva Cardioangiol* 42(6):299-304, 1994.

33 Belcaro GV, Grimaldi R, Guidi G: *Angiology* 41(7):533-540, 1990.

34 Belcaro G et al: *Curr Ther Res* 46:1015-1026, 1989.

35 Belcaro GV, Rulo A, Grimaldi R: *Angiology* 41(1):12-18, 1990.

36 Cesarone MR et al: *Angiology* 52(supp 2):S49-S54, 2001.

37 Pointel JP et al: *Angiology* 38(1, pt 1):46-50, 1987.

38 Capelli R: *Giorn Ital Angiol* 1:44-48, 1983.

39 Monteverde A et al: *Acta Therapeut* 13:629-636, 1987.

40 Cospite M et al: *Giorn Ital Angiol* 4(3):200-205, 1984.

41 Allegra C: *Clin Ter* 110(6):555-559, 1984.

42 Arpaia MR et al: *Int J Clin Pharmacol Res* 10(4):229-233, 1990.

43 Montecchio GP et al: *Haematologica* 76(3):256-259, 1991.

44 Guarerio F et al: *Giorn Ital Angiol* 6(1):46-52, 1986.

45 Shin HS et al: *Korean J Gastroenterol* 14:49-56, 1982.

46 Rhee JC, Choi KW: *Korean J Gastroenterol* 13:35-40, 1981.

47 Chung JM, Chung KS: *Korean J Gastroenterol* 13:41, 1981.

48 Fam A: *Int Surg* 58(7):451-452, 1973.

49 Mayall RC et al: *Rev Bras Med* 32:26-29, 1975.

50 Huriez CL, Martin P: *Lille Med* 44(9):463-464, 1972.

Gotu Kola continued on page 260

51 Bourguignon D: *Gaz Med Fr* 82:4579-4583, 1975.

52 Hachen A, Bourgoin JY: *Med Prat* 738(suppl):7, 1979.

53 Bosse JP et al: *Ann Plast Surg* 3(1):13-21, 1979.

54 Darnis F et al: *Sem Hop* 55(37-38):1749-1750, 1979.

55 Appa Rao MVR, Srinivasan K, Koteswara Rao T: *J Res Indian Med* 8(4):9-15, 1973.

56 Singh RH, Shukla SP, Misra BK: *J Res Ayurv Siddha* 2(1):1-10, 1981.

57 Appa Rao MVR et al: *J Res Indian Med* 2:79-85, 1967.

58 Appa Rao MVR et al: *Nagarjun* 12:33, 1969.

59 Herbert D et al: *Indian J Lepr* 66(1):65-68, 1994.

60 Boiteau P et al: *Nature* 163:258, 1949.

61 Kakkar KK: *Indian Drugs* 26(3):92-97, 1988.

62 Chakrabarty T, Deshmukh S: *Sci Culture* 11:573, 1976

63 Frati Munari AC et al: *Bol Med Hosp Infant Mex* 36(2):201-214, 1979.

64 Sasaki S, Shinkai YA, Kishinara Y: *Acta Derm Venereol* 52(2):141-150, 1972.

65 Szczepanski A, Dabrowska H, Blaszczyk M: *Przegl Dermatol* 61(5):701-703, 1974.

66 Young GL, Jewell MD: *Cochrane Database Syst Rev* (2):CD000066, 2000.

67 Allegra C et al: *Clin Terap* 99(5):507-513, 1981.

68 Marastoni F et al: *Minerva Cardioangiol* 4:201-207, 1982.

69 Natarajan S, Paily PP: *Indian J Dermatol* 18(4):82-85, 1973.

70 Apperti M et al: *Quad Chir Prat* 3:115, 1982.

71 Nebout M: *Bull Soc Pathol Exot* 67(5):471-478, 1974.

72 Morisset R, Cote NG, Panisset JC: *Phytother Res* 1(3):117-121, 1987.

73 Boiteau P, Ratsimamanga AR: *Bull Soc Sci Bretagne* 34:307-315, 1959.

74 Gravel JA: *Laval Med* 36(5):413-415, 1965.

75 Carraro Pereira I: *Folha Med* 79(5):401-414, 1979.

GREATER CELANDINE

Other Common Name:	Chelidonium
Botanical Name:	*Chelidonium majus*
Family:	Papaveraceae
Plant Part Used:	Aerial parts

PRESCRIBING INFORMATION

Actions

Choleretic, cholagogue, spasmolytic, mild laxative, antiinflammatory, antiviral (topically), vulnerary (topically)

Potential Indications

Based on appropriate evaluation of the patient, practitioners should consider prescribing greater celandine in formulations in the context of:
- Biliary dyskinesia, in combination with turmeric (2)
- Increasing bile flow and pancreatic secretion, in combination with milk thistle and turmeric (3)
- Cholangitis, gallstones, cholecystitis without stones (3,5)
- Cramping pain of the gastrointestinal tract and gall ducts (4,5)
- Liver disease, jaundice, bilious dyspepsia, bilious headache, migraine, supraorbital neuralgia, skin conditions, especially psoriasis (5)
- Chronic bronchitis, whooping cough (4)
- An enema for colonic polyposis (4)
- Topical treatment for warts (4,5)

Contraindications

None known.

Warnings and Precautions

Given the nature of the alkaloid content of this herb and the reported cases of hepatotoxicity (see the "Side Effects" section in this monograph), long-term use of higher doses (except topical) is not recommended.

Interactions

None known.

Use in Pregnancy and Lactation

No adverse effects expected.

Side Effects

Several cases of hepatotoxicity[1-4] and one case of hemolytic anemia have been reported after ingesting greater celandine or preparations containing the herb.

Intense itching and erythema with papules was reported after topical application of the juice in a 64-year-old woman. The patient reacted positively to patch tests of the juice and extract, whereas no reactions were observed in 10 control volunteers.[5]

When greater celandine was used in TCM, various degrees of adverse reactions such as dry mouth, dizziness, gastric discomfort, diarrhea, abdominal distension, nausea, and mild leukopenia were reported in a minority of patients. Symptoms generally disappeared within 3 to 5 days without discontinuing the treatment.

Greater Celandine *continued on page 262*

Dosage

Dose per day*	Dose per week*
1-2 ml of 1:2 liquid extract	7-15 ml of 1:2 liquid extract

Short-term use of higher doses up to the equivalent of 3 g per day may be necessary to alleviate gastrointestinal or gall duct cramping pains.

SUPPORTING INFORMATION

Traditional Prescribing

Traditional Western herbal medicine uses include:
- Liver and gallbladder inflammation and pain,[6] gallstones,[6,7] cholecystitis[7]
- Gastrointestinal conditions resulting from poor liver function[7]
- Jaundice, hemorrhoids, bilious dyspepsia[7]
- Bilious headache, migraine, supraorbital neuralgia[7]
- Skin conditions[7]
- Topically for warts, indolent ulcers, fungal growths, traumatic inflammations, hemorrhoids, skin conditions[7]

Uses from TCM include abdominal pain, peptic ulcers, chronic bronchitis, and whooping cough.[8]

Pharmacologic Research

Key constituents of greater celandine aerial parts include the isoquinoline alkaloids (0.4% to 1.3%), especially chelidonine.
- Oral administration of an alcohol extract of dried greater celandine decreased chemically induced liver injury in experimental models, indicating a hepatoprotective activity.
- Greater celandine extract induced bile flow without increasing the total output of bile acids in the isolated perfused liver (in other words, the flow of additional dilute bile was increased).
- Oral administration of greater celandine extract significantly reduced stomach tumor incidence in experimental models. Intraperitoneal injection demonstrated high tumor inhibition with relatively mild cytotoxic side effects. Greater celandine also exerted an antimutagenic effect *in vitro* against several mutagens in the Ames test.
- Greater celandine extract inhibited 5-lipoxygenase *in vitro*. The alkaloids sanguinarine and chelerythrine are potent inhibitors of 5-lipoxygenase and 12-lipoxygenase and have demonstrated antiinflammatory activity in the carrageenan rat paw edema test (after oral administration and subcutaneous injection).
- Chelerythrine chloride exerted an *in vitro* antiplatelet effect that is believed to be caused by the inhibition of both thromboxane formation and phosphoinositide breakdown.
- Greater celandine extract inhibited human keratinocyte proliferation *in vitro*, indicating possible topical application for psoriasis.

Greater Celandine *continued on page 263*

*This dose range is extrapolated from the British Herbal Pharmacopoeia 1983 and the author's education and experience.

- Extracts of greater celandine were shown to have *in vitro* antiviral activity and antifungal activity against Fusarium strains.[9] Fusarium strains have a high resistance to conventional fungicides. Greater celandine alkaloids had significant antimicrobial activity against fungal species and gram-positive bacteria (but not gram-negative bacteria) and inhibited the growth of *Trichomonas vaginalis in vitro*. The alkaloids sanguinarine and chelerythrine were active against gram-positive bacteria and *Candida albicans*.

Clinical Studies

- In a controlled trial, greater celandine extract exerted good to very good results in two thirds of patients treated for cholangitis, gallstones, and cholecystitis without stones. Greater celandine treatment was as effective as treatment with unspecified proprietary preparations commonly used for treating these gallbladder conditions. The administered daily dose was 3 ml of fresh plant tincture standardized to 0.6 mg/day alkaloids and taken for 43 to 50 days.
- Greater celandine, in combination with milk thistle and turmeric, increased bile flow and pancreatic secretion in a placebo-controlled trial.
- In an uncontrolled, multicenter trial, a high dose of greater celandine extract had a good to very good effect on gastrointestinal or gall duct cramping pains, with quick response (30 minutes). The administered daily dose contained 14.25 mg of total alkaloids initially. The dose was then reduced and contained 8.55 mg per day of total alkaloids.
- A combination of greater celandine and turmeric dried extracts reduced right upper quadrant pain resulting from biliary dyskinesia in a randomized, placebo-controlled, multicenter study.[10]
- Greater celandine decoction taken for 2 weeks (made from 60 g of herb per day) caused degeneration of cancerous tissue in patients with squamous cell carcinoma of the esophagus. The trial compared patients treated preoperatively with one of three traditional Chinese herbs, herbs combined with cyclophosphamide, and control patients who received no treatment. The degeneration was less clear in patients treated with herbs plus cyclophosphamide and the controls.
- Greater celandine (equivalent to 15 g of herb per day) given as an extract or syrup had an 80% effective rate in an uncontrolled trial involving patients with chronic bronchitis. Greater celandine syrup or decoction cured 71% and improved 23% of 500 cases of whooping cough in infants and children in another uncontrolled trial.
- Greater celandine administered as an enema reduced, and in some cases cleared, nonmalignant colonic polyposis in uncontrolled trials. Treatment frequency ranged from one to three courses of 10 to 20 enemas each.
- In an uncontrolled trial, topical application of greater celandine extract completely resolved warts, papillomas, condylomas, and nodules within 15 to 20 days in 135 of 200 nursing mothers. The extract was applied approximately 200 times per day for 2 to 3 weeks or until improvement was observed.

Greater Celandine *continued on page 264*

- In Germany, the Commission E supports using greater celandine to treat spastic discomfort of the bile ducts and gastrointestinal tract.[11]

REFERENCES

Except when specifically referenced, the following book was referred to in the compilation of the pharmacological and clinical information that has not been referenced here: Mills S, Bone K: *Principles and Practice of Phytotherapy: Modern Herbal Medicine,* Edinburgh, 2000, Churchill Livingstone.

1 de Smet PA et al: *BMJ* 313(7049):92, 1996.
2 Greving I et al: *Pharmacoepidemiol Drug Saf* 7:S66-S69, 1998.
3 Benninger J et al: *Gastroenterol* 117(5):1234-1237, 1999.
4 Strahl S et al: *Deutsche Medizinische Wochenschrift* 123(47):1410-1414, 1998.
5 Etxenagusia MA, Anda A, Gonzalez-Mahave I: *Contact Dermatitis* 43(1):47, 2000.
6 Felter HW, Lloyd JU: *King's American dispensatory,* ed 18, rev 3, Portland, 1905, reprinted 1983, Eclectic Medical Publications.
7 British Herbal Medicine Association's Scientific Committee: *British herbal pharmacopoeia,* Bournemouth, 1983, BHMA.
8 Huang KC: *The pharmacology of Chinese herbs,* Boca Raton, Fla, 1993, CRC Press.
9 Matos OC et al: *J Ethnopharmacol* 66(2):151-158, 1999.
10 Niederau C, Gopfert E: *Med Klin* 94(8):425-430, 1999.
11 Blumenthal M et al, eds: *The complete German Commission E monographs: therapeutic guide to herbal medicines,* Austin, 1998, American Botanical Council.

GRINDELIA

Botanical Names: *Grindelia camporum, Grindelia robusta*[+]
Family: Compositae
Plant Part Used: Aerial parts

PRESCRIBING INFORMATION

Actions

Expectorant, spasmolytic, bronchospasmolytic

Potential Indications

Based on appropriate evaluation of the patient, practitioners should consider prescribing Grindelia in formulations in the context of respiratory conditions marked by spasm, asthma, whooping cough, bronchitis, dry and irritable cough, and upper respiratory catarrh. *(5)*

Contraindications

None known.

Warnings and Precautions

None required.

Interactions

None known.

Use in Pregnancy and Lactation

No adverse effects expected.

Side Effects

None expected if taken within the recommended dose range. The *British Herbal Pharmacopoeia* 1983 notes that large doses are reported to cause renal irritation.[1] This warning may be the result of the presence of saponins.

Dosage

*Dose per day**	*Dose per week**
1.5-3.0 ml of 1:2 liquid extract	10-20 ml of 1:2 liquid extract

SUPPORTING INFORMATION

Traditional Prescribing

Traditional Western herbal medicine uses include:
- Bronchitis, asthma, upper respiratory catarrh, whooping cough; harsh and dry cough, difficult breathing resulting from heart disease[1,2]
- Cystitis[1,2]

Native Americans used Grindelia species for a variety of therapeutic purposes, including coughs, the common cold, tuberculosis, skin infections, and colic in children. The dried leaf and flowering tops of Grindelia were official in the USP from 1882 to 1926 and the NF from 1926 to 1960. Several species have been official under this name and have been used as sedatives, antispasmodics, expectorants, and as remedies for poison ivy, a liquid extract being used in the last case.[3]

Grindelia continued on page 266

[+]Medicinally interchangeable species.
*This dose range is extrapolated from the *British Herbal Pharmacopoeia* 1983 and the author's education and experience.

Pharmacologic Research

The aerial parts of Grindelia contain resin and saponins. An antimicrobial activity has been demonstrated *in vitro*, which is not the result of the saponins but is at least partially caused by the resin fraction.[4]

Clinical Studies

No clinical studies using Grindelia have been found.

REFERENCES

1 British Herbal Medicine Association's Scientific Committee: *British herbal pharmacopoeia*, Bournemouth, 1983, BHMA.

2 Felter HW, Lloyd JU: *King's American dispensatory*, ed 18, rev 3, Portland, 1905, reprinted 1983, Eclectic Medical Publications.

3 Vogel VJ: *American Indian medicine*, Norman, Okla, 1970, University of Oklahoma Press.

4 Kreutzer S, Schimmer O, Waibel R: *Planta Med* 56(4):392-394, 1990.

GYMNEMA

Botanical Name: *Gymnema sylvestre*
Family: Asclepiadaceae
Plant Part Used: Leaf

PRESCRIBING INFORMATION

Actions	Antidiabetic, hypoglycemic, hypocholesterolemic, weight reducing
Potential Indications	Based on appropriate evaluation of the patient, practitioners should consider prescribing Gymnema in formulations in the context of: • Diabetes mellitus (both insulin-dependent and non-insulin–dependent) *(3,5)* • Reducing the sense of taste for sweet foods *(3,5)* • Reducing appetite and calorie intake *(3,5)*
Contraindications	None known.
Warnings and Precautions	None required.
Interactions	None known.
Use in Pregnancy and Lactation	No adverse effects expected.
Side Effects	As with all saponin-containing herbs, oral use may cause irritation of the gastric mucous membranes and reflux.

Dosage

*Dose per day**^	*Dose per week**
3.5-11.0 ml of 1:1 liquid extract	25-75 ml of 1:1 liquid extract

One to two ml per day is all that is necessary for reducing sweet-craving and the sweet taste. In the latter case, the extract should be applied directly to the tongue, rinsed off, and swallowed after 1 minute. This procedure can be done at 2- to 3-hour intervals.

SUPPORTING INFORMATION

Traditional Prescribing	Traditional Ayurvedic uses include: • Glycosuria, diabetes (known as the "sugar destroyer")[1,2] • Urinary disorders, fever, cough[3] Ayurvedic texts note that chewing Gymnema leaf removes the ability to taste sweet or bitter substances.[2]

Gymnema *continued on page 268*

---

*This dose range is extrapolated from traditional Ayurvedic medicine[1,3] and the author's education and experience.
^Less may be needed if combined with other antidiabetic herbs. Some cases of diabetes will respond quickly, but best results come after 6 to 12 months of continuous use.

Pharmacologic Research

Key constituents of Gymnema leaves include saponins, which are present as both nonacylated glycosides known as gymnemasaponins and the acylated gymnemic acids.[4] Gymnemic acid referred to in the literature is often not defined and most likely refers to the crude saponin fraction or to a mixture of gymnemic acids.

- The antisweet principles of Gymnema include the gymnemic acids,[5] gymnemasaponins,[6] and gurmarin (a peptide).[7] Gymnemic acid suppressed the sweet taste of sweeteners in chimpanzees. Gymnemic acid had no effect on the responses to bitter, salty, or sour compounds.[8,9]
- Oral administration of Gymnema demonstrated hypoglycemic activity in experimental models of diabetes. Gymnema treatment:
  - Regulated blood sugar and increased the activity of the enzymes that facilitate the use of glucose by insulin-dependent pathways[10]
  - Increased the uptake of glucose into glycogen and protein in liver, kidney, and muscle[10]
  - Corrected hyperglycemia in mild diabetic models and significantly prolonged life span in models of severe diabetes (with completely destroyed pancreatic tissue)[11]
  - Reduced postprandial serum glucose and improved glucose tolerance. (Pancreas weight and content of insulin were not changed.)[12]
  - Returned fasting blood glucose levels to normal after 20 days. (A rise in insulin and pancreatic islet regeneration occurred to some extent.)[13]
  - Produced hypoglycemic activity in a slow and steady manner, with 12 to 24 weeks of treatment required in mild diabetes[14]
  - Lowered blood sugar levels in normal and diabetic models but was six times less potent than tolbutamide in diabetic animals[15]
- The mechanism of action may also include inhibition of glucose absorption in the intestine.[16]
- Feeding with Gymnema aqueous extract decreased body weight in fat and lean rats compared with those consuming only the test diet. In addition to lowering blood glucose levels, Gymnema also improved hypertriglyceridemia but not hypercholesterolemia.[17] In another study, oral administration of Gymnema extract fractions decreased body weight gain and food intake and increased fecal excretion of cholesterol, total neutral steroids, total bile acids, and cholic acid–derived bile acid.[18] Gymnema ingestion produced a significant lowering of cholesterol in a hypertension model.[19]

Clinical Studies

- Several clinical studies verify that pretreatment with Gymnema extract, Gymnema infusion, and gymnemic acid solution reduced the sweet taste of sweeteners.[20-23] A period of at least 30 seconds was required after tasting the Gymnema infusion for the full sweet-suppression effect to appear.[23]
- Gymnema powder (10 g/day for 7 days) demonstrated a hypoglycemic effect in mild diabetic models in an uncontrolled trial. Serum triglycerides, free fatty acid and cholesterol levels, and creatinine excretion, were also decreased.[24]

Gymnema *continued on page 269*

- A controlled study involving patients with insulin-dependent diabetes found that Gymnema extract reduced insulin requirements, fasting blood glucose, glycosylated hemoglobin, and glycosylated plasma protein levels compared with patients receiving insulin therapy alone. Cholesterol, triglycerides, free fatty acids, and serum amylase were also lowered. Some suggestion of enhancing endogenous insulin production, possibly by pancreatic regeneration, was demonstrated. Gymnema extract (400 mg/day, equivalent to 10 to 13 g/day of dried leaf) was administered for 6 to 30 months.[25]

- A second study by the same research group found that the same Gymnema extract (400 mg/day for 18 to 20 months) produced similar results for patients with non-insulin–dependent diabetes with a reduction of similar biochemical parameters and hypoglycemic drug requirements. Fasting and postprandial serum insulin levels were elevated in the Gymnema group compared with controls taking only conventional drugs. Administering Gymnema to healthy volunteers did not produce any acute reduction in fasting blood glucose levels.[26]

- Clinical research under double-blind, placebo-controlled conditions found that a concentrated Gymnema extract (gymnemic acid content not defined) considerably diminished the sweet taste and significantly decreased appetite and the amount of calories consumed for up to 90 minutes after the sweet-numbing effect.[27]

REFERENCES

1 Thakur RS, Puri HS, Husain A: *Major medicinal plants of India,* Lucknow, India, 1989, Central Institute of Medicinal and Aromatic Plants.

2 Chopra RN et al: *Chopra's indigenous drugs of India,* ed 2, Calcutta, 1958, reprinted 1982, Academic Publishers.

3 Kapoor LD: *CRC handbook of Ayurvedic medicinal plants,* Boca Raton, Fla, 1990, CRC Press.

4 Hostettmann K, Marston A: *Chemistry & pharmacology of natural products: saponins,* Cambridge, 1995, Cambridge University Press.

5 Liu HM, Kiuchi F, Tsuda Y: *Chem Pharm Bull (Tokyo)* 40(6):1366-1375, 1992.

6 Yoshikawa K: *Tetrahedron Lett* 32(6):789-792, 1991.

7 Imoto T et al: *Comp Biochem Physiol* 100(2):309-314, 1991.

8 Hellekant G et al: *Physiol Behav* 60(2):469-479, 1996.

9 Hellekant G, Ninomiya Y, Danilova V: *Physiol Behav* 65(2):191-200, 1998.

10 Shanmugasundaram KR et al: *J Ethnopharmacol* 7(2):205-234, 1983.

11 Srivastava Y et al: *Int J Crude Drug Res* 24(4):171-176, 1986.

12 Okabayashi Y et al: *Diabetes Res Clin Pract* 9(2):143-148, 1990.

13 Shanmugasundaram ER et al: *J Ethnopharmacol* 30(3):265-279, 1990.

14 Shanmugasundaram KR et al: *Pharmacol Res Commun* 13(5):475-486, 1981.

15 Chattopadhyay RR: *J Ethnopharmacol* 67(3):367-372, 1999.

16 Wang LF et al: *Can J Physiol Pharmacol* 76(10-11):1017-1023, 1998.

17 Teresawa H, Miyoshi M, Imoto T: *Yonago Acta Med* 37(2):117-127, 1994.

18 Nakamura Y et al: *J Nutr* 129(6):1214-1222, 1999.

19 Preuss HG et al: *J Am Coll Nutr* 17(2):116-123, 1998.

20 Min BC, Sakamoto K: *Appl Human Sci* 17(1):9-17, 1998.

21 Frank RA et al: *Chem Senses* 17(5):461-479, 1992.

22 Gent JF et al: *Chem Senses* 24(4):393-403, 1999.

23 Meiselman HL, Halperin BP: *Physiol Behav* 5(8):945-948, 1970.

24 Balasubramaniam KB et al: *J Natl Sci Counc Sri Lanka* 20(1):81-89, 1992.

25 Shanmugasundaram ER et al: *J Ethnopharmacol* 30(3):281-294, 1990.

26 Baskaran K et al: *J Ethnopharmacol* 30(1):1-9, 1983.

27 Brala PM, Hagen RL: *Physiol Behav* 30(1):1-9, 1983.

HAWTHORN

Botanical Names: *Crataegus monogyna, Crataegus laevigata*+ *(Crataegus oxyacantha*#*)*
Family: Rosaceae
Plant Parts Used: Leaf, berry

PRESCRIBING INFORMATION

Actions

Hawthorn leaf and berry: cardioprotective, mild cardiotonic, hypotensive, peripheral vasodilator, antiarrhythmic, antioxidant, mild astringent, collagen stabilizing

Potential Indications

Based on appropriate evaluation of the patient, practitioners should consider prescribing hawthorn leaf and berry in formulations in the context of:
- Cardiac insufficiency, particularly corresponding to New York Heart Association (NYHA) stages I and II *(1,4,5)*
- Other mild heart conditions, such as minor angina pectoris *(2,5)*
- Low heart rate variability *(2)*
- Hypertension *(3,5)*
- Cardiac arrhythmias, tachycardia, nervous heart complaints, circulatory support *(4)*
- Arteriosclerosis, Buerger's disease *(5)*

Contraindications

None known.

Warnings and Precautions

None required.

Interactions

Hawthorn may act in synergy with digitalis glycosides, beta-blockers, and other hypotensive drugs. Modification of drug dosage may be required.

Use in Pregnancy and Lactation

No adverse effects expected.

Side Effects

None expected if taken within the recommended dose range.

In a postmarketing surveillance study involving 3664 patients with cardiac insufficiency corresponding to NYHA stages I and II, hawthorn extract (corresponding to 2.7 g/day of dried leaf and flower, containing 19.8 mg flavonoids) was well tolerated. Adverse reactions with a causal relationship to hawthorn therapy were confirmed in 22 cases and probable in another 4 (a total of 0.7%). Reported side effects included gastrointestinal disorders, palpitations, headache, dizziness, circulatory disturbances, sleeplessness, and inner agitation.

Hawthorn *continued on page 271*

+Medicinally interchangeable species.
#Alternative name.

Dosage

Hawthorn berry:

Dose per day*	*Dose per week**
3-7 ml of 1:2 liquid extract	20-50 ml of 1:2 liquid extract

Extracts providing quantified levels of oligomeric procyanidins (OPCs) are recommended. Ideally, aqueous ethanol extracts should contain not less than 4 mg/ml of OPCs.

Hawthorn leaf:

Dose per day**	*Dose per week***
3-6 ml of 1:2 liquid extract	20-40 ml of 1:2 liquid extract

Extracts providing quantified levels of OPCs are recommended. Ideally, aqueous ethanol extracts should contain not less than 10 mg/ml of OPCs.

Higher doses than those outlined here may be necessary for effective control of hypertension.

SUPPORTING INFORMATION

Traditional Prescribing

Traditional Western herbal medicine uses of hawthorn berry include myocardial weakness, hypertension, angina pectoris, tachycardia, and other circulatory disorders, such as arteriosclerosis and Buerger's disease.[1]

Traditional Western herbal medicine uses of hawthorn leaf include as an astringent and tonic.[2]

Native Americans used Hawthorn fruit and bark for women's medicine, and the chewed leaves were used as a poultice for swellings.[3] Eclectic physicians used hawthorn fruit and bark for cardiac problems, particularly those of a functional nature, and as a general tonic as well.[2]

Pharmacologic Research

Key constituents of hawthorn include OPCs, especially procyanidin B-2, and flavonoids. The levels vary with the species of hawthorn and also within the plant part. The flowers contain the highest levels of flavonoids, and the leaves contain the highest levels of OPCs. The ripe berries are the lowest in OPCs and flavonoids. Therefore a fair assumption would be that the leaf is more active than the traditionally preferred berry.

- Studies have shown (many *in vitro*) hawthorn extracts or fractions to increase coronary blood flow, to be positively inotropic (increasing

Hawthorn *continued on page 272*

*This dose range is extrapolated from British Herbal Pharmacopoeia 1983 and the author's education and experience.
**This dose range is extrapolated from clinical studies.

the force of contraction), negatively chronotropic (decreasing the heart rate), and cardioprotective. Oral administration also found an increase in coronary blood flow in an experimental model.

- Purified flavonoids from hawthorn leaf produced a smaller necrotic focus and improved revascularization of finer vessels (after myocardial infarction) when compared with controls.
- In experimental models, the following has been observed:
  - Improved myocardial performance (OPCs, by injection)
  - Increased coronary blood flow (OPCs, by both oral and injected routes)
  - Decreased blood pressure (extract, OPCs, by both oral and injected routes)
  - Antiarrhythmic effect (extract, oral route)
- In laboratory studies, when compared with a digoxin preparation, hawthorn extract increased the erythrocyte flow rate in all the vascular networks examined and reduced both leukocyte endothelial adhesion and diapedesis in the venular network of mesenteric vessels.
- Hawthorn leaf and berry extracts exhibited antioxidant activity *in vitro*. Hawthorn tincture inhibited *in vitro* oxidation of LDL and VLDL from the plasma of patients with non-insulin–dependent diabetes mellitus.[4]
- Although studies have not been conducted specifically on the OPCs found in hawthorn, hawthorn OPCs will likely share many of the known pharmacological properties of OPCs. These indications might include prevention of cancer, atheroma, and any cell damage occurring under hypoxic conditions. Hawthorn OPCs have also stabilized collagen *in vitro*.

Clinical Studies

The NYHA classifies loss of cardiac output: for stage I, the patient is symptom-free when at rest and on treatment; for stage II, patients have loss of capacity with medium effort.

- A meta-analysis reviewing eight clinical trials from 1989 to 1994 found standardized hawthorn leaf and flower extract to be efficacious for treating heart failure (mostly of NYHA stage II). A significant effect was observed for subjective findings in all but one trial, for pressure-rate product (which measures cardiac work performance) in four trials, and for work tolerance in three trials. Two trials were open, five were randomized, double-blind, and placebo-controlled, and one was a multicenter, double-blind, comparative trial with the drug captopril. Information available indicates that for four trials, a dose range equivalent to 0.9 to 2.7 g per day of dried leaf and flower standardized to 6.6 to 19.8 mg per day of flavonoids was administered. In two trials, a dose range equivalent to 0.8 to 1.2 g per day of dried leaf and flower standardized to 30 to 45 mg per day of OPC was administered. The randomized, double-blind, placebo-controlled trial that failed to find significant improvement for pressure-rate product had used a lower dose of hawthorn extract (equivalent to 0.9 g/day of leaf and flower and containing 6.6 mg/day of flavonoids).

Hawthorn *continued on page 273*

- In a randomized, double-blind, placebo-controlled study, hawthorn leaf and flower extract (equivalent to 1.2 g/day leaf and flower standardized to 45 mg/day OPC) administered for 12 weeks increased exercise tolerance in patients with NYHA class II congestive heart failure. Exercise tolerance was reduced in the placebo group. No adverse reactions were reported in the hawthorn group. A number of biochemical indices were monitored, and these either remained within their normal ranges or did not differ in a clinically significant manner during therapy.[5]

- Significant benefit in cardiac parameters was achieved in a multicenter, double-blind, placebo-controlled trial using hawthorn leaf and berry extract in 80 patients with mild congestive heart disease resulting from ischemia or hypertension. No adverse interactions with conventional medication were observed.

- In a randomized, double-blind, placebo-controlled study, hawthorn extract significantly increased heart rate variability (HRV) in geriatric patients compared with placebo. (Low HRV is a risk factor in coronary heart disease, and a positive correlation exists between HRV and life expectancy.)

- In a randomized, double-blind, placebo-controlled clinical study, hawthorn extract (equivalent to 900 mg/day of dried herb for 3 weeks) was shown to improve pathology in patients with angina pectoris.

- In a postmarketing surveillance study, standardized hawthorn leaf and flower extract (equivalent to 2.7 g/day leaf and flower standardized to 19.8 mg/day of flavonoids for 8 weeks) was shown to be well tolerated and improved the symptom score on average by 66.6% in patients with heart disease (NYHA stages I and II). Clinicians rated overall efficacy as better than 90%. Patients with borderline hypertension, tachycardia, and cardiac arrhythmias exhibited excellent results, with blood pressure, heart rate, and incidence of arrhythmias being reduced. A large number of patients previously unsuccessfully treated with digoxin alone were compensated for rest and slight stress with relatively low oral doses of the glycoside in combination with hawthorn.

- In an uncontrolled trial, hawthorn berry tincture (equivalent to 4.3 g/day of berry) significantly reduced systolic and diastolic blood pressure. When treatment was stopped, blood pressures returned to their initial values over a 2-week period.

- In a randomized, double-blind, placebo-controlled study, hawthorn leaf and flower extract in combination with passion flower was efficacious in treating patients with dyspnea commensurate with NYHA stage II. The dosage of hawthorn corresponded to 1.6 g per day of leaf and flower and contained 15 mg per day of flavonoids and 28 mg per day of OPCs. The preparation was administered for 6 weeks.

- In a placebo-controlled, crossover study, the effect of a single dose of standardized hawthorn leaf and flower extract (equivalent to 2.7 g of leaf and flower, standardized to 19.8 mg/day of flavonoids) on the

Hawthorn *continued on page 274*

cutaneous microcirculation was compared with 0.3 mg medigoxin. Six hours after taking hawthorn, the hemocrit had dropped by a mean of 3.2%, whereas, 3 hours after taking the digoxin, erythrocyte aggregation increased significantly by a mean of 19%.

- In Germany, the Commission E supports using hawthorn leaf with flower to treat decreased cardiac output as described in NYHA stage II.[6]
- ESCOP recommends hawthorn leaf and flower extract for treating declining cardiac performance corresponding to NYHA stage II. Other preparations, including herbal teas, are indicated for nervous heart complaints and circulatory support.[7]

REFERENCES

Except when specifically referenced, the following book was referred to in the compilation of the pharmacological and clinical information: Mills S, Bone K: *Principles and Practice of Phytotherapy: Modern Herbal Medicine,* Edinburgh, 2000, Churchill Livingstone.

1 British Herbal Medicine Association's Scientific Committee: *British herbal pharmacopoeia,* Bournemouth, 1983, BHMA.

2 Felter HW: *The eclectic materia medica, pharmacology and therapeutics,* Portland, 1922, reprinted 1983, Eclectic Medical Publications.

3 Vogel VJ: *American Indian medicine,* Norman, Okla, 1970, University of Oklahoma Press.

4 Rajalakshmi K, Gurumurthi P, Devaraj SN: *Indian J Exp Biol* 38(5):509-511, 2000.

5 Zapfe jun. G: *Phytomed* 8(4):262-266, 2001.

6 Blumenthal M et al, editors: *The complete German Commission E monographs: therapeutic guide to herbal medicines,* Austin, 1998, American Botanical Council.

7 Scientific Committee of the European Scientific Cooperative on Phytotherapy [ESCOP]: *ESCOP monographs: Crataegi folium cum flore.* European Scientific Cooperative on Phytotherapy, ESCOP Secretariat, Argyle House, Gandy Street, Exeter, Devon, EX4 3LS, United Kingdom, October 1999.

HEMIDESMUS

Other Common Name: Indian sarsaparilla
Botanical Name: *Hemidesmus indicus*
Family: Asclepiadaceae
Plant Part Used: Root

PRESCRIBING INFORMATION

Actions

Depurative, diaphoretic, immune depressant

Potential Indications

Based on appropriate evaluation of the patient, practitioners should consider prescribing Hemidesmus in formulations in the context of:
- Autoimmune diseases such as rheumatoid arthritis (7)
- Diseases of the genitourinary tract (5)
- Skin diseases, fever (5)

Contraindications

None known.

Warnings and Precautions

None required.

Interactions

None known.

Use in Pregnancy and Lactation

No adverse effects expected.

Side Effects

None expected if taken within the recommended dose range.

Dosage

Dose per day*	Dose per week*
3.5-8.5 ml of 1:2 liquid extract	25-60 ml of 1:2 liquid extract

SUPPORTING INFORMATION

Traditional Prescribing

Traditional Ayurvedic uses include:
- Diseases of the genitourinary system[2]
- Loss of appetite, fever, skin diseases, chronic cough[1]
- Topically as an antiinflammatory remedy[2]

Hemidesmus is regarded in Ayurvedic medicine as a depurative and tonic and is used as a substitute for sarsaparilla (*Smilax* spp.).[3]

Pharmacologic Research

- Hemidesmus has demonstrated antifungal activity *in vitro*.[4]
- Oral administration of Hemidesmus has been found to depress both the cell-mediated and humoral components of the immune system.[5]
- An inhibiting effect on leprosy was found in an experimental model (dose route unknown).[6]
- An organic acid isolated from the root of Hemidesmus inhibited the activity of snake venom in experimental models (by injection).

Hemidesmus *continued on page 276*

*This dose range is extrapolated from traditional Ayurvedic medicine[1] and the author's education and experience.

The acid inhibited the lethal hemorrhagic, coagulant, and anticoagulant activities that the viper venom induced.[7,8] The same compound demonstrated antiinflammatory activity in an experimental model (most likely by injection) and *in vitro* antioxidant activity.[9]

- Oral administration of Hemidesmus extract prevented experimentally induced hepatotoxicity in two models.[10]

Clinical Studies

No clinical studies using Hemidesmus have been found.

REFERENCES

1 Kapoor LD: CRC *handbook of Ayurvedic medicinal plants,* Boca Raton, Fla, 1990, CRC Press.

2 Thakur RS, Puri HS, Husain A: *Major medicinal plants of India,* Lucknow, India, 1989, Central Institute of Medicinal and Aromatic Plants.

3 Chopra RN et al: *Chopra's indigenous drugs of India,* ed 2, Calcutta, 1958, reprinted 1982, Academic Publishers.

4 Hiremath SP, Rudresh K, Badami S: *Indian J Pharm Sci* 59(3):145-147, 1997.

5 Atal CK et al: *J Ethnopharmacol* 18(2):133-141, 1986.

6 Gupta PN: *Lepr India* 53(3):354-359, 1981.

7 Alam MI, Auddy B, Gomes A: *Toxicon* 32(12):1551-1557, 1994.

8 Alam MI, Gomes A: *Toxicon* 36(10):1423-1431, 1998.

9 Alam MI, Gomes A: *Toxicon* 36(1):207-215, 1998.

10 Prabakan M, Anandan R, Devaki T: *Fitoterapia* 71:55-59, 2000.

HOPS

Botanical Name: *Humulus lupulus*
Family: Cannabaceae
Plant Part Used: Strobile (cones or female inflorescences)

PRESCRIBING INFORMATION

Actions

Hypnotic, mild sedative, spasmolytic, bitter tonic

Potential Indications

Based on appropriate evaluation of the patient, practitioners should consider prescribing hops in formulations in the context of:
- Sleep disorders,* in combination with valerian *(2)*
- Mood disturbances such as anxiety, restlessness *(4,5)*
- Disorders of the nervous system such as neuralgia, headache *(5)*
- Indigestion, dyspepsia *(5)*
- Sexual activity in men *(5)*
- Bath for sleep disorders *(2)*

Contraindications

Traditionally contraindicated in depression.[1,2]

Warnings and Precautions

None required.

Interactions

None known.

Use in Pregnancy and Lactation

No adverse effects expected, although profound estrogenic effects have been recorded in women harvesting the plant by hand. The polyphenol xanthohumol has estrogenic activity, and although present in freshly harvested hops, it disappears rapidly through oxidation, even on cold storage.[3] Hops also contains estrogenic flavonoid derivatives (see the "Pharmacologic Research" section in this monograph).

Side Effects

None expected if taken within the recommended dose range.

Dosage

Dose per day**	Dose per week**
1.5-3.0 ml of 1:2 liquid extract	10-20 ml of 1:2 liquid extract

SUPPORTING INFORMATION

Traditional Prescribing

Traditional Western herbal medicine uses include:
- Insomnia, excitability, neuralgia, headache, delirium tremens[1,4]
- Hysteria[5]
- Indigestion, dyspepsia, mucous colitis; kidney stones[1,4]
- Topically for leg ulcers, swellings, inflammation of internal organs (such as pleurisy, enteritis)[1,4]

Hops continued on page 278

*Hops has also been used in traditional herbal medicine and is recommended by both the Commission E and ESCOP for treating sleep disorders. (4,5)

**This dose range is extrapolated from the British Herbal Pharmacopoeia 1983, the British Herbal Compendium 1992, and the author's education and experience.

Native Americans used hops as a sedative and diuretic and for insomnia, fevers, and intestinal pains. Topically, hops was applied to toothache and earache. Hops was official in the USP from 1820 to 1926, the NF from 1916 to 1947, and was used as a stomachic, sedative, and tonic.[6]

Pharmacologic Research

- A potent phytoestrogen was determined in hops using sensitive and specific *in vitro* bioassays. 8-Prenylnaringenin had an activity greater than that of other established plant estrogens.[7] In an earlier *in vitro* study, polyphenolic extracts demonstrated activity, but isolated constituents, including the bitter acids, lacked activity.[8]
- Water-soluble substances isolated from hops demonstrated antigonadotropic activity *in vitro* and in experimental models (by injection).[9-11]
- Sedative, anticonvulsant, analgesic, and hypothermic activities have been demonstrated for a hops extract administered by intraperitoneal injection in experimental models.[12,13] No sedative activity was observed after oral administration of hops extract or lupulone in an early study that used a number of experimental models.[14] Oral administration of hops extract (400 mg/kg) decreased motor activity for 4 hours in rats and mice.[15]
- 2-Methyl-3-butene-2-ol, a constituent of hops volatile oil, and stored hops produced a central nervous system–depressant effect when administered in high doses by intraperitoneal injection. The effect was similar to that from the sedative drug methylpentynol at the same dosage.[16,17] This constituent is present in small amounts but may be formed from the metabolism of other hops constituents.[18,19] The constituent might also explain the sedative effect of the hops pillow.
- Hops extract stimulated gastric secretions *in vivo* (route unknown).[20]
- Prenylated flavonoids isolated from hops demonstrated potent and selective inhibition of cytochrome P-450 enzymes and antiproliferative activity in human cancer cell lines *in vitro*.[21,22] Colupulone, a constituent of hops, induced the cytochrome P-450 system but without promutagen activation (measured *ex vivo*).[23,24]
- Hops essential oil demonstrated activity against gram-positive bacteria (e.g., *Bacillus subtilis*, *Staphylococcus aureus*) and the fungus *Trichophyton mentagrophytes* var. *interdigitalis in vitro* but not against *Escherichia coli* or *Candida albicans*.[25]

Clinical Studies

- In an early study, a lipophilic hops concentrate had no sleep-inducing activity on 15 volunteers.[26]
- A quantitative topographic EEG showed slight but clearly visible effects on the central nervous system of healthy volunteers consuming a combination of valerian and hops extracts (1500 mg and 360 mg, respectively) compared with placebo in a single-blind, crossover design.[27]
- The combination of hops and valerian reduced the noise-induced disturbance of sleep stage patterns (slow-wave sleep and rapid eye movement [REM] sleep) in sleep-disturbed volunteers compared with

Hops continued on page 279

baseline values. The daily dose of the herbal product contained the dried herb equivalent of 2 g of hops and 1 g of valerian. The preparation was taken for several days.[28]

- A randomized, double-blind, parallel trial demonstrated equivalent efficacy and tolerability for a hops-valerian preparation compared with a benzodiazepine in patients experiencing temporarily sleep onset and sleep interruption disorders.[29] A surveillance study involving 484 patients found a hops-valerian preparation to be a safe and effective combination that exerted relevant effects on sleep latency, sleep quality, and psychovegetative symptoms. The combination did not have a negative impact on daytime vigilance. The average daily dose taken corresponded to approximately 1.3 g of hops and 5 g of valerian root and was taken on average for 21 days.[30] EEG measurements indicated that a high dose of a hops-valerian combination had an effect on the central nervous system of healthy volunteers. The daily dose was equivalent to approximately 2.2 g of hop strobiles and 7.5 g of valerian root.[31]

- A postmarketing surveillance study in Germany involving 518 patients found an herbal combination of valerian, hops, and lemon balm to be a highly effective treatment for nervous insomnia and restlessness, with very few side effects. The dose administered ranged from one to nine tablets. One tablet contained valerian dried root (450 mg), dried hop strobiles (126.5 mg), and lemon balm dried leaf (225 mg).[32]

- A randomized, double-blind, crossover study involving alcoholic patients with sleep disturbances found consumption of an herbal tablet produced improvement in sleep parameters. The tablet, which was taken for one night and compared with placebo (also one night), contained the following weights of dried herb: valerian root (170 mg), hop strobiles (50 mg), lemon balm leaf (50 mg), and motherwort herb (50 mg).[33]

- The calming effect of a hops bath taken on three successive days was evaluated on 40 patients with sleep disturbances in a randomized, double-blind, placebo-controlled, clinical trial. The hops bath consisted of a solution of concentrated hops extract equivalent to approximately 4 g of hops. The placebo solution had the same appearance and foaming as the hops bath solution. The baseline used was the average sleep quality on two nights before the baths. Results yielded a significant improvement in sleep quality with the hops extract baths as compared with the placebo baths.[34]

- In Germany, the Commission E supports using hops to treat mood disturbances such as restlessness and anxiety and sleep disorders.[35]

- ESCOP recommends hops for treating tenseness, restlessness, and difficulty in falling asleep.[36]

REFERENCES

1 British Herbal Medicine Association's Scientific Committee: *British herbal pharmacopoeia*, Bournemouth, 1983, BHMA.

2 British Herbal Medicine Association: *British herbal compendium*, vol 1, Bournemouth, 1992, BHMA.

3 Verzele M: *J Inst Brew* 92:32-48, 1986.

Hops continued on page 280

4 Felter HW, Lloyd JU: *King's American dispensatory,* ed 18, rev 3, Portland, 1905, reprinted 1983, Eclectic Medical Publications.

5 Osol A et al: *The dispensatory of the United States of America,* ed 24, Philadelphia, 1947, Lippincott.

6 Vogel VJ: *American Indian medicine,* Norman, Okla, 1970, University of Oklahoma Press.

7 Milligan SR et al: *J Clin Endocrinol Metab* 83(6):2249-2252, 1999.

8 de Keukeleire D et al: *Pharm Pharmacol Lett* 7(2-3):83-86, 1997.

9 Kumai A, Okamoto R: *Toxicol Lett* 21(2):203-208, 1984.

10 Okamoto R, Kumai A: *Acta Endocrinol* 127(4):371-377, 1992.

11 Kumai A et al: *Nippon Naibunpi Gakkai Zasshi* 60(10):1202-1213, 1984.

12 Lee KM et al: *Planta Med* 59(suppl):A691, 1993.

13 Bravo L et al: *Boll Chim Farm* 113:310-315, 1974.

14 Hansel R, Wagener HH: *Arzneim Forsch* 17(1):79-81, 1967.

15 Schiller H et al. Presented at the International Congress and 48th Annual Meeting of the Society for Medicinal Plant Research and the 6th International Congress on Ethnopharmacology of the International Society for Ethnopharmacology, Zurich, September 3-7, 2000, abstract P4B/18.

16 Hansel R, Wohlfart R, Coper H: *Z Naturforsch [C]* 35(11-12):1096-1097, 1980.

17 Wohlfart R, Hansel R, Schmidt H: *Planta Med* 48(2):120-123, 1983.

18 Hansel R, Wohlfart R, Schmidt H: *Planta Med* 45:224-228, 1982.

19 Wohlfart R et al: *Arch Pharm* 316:132-137, 1983.

20 Tamasdan S, Cristea E, Mihele D: *Farmacia* 29:71-75, 1981.

21 Henderson MC et al: *Xenobiotica* 30(3):235-251, 2000.

22 Miranda CL et al: *Food Chem Toxicol* 37(4):271-285, 1999.

23 Shipp EB, Mehigh CS, Helferich WG: *Food Chem Toxicol* 32(11):1007-1014, 1994.

24 Mannering GJ, Shoeman JS, Shoeman DW: *Biochem Biophys Res Commun* 200(3):1455-1462, 1994.

25 Langezaal CR, Chandra A, Scheffer JJ: *Pharm Weekbl Sci* 14(6):353-356, 1992.

26 Stocker HR: *Schweizer Brauerei Rundschau* 78:80-89, 1967.

27 Vonderheid-Guth B et al: *Eur J Med Res* 5(4):139-144, 2000.

28 Muller-Limmroth W, Ehrenstein W: *Med Klin* 72:1119-1125, 1977.

29 Schmitz M, Jackel M: *Wien Med Wochenschr* 148(13):291-298, 1998.

30 Petrowicz O, Deitelhoff P, Lange P: *Phytomed* 7(supp 2):106-114, 2000.

31 Vonderheid-Guth B et al: *Eur J Med Res* 5:139, 2000.

32 Friede M et al: 2nd International Congress on Phytomedicine, Munich, September 11-14, 1996, abstract P-75.

33 Widy-Tyszkiewicz E, Schminda R: *Herba Polonica* 43(2):154-159, 1997.

34 von Rosen M et al: *Z Phytother Abstractband*, p26, 1995.

35 Blumenthal M et al, eds: *The complete German Commission E monographs: therapeutic guide to herbal medicines,* Austin, 1998, American Botanical Council.

36 Scientific Committee of the European Scientific Cooperative on Phytotherapy [ESCOP]: *ESCOP monographs: Lupuli flos.* European Scientific Cooperative on Phytotherapy, ESCOP Secretariat, Argyle House, Gandy Street, Exeter, Devon, EX4 3LS, United Kingdom, July 1997.

HORSECHESTNUT

Botanical Name: _Aesculus hippocastanum_
Family: Hippocastanaceae
Plant Part Used: Seed

PRESCRIBING INFORMATION

Actions	Venotonic, antiedematous, antiinflammatory, antiecchymotic (against bruises)
Potential Indications	Based on appropriate evaluation of the patient, practitioners should consider prescribing horsechestnut in formulations in the context of:

- Varicose veins _(2,4,5)_
- Chronic venous insufficiency, edema of the lower limbs _(1,4,5)_
- Restless leg syndrome _(4)_
- Hemorrhoids, rectal complaints, neuralgia, rheumatism _(5)_
- Improving capillary resistance in healthy individuals _(4a)_
- Reducing the risk of deep vein thrombosis following surgery _(3, by injection)_
- Disorders where local tissue edema may be involved _(4a,7)_
- Topical treatment for hematoma, contusions, nonpenetrating wounds and sports injuries resulting in edema _(4a, often in combination with other treatments)_

Contraindications	Because of the irritant effect of the saponins, horsechestnut should not be applied to broken or ulcerated skin.
Warnings and Precautions	None required.
Interactions	None known.
Use in Pregnancy and Lactation	No adverse effects expected.
Side Effects	As with all saponin-containing herbs, oral use may cause irritation of the gastric mucous membranes and reflux. This irritation can be avoided by using enteric-coated preparations. From 1968 until 1989, nearly 900 million individual doses of one brand of standardized horsechestnut extract were prescribed. In that time, only 15 patients reported side effects. The Commission E advises that pruritis, nausea, and gastric complaints may occur in isolated cases.

Dosage

Dose per day*	Dose per week*
2-5 ml of 1:2 liquid extract	15-35 ml of 1:2 liquid extract

Horsechestnut _continued on page 282_

*This dose range is extrapolated from ESCOP.[1]

Traditional Prescribing

Traditional Western herbal medicine uses include:
- Conditions involving venous congestion, particularly with dull, aching pain and fullness[2]
- Rectal irritation, rectal neuralgia, proctitis, hemorrhoids[2]
- Reflex conditions attributed to rectal irritation: dyspnea, spasmodic asthma, dizziness, headache, backache, and dyspepsia[2]
- Rheumatism, neuralgia[2]

Pharmacologic Research

The major constituents of horsechestnut seeds are saponins (3% to 6%), collectively referred to as escin. Escin is a complex mixture of over 30 individual pentacyclic triterpene diester glycosides.
- Horsechestnut extract and escin have been shown to have anti-exudative and antiinflammatory activity *in vitro* and *in vivo* by oral, parenteral, and topical routes. Both substances act to reduce capillary permeability and the localized edema associated with inflammation.
- Horsechestnut extract caused contraction of venous valves, increased venous pressure and flow, and increased lymphatic flow in isolated tissue samples.
- Oral administration of horsechestnut extract improved the tone of connective tissue and improved circulation by toning the veins in experimental models.
- Standardized horsechestnut extract reduced cutaneous capillary hyperpermeability, increased skin capillary resistance, decreased the formation of edema of lymphatic or inflammatory origin, and decreased connective tissue formation in subchronic inflammatory granuloma after oral and subcutaneous administration.
- Saponin constituents from horsechestnut showed inhibitory effects on the connective tissue enzyme hyaluronidase *in vitro*.

Clinical Studies

- A review of randomized, double-blind, placebo-controlled trials published up to December 1996 concluded that horsechestnut extract is superior to placebo and is as efficacious as other medications in alleviating the objective signs and subjective symptoms in patients with chronic venous insufficiency. Horsechestnut treatment was associated with reduced edema, pain, itchiness, and feeling of fatigue. A dosage of 600 mg/day of horsechestnut extract (containing 100 mg escin) was used for 4 to 12 weeks in the majority of these trials. Results from one comparative trial indicated that edema reduction from horsechestnut treatment was equivalent to that achieved by compression therapy with elastic stockings.[3] An updated review of the literature up to November 2000 found that all of the 14 randomized, controlled trials scored at least 3 out of 5 points for methodological quality. In addition to these results, horsechestnut treatment was as beneficial as treatment with O-β-hydroxyethylrutosides. Adverse effects reported from horsechestnut treatment were mild and infrequent.[4]

Horsechestnut *continued on page 283*

- A case observation study (published in 1996) that involved more than 800 German general practitioners and more than 5000 patients with chronic venous insufficiency found that horsechestnut extract improved subjective symptoms markedly. Horsechestnut was considered an economical, practice-relevant, therapeutic tool that had better compliance than compression therapy.
- Horsechestnut significantly lowered blood viscosity in patients with varicose veins of the lower extremities in an uncontrolled trial. The daily dose of 1800 mg of extract contained 300 mg of escin and was administered for 12 days. Horsechestnut extract (600 mg/day standardized to 100 mg escin) increased vascular flow in healthy volunteers in a double-blind, placebo-controlled trial. Significant reduction in leg volume was recorded after horsechestnut treatment was taken for 4 weeks in a randomized, double-blind, placebo-controlled, crossover trial involving women with pregnancy-induced varicose veins.
- Oral treatment of healthy volunteers with standardized horsechestnut extract (containing 300 mg/day of escin) for 14 days was shown to significantly improve capillary resistance in a randomized, double-blind, placebo-controlled, crossover study.
- In a controlled trial, intravenous injection of a combination of horsechestnut extract with vitamin B complex, vitamin C, and either strophanthin or Digitalis significantly reduced the incidence of deep venous thrombosis following surgery, compared with the same injection without horsechestnut.
- Injected escin has been efficacious in treating cerebral edemas following cranial fractures and traumas, cerebral tumors, intracranial aneurysms, cerebral sclerosis, subdural hematomas, encephalitis, meningitis, and cerebral abscesses.
- Topical preparations containing escin have been successfully used:
  - For treating edema and hematoma in surgical practice
  - For preventing and treating sports injuries (gel containing escin and salicylate)
  - For inflammation of veins, venous insufficiency, varicose veins (escin combined with buphenine, heparin, benzydamine, and lecithin)
  - For hypertrophic scars, keloid scars, stretch marks, lymphodema after mastectomy (escin combined with thyroxine), and anorectal varicose pathologic conditions
- Topical treatment of trauma cases with limb bruising using a gel containing escin and salicylate for 9 days significantly increased the mobility of the injured limb and reduced lower leg swelling, subjective complaints, and relapse frequencies in a randomized, double-blind, placebo-controlled trial. In a study of similar design, escin gel significantly reduced tenderness to pressure in experimentally induced hematoma in volunteers.
- In Germany, the Commission E supports using horsechestnut to treat chronic venous insufficiency. This syndrome may involve pain and a sensation of heaviness in the legs, nocturnal cramping in the calves, pruritis, and swelling of the legs.[5]

Horsechestnut *continued on page 284*

- ESCOP recommends horsechestnut for treating chronic venous insufficiency and varicosis.[1]

REFERENCES

Except when specifically referenced, the following book was referred to in the compilation of the pharmacological and clinical information: Mills S, Bone K: *Principles and Practice of Phytotherapy: Modern Herbal Medicine,* Edinburgh, 2000, Churchill Livingstone.

1 Scientific Committee of the European Scientific Cooperative on Phytotherapy [ESCOP]: *ESCOP monographs: Hippocastani semen.* European Scientific Cooperative on Phytotherapy, ESCOP Secretariat, Argyle House, Gandy Street, Exeter, Devon, EX4 3LS, United Kingdom, October 1999.
2 Felter HW: *The eclectic materia medica, pharmacology and therapeutics,* Portland, 1922, reprinted 1983, Eclectic Medical Publications.
3 Pittler MH, Ernst E: *Arch Dermatol* 134(11):1356-1360, 1998.
4 Pittler MH, Ernst E: *Altern Ther Health Med* 7(3):108, 2001.
5 Blumenthal M et al, editors: *The complete German Commission E monographs: therapeutic guide to herbal medicines,* Austin, 1998, American Botanical Council.

HORSETAIL

Botanical Name: Equisetum arvense
Family: Equisetaceae
Plant Part Used: Aerial parts

PRESCRIBING INFORMATION

Actions   Diuretic, astringent, styptic (hemostatic)

Potential Indications   Based on appropriate evaluation of the patient, practitioners should consider prescribing horsetail in formulations in the context of:
- Posttraumatic and static edema, bacterial and inflammatory diseases of the lower urinary tract, renal gravel (4,5)
- Nocturnal enuresis, renal colic, hematuria, enlarged prostate, prostatitis (5)
- Hemorrhage, hematemesis (6)
- Topical treatment for poorly healing wounds (4)

Contraindications   The Commission E recommends copious fluid intake to assist in reducing microorganisms in the urinary tract, but this should not be undertaken if edema resulting from impaired cardiac or renal function exists.[1]

Warnings and Precautions   None required.

Interactions   None known.

Use in Pregnancy and Lactation   No adverse effects expected.

Side Effects   None expected if taken within the recommended dose range.

Dosage

Dose per day*	Dose per week*
2-6 ml of 1:2 liquid extract	15-40 ml of 1:2 liquid extract

SUPPORTING INFORMATION

Traditional Prescribing   Traditional Western herbal medicine uses include:
- Cystitis, urethritis, frequent urination, nocturnal enuresis, urinary calculi, renal colic, hematuria, enlarged prostate, prostatitis[2,3]
- Edema, gonorrhea, gleet (gonorrheal urethritis)[3]
- Ulceration of the urinary tract, hematemesis, hemorrhage[4]

Pharmacologic Research   The main phenolic compounds in the aerial parts of horsetail are hydroxycinnamic acid derivatives such as caffeic acid esters and flavonoids such as quercetin and kaempferol glycosides.[5] The herb is also rich in silica.

Horsetail continued on page 286

*This dose range is extrapolated from the British Herbal Compendium 1992 and the author's education and experience.

- Chloroform extracts of several species of horsetail demonstrated diuretic activity *in vivo*.[6]
- Horsetail contains from 1.2% to 6.9% silica. The solubility of the silicon in horsetail was investigated in a Polish study.[7] Fresh and dried samples of horsetail were extracted with water under various conditions. The extraction of soluble silicon was slow and only occurred significantly with the application of heat. The rate of extraction was much faster from the fresh herb but was still significant for the dried herb. In both cases, several hours of decoction were required to extract a significant percentage of silicon from the plant.

Clinical Studies

- To examine the metabolism and renal excretion of compounds in horsetail, a standardized extract was administered to 11 volunteers following a flavonoid-free diet for 8 days. Quercetin metabolites 3,4-dihydroxyphenylacetic acid or 3,4-dihydroxytoluene was undetectable, and homovanillic acid excretion did not increase. Hippuric acid, the glycine conjugate of benzoic acid, increased twofold after intake. Therefore degradation to benzoic acid derivatives rather than phenylacetic acid derivatives appears to be a predominant route of metabolism.[8]
- In Germany, the Commission E supports using horsetail to treat post-traumatic and static edema, with copious fluid intake for bacterial and inflammatory diseases of the lower urinary tract and renal gravel. Externally, horsetail can be recommended as supportive treatment for poor healing wounds.[1]

REFERENCES

1 Blumenthal M et al, editors: *The complete German Commission E monographs: therapeutic guide to herbal medicines*, Austin, 1998, American Botanical Council.
2 British Herbal Medicine Association's Scientific Committee: *British herbal pharmacopoeia*, Bournemouth, 1983, BHMA.
3 Felter HW, Lloyd JU: *King's American dispensatory*, ed 18, rev 3, Portland, 1905, reprinted 1983, Eclectic Medical Publications.
4 Grieve M: *A modern herbal*, New York, 1971, Dover Publications.
5 Veit M et al: *Phytochem* 38(4):881-891, 1995.
6 Perez Gutierrez RM, Laguna GY, Walkowski A: *J Ethnopharmacol* 14(2-3):269-272, 1985.
7 Piekos R, Paslawska S: *Planta Med* 27(2):145-150, 1975.
8 Graefe EU, Veit M: *Phytomed* 6(4):239-246, 1999.

HYDRANGEA

Other Common Name:	Seven barks
Botanical Name:	*Hydrangea arborescens*
Family:	Hydrangeaceae
Plant Part Used:	Root

PRESCRIBING INFORMATION

Actions

Diuretic, antilithic

Potential Indications

Based on appropriate evaluation of the patient, practitioners should consider prescribing Hydrangea in formulations in the context of:
- Disorders of the prostate, including prostatitis and enlarged prostate (5)
- Urinary, bladder or kidney stones; inflammatory conditions of the urinary system (5)

Contraindications

None known.

Warnings and Precautions

None required.

Interactions

None known.

Use in Pregnancy and Lactation

No adverse effects expected.

Side Effects

None expected if taken within the recommended dose range.

Dosage

Dose per day*	*Dose per week**
2-7 ml of 1:2 liquid extract	15-50 ml of 1:2 liquid extract

SUPPORTING INFORMATION

Traditional Prescribing

Traditional Western herbal medicine uses include:
- Cystitis, urethritis, urinary calculi, difficult urination, bladder gravel, prostatitis, enlarged prostate gland, chronic gleet (gonorrheal urethritis)[1,2]
- Improving the nutrition of the urinary mucous membranes[2]

Native Americans used Hydrangea for calculous complaints and as a decoction with other plants for women "who had strange dreams during their menstrual period." Hydrangea was official in the NF from 1916 to 1926 and was used for diuretic and diaphoretic purposes.[3]

Pharmacologic Research

No pharmacologic information has been found for Hydrangea.

Hydrangea *continued on page 288*

*This dose range is extrapolated from the British Herbal Pharmacopoeia 1983 and the author's education and experience.

Clinical Studies   No clinical studies using Hydrangea have been found.

REFERENCES

1 British Herbal Medicine Association's Scientific Committee: *British herbal pharmacopoeia,* Bournemouth, 1983, BHMA.

2 Felter HW, Lloyd JU: *King's American dispensatory,* ed 18, rev 3, Portland, 1905, reprinted 1983, Eclectic Medical Publications.

3 Vogel VJ: *American Indian medicine,* Norman, Okla, 1970, University of Oklahoma Press.

JAMAICA DOGWOOD

Other Common Name:	Jamaican dogwood
Botanical Names:	*Piscidia erythrina, Piscidia piscipula*[#^]
Family:	Leguminosae
Plant Part Used:	Root bark

PRESCRIBING INFORMATION

Actions

Analgesic, spasmolytic, mild sedative

Potential Indications

Based on appropriate evaluation of the patient, practitioners should consider prescribing Jamaica dogwood in formulations in the context of:
- Insomnia, anxiety *(5,7)*
- Painful conditions, neuralgia, sciatica, headache, toothache *(5)*
- Dysmenorrhea, muscular spasm, rheumatism *(5)*

Contraindications

Pregnancy, bradycardia, cardiac insufficiency[2]

Warnings and Precautions

The recommended dose must not be exceeded. Although Jamaica dogwood has been used as a fish and insect poison (the component rotenone impairs oxygen consumption in these species), the herb has been found to have negligible toxicity in rodents.[3,4]

Interactions

None known.

Use in Pregnancy and Lactation

Contraindicated in pregnancy.

Side Effects

Traditional texts suggest that Jamaica dogwood may cause nausea, vomiting, and headache in some patients prescribed even small, therapeutic doses and that overdose produces toxic effects.[5,6]

Dosage

Dose per day[*]	**Dose per week**[*]
3-6 ml of 1:2 liquid extract	20-40 ml of 1:2 liquid extract

SUPPORTING INFORMATION

Traditional Prescribing

Traditional Western herbal medicine uses include:
- Pain relief, spasm, nervous excitability and to induce sleep[6]
- Neuralgia, particularly sciatica; painful conditions of the mouth, migraine, dysmenorrhea, muscular spasm, rheumatism, asthma[6,7]
- Insomnia, nervous tension[6,7]

Pharmacologic Research

Jamaica dogwood root bark contains nearly 60 isoflavonoid constituents and rotenoids.[2,8]

Jamaica Dogwood *continued on page 290*

[#]Alternative name.

[^]Adopted by the American Herbal Products Association as the new botanical name.[1]

[*]This dose range is extrapolated from the British Pharmaceutical Codex 1934, the British Herbal Pharmacopoeia 1983, the British Herbal Compendium 1992, and the author's education and experience.

- Oral administration of Jamaica dogwood extract demonstrated central nervous system activity in an experimental model. Activity was intermediate between the anxiolytic activity of passion flower and the sedative activity of valerian and hawthorn.[9]
- The isoflavones may be responsible for the antispasmodic activity, as demonstrated with isolated tissue.[10] In addition to sedative and antispasmodic activity, the following activities have been demonstrated in experimental models: antipyretic, antiinflammatory, hypotensive, and antitussive.[3]
- In an early study, Jamaica dogwood extract given by injection did not influence uterine tone or contractions *in vivo*,[11] although a later study found it to exert appreciable spasmolytic activity.[4]

Clinical Studies

No clinical studies using Jamaica dogwood have been found; however, anecdotal clinical reports of the late nineteenth century and early twentieth century indicate its usefulness in treating tuberculosis, neuralgia, and whooping cough.[4]

REFERENCES

1 McGuffin M, editor: *Herbs of commerce*, ed 2 [draft 3.3], Bethesda, Md, 1998, American Herbal Products Association.

2 British Herbal Medicine Association: *British herbal compendium*, Bournemouth, 1992, BHMA.

3 Aurousseau M, Berny C, Albert O: *Ann Pharm Franc* 23:251-257, 1965.

4 Costello CH, Butler CL: *J Am Pharm Assoc* 37(3):89-97, 1948.

5 Grieve M: *A modern herbal*, New York, 1971, Dover Publications.

6 Felter HW, Lloyd JU: *King's American dispensatory*, ed 18, rev 3, Portland, 1905, reprinted 1983, Eclectic Medical Publications.

7 British Herbal Medicine Association's Scientific Committee: *British herbal pharmacopoeia*, Bournemouth, 1983, BHMA.

8 Tahara S et al: *Phytochem* 34(1):303-315, 1993.

9 Della Loggia R, Tubaro A, Redaelli C: *Riv Neurol* 51(5):297-310, 1981.

10 Della Loggia R et al: *Prog Clin Biol Res* 280:365-368, 1988.

11 Pilcher JD, Mauer RT: *Surg Gynecol Obstet* 27:97-99, 1918.

KAVA

Other Common Name:	Kava kava
Botanical Name:	*Piper methysticum*
Family:	Piperaceae
Plant Part Used:	Root (rootstock)

PRESCRIBING INFORMATION

Actions

Anxiolytic, hypnotic, anticonvulsant, mild sedative, skeletal muscle relaxant, spasmolytic, local anesthetic, mild analgesic, antipruritic (topically)

Potential Indications

Based on appropriate evaluation of the patient, practitioners should consider prescribing kava in formulations in the context of:

- Anxiety *(1,4,5)*
- Stress *(3)*
- Insomnia,* in combination with valerian *(3)*
- Menopausal symptoms, mild depression *(2)*
- Muscle tension *(4,5)*
- Improving cognitive performance in healthy individuals and patients with anxiety *(2)*
- Headache, neuralgia, general debility, inflammation and infection of the genitourinary tract *(5)*

Given that kava has been shown to have similar efficacy to certain benzodiazepine drugs in treating anxiety *(3)*, it may be useful to assist in withdrawal from benzodiazepines.

Contraindications

The German Commission E lists the following contraindications: pregnancy, lactation, and endogenous depression. However, these contraindications have resulted from a lack of positive data to show that use is safe under these circumstances rather than any published safety concerns.

Kava extract is contraindicated in patients with preexisting liver conditions. Patients prescribed kava should be closely monitored for any signs of a rare liver toxicity.

Warnings and Precautions

Because of possible dopamine antagonism, kava should be used cautiously in elderly patients, especially those with Parkinson's disease (refer to the "Side Effects" section in this monograph).

Interactions

According to the Commission E, a synergistic effect is possible for substances acting on the central nervous system, such as alcohol, barbiturates, and psychopharmacological agents. A case of possible interaction between kava and a benzodiazepine drug (alprazolam) has been reported.

Kava continued on page 292

---

*Kava has also been used in traditional herbal medicine for treating insomnia. (6)

Use in Pregnancy and Lactation

No adverse effects expected at normal therapeutic doses, despite the caution from the Commission E.

Side Effects

Two postmarketing surveillance studies involving 3029 and 4049 patients found adverse events occurred in 2.3% and 1.5%, respectively, of patients during treatment with standardized kava extract. The doses of kava contained 120 to 240 mg and 105 mg of lactones, respectively. A meta-analysis noted that standardized kava extract is relatively safe with two studies, representing 31% of the studied patients, not reporting any adverse events in those treated with kava.[1]

A dry, scaly, pigmented skin condition known as kava dermopathy is a well-known side effect of excessive and chronic use of kava but is unlikely to occur after normal therapeutic use. The rash quickly regresses if kava intake is ceased. Dermatitis after oral administration of kava at the lower therapeutic doses has been reported.

A group of German neurologists described four cases of patients who developed clinical signs suggestive of dopamine antagonism after taking kava. Overdose of kava (without concurrent alcohol use or petrol sniffing) causing generalized choreoathetosis (involuntary movement disorder) has been reported in an Aboriginal Australian.[2]

Associations with heavy kava use reported in the Australian medical literature from 1988 to 1999 include ischemic cardiac events and sudden cardiac death.[2,3] These events have not been definitively linked to excessive kava use and the possibility of concurrent alcohol abuse, and the involvement of other socioeconomic factors cannot be ruled out. A pilot survey investigating the effects of heavy kava use published in 1988 indicated that no epidemiological evidence was found to link sudden deaths with kava use.[4]

A report published in 2000 by a Swiss government regulatory agency described nine cases of hepatotoxicity attributed to kava. All cases involved the consumption of a high dose acetone extract standardized to 70% kava lactones. The product has been subsequently banned. The author rated the risk of hepatotoxicity as rare but serious.[5] German regulatory authorities reported cases of hepatotoxicity involving ethanolic kava extracts,[6] and kava products were subsequently removed from the market in this and several other countries. Good evidence exists that the hepatotoxicity was immune-mediated. A deficiency of the drug-metabolizing enzyme CYP2D6 (which occurs in 9% of the population) might be a predisposing factor.[7] The rare cases of hepatotoxicity resulting from kava consumption are therefore likely to be an immunoallergic reaction, perhaps exaggerated by the type of extract consumed and deficiencies in detoxifying enzymes.

Kava continued on page 293

Dosage

<table>
<tr><td>*Dose per day***
3.0-8.5 ml of 1:2 liquid extract</td><td>*Dose per week***
20-60 ml of 1:2 liquid extract</td></tr>
</table>

Extracts providing quantified levels of kava lactones are recommended. Ideally, aqueous ethanol extracts should contain not less than 20 mg/ml of kava lactones.

SUPPORTING INFORMATION

Traditional Prescribing

Traditional Western herbal medicine uses include:
- Neuralgia (especially toothache, earache, and ocular pain), dizziness, chronic catarrh, bronchitis[8]
- Cystitis, urethritis, dysuria, renal colic, nocturnal incontinence[8,9]
- Dysmenorrhea, vaginitis, leukorrhea, gonorrhea[8,9]
- Anorexia, dyspepsia, intestinal catarrh, hemorrhoids[8]
- Rheumatism, gout, topically for joint pain[8,9]

Uses according to other traditional systems such as those of the Pacific region include:
- To soothe nerves and to induce relaxation and sleep[10]
- To counteract fatigue; for general debility, weary muscles, chills, the common cold, dysuria, headache[10]
- Skin diseases, leprosy, to prevent suppuration[11]
- Filariasis (systemic worm infestation)[11,12]
- Sore throat, toothache[13]
- As a contraceptive for women who have recently given birth;[11,12] topically for vaginal prolapse[11]

Pharmacologic Research

Key constituents of kava root include the kava lactones (also known as kava pyrones) and flavonoids (flavokawains). Extracts are often standardized to the lactones.
- Kava extracts or purified lactones demonstrated sedative effects and induced sleep in a variety of *in vivo* experimental models. The combination of kava and passion flower *(Passiflora incarnata)* produced a synergistic effect on sedation.
- Kava extract and lactones produced relaxation of skeletal muscle *in vitro* and *in vivo*. A synergistic effect was noted when a mixture of lactones (similar to that found in the root) was administered orally in an epilepsy model.
- Kava lactones have demonstrated analgesic activity via nonopiate pathways in several experimental models and have potencies similar to cocaine and procaine as local anesthetics.
- Kava lactones exhibited potent fungistatic activity *in vitro* against a wide variety of pathogenic fungi, excluding species of Candida.

Kava continued on page 294

**This dose range is extrapolated from British *Pharmaceutical Codex* 1934, the British *Herbal Pharmacopoeia* 1983, and the author's education and experience.

- Kava extract protected brain tissue against ischemic damage in experimental models.
- Kava lactones demonstrated antithrombotic activity *in vitro*.

Clinical Studies

- A meta-analysis assessing seven randomized, double-blind, placebo-controlled trials found that kava extract significantly reduced anxiety (compared with placebo). The dosage of standardized kava extract prescribed varied and contained 60 to 240 mg per day of kava lactones. The duration of treatment ranged from 1 to 24 weeks. One trial investigated the reduction in anxiety for preoperative patients who received kava extract the night before and 1 hour before surgery.[1] The authors of one of the trials[14] included in this meta-analysis concluded that the efficacy and tolerability of standardized kava extract recommend it as an alternative to tricyclic antidepressants and benzodiazepines for treating anxiety.
- Kava lactones and standardized kava extracts demonstrated activity equivalent to oxazepam and bromazepam (benzodiazepine drugs) in patients with anxiety in double-blind, placebo-controlled trials. The daily dose ranged from 210 to 400 mg of kava lactones. Side effects were higher in the patient groups assigned the conventional drugs.
- Kava has also been shown to have therapeutic benefit in cases of situational anxiety. In a randomized, double-blind, placebo-controlled trial, standardized kava extract taken for 1 week significantly reduced anxiety compared with placebo in patients awaiting the results of medical diagnostic tests for suspected breast carcinoma. Fatigue, introverted behavior, excitability, and depression were decreased, and alertness was increased in patients receiving kava extract. The administered daily dose of kava contained 150 mg of kava lactones and corresponded to approximately 2.5 g of dried root.[15]
- Preliminary findings suggest a beneficial effect of kava on baroreflex control of heart rate (BRC). Significantly more patients with generalized anxiety disorder exhibited improved BRC following treatment with kava compared with a placebo. No effect was observed on respiratory sinus arrhythmia, a measure of the heart rate changes occurring with respiration. Patients in the study were a subgroup of a larger randomized, double-blind trial and received standardized kava extract or placebo for 4 weeks.[16]
- Two postmarketing surveillance studies involving over 3000 patients each found standardized kava extract improved nervousness, restlessness, anger, sleep disturbances, menopausal complaints, muscle tension, and sexual disturbances. Undesirable side effects included allergic reactions, gastrointestinal complaints, headache, and dizziness. The daily dose of extract ranged from that containing 105 mg to 240 mg of kava lactones for 4 and 7 weeks, respectively.
- In a placebo-controlled trial, standardized kava extract (containing 105 to 210 mg kava lactones for 1 day) improved several aspects of the sleep cycle. The measurements were favorable when compared with orthodox sedatives such as benzodiazepines and barbiturates.

Kava continued on page 295

- In a pilot study, patients with stress-induced insomnia were treated in each phase for 6 weeks with kava, then valerian, then a combination of kava and valerian, with washout periods between each treatment phase of 2 weeks. Total stress severity was significantly relieved by the kava and valerian single treatments (stress was measured in three areas: social, personal, and life events). Insomnia was significantly relieved by the combination of kava and valerian.[17]
- A randomized, placebo-controlled, double-blind trial of patients with neurovegetative symptoms associated with menopause found standardized kava extract for 8 weeks (containing 210 mg/day of kava lactones) produced a significant reduction in anxiety (symptoms and severity of symptoms), depression, and menopausal symptoms. (This trial was included in the previously mentioned meta-analysis.)
- Kava plus HRT significantly reduced menopausal anxiety compared with HRT alone in a controlled trial.[18]
- In a single-blind, placebo-controlled study with healthy volunteers, kava improved cognitive performance and stabilized emotional disposition without causing sedation. The study was conducted over 5 weeks and included washout, placebo, kava, and rebound placebo phases. Volunteers were administered a daily dose of standardized extract containing 210 mg of kava lactones, increasing to 420 mg over a 2-week period.
- Despite its relaxing properties, a single dose of standardized kava extract (containing 120 mg of kava lactones) was shown to increase performance in mental alertness tests compared with diazepam (10 mg) and placebo in a randomized, double-blind, crossover, clinical study involving healthy volunteers. In other studies of similar design, conflicting results have been obtained. Standardized kava extract (containing 420 mg/day of kava lactones) for 5 days did not significantly change the quality and speed of responses to psychometric tests, whereas oxazepam (3 days of placebo, 15 mg on the day before testing and 75 mg on the morning of testing) significantly decreased responses. However, standardized kava extract had a positive effect on the allocation of attention and processing capacity, compared with a reduced response produced by oxazepam in healthy volunteers.
- A double-blind study involving healthy volunteers concluded that patients are not exposed to additional side effects or risks (in terms of mental performance and general well being) while taking kava extract (containing 240 mg/day of kava lactones) plus a benzodiazepine, as compared with taking the benzodiazepine alone (9 mg/day bromazepam).
- In a placebo-controlled, double-blind study, no negative effects on safety-relevant performance were caused by combining standardized kava extract with ethanol. In fact, kava tended to counter the adverse effect of alcohol on mental concentration. No significant changes were found in performance capability (in terms of operating machines and driving) in the healthy volunteers studied. The daily dose of kava administered contained 210 mg of kava lactones and the trial

Kava continued on page 296

was 8 days in length. In a more recent randomized, placebo-controlled trial, acute administration of a very high dose of kava combined with alcohol potentiated both the perceived and measured impairment of motor and cognitive function produced by alcohol alone. Kava was administered as the traditional aqueous extract (1 g/kg body weight); the dose of lactones was not defined.[19]

- Clinical trial results indicated that kava extracts and lactones are not suitable alone for treating epilepsy.
- An epidemiological study analyzing data obtained in the 1980s from the South Pacific region suggests a close inverse relationship between cancer incidence and kava consumption (the more kava is consumed by the population, the lower the cancer incidence will be). The results imply that kava may be an effective cancer chemoprotective agent, but no other conclusions can be made until further research is completed. Kava consumption is unlikely to be solely responsible for the low cancer rate in these islands.[20]
- In Germany, the Commission E supports using kava to treat conditions of nervous anxiety, stress, and restlessness.[21]

REFERENCES

Except when specifically referenced, the following book was referred to in the compilation of the pharmacologic and clinical information: Mills S, Bone K: *Principles and Practice of Phytotherapy: Modern Herbal Medicine,* Edinburgh, 2000, Churchill Livingstone.

1 Pittler MH, Ernst E: *J Clin Psychopharmacol* 20:84-89, 2000.
2 Spillane PK, Fisher DA, Currie BJ: *Med J Aust* 167(3):172-173, 1997.
3 Young MC et al: *Med J Aust* 170(9):425-428, 1999.
4 Mathews JD et al: *Med J Aust* 148(11):548-555, 1988.
5 Stoller R: *Schweiz Arztezeit* 81(24):1335-1336, 2000.
6 Stafford N: *Germany may ban kava kava herbal supplement,* Yahoo News, Nov 19, 2001. URL: http://dailynews.yahoo.com.
7 Russmann S, Lauterburg BH, Helbling A: *Ann Intern Med* 135(1):68-69, 2001.
8 Felter HW, Lloyd JU: *King's American dispensatory,* ed 18, rev 3, Portland, 1905, reprinted 1983, Eclectic Medical Publications.
9 British Herbal Medicine Association's Scientific Committee: *British herbal pharmacopoeia,* Bournemouth, 1983, BHMA.
10 Titcomb M: *J Polynes Soc* 57:105-171, 1948.
11 Lebot V, Merlin M, Lindstrom L: *Kava—the Pacific elixir: the definitive guide to its ethnobotany, history and chemistry,* New Haven, 1992, Yale University Press.
12 Cambie RC, Ash J: *Fijian medicinal plants,* Melbourne, Australia, 1994, CSIRO Publishing.
13 World Health Organization: *Medicinal plants in the South Pacific,* Manilla, 1998, WHO Regional Office for the Western Pacific.
14 Volz HP, Kieser M: *Pharmacopsychiatry* 30:1-5, 1997.
15 Neuhaus W et al: *Zentralbl Gynakol* 122(11):561-565, 2000.
16 Watkins LL, Connor KM, Davidson JRT: *J Psychopharmacol* 15(4):283-286, 2001.
17 Wheatley D: *Human Psychopharmacol* 16(4):353-356, 2001.
18 De Leo V et al: *Maturitas* 39(2):185-188, 2001.
19 Foo H, Lemon J: *Drug Alcohol Rev* 16:147-155, 1997.
20 Steiner GG: *Hawaii Med J* 59(11):420-422, 2000.
21 Blumenthal M et al, eds: *The complete German Commission E monographs: therapeutic guide to herbal medicines,* Austin, 1998, American Botanical Council.

KOREAN GINSENG

Botanical Name: *Panax ginseng*
Family: Araliaceae
Plant Part Used: Root

PRESCRIBING INFORMATION

Actions

Adaptogenic, tonic, immune modulating, cardiotonic, male tonic, cancer preventative, cognition enhancing

Potential Indications

Based on appropriate evaluation of the patient, practitioners should consider prescribing Korean ginseng in formulations in the context of:
- Improving physical and mental performance and well being; improving general performance under stress (2,4,5)
- Improving immune function (2,5)
- Non-insulin–dependent diabetes (2)
- Congestive heart failure (3,5)
- Raising HDL cholesterol, cerebrovascular deficit (3)
- Impotence, male fertility problems (2,5)
- Preventing cancer (excluding cancers of the breast, cervix, bladder, and thyroid); adjuvant therapy while undergoing radiation therapy (3)
- Antioxidant activity (2)
- Improving memory in healthy, middle-aged individuals, in combination with Ginkgo (3)
- Improving recovery from bacterial infection in chronic bronchitis (2)
- Psychological symptoms of menopause (2)
- Fatigue, debility, convalescence (4,5)
- A tonic for older adults (3,4,5)
- Prostration, neuralgia, convulsions, neurosis, anxiety, palpitations, cold limbs, spontaneous sweating, organ prolapse, dyspnea, asthma (5)

Contraindications

Korean ginseng is contraindicated in acute asthma, signs of heat, excessive menstruation, or nose bleeds. Korean ginseng is best not used during acute infections.

Given that the clinical implications of the effect of Korean ginseng on blood pressure are not clear, Korean ginseng should be avoided in hypertension.

Warnings and Precautions

Concurrent use with stimulants such as caffeine and amphetamines should be avoided. Overstimulation may occur in susceptible patients, especially at higher doses.

Interactions

Korean ginseng may interact with the monoamine oxidase inhibitor phenelzine and with warfarin. An experimental study using rats as the model found no significant interaction between warfarin and Korean ginseng,[1] thus any such interaction is likely to be rare.

Use in Pregnancy and Lactation

No adverse effects expected.

Korean Ginseng *continued on page 298*

Side Effects

Excessive doses of Korean ginseng can cause overstimulation, and symptoms of ginseng abuse syndrome (GAS) have been reported in independent studies. GAS is defined as hypertension together with nervousness, euphoria, insomnia, skin eruptions, and morning diarrhea and is thought to be related to Korean ginseng's interaction with glucocorticoid production in the body.

Korean ginseng may cause side effects related to an estrogenlike activity in women, and cases of mastalgia and postmenopausal bleeding have been reported.

Ginseng is widely used, and several other rare adverse reactions have been reported that are, at best, possibly related to ginseng or may otherwise reflect contamination, adulteration, or coincidence. These conditions include Stevens-Johnson syndrome, diuretic resistance, cerebral arteritis, mania, and mydriasis.

Dosage

Dose per day*	Dose per week*
1-6 ml of 1:2 liquid extract	7-40 ml of 1:2 liquid extract

Extracts providing standardized levels of ginsenosides are recommended. Ideally, aqueous ethanol extracts should contain 11 mg/ml of ginsenosides, with the ratio of ginsenoside Rg_1 to ginsenoside Rb_1 greater than or equal to 0.5 (indicating that the product was made from main roots, lateral roots, or both).

The Commission E advises that Korean ginseng can be used for up to 3 months with a repeat course if necessary. Continuous use in the unwell and in older adults is appropriate. Doses in excess of 2 ml per day of a 1:2 liquid extract may cause overstimulation.

SUPPORTING INFORMATION

Traditional Prescribing

Uses and properties from TCM include:
- To reinforce the *vital energy*, diminished function of the *spleen* or *lung*[2]
- Prostration with impending collapse marked by cold limbs, faint pulse, sweating; heart failure, shock; palpitation with anxiety, forgetfulness, restlessness[2,3]
- General weakness with irritability and insomnia in chronic diseases[2]
- Impotence or frigidity[2]
- Wheezing, shortness of breath, organ prolapse[3]

Traditional Western herbal medicine uses include:
- Physical or mental exhaustion, neurasthenia, stress, inadequate resistance to infections[4,5]

Korean Ginseng continued on page 299

*This dose range is also extrapolated from British Herbal Pharmacopoeia 1983, the British Herbal Compendium 1992, and from clinical trials.

- Neuralgia, insomnia, hypotonia[5]
- Depressive states associated with sexual inadequacy[5]
- Loss of appetite, nervous dyspepsia; convulsions, paralysis[6]

Pharmacologic Research

Key constituents of Korean ginseng root include a complex mixture of dammarane saponins called ginsenosides.

- The ability of ginsenosides to independently target multireceptor systems at the plasma membrane, as well as to activate intracellular steroid receptors, may explain some of the pharmacological effects of Korean ginseng.[7]
- The positive effects of Korean ginseng in promoting the longevity, metabolism, and growth of normal cells have been demonstrated by many studies, both *in vitro* and *in vivo*. Many investigating scientists have seen these effects as confirming the tonic activity of Korean ginseng.
- Countless animal studies have demonstrated that Korean ginseng increases the resistance to a wide variety of physical, chemical, and biological stressors. Oral doses of Korean ginseng increased organ and muscle weights and countered some of the effects of aging in experimental models.
- Oral doses of Korean ginseng extract significantly improved learning and memory in experimental models. Oral ginsenosides accelerated brain and body development in young animals.
- Korean ginseng extract enhanced B- and T-lymphocyte and natural killer cell activities, increased production of interferon, and improved antibody formation in experimental models after oral doses.
- Oral administration of Korean ginseng extract suppressed experimental Semliki Forest viral infection and protected against *Candida albicans* infection *in vivo*.
- Korean ginseng extract and ginsenosides have demonstrated anticancer activity, both *in vitro* and *in vivo* via the oral route, by inhibiting growth of cancers, inducing differentiation, exhibiting antimutagenic activity against genotoxic agents, inhibiting metastasis, potentiating the activity of anticancer drugs, and improving survival in experimental cancer models.
- Injecting Korean ginseng extract or ginsenosides countered the deleterious effects of repeated administration of narcotic drugs such as morphine, cocaine, methamphetamine, or apomorphine. Morphine-induced tolerance and physical dependence were reduced after oral administration of Korean ginseng. Accelerated ethanol clearance from the blood, but not the brain, was achieved in experimental models after oral doses of Korean ginseng.
- Experimental studies suggest that the antioxidant and organ-protective actions of Korean ginseng are linked to enhanced nitric oxide synthesis in the endothelium of the lungs, heart, kidney, and corpus cavernosum. Enhanced nitric oxide synthesis might contribute to the vasodilation and aphrodisiac actions attributed to Korean ginseng.

Korean Ginseng *continued on page 300*

Clinical Studies

When referred to in the following points, red ginseng is *Panax ginseng* that has been steamed before drying.

- Although some negative findings have been reported, the majority of clinical trials have found that Korean ginseng increases physical performance. Physical performance and visual and auditory reaction times were significantly increased in a randomized, double-blind, placebo-controlled trial using Korean ginseng extract administered for 12 weeks to people aged 22 to 80 years. Male athletes significantly increased their aerobic capacity and significantly reduced their blood lactate levels and heart rate while taking Korean ginseng in randomized and nonrandomized, double-blind, placebo-controlled trials and in uncontrolled trials. These trials were conducted by the same research group over a 9-week period. The daily dose of Korean ginseng extract administered was 200 mg/day (containing 4% ginsenosides and equivalent to approximately 1 g/day of dried root).

- Randomized, double-blind, controlled trials have shown that Korean ginseng significantly improves quality of life and well being measures while under stress, including alertness, relaxation, appetite, fatigue levels, sleep quality, recovery from the common cold and bronchitis, and significantly decreases systolic blood pressure compared with controls. Two of these trials compared Korean ginseng combined with vitamins and minerals against placebo. One trial compared this combination against vitamins and minerals, and another trial compared Korean ginseng on its own against placebo. The Korean ginseng, vitamin, and mineral combination was superior to the vitamins and minerals alone. In two of these trials, the daily dose was equivalent to between 0.4 and 1.0 g of dried root, which was administered for up to 4 months.

- The Korean ginseng, vitamin, and mineral combination improved REM sleep in elderly volunteers in a double-blind, placebo-controlled trial. Reaction time and decision-making were improved in elderly volunteers taking red ginseng (1.5 g/day) in a double-blind crossover trial.

- A combination containing Ginkgo extract (120 mg/day standardized to 24% ginkgo flavone glycosides) and Korean ginseng extract (200 mg/day standardized to 4% ginsenosides) demonstrated improvement in the working and long-term memory of healthy, middle-aged volunteers over 14 weeks in a multicenter, double-blind, placebo-controlled trial.[8] Three single, increasing doses of standardized Korean ginseng extract produced a dose-dependent improvement in several aspects of memory when compared with placebo in healthy young volunteers. The trial was of randomized, double-blind, crossover design.[9]

- Korean ginseng extracts significantly improved cell-mediated immune function (chemotaxis, phagocytic activity, and intracellular killing) in a double-blind, placebo-controlled trial involving healthy volunteers. A standardized extract (200 mg/day, equivalent to approximately 1 g/day of root and containing 4% ginsenosides) was compared with 200 mg/day of aqueous extract for 8 weeks. A randomized,

Korean Ginseng *continued on page 301*

double-blind, placebo-controlled study demonstrated significant prevention of influenza and the common cold for Korean ginseng over placebo in volunteers also receiving an antiinfluenza vaccination. The Korean ginseng group demonstrated significantly higher antibody titers and natural killer cell activity. Extract doses equivalent to approximately 1 g per day of root containing 4% ginsenosides were given for 12 weeks. In a more recent randomized, double-blind, placebo-controlled trial, treatment with Korean ginseng extract for 4 months improved the immune response (IgM and IgA antibody levels) to influenza vaccination in healthy volunteers.[10]

- Korean ginseng extract (equivalent to approximately 1 g/day of root) improved the immune response of alveolar macrophages isolated from chronic bronchitis patients in a placebo-controlled, single-blind trial. In a randomized, controlled trial involving patients with chronic bronchitis, Korean ginseng combined with antibacterial drugs reduced the bronchial bacterial count faster than antibacterial drugs alone. The daily dose of Korean ginseng extract was 200 mg standardized to contain 4% ginsenosides. The duration of the trial was 9 days.[11]

- Controlled and uncontrolled trials have found ginseng may be of value in treating HIV infection. The dosage used in one of the uncontrolled studies was 5.4 g per day of red ginseng powder.

- Significant improvement in cerebrovascular circulation was observed in patients with moderate cerebrovascular deficit treated with either Korean ginseng extract (containing 4% ginsenosides and equivalent to approximately 1 g/day of root) or the drug hydergine (3 mg/day) when compared with placebo under double-blind conditions over a period of 3 months.

- A combined Korean ginseng and Ginkgo product (containing 4 mg/day ginsenosides and 28.8 mg/day ginkgo flavone glycosides) improved circulation and lowered blood pressure in a small, placebo-controlled, single-dose study in healthy volunteers. A controlled trial involving patients with congestive heart failure found red ginseng improved biochemical and hemodynamic parameters. Greater improvement was noted when the herb was combined with digoxin. Erectile function and HDL cholesterol were significantly improved in elderly men with psychogenic impotence treated with red ginseng (1.8 g or 2.7 g for 2 months) in a placebo-controlled study.

- Red ginseng (6 g/day) improved psychological test scores in postmenopausal women with symptoms of fatigue, insomnia, and depression when compared with baseline values. The improvement was at least partially the result of an antistress effect, as demonstrated by a decrease in the cortisol/dehydroepiandrosterone (DHEA) ratio.[12] In a randomized, double-blind, placebo-controlled trial, postmenopausal women reported improvement in quality-of-life measures, including depression and well being, after treatment with standardized Korean ginseng extract (containing 4% ginsenosides, equivalent to approximately 1 g/day of root). No benefit over placebo was observed for physiological parameters, including FSH and estradiol levels and endometrial thickness.[13]

Korean Ginseng continued on page 302

- Epidemiological studies have found an inverse relationship between Korean ginseng intake and cancer in South Korea, where Korean ginseng tea is consumed as frequently as coffee. A case-controlled study on 1987 pairs found that the relative risk for cancer for Korean ginseng users was 50% lower than for those who did not use Korean ginseng. The incidence of cancers of the lung, lip, oral cavity, and pharynx were substantially lower in smokers who were Korean ginseng users compared with smokers who were not. The incidences of cancers of the breast, cervix, bladder, and thyroid gland were not affected by Korean ginseng. Prospective cohort studies found decreased risk of cancer for participants who had consumed Korean ginseng compared with nonconsumers. Ginseng consumption was also linked to decreased risk for gastric and lung cancers.[14,15]
- Daily supplementation of red ginseng (1.8 g) for 4 weeks in smokers resulted in a linear increase in plasma antioxidant concentration compared with values obtained from smokers administered a placebo. In this randomized trial, Korean ginseng treatment also decreased markers of DNA oxidative damage.[16]
- A randomized, double-blind, placebo-controlled study involving patients with cervical cancer who were undergoing radiation therapy found that Korean ginseng (5 g/day for 5 weeks) exerted a protective effect on bone marrow depression and significantly elevated platelet count.
- Sperm count, sperm motility, total testosterone, free testosterone, and dihydrotestosterone (DHT) rose substantially, and prolactin levels decreased after 3 months of ginseng treatment in men with idiopathic low sperm count and low sperm count associated with varicocele. The control group mirrored these responses on a smaller scale. Red ginseng extract significantly improved erectile dysfunction compared with the drug trazodone, which demonstrated a similar effect to placebo in a randomized trial.
- Pregnant women taking ginseng had a significantly lower incidence of preeclampsia than their matched controls. The control group had higher mean blood pressures in the second and third trimesters.
- In a randomized, double-blind, placebo-controlled study involving patients with non-insulin–dependent diabetes, Korean ginseng extract taken for 8 weeks significantly improved patients' fasting blood glucose, mood, vigor, well being, and psychomotor performance.
- Only minor benefit was observed in a single-blind, placebo-controlled trial involving patients with essential hypertension treated with red ginseng root (4.5 g/day for 8 weeks).[17] In a small, controlled trial, red ginseng improved the vascular endothelial dysfunction in patients with hypertension, possibly through increasing the synthesis of nitric oxide.[18]
- In Germany, the Commission E supports using Korean ginseng as a tonic for invigoration and fortification in times of fatigue and debility, for declining capacity for work and concentration, and during convalescence.[19]
- Korean ginseng is official in the USP24-NF19.

Korean Ginseng *continued on page 303*

REFERENCES

Except when specifically referenced, the following book was referred to in the compilation of the pharmacological and clinical information: Mills S, Bone K: *Principles and Practice of Phytotherapy: Modern Herbal Medicine,* Edinburgh, 2000, Churchill Livingstone.

1 Zhu M et al: *J Pharm Pharmacol* 51:175-180, 1999.
2 Pharmacopoeia Commission of the People's Republic of China: *Pharmacopoeia of the People's Republic of China,* English ed, Beijing, 1997, Chemical Industry Press.
3 Bensky D, Gamble A: *Chinese herbal medicine materia medica,* Seattle, 1986, Eastland Press.
4 British Herbal Medicine Association: *British herbal compendium,* Bournemouth, 1992, BHMA.
5 British Herbal Medicine Association's Scientific Committee: *British herbal pharmacopoeia,* Bournemouth, 1983, BHMA.
6 Felter HW, Lloyd JU: *King's American dispensatory,* ed 18, rev 3, Portland, 1905, reprinted 1983, Eclectic Medical Publications.
7 Attele AS, Wu JA, Yuan CS: *Biochem Pharmacol* 58(11):1685-1693, 1999.
8 Wesnes KA et al: *Psychopharmacology* 152(4):353-361, 2000.
9 Kennedy DO, Scholey A, Wesnes KA: *Phytomed* 7(supp 2):105, 2000.
10 Gundling K et al: *Altern Ther Health Med* 7(3):104, 2001.
11 Scaglione F, Weiser K, Alessandria M: *Clin Drug Invest* 21(1):41-45, 2001.
12 Tode T et al: *Int J Gynaecol* 67:169-174, 1999.
13 Wiklund IK et al: *Int J Clin Pharmacol Res* 19(3):89-99, 1999.
14 Yun TK, Choi SY, Lee YS: Second International Cancer Chemo Prevention Conference, Berlin, April 28-30, 1993.
15 Yun TK, Choi SY: *Proc Annu Meet Am Assoc Cancer Res* 37:1906, 1996.
16 Lee BM, Lee SK, Kim HS: *Cancer Lett* 132(1-2):219-227, 1998.
17 Han KH et al: *Am J Chin Med* 26:199-209, 1988.
18 Sung J et al: *Am J Chin Med* 28(2):205-216, 2000.
19 Blumenthal M et al, editors: *The complete German Commission E monographs: therapeutic guide to herbal medicines,* Austin, 1998, American Botanical Council.

LAVENDER

Botanical Names: *Lavandula officinalis, Lavandula angustifolia,*[#^] *Lavandula angustifolia* subsp. *angustifolia,*[#] *Lavandula vera*[#]
Family: Labiatae
Plant Part Used: Flower

PRESCRIBING INFORMATION

Actions

Carminative, spasmolytic, antidepressant, anxiolytic

Potential Indications

Based on appropriate evaluation of the patient, practitioners should consider prescribing lavender in formulations in the context of:
- Restlessness, insomnia *(4)*
- Anxiety, to elevate mood *(4a*)*
- Depression, headache *(5)*
- Functional abdominal complaints, such as nervous stomach irritations and meteorism (i.e., gaseous distension of the abdomen or intestine) *(4)*
- Flatulent dyspepsia, colic, digestive dysfunction, rheumatism *(5)*
- As a bath for functional circulatory disorders *(4)*

Contraindications

None known.

Warnings and Precautions

None required.

Interactions

None known.

Use in Pregnancy and Lactation

No adverse effects expected.

Side Effects

None expected if taken within the recommended dose range. High (undefined) doses are said to cause abdominal pain and colic.[2,3]

Dosage

Dose per day**	Dose per week**
2.0-4.5 ml of 1:2 liquid extract	15-30 ml of 1:2 liquid extract

SUPPORTING INFORMATION

Traditional Prescribing

Traditional Western herbal medicine uses include:
- Flatulent dyspepsia, colic, digestive dysfunction, headache, depressive states[2,4]
- Internally as an infusion or extract to treat rheumatism[4]
- As a stimulant for children[2]
- Topically (heated) for painful local affections[2]
- Regarded as a mild sedative and having slight cholagogue activity[5]

Lavender *continued on page 305*

[#]Alternative name.

[^]Adopted by the American Herbal Products Association as the new botanical name.[1]

*Based on the assumption that oral dosage of lavender infusion or liquid extract would deliver a similar concentration of active constituents to the bloodstream as would topical use (or inhalation) of lavender essential oil.

**This dose range is extrapolated from the British Herbal Pharmacopoeia 1983 and the author's education and experience.

- As a bath for vegetative dystonia[5]
- As a gargle for hoarseness and loss of voice[3]

Pharmacologic Research

Lavender flowers contain 1% to 3% essential oil (consisting mainly of linalyl acetate and linalool),[6] phenolic compounds (probably derivatives of rosmarinic acid), and flavonoids.[7] The percentage of essential oil present in a liquid extract depends on the percentage of ethanol used in the extraction with approximately 30% of the essential oil extracted by 45% ethanol.

- Dried lavender straw as bedding material decreased the incidence and severity of travel sickness in pigs but not overall levels of stress.[8]
- An aqueous methanolic extract of lavender and its isolated phenolic components produced concentration-dependent inhibition of lipid peroxidation in vitro.[9]
- The spasmolytic activity of an aqueous methanolic extract of lavender was demonstrated for experimentally induced contractions of isolated circular and longitudinal smooth muscle.[10] Lavender oil decreased tone in skeletal muscle tissue.[11] The mechanism of the spasmolytic action of lavender oil is postsynaptic and not atropinelike and is most likely to be mediated through cAMP. The activity of linalool reflected that of the whole oil.[12]
- Lavender oil demonstrated sedative activity after inhalation in an experimental model. The activity correlated to the presence of linalool in the blood. Lavender oil, linalool, and linalyl acetate inhibited stimulation by caffeine.[13] Oral administration of lavender oil (1.6%) produced sedative and anxiolytic activities in experimental models.[14,15]
- Inhaling lavender oil reduced the content of cholesterol in aortic tissue and decreased atherogenesis in an experimental model. Serum cholesterol levels were unchanged.[16]
- An anticonvulsive activity for inhaled lavender oil was demonstrated in several experimental models using drug-induced convulsion.[17]
- Lavender oil has also demonstrated the following activities:
  - Antimicrobial activity in vitro for the vapor was observed, particularly in relation to filamentous fungi.[18,19] No antisporulating effect was observed when the oil was applied in solution, indicating that the vapor was specifically active.[19] Antifungal activity has been demonstrated towards human pathogenic fungi, including Trichophyton rubrum after direct contact in vitro.[20]
  - Inhibition of immediate-type allergic reactions via inhibition of mast cell degranulation was observed following topical or intradermal administration in several experimental models.[21]
  - Moderate immunostimulatory activity was exhibited in the modified carbon clearance test in vivo (usually by injection).[22]

Clinical Studies

No clinical studies using lavender dried flower or lavender extracts have been found.

- A study of percutaneous absorption of lavender oil following massage found that the main constituents of the oil were detected in the

Lavender continued on page 306

blood within 5 minutes after application. Following this rapid absorption, most of the lavender oil was excreted within 90 minutes.[23]

- Inhaling lavender oil by volunteers decreased vigilance by approximately 20% from baseline values, indicating a sedative effect.[24]

- An open, controlled trial investigating the effect of aromatherapy on patients with chronic hemodialysis found lavender aroma alleviated anxiety (by significantly reducing anxiety mean scores).[25] In a controlled study using volunteers and designed to link the effect of odors with the emotional process, inhaling lavender odor elicited mostly "happiness" as measured by evaluation and autonomic nervous system parameters.[26] Inhaling lavender oil for 3 minutes by volunteers produced increased frontal beta power (suggesting increased drowsiness), less depressed mood, relaxed feelings, and faster and more accurate mathematic computations compared with baseline values. The trial was randomized and controlled (compared with rosemary oil).[27]

- A randomized, controlled trial compared the use of aromatherapy with lavender oil, massage, and periods of rest in an intensive care environment. No significant differences were observed in the physiological stress indicators or patients' ability to cope following any of the three treatments. However, patients who received aromatherapy reported greater improvement in their mood. These patients also felt less anxious and were more positive immediately following therapy, although this effect was not sustained or cumulative.[28]

- Lavender oil aromatherapy resulted in a near statistically significant reduction in diastolic blood pressure during recovery from exercise in a randomized, controlled trial involving 20 healthy men. (The control group received no aromatherapy.)[29] In an open trial, inhaling lavender oil had an antistress effect and reduced arousal in volunteers subjected to noise stress. The treatment had no effect on blood pressure or heart rate.[30]

- Six drops of pure lavender oil in bath water, repeated for 10 days, produced lower mean discomfort scores in women with perineal discomfort subsequent to childbirth. However, no statistically significant difference was observed among the groups (pure lavender oil, synthetic lavender oil, and an inert substance) in this randomized, placebo-controlled trial.[31] The authors suggested that further studies should explore varying the dose and mode of application.[32]

- A survey of hospital staff found an improvement in the work environment following the use of lavender oil burners for 3 months.[33]

- Lavender oil inhalation lengthened sleep time in four geriatric patients with sleep disorders, three of whom had been taking benzodiazepines and neuroleptic drugs for some time. In this open trial, the drugs were discontinued, and lavender oil was then administered after a washout period.[34]

- In a randomized, double-blind, placebo-controlled trial using lavender baths, a mild improvement in sleep quality was observed for patients with sleep disorders. (Low and high strength baths were compared.)[35]

Lavender *continued on page 307*

- In a randomized, crossover trial, a 10-minute hot footbath with or without lavender oil produced an increase in blood flow and parasympathetic nerve activity in volunteers. The footbath with the addition of lavender oil produced changes in autonomic activity characteristic of relaxation.[36]
- In Germany the Commission E supports oral use of lavender to treat mood disturbances, such as restlessness or insomnia, and functional abdominal complaints (e.g., nervous stomach irritations, meteorism, nervous intestinal discomfort). The Commission E also supports using lavender for "functional circulatory disorders."[37]

REFERENCES

1 McGuffin M, editor: *Herbs of commerce*, ed 2 [draft 3.3], Bethesda, Md, 1998, American Herbal Products Association.
2 Felter HW, Lloyd JU: *King's American dispensatory*, ed 18, rev 3, Portland, 1905, reprinted 1983, Eclectic Medical Publications.
3 Grieve M: *A modern herbal*, New York, 1971, Dover Publications.
4 British Herbal Medicine Association's Scientific Committee: *British herbal pharmacopoeia*, Bournemouth, 1983, BHMA.
5 Weiss RF: *Herbal medicine*, English ed, Beaconsfield, UK, 1988, Beaconsfield Publishers.
6 Wagner H, Bladt S: *Plant drug analysis: a thin layer chromatography atlas*, ed 2, Berlin, 1996, Springer-Verlag.
7 Bisset NG, editor: *Herbal drugs and phytopharmaceuticals*, Stuttgart, 1994, Medpharm Scientific Publishers.
8 Bradshaw RH et al: *J Altern Complement Med* 4(3):271-275, 1998.
9 Hohmann J et al: *Planta Med* 65(6):576-578, 1999.
10 Izzo AA et al: *Phytother Res* 10(suppl 1):S107-S108, 1996.
11 Lis-Balchin M, Hart S: *J Ethnopharmacol* 58(3):183-187, 1997.
12 Lis-Balchin M, Hart S: *Phytother Res* 13(6):540-542, 1999.
13 Buchbauer G et al: *Z Naturforsch [C]* 46(11-12):1067-1072, 1991.
14 Guillemain J, Rousseau A, Delaveau P: *Ann Pharm Fr* 47(6):337-343, 1989.
15 Delaveau P et al: *C R Seances Soc Biol Fil* 183(4):342-348, 1989.
16 Nikolaevskii VV et al: *Patol Fiziol Eksp Ter* (5):52-53, 1990.
17 Yamada K, Mimaki Y, Sashida Y: *Biol Pharm Bull* 17(2):359-360, 1994.
18 Larrondo JV, Agut M, Calvo-Torras MA: *Microbios* 82(332):171-172, 1995.
19 Inouye S et al: *Mycoses* 41(9-10):403-410, 1998.
20 Adam K et al: *J Agri Food Chem* 46(5):1739-1745, 1998.
21 Kim HM, Cho SH: *J Pharm Pharmacol* 51(2):221-226, 1999.
22 Kedzia B et al: *Herba Polon* 44(2):126-135, 1998.
23 Jager W et al: *J Soc Cosm Chem* 43:49-54, 1992.
24 Buchbauer B et al. Cited in Teranishi R, Buttery RG, Sugisawa H, editors: *Bioactive volatile compounds from plants. ACS Symposium series*, Washington, DC, 1993, American Chemical Society.
25 Itai T et al: *Psychiatry Clin Neurosci* 54(4):393-397, 2000.
26 Vernet-Maury E et al: *J Auton Nerv Syst* 75(2-3):176-183, 1999.
27 Diego MA et al: *Int J Neurosci* 96(3-4):217-224, 1998.
28 Dunn C, Sleep J, Collett D: *J Adv Nurs* 21(1):34-40, 1995.
29 Romine IJ, Bush AM, Geist CR: *Percept Mot Skills* 88(3, pt 1):756-758, 1999.
30 Motomura N, Sakurai A, Yotsuya Y: *Memoir Osaka Kyoiku Univ III Nat Sci Appl Sci* 47(2):281-287, 1999.
31 Dale A, Cornwell S: *J Adv Nurs* 19(1):89-96, 1994.
32 Cornwell S, Dale A: *Mod Midwife* 5(3):31-33, 1995.
33 Tysoe P: *Int J Nurs Pract* 6(2):110-112, 2000.
34 Hardy M, Kirk-Smith MD, Stretch DD: *Lancet* 346(8976):701, 1995.
35 Emmerling M et al: *Z Phytother Abstractband*, p25, 1995.
36 Saeki Y: *Complement Ther Med* 8(1):2-7, 2000.
37 Blumenthal M et al, editors: *The complete German Commission E monographs: therapeutic guide to herbal medicines*, Austin, 1998, American Botanical Council.

LEMON BALM

Other Common Name: Melissa
Botanical Name: *Melissa officinalis*
Family: Labiatae
Plant Part Used: Aerial parts

PRESCRIBING INFORMATION

Actions

Carminative, spasmolytic, mild sedative, diaphoretic, TSH antagonist, antiviral (topically)

Potential Indications

Based on appropriate evaluation of the patient, practitioners should consider prescribing lemon balm in formulations in the context of:
- Sleep disturbances, in combination with valerian, hops, and motherwort (2)
- Nervous sleeping disorders (4)
- Infantile colic, in combination with chamomile, vervain, licorice, and fennel (3)
- Indigestion, flatulence, colic (4,5)
- Tenseness, irritability (4)
- Depression, nervous breakdown (5)
- Fevers (5)
- The common cold, influenza (6)
- Topical treatment for herpes simplex virus infection (2,4)

Contraindications

None known.

Warnings and Precautions

None required.

Interactions

None known.

Use in Pregnancy and Lactation

No adverse effects expected.

Side Effects

None expected if taken within the recommended dose range.

Dosage

Dose per day*	**Dose per week***
3-6 ml of 1:2 liquid extract	20-40 ml of 1:2 liquid extract

SUPPORTING INFORMATION

Traditional Prescribing

Traditional Western herbal medicine uses include:
- Flatulent dyspepsia; depression, nervous breakdown[1]
- As a diaphoretic in febrile diseases, painful menstruation,[2] the common cold and influenza[3]

Lemon Balm *continued on page 309*

*This dose range is extrapolated from the British Herbal Pharmacopoeia 1983 and the author's education and experience.

Pharmacologic Research

The aerial parts of lemon balm contain an essential oil that contains a large number of monoterpenes and sesquiterpenes, predominantly citronellal and citral.[4] In addition, lemon balm contains phenolic acid derivatives, which contribute to the antiviral activity.

- Aqueous freeze-dried extract of lemon balm inhibited the binding of TSH and the deiodination of thyroid hormone T_4 to T_3 and other products *in vitro*.[5,6] Lemon balm also inhibited the binding of thyroid-stimulating autoantibodies to TSH receptors *in vitro*.[5,7] Injecting a freeze-dried aqueous ethanol extract of lemon balm reduced serum TSH concentration in a normal thyroid model. Pituitary TSH concentration was reduced, but thyroid hormone levels remained unchanged. Despite administering a higher dose, lemon balm did not lower TSH levels in a goiter (hypothyroid) model.[8]
- A strong prolactin-lowering effect was observed after a single intravenous injection of aqueous freeze-dried lemon balm extract *in vivo*.[9]
- Lemon balm extract demonstrated sedative and sleep-promoting activity *in vivo* (route unknown) and analgesic activity at high dose.[10] The essential oil exerted on antispasmodic activity on isolated tissue,[11,12] but in another study, the extract was devoid of activity.[13]
- An aqueous ethanol extract of lemon balm strongly displaced nicotine and scopolamine from human brain cell membranes containing acetylcholine receptors *in vitro*.[14] (Acetylcholine receptor agonists have potential for use in neurodegenerative diseases associated with aging, such as Alzheimer's disease.)
- Lemon balm extract demonstrated antioxidant activity *in vitro*.[15,16]
- Lemon balm ethanolic extract, essential oil, and oil constituents (citral, geraniol, nerol) inhibited the formation of the proinflammatory eicosanoids, leukotriene B_4, and thromboxane B_2 *in vitro*. The aqueous extract was devoid of activity.[17]
- Lemon balm extract demonstrated antiviral activity against a number of viruses, including HSV *in vitro*.[18] This finding has relevance for the topical use of the herb. The essential oil has demonstrated antimicrobial activity *in vitro*.[19]

Clinical Studies

- A single administration of lemon balm extract to volunteers resulted in a quantitative EEG recording that was distinguishable from that obtained for placebo. However, results from the self-rating of alertness did not differ from placebo. The dose was equivalent to 6.2 g of dried herb.[20] An acute sedative effect was not demonstrated, but analysis after ongoing administration may yet demonstrate a sedative effect.
- The effect of an herbal preparation containing valerian and lemon balm on objective sleep parameters was compared with an orthodox sedative (triazolam) and placebo in 20 volunteers composed of both good and poor sleepers. The herbal preparation induced a significant increase in sleep efficiency in stages 3 and 4, and poor sleepers benefitted more from the treatment. No shortening of sleep latency and wake time were observed, and no rebound effects were observed.

Lemon Balm *continued on page 310*

The herbal combination and triazolam were tested on day 3 and day 6, respectively, with baseline and placebo evaluated on days 1, 2, 4, 5, and 7. The daily dose corresponded to 1.4 g of dried valerian root and 0.9 g of dried lemon balm herb. The trial was of double-blind, placebo-controlled, crossover design.[21]

- In a randomized, double-blind, placebo-controlled, multicenter trial, a lemon balm (equivalent to 1.7 g/day) and valerian (equivalent to 2.9 g/day) preparation taken for 3 weeks produced an improvement in sleep parameters in ambulatory patients with light insomnia.[22] A later trial with the same design produced a significantly higher quality of sleep in healthy volunteers compared with placebo. The preparation was administered 30 minutes before bed and contained the equivalent of 1.2 g per day lemon balm and 1.6 g per day of valerian, taken for 30 days.[23]

- A postmarketing surveillance study in Germany involving 518 patients found an herbal combination of valerian, hops, and lemon balm to be a highly effective treatment for nervous insomnia and restlessness, with very few side effects. The dose administered ranged from one to nine tablets. One tablet contains 450 mg of valerian dried root, 126.5 mg of dried hop strobiles, and 225 mg of lemon balm dried leaf.[24]

- A randomized, double-blind, crossover study involving alcoholics with sleep disturbances found that consumption of an herbal tablet produced improvement in sleep parameters. The tablet that was taken for one night and compared with placebo (also one night) contained the following weights of dried herb: valerian root (170 mg), hop strobiles (50 mg), lemon balm leaf (50 mg), and motherwort herb (50 mg).[25]

- A double-blind study on babies approximately 3 weeks of age with infantile colic investigated the effect of an instant herbal tea preparation containing lemon balm, chamomile, vervain, licorice, and fennel. After 7 days, the colic improvement scores were significantly better in the herbal tea group, and more babies in this treatment group had their colic eliminated. The tea preparation was offered with every episode of colic, up to 150 ml per dose, but not more than three times per day. The exact composition of the preparation was not defined.[26]

- In a double-blind, placebo-controlled crossover study, a citronellol bath produced a dose-dependent, sedative, and sleep-promoting effect in both healthy volunteers and in patients with nervous or sleep disorders.[27]

- Randomized, controlled clinical trials with lemon balm have yielded conclusive results for the topical treatment of recurrent herpes simplex virus type I infection.[28-33] These trials used a cream containing 1% lemon balm extract (70:1). In one trial, the cream was used on the affected area two to four times daily for 5 to 10 days.[31]

- In Germany, the Commission E supports using lemon balm to treat nervous sleeping disorders and functional gastrointestinal complaints.[34]

Lemon Balm *continued on page 311*

- ESCOP recommends lemon balm internally for treating tenseness, restlessness and irritability, as well as symptomatic treatment of digestive disorders such as minor spasms. Externally, lemon balm is recommended for treating herpes labialis (cold sores).[35]

REFERENCES

1 British Herbal Medicine Association's Scientific Committee: *British herbal pharmacopoeia,* Bournemouth, 1983, BHMA.
2 Felter HW, Lloyd JU: *King's American dispensatory,* ed 18, rev 3, Portland, 1905, reprinted 1983, Eclectic Medical Publications.
3 Grieve M: *A modern herbal,* New York, 1971, Dover Publications.
4 Wagner H, Bladt S: *Plant drug analysis: a thin layer chromatography atlas,* ed 2, Berlin, 1996, Springer-Verlag.
5 Auf'mkolk M et al: *Endocrinology* 115(2):527-534, 1984.
6 Auf'mkolk M et al: *Horm Metab Res* 16(4):188-192, 1984.
7 Auf'mkolk M et al: *Endocrinology* 116(5):1687-1693, 1985.
8 Sourgens H et al: *Planta Med* 45:78-86, 1982.
9 Sourgens H et al: *Int J Crude Drug Res* 24(2):53-61, 1986.
10 Soulimani R et al: *Planta Med* 57(2):105-199, 1991.
11 Wagner H, Sprinkmeyer L: *Dtsch Apoth Ztg* 113:1159-1166, 1973.
12 Debelmas AM, Rochat J: *Plantes Med Phytother* 1:23-27, 1967.
13 Forster HB, Niklas H, Lutz S: *Planta Med* 40:309-319, 1980.
14 Wake G et al: *J Ethnopharmacol* 69:105-114, 2000.
15 Hohmann J et al: *Planta Med* 65(6):576-578, 1999.
16 Lamaison JL, Petitjean-Freytet C, Carnat A: *Pharm Acta Helv* 66(7):185-188, 1991.
17 Howes M, Houghton PJ, Hoult J. Presented at the International Congress and 48th Annual Meeting of the Society for Medicinal Plant Research and the 6th International Congress on Ethnopharmacology of the International Society for Ethnopharmacology, Zurich, September 3-7, 2000, abstract SL16.
18 Kucera LS, Cohen RA, Herrmann EC Jr: *Ann N Y Acad Sci* 130(1):474-482, 1965.
19 Larrondo JV, Agut M, Calvo-Torras MA: *Microbios* 82(332):171-172, 1995.
20 Schulz H, Jobert M, Hubner WD: *Phytomed* 5(6):449-458, 1998.
21 Dressing H et al: *Therapiewoche* 42(12):726-736, 1992.
22 Dressing H, Kohler S, Muller WE: *Psychopharmakother* 3(3):123-130, 1996.
23 Cerny A, Schmid K: *Fitoterapia* 70:221-228, 1999.
24 Friede M et al. Presented at the 2nd International Congress on Phytomedicine, Munich, September 11-14, 1996, abstract P-75.
25 Widy-Tyszkiewicz E, Schminda R: *Herba Polonica* 43(2):154-159, 1997.
26 Weizman Z et al: *J Pediatrics* 122(4):650-652, 1993.
27 Pischel B, Uehleke B: *Z Phytother Abstractband,* p25, 1995.
28 Wolbling RH, Rapprich K: *Dtsch Dermatol* 10:1318-1328, 1983.
29 Wolbling RH, Milbradt R: *Therapiewoche* 34:1193-1200, 1984.
30 Vogt H et al. Presented at the 4th International Congress on Phytotherapy, Munich, September 10-13, 1992, abstract SL 15.
31 Wolbling RH, Leonhardt K: *Phytomed* 1(1):25-31, 1994.
32 Koytchev R, Alken RG, Dundarov S: *Phytomed* 6(4):225-230, 1999.
33 Mohrig A: *Dtsch Apoth Ztg* 136:109-114, 1996.
34 Blumenthal M et al, editors: *The complete German Commission E monographs: therapeutic guide to herbal medicines,* Austin, 1998, American Botanical Council.
35 Scientific Committee of the European Scientific Cooperative on Phytotherapy [ESCOP]: *ESCOP monographs: Melissae folium.* European Scientific Cooperative on Phytotherapy, ESCOP Secretariat, Argyle House, Gandy Street, Exeter, Devon, EX4 3LS, United Kingdom, March 1996.

LICORICE

Other Common Name: Liquorice
Botanical Name: *Glycyrrhiza glabra*
Family: Leguminosae
Plant Part Used: Root and stolon

PRESCRIBING INFORMATION

Actions

Antiinflammatory, mucoprotective, demulcent, antiulcer (peptic), adrenal tonic, expectorant, antitussive, mild laxative, anticariogenic

Potential Indications

Based on appropriate evaluation of the patient, practitioners should consider prescribing licorice in formulations in the context of:
- Gastric and duodenal ulceration, gastroesophageal reflux *(4,5)*
- Polycystic ovary syndrome, infertility, muscle cramps, dysmenorrhea, in combination with white peony *(4)*
- Adrenal insufficiency and withdrawal from corticosteroid drugs *(5,7)*
- Inflammatory conditions, rheumatoid arthritis, urinary tract inflammation *(5,7)*
- Upper respiratory tract catarrh *(4,5)*
- Cough, bronchitis *(5,7)*
- Addison's disease *(4,5)*
- Topical treatment for eczema, melasma (increased melanin pigmentation) *(4)*
- Topical treatment for recurrent mouth ulcers and herpes lesions *(4a)*

Contraindications

Contraindications listed by the Commission E include cholestatic liver disorders, liver cirrhosis, hypertension, hypokalemia, severe kidney insufficiency, and pregnancy. Licorice is also contraindicated if edema or congestive heart failure is present. However, licorice has been safely used in combination with white peony *(Paeonia lactiflora)* in a clinical study involving pregnant women. The women were successfully treated with the combination (equivalent to 6 g/day of each herb for 24 weeks) for infertility resulting from polycystic ovary syndrome. A number of pregnancies were recorded at the 12-week mark. Additionally, a study of licorice intake during pregnancy found no substantial health risks associated with its use.[1]

Warnings and Precautions

Patients who are prescribed high glycyrrhizin licorice preparations for prolonged periods should be placed on a high-potassium, low-sodium diet and closely monitored for blood pressure increases and weight gain. Hypokalemia is the greatest threat and can occur at relatively low doses. Special precautions should be taken with elderly patients and patients with hypertension or cardiac, renal, or hepatic disease. These individuals should not receive licorice preparations high in glycyrrhizin (GL) for prolonged periods.

Interactions

A slight chance exists that GL or glycyrrhetinic acid (GA) may counteract the contraceptive pill.

Licorice *continued on page 313*

Potassium loss may be severe if licorice is taken in conjunction with potassium-depleting drugs (e.g., thiazide diuretics, laxatives) leading to undesirable side effects. With potassium loss, sensitivity to cardioactive glycosides increases, with potential toxic effects. The intake of licorice may exaggerate the effects of a high-salt diet.

Oral administration of GL increases plasma prednisolone concentrations by inhibiting its metabolism. Licorice may thereby potentiate the pharmacologic effects of prednisolone and other corticosteroid drugs.

Use in Pregnancy and Lactation

The Commission E advises that licorice is contraindicated in pregnancy. However, doses up to 3 g per day (i.e., up to 3 ml of 1:1 liquid extract or 3 ml of 1:1 high glycyrrhizin liquid extract) are likely to be safe.

Side Effects

Licorice has been known to cause hypertension, sodium and water retention, and hypokalemia through the mineralocorticoid effect of GL. Individual variation in susceptibility to GL is highly varied: in the most sensitive individuals, a regular daily intake (over several weeks) of no more than 100 mg GL (corresponding to approximately 50 g of licorice candies) can produce symptoms; most individuals who consume 400 mg GL daily experience side effects.

Excessive consumption of licorice confectionery has been associated with congestive heart failure, pulmonary edema, myopathy, pseudoaldosteronism, hypokalemic rhabdomyolysis (secondary to chronic glycyrrhizic acid intoxication), and generalized edema.

In a trial designed to study the effect of prolonged ingestion, graded doses of dried, aqueous extract of licorice root (corresponding to 108 to 814 mg GA/day) were administered to healthy volunteers of both sexes for 4 weeks. Only the highest doses of licorice (corresponding to 380 and 814 mg GA) led to adverse effects, and in most of these cases, subclinical disease (arterial hypertension) or oral contraceptive use was also involved. The adverse effects were less common and less pronounced than what had been previously reported after taking GL alone or in confectionery products.

Dosage

Dose per day	Dose per week
2-6 ml of 1:1 liquid extract*	15-40 ml of 1:1 liquid extract*
1.5-4.5 ml of 1:1 high-GL liquid extract (3% to 4% glycyrrhizin)**	10-30 ml of 1:1 high-GL liquid extract (3% to 4% glycyrrhizin)**

Extracts providing quantified levels of GL are recommended. Ideally, high-grade extracts should contain not less than 30 mg/ml of GL.

Licorice *continued on page 314*

*This dose range is extrapolated from the British Pharmacopoeia 1973, the British Herbal Pharmacopoeia 1983, and the author's education and experience.
**This dose range is extrapolated from the licorice extract dosage and literature on the pharmacologic activity of the constituent GL.

Higher doses of licorice should not be consumed long term. The Commission E advises that licorice should not be taken for longer than 6 to 8 weeks without professional supervision.

SUPPORTING INFORMATION

Traditional Prescribing

Traditional Western herbal medicine uses include:
- Reducing the irritation of mucous surfaces of the urinary, respiratory, and digestive tracts[2]
- Bronchial catarrh, bronchitis, chronic gastritis, gastric or duodenal ulcer, colic[3]
- Adrenal insufficiency, Addison's disease[3]
- Rheumatism, arthritis[4]

Uses and properties from TCM include:
- Deficiency of *spleen* and *stomach* marked by fatigue and weakness[5]
- Palpitations, arrhythmia[5]
- Coughing, wheezing[6]
- Painful spasms in the abdomen and legs[6]
- Reducing the toxic or drastic actions of other herbs[6]

Traditional Ayurvedic uses include:
- As a tonic and expectorant; coughs[7]
- As a demulcent for catarrhal conditions of the genitourinary tract[7]
- Stomach pain and discomfort; also as a mild laxative[7]

Pharmacologic Research

Key constituents of licorice dried root include triterpenoid saponins, especially GL, in the form of potassium and calcium salts, GA, and a wide range of flavonoids and sterols. Higher grades of licorice extracts contain a higher proportion of the GL than is contained within standard grade products. Deglycyrrhinized licorice (DGL) is a licorice preparation from which most of the GL has been removed. Carbenoxolone is a semisynthetic derivative of GA developed in the 1960s.
- In animal studies, DGL prevented ulcer development, inhibited gastric acid secretion, and protected the gastric mucosa against damage from aspirin and bile. Licorice and licorice derivatives protected against gastric ulcer induced by aspirin, ibuprofen, and ethanol in experimental models.
- GA and GL exhibited antiinflammatory effects *in vivo* after oral administration in several experimental models, including arthritis. Licorice and GL also demonstrated topical antiinflammatory activity that was comparable to prednisolone and dexamethasone in animal studies.
- GL and GA exert a powerful influence on human steroid hormone function. Oral GL inhibited the activity and production of the enzyme that converts cortisol into its inactive metabolites, which leads to significantly increased cortisol levels. Both GL and GA increase the antiinflammatory action of cortisol *in vivo*. GL has also been

Licorice *continued on page 315*

shown to antagonize some of the side effects of cortisol, such as its antigranulomatous action and its suppressive effect on ACTH synthesis and secretion and on adrenal weight. Licorice has well-documented aldosterone-like effects. Strong evidence suggests that licorice and its derivatives act in this way by altering the metabolism of certain steroid hormones.

- Oral doses of licorice helped in the recovery of total leukocyte count, lymphocyte count, and cellular immunity after irradiation in experimental models. Oral administration of *Glycyrrhiza uralensis* countered the carrageenan-induced decrease in immune complex clearance.
- Licorice extract decreased mutation frequencies induced by a series of well-known mutagens and carcinogens *in vitro* over a range of concentrations that were well below its toxic level. Oral administration of 1% aqueous extract of licorice protected against chemical carcinogen-induced lung and forestomach tumorigenesis *in vivo*.
- Licorice and its derivatives demonstrated hepatoprotective activity *in vivo* after oral administration. Oral doses of licorice exhibited choleretic activity in experimental models.
- GL has antiviral effects *in vitro* and *in vivo* by intraperitoneal injection, but GA does not. As GL is converted to GA after oral ingestion, only topical antiviral uses, rather than systemic, are indicated. GL was particularly active against HSV, varicella-zoster virus, and HIV *in vitro*.
- Licorice flavonoids demonstrated significant antimicrobial activity *in vitro*. Oral administration of a licorice flavonoid conferred protection against *Plasmodium yoelii* infection.
- Carbenoxolone enhanced the defense mechanism of the bladder and inhibited bacterial adherence to the injured epithelium *in vivo* by intramuscular injection.
- Oral doses of GA demonstrated an antitussive effect similar to codeine.
- Oral intake of licorice reduced hyperphagia, polydipsia, and sorbitol levels in diabetic experimental models.

Clinical Studies

- Well-controlled clinical trials have shown DGL (2.3 to 3.8 g/day for 12 to 16 weeks) combined with antacids is as efficacious at healing gastric and duodenal ulcers as carbenoxolone, cimetidine, and ranitidine.
- Early uncontrolled trials demonstrated the curative effects of licorice on peptic ulcers. Unfortunately, a high percentage of patients developed side effects associated with sodium retention. In one trial, approximately 7 g of licorice juice-paste was administered daily. Side effects might have been countered by a low-sodium diet, unless the patient was taking doses in excess of 40 g of licorice daily.
- Licorice extract demonstrated a dramatic effect in maintaining electrolyte equilibrium in patients with Addison's disease. The daily dose ranged from 10 to 30 g of licorice extract. If adrenal cortex function was severely impaired, licorice was not a suitable treatment on its own but had a synergistic action with cortisone.

Licorice continued on page 316

- In uncontrolled studies, licorice combined with white peony lowered the LH/FSH ratio, reduced ovarian testosterone production, and induced regular ovulation in patients with polycystic ovary syndrome. This combination contained equal amounts of licorice and white peony. Doses equivalent to 4 to 8 g per day of each herb were prescribed for 2 to 24 weeks.

- Licorice and white peony combination is approved for use in clinical practice in Japan and has been used to treat acute muscle cramps and dysmenorrhea. Doses equivalent to 6 g per day of each herb are prescribed.[8]

- A substantial and significant drop in serum testosterone and a smaller significant increase in 17-hydroxyprogesterone was observed in a clinical study in which seven normal men received 7 g per day of a licorice extract containing 0.5 g of GL. Serum androstenedione was also raised, but the difference did not achieve statistical significance.[9] The possibility exists that excessive intake of licorice may cause decreased libido, but this is unlikely to result from its informed use as a therapeutic agent at the doses recommended in this monograph. In a more recent clinical trial, researchers twice failed to replicate the previously listed results. The authors identified differences between their methods and those of the previous study and possible statistical anomalies (including inappropriate use of statistical tests) in the earlier report.[10]

- In an uncontrolled trial, Glyke (a patented preparation made from *G. uralensis*) improved the T-lymphocyte CD4/CD8 ratio and CD4 counts in patients with HIV. An oral dose of 120 mg per day was given for 3 to 6 months. In an open study, HIV-positive hemophiliacs treated with GL (150 to 225 mg/day for 3 to 7 years) remained asymptomatic, but untreated controls showed decreases in T-lymphocyte counts.

- Results of a clinical trial in which GL was administered intravenously to hemophiliacs with AIDS suggest that GL by this route might inhibit HIV-1 replication *in vivo*.

- In a small uncontrolled study, GL (150 mg/day) was observed to be a safe treatment for hyperkalemia resulting from selective hypoaldosteronism in non-insulin–dependent diabetes mellitus. This dose of GL correlates to approximately 3 to 5 g per day of licorice.

- The successful treatment of chronic fatigue syndrome by licorice was reported in a case study. The daily dose of licorice was dissolved in milk (2.5 g/500 ml).

- Improvement of mouth ulcers was seen after 1 day, with complete healing in 3 days, when DGL was used in an uncontrolled trial. Patients were advised to gargle four times daily for 7 days with powdered DGL (200 mg per capsule) dissolved in 200 ml of warm water. In a double-blind, crossover trial, a carbenoxolone mouthwash significantly reduced the number of recurrent ulcers and associated discomfort.

- A controlled trial found GL application after 3 days reduced dental plaque. One side of the mouth was treated, and the other side served as the control.

Licorice *continued on page 317*

- The antiviral drug idoxuridine (0.2%) incorporated in a GL gel was significantly better than a regular 0.5% idoxuridine ointment at reducing pain and increasing healing in patients with herpes lesions of the lips and nose. Carbenoxolone cream was better than placebo for treating initial and recurrent herpes genitalis in a double-blind study.
- An ointment containing crude licorice powder yielded good results in treating chronic eczema. Topical application of licorice extract demonstrated appreciable activity in patients with melasma (increased melanin pigmentation).
- In Germany, the Commission E supports using licorice to treat catarrh of the upper respiratory tract and gastric and duodenal ulcers.[11]

REFERENCES

Except when specifically referenced, the following book was referred to in the compilation of the pharmacologic and clinical information: Mills S, Bone K: *Principles and Practice of Phytotherapy: Modern Herbal Medicine,* Edinburgh, 2000, Churchill Livingstone.

1 Strandberg TE et al: Birth outcome in relation to licorice consumption during pregnancy, *Am J Epidemiol* 153:1085, 2001.
2 Felter HW, Lloyd JU: *King's American dispensatory,* ed 18, rev 3, Portland, 1905, reprinted 1983, Eclectic Medical Publications.
3 British Herbal Medicine Association's Scientific Committee: *British herbal pharmacopoeia,* Bournemouth, 1983, BHMA.
4 British Herbal Medicine Association: *British herbal compendium,* Bournemouth, 1992, BHMA.
5 Pharmacopoeia Commission of the People's Republic of China: *Pharmacopoeia of the People's Republic of China,* English ed, Beijing, 1997, Chemical Industry Press.
6 Bensky D, Gamble A: *Chinese herbal medicine materia medica,* Seattle, 1986, Eastland Press.
7 Chopra RN et al: *Chopra's indigenous drugs of India,* ed 2, Calcutta, 1958, reprinted 1982, Academic Publishers.
8 Yamada K et al: *J Clin Psychopharmacol* 19(4):380-381, 1999.
9 Armanini D, Bonanni G, Palermo M: *N Engl J Med* 341(15):1158, 1999.
10 Josephs RA et al: *Lancet* 358(9293):1613-1614, 2001.
11 Blumenthal M et al, eds: *The complete German Commission E monographs: therapeutic guide to herbal medicines,* Austin, 1998, American Botanical Council.

LIME FLOWERS

Other Common Names:	Linden flower, lime blossom
Botanical Name:	*Tilia* spp.
Family:	Tiliaceae
Plant Part Used:	Flower

PRESCRIBING INFORMATION

Actions

Spasmolytic, peripheral vasodilator, mild sedative, diaphoretic

Potential Indications

Based on appropriate evaluation of the patient, practitioners should consider prescribing lime flowers in formulations in the context of:

- The common cold, cold-related coughs *(4,5)*
- Catarrhal respiratory conditions, feverish conditions *(5)*
- Anxiety, restlessness, insomnia, headache, hypertension *(5)*
- Palpitations *(6)*

Contraindications

None known.

Warnings and Precautions

None required.

Interactions

Lime flowers infusion reduced the absorption of iron by 52% from a bread meal (compared with a water control) in adult volunteers. The inhibition was dose-dependent and related to its polyphenol content (phenolic acids, monomeric flavonoids, polymerized polyphenols). Inhibition by black tea was 79% to 94%.[1] This finding indicates a potential interaction for concomitant administration of lime flowers during iron intake. In anemia and cases for which iron supplementation is required, lime flowers should not be taken simultaneously with meals or iron supplements.

Use in Pregnancy and Lactation

No adverse effects expected.

Side Effects

Allergic contact sensitivity to lime flowers extract has been reported.[2,3]

Dosage

Dose per day*	Dose per week*
2.0-4.5 ml of 1:2 liquid extract	15-30 ml of 1:2 liquid extract

SUPPORTING INFORMATION

Traditional Prescribing

Traditional Western herbal medicine uses include:

- Hypertension; headache, migraine; the common cold, fever, catarrhal conditions; nervous conditions, restlessness; dyspepsia, indigestion[4,5]
- To promote rest and sleep[5]; palpitations[6]

Lime Flowers continued on page 319

*This dose range is extrapolated from the British Herbal Pharmacopoeia 1983, the British Herbal Compendium 1992, and the author's education and experience.

Pharmacologic Research

The most commonly used species of Tilia in Western herbal medicine are *T. cordata* and *T. platyphyllos*.[7] *Tilia europaea,* also referenced, is listed as a variety and subspecies of *T. platyphyllos,* among other species. Other species of Tilia may also be appropriate; for example, the Eclectics used *T. tomentosa* (Latin American) and *T. americana.*

Lime flowers contain essential oil and flavonoids.[8]

- Polysaccharides from *Tilia cordata* showed moderate bioadhesion to isolated epithelial tissue.[9] The mucilage in lime flowers has emollient activity.[10]
- A complex fraction isolation from the aqueous extract of *Tilia tomentosa* demonstrated an anxiolytic effect in an experimental model after intraperitoneal injection. The fraction most likely contained flavonoids.[11] Inhalation of essential oil of lime flowers produced sedative effects in an experimental model.[12]
- Lime flowers extract mildly promoted iron absorption in isolated intestinal segment, which contrasts with the study quoted in the "Interactions" section.[13]
- Aqueous extract of *Tilia europaea* inhibited muscimol binding to synaptic membranes and stimulated chloride uptake by synaptoneurosomes. These results suggest that the extract contained a compound with affinity for the competitive binding site of the $GABA_A$ receptor-complex. At high concentrations, the extract displaced flunitrazepam (a benzodiazepine drug) bound to synaptic membranes. Benzodiazepine-like substances may be responsible for this activity. Although the GABA content of the extract might explain the displacement of muscimol, it does not explain the decrease in flunitrazepam binding or the *in vivo* sedative effect demonstrated for lime flowers.[14]
- In an earlier study, lime flowers extracts that inhibited the binding of flunitrazepam to synaptic membrane were found to contain benzodiazepine-like compounds, as evidenced by their specific interaction with a monoclonal antibody against benzodiazepines.[15]

Clinical Studies

- *Tilia sylvestris* extract accelerated the healing time of artificially induced skin abrasion in volunteers.[16]
- In Germany, the Commission E supports using lime flowers to treat the common cold and cold-related coughs.[17]

REFERENCES

1 Hurrell RF, Reddy M, Cook JD: *Br J Nutr* 81(4):289-295, 1999.
2 Picardo M et al: *Contact Dermatitis* 19(1):72-73, 1988.
3 de Smet PAGM et al, eds: *Adverse effects of herbal drugs,* Berlin, 1993, Springer-Verlag.
4 British Herbal Medicine Association's Scientific Committee: *British herbal pharmacopoeia,* Bournemouth, 1983, BHMA.
5 Felter HW, Lloyd JU: *King's American dispensatory,* ed 18, rev 3, Portland, 1905, reprinted 1983, Eclectic Medical Publications.
6 Grieve M: *A modern herbal,* New York, 1971, Dover Publications.
7 British Herbal Medicine Association: *British herbal compendium,* Bournemouth, 1992, BHMA.
8 Bisset NG, ed: *Herbal drugs and phytopharmaceuticals,* Stuttgart, 1994, Medpharm Scientific Publishers.

Lime Flowers *continued on page 320*

9 Schmidgall J, Schnetz E, Hensel A: *Planta Med* 66(1):48-53, 2000.

10 Kanschat H, Lander C: *Pharm Ztg* 129:370-373, 1984.

11 Viola H et al: *J Ethnopharmacol* 44(1):47-53, 1994.

12 Buchbauer G, Jirovetz L, Jager W: *Arch Pharm* 325(4):247-248, 1992.

13 el-Shobaki FA, Saleh ZA, Saleh N: *Z Ernahrungswiss* 29(4):264-269, 1990.

14 Cavadas C et al: *Phytother Res* 11(1):17-21, 1997.

15 Medina JH et al: *Biochem Biophys Res Commun* 165(2):547-553, 1989.

16 Fleischner AM: *Cosmet Toiletries* 100:54-55, 1985.

17 Blumenthal M et al, eds: *The complete German Commission E monographs: therapeutic guide to herbal medicines,* Austin, 1998, American Botanical Council.

MARSHMALLOW

Botanical Name: *Althaea officinalis*
Family: Malvaceae
Plant Parts Used: Root, leaf

PRESCRIBING INFORMATION

Actions

Marshmallow root and leaf: demulcent, urinary demulcent, emollient

Potential Indications

Based on appropriate evaluation of the patient, practitioners should consider prescribing marshmallow root in formulations in the context of:
- Irritations of the oral, pharyngeal, or gastric mucosa, dry cough *(4,5)*
- Gastric or peptic ulcer, enteritis *(5)*
- Cystitis, urinary tract infections in general *(5)*
- Topical treatment for varicose ulcers, wounds, burns *(5)*

Based on appropriate evaluation of the patient, practitioners should consider prescribing marshmallow leaf in formulations in the context of:
- Irritations of the oral and pharyngeal mucosa, dry cough *(4)*
- Bronchitis, respiratory tract catarrh *(5)*
- Cystitis, urethritis, urinary gravel or calculus *(5)*
- Topical treatment for abscesses, boils, and ulcers *(5)*

Contraindications

None known.

Warnings and Precautions

The absorption of other medications taken simultaneously with marshmallow root may be retarded.[1] Simultaneous ingestion of drug medications and marshmallow root should therefore be avoided.

Interactions

None known.

Use in Pregnancy and Lactation

No adverse effects expected.

Side Effects

None expected if taken within the recommended dose range.

Dosage

Root:

Dose per day*	Dose per week*
3-6 ml of 1:5 tincture	20-40 ml of 1:5 tincture
3-6 ml of 1:5 glycetract	20-40 ml of 1:5 glycetract

Leaf:

Dose per day**	Dose per week**
3-6 ml of 1:2 liquid extract	20-40 ml of 1:2 liquid extract

Marshmallow *continued on page 322*

---

*This dose range is extrapolated from the British *Pharmaceutical Codex* 1949, the British *Herbal Pharmacopoeia* 1983, the British *Herbal Compendium* 1992, and the author's education and experience.
**This dose range is extrapolated from the British *Herbal Pharmacopoeia* 1983 and the author's education and experience.

Traditional Prescribing

Traditional Western herbal medicine uses of marshmallow root include:
- Diseases of the mucous membranes, such as hoarseness, catarrh, pneumonia, and other respiratory complaints, gonorrhea, vesical catarrh, renal irritation, acute dysentery, diarrhea[2]
- Strangury (pain in the urethra), inflammation of the bladder, hematuria, retention of urine, some forms of gravel, and most kidney or bladder infections[2]
- Gastrointestinal irritation and inflammation,[2] specially gastric or duodenal ulcer[3]
- Topically for varicose ulcers,[3] inflammatory lesions, swellings, wounds, bruises, and scalds[2]

Traditional Western herbal medicine uses of marshmallow leaf include:
- Bronchitis, respiratory catarrh[3]
- Cystitis, urethritis, urinary gravel or calculus[3]
- Topically for abscesses, boils, ulcers[3]

Pharmacologic Research

The roots and leaves of marshmallow contain mucilage, consisting of acidic polysaccharides.[4] Ethanol-water extracts of both marshmallow leaf and root will extract some of the mucilage in the starting herb, although mucilage is sparingly soluble in such mixtures. In the case of the root, which contains a much higher concentration of mucilage than the leaf, a glycerol-water combination is preferable for extraction given that mucilage is more soluble in this medium.
- The results of an *in vitro* study suggest that the adhesive effects of certain plant-derived polysaccharides to mucous membranes may account, in part, for the therapeutic effects of mucilage-containing plants in treating irritated buccal membranes. Polysaccharides from marshmallow root demonstrated moderate bioadhesion to epithelial tissue.[5]
- Cold macerate of marshmallow root inhibited esophageal mucociliary transport *in vitro*.[6]
- In an experimental model, oral administration of an extract of marshmallow root or the polysaccharide fraction demonstrated significant antitussive activity, depressing the cough resulting from both laryngopharyngeal and tracheobronchial stimulation. This study provides indirect evidence that a soothing action on the upper gastrointestinal mucosa causes reflex soothing of the respiratory tract, leading to bronchodilation and reduced tendency to cough.[7]
- Extracts of marshmallow root demonstrated potential antiinflammatory and immunomodulatory effects *in vitro*,[8] but lack of antiinflammatory activity was observed after oral administration of marshmallow root in carrageenan-induced rat paw edema.[9] The *in vivo* antiinflammatory effect of an ointment containing both marshmallow root extract and dexamethasone was superior to that of the individual ingredients.[10]

Marshmallow *continued on page 323*

Clinical Studies

No clinical studies using marshmallow root or leaf have been found.
- In Germany, the Commission E supports using marshmallow root and leaf to treat irritation of the oral and pharyngeal mucosa and associated dry cough and marshmallow root to treat mild inflammation of the gastric mucosa.[11]
- ESCOP recommends marshmallow root for treating dry cough and irritations of the oral, pharyngeal, or gastric mucosa.[1]

REFERENCES

1 Scientific Committee of the European Scientific Cooperative on Phytotherapy [ESCOP]: *ESCOP monographs: Althaeae radix*. European Scientific Cooperative on Phytotherapy, ESCOP Secretariat, Argyle House, Gandy Street, Exeter, Devon, EX4 3LS, United Kingdom, March 1996.

2 Felter HW, Lloyd JU: *King's American dispensatory*, ed 18, rev 3, Portland, 1905, reprinted 1983, Eclectic Medical Publications.

3 British Herbal Medicine Association's Scientific Committee: *British herbal pharmacopoeia*, Bournemouth, 1983, BHMA.

4 Bisset NG, ed: *Herbal drugs and phytopharmaceuticals*, Stuttgart, 1994, Medpharm Scientific Publishers.

5 Schmidgall J, Schnetz E, Hensel A: *Planta Med* 66(1):48-53, 2000.

6 Muller-Limmroth W, Frohlich HH: *Fortschr Med* 98:95-101, 1980.

7 Nosal'ova G et al: *Pharmazie* 47:224-226, 1992.

8 Scheffer J, Konig W: 3rd Phytotherapy Congress, Lubeck-Travemunde, October 3-6, 1991, abstract P9.

9 Mascolo N et al: *Phytother Res* 1:28-31, 1987.

10 Beaune A, Balea T: *Therapie* 21:341-347, 1966.

11 Blumenthal M et al, eds: *The complete German Commission E monographs: therapeutic guide to herbal medicines*, Austin, 1998, American Botanical Council.

MEADOWSWEET

Botanical Name: *Filipendula ulmaria*
Family: Rosaceae
Plant Part Used: Aerial parts

Actions

Antacid, antiinflammatory, mild urinary antiseptic, astringent

Potential Indications

Based on appropriate evaluation of the patient, practitioners should consider prescribing meadowsweet in formulations in the context of:
- Gastric ulcer *(5,7)*
- Dyspepsia, hyperacidity, heartburn, diarrhea, irritable bowel syndrome *(5)*
- Genitourinary tract disorders, such as cervicitis, vaginitis, leukorrhea, cystitis, and *dysuria (5)*
- Fever; arthritic and rheumatic *conditions (5)*
- Possible benefit by topical application for cervical dysplasia and to protect and repair the mucosa of the vagina and cervix *(4)*

Contraindications

None known.

Warnings and Precautions

Meadowsweet contains salicylates and should be avoided or used with caution in patients with salicylate sensitivity.

Interactions

None known. Given the experimental anticoagulant effect, meadowsweet should be used with caution if patients are taking warfarin.

Use in Pregnancy and Lactation

No adverse effects expected.

Side Effects

None expected if taken within the recommended dose range.

Dosage

Dose per day*	Dose per week*
3-6 ml of 1:2 liquid extract	20-40 ml of 1:2 liquid extract

Traditional Prescribing

Traditional Western herbal medicine uses include:
- Atonic dyspepsia with heartburn and hyperacidity; gastric ulcer (prophylaxis and treatment), diarrhea[1]
- Fevers; genitourinary tract irritation, acute catarrhal cystitis, retention of urine resulting from enlarged prostate, chronic cervicitis, chronic vaginitis with leukorrhea[1,2]
- Rheumatic muscle and joint pains[1]

Maedowsweet *continued on page 325*

*This dose range is extrapolated from the British Herbal Pharmacopoeia 1983, the British Herbal Compendium 1992, and the author's education and experience.

Pharmacologic Research

- An *in vitro* study demonstrated that the ethyl acetate extract of meadowsweet flowers strongly inhibited the classical pathway of complement activation. This activity was also observed using methanol extracts of the herb and flower.
- The authors of an *in vitro* study suggested that the observed immunomodulatory activity may explain the therapeutic benefit of meadowsweet preparations in inflammatory diseases.
- *In vitro* studies have demonstrated antimicrobial activity against *Staphylococcus aureus haemolyticus*, *Streptococcus pyogenes haemolyticus*, *Escherichia coli*, *Shigella flexneri*, *Klebsiella pneumoniae*, and *Bacillus subtilis*. Another study suggested that water extracts of various parts of meadowsweet showed antibacterial activity and may be used on wounds.
- Decoctions of meadowsweet flowers demonstrated antiulcerogenic activity in an experimental model. Alcohol extracts and water decoctions of the flowers decreased the development of experimental erosion and ulcers *in vivo*.
- Anticoagulant activity for extracts of both meadowsweet flower and seed have been demonstrated *in vitro* and *in vivo* (orally). This action is thought to be the result of a heparinlike anticoagulant found in the plant.
- In an experimental study, local administration of a decoction of the flowers resulted in a 39% drop in the frequency of squamous cell carcinoma of the cervix and vagina.

Clinical Studies

In 48 cases of cervical dysplasia treated with an ointment containing meadowsweet, a positive result was recorded in 32 patients and complete remission in 25 cases. No recurrence was observed in 10 of the completely cured patients within 12 months.

REFERENCES

The following book was referred to in the compilation of the pharmacologic and clinical information: Mills S, Bone K: *Principles and Practice of Phytotherapy: Modern Herbal Medicine,* Edinburgh, 2000, Churchill Livingstone.

1 British Herbal Medicine Association's Scientific Committee: *British herbal pharmacopoeia,* Bournemouth, 1983, BHMA.
2 Felter HW, Lloyd JU: *King's American dispensatory,* ed 18, rev 3, Portland, 1905, reprinted 1983, Eclectic Medical Publications.

MILK THISTLE

Other Common Name: St. Mary's thistle
Botanical Name: *Silybum marianum, Carduus marianus#*
Family: Compositae
Plant Part Used: Fruit (sometimes referred to as seed)

PRESCRIBING INFORMATION

Actions

Hepatoprotective, hepatic trophorestorative, antioxidant, choleretic

Potential Indications

Based on appropriate evaluation of the patient, practitioners should consider prescribing milk thistle in formulations in the context of:
- Hepatitis, particularly for the hepatoprotective *activity (4a,6)*
- Nonalcoholic and alcoholic liver damage or disease, including abnormal liver function and fatty liver *(4a)*
- Exposure to chemical pollutants and conventional drugs *(4a)*
- Skin conditions involving liver dysfunction *(4a)*
- Dyspeptic complaints *(4)*
- Preventing gallstone formation *(4a,6)*
- Gallbladder problems *(6)*

Contraindications

None known.

Warnings and Precautions

None required.

Interactions

None known.

Use in Pregnancy and Lactation

No adverse effects expected.

Side Effects

Drug monitoring studies in 1995 investigating the concentrated extract (silymarin) indicated that adverse effects were recorded in 1% of patients, mainly as mild gastrointestinal complaints. A mild laxative effect was occasionally observed with milk thistle preparations. Two cases of anaphylactic shock have been reported.

Dosage

Dose per day*	Dose per week*
4.5-8.5 ml of 1:1 liquid extract	30-60 ml of 1:1 liquid extract
4.5-8.5 ml of 1:1 glycetract	30-60 ml of 1:1 glycetract

Extracts providing quantified levels of silymarin-silybin are recommended. Ideally, aqueous ethanol extracts should contain not less than 25 mg/ml silymarin, and aqueous glycerol extracts should contain not less than 10 mg/ml silymarin.

Higher doses should be used in more severe cases of liver damage. Milk thistle glycetract would be appropriate for patients with liver

Milk Thistle *continued on page 327*

#Alternative name.
*This dose range is extrapolated from the German Commission E monograph.[1]

damage in whom additional alcohol is not advisable. Because the absorption of silymarin is enhanced by lecithin, simultaneous lecithin supplementation is recommended.

SUPPORTING INFORMATION

Traditional Prescribing

Traditional Western herbal medicine uses include liver and gallbladder problems, including jaundice, hepatitis, and gallstones.[2,3]

Pharmacologic Research

Silymarin is a highly concentrated extract of milk thistle seed that contains up to 80% flavanolignans, such as silybin, silychristin, and silydianin (collectively described as silymarin). Standardized or quantified extracts of milk thistle often express the level of flavanolignans as "calculated as silybin." Almost all of the pharmacologic and clinical research has been conducted using this preparation. However, based on dosage considerations, extrapolating this data to the use of the galenical liquid extract (provided that the extract contains at least 25 mg of flavanolignans as silymarin per ml) is reasonable.

- Intraperitoneal administration of silymarin increased the redox state and the total glutathione content of the liver, stomach, and intestine.
- Silymarin and silybin demonstrated both prophylactic and curative hepatoprotective activity against liver damage (chemicals, heavy metals, death cap mushroom *[Amanita phalloides]*, irradiation, and viruses) in numerous *in vitro* and *in vivo* studies, via intraperitoneal and oral routes. Activity at the nuclear level (involving RNA and DNA) is probably the predominant mechanism. Antioxidant activity by scavenging free radicals is also involved.
- Silybin countered the acetaminophen (paracetamol)-induced reduction in bile flow and bile salt output.
- Silybin inhibited the growth of human ovarian and breast cancer cell lines *in vitro* and demonstrated a synergistic action with the antineoplastic drugs cisplatin and doxorubicin. Topical application of silymarin protected against carcinogen and ultraviolet light B (UVB)–induced skin tumors.
- Oral doses of silymarin resulted in antiinflammatory activity in carrageenan-induced rat paw edema. Silybin inhibited arachidonic acid metabolites *in vitro*.
- Treatment of diabetic rats with silybin did not affect hyperglycemia but prevented the inhibition of protein mono-ADP-ribosylation. Silybin treatment helped prevent substance P–like immunoreactivity loss in the sciatic nerve, typical of diabetic neuropathy.

Clinical Studies

The oral dosages used in the following clinical studies ranged from 140 to 800 mg per day of silymarin, with 420 mg per day the most commonly administered dose.

- Silymarin treatment significantly reduced serum levels of hepatic enzymes, significantly improved platelet counts, and improved nausea, discomfort, and skin itching in patients with toxic liver damage of differing origins in uncontrolled trials.

Milk Thistle *continued on page 328*

- Silymarin improved biochemical, functional, and morphologic alterations in the livers of patients with slight acute and subacute liver disease in a double-blind, placebo-controlled, clinical trial.
- Silymarin reduced lipoperoxidation of cell membranes and insulin resistance and significantly decreased insulin overproduction and the need for insulin in a controlled study involving patients with insulin-dependent diabetes and alcoholic cirrhosis.
- In other controlled studies involving patients with alcoholic liver disease, silymarin demonstrated significant reduction of hepatic enzymes and bilirubin and improvements in antioxidant and lipid peroxidation parameters. Other studies reported statistically insignificant improvements, but continuing alcohol consumption may have confounded the experimental results.
- Silymarin treatment significantly increased survival rates in patients with cirrhosis of different causes (especially alcoholic cirrhosis) in long-term, randomized, double-blind trials.
- Well-controlled clinical studies of the treatment of various types of hepatitis with silymarin have produced mixed results, with some studies demonstrating significant reductions in serum liver enzymes and bilirubin and others not.
- Silymarin, given preoperatively and postoperatively, prevented the increase of serum hepatic enzymes induced by the toxic effect of general anesthesia.
- In a randomized, double-blind, placebo-controlled study, silymarin reduced the lipoperoxidative hepatic damage that occurs during psychotropic drug treatment.
- Silymarin improved liver function in patients with occupational toxic liver damage caused by exposure to halogenated hydrocarbons, solvents, paints, and glues in uncontrolled and placebo-controlled trials.
- Silymarin protected against histologic changes in the livers of pregnant women and those taking oral contraceptives.
- In both cholelithiasis and cholecystectomized patients, silymarin reduced biliary cholesterol concentration and bile saturation compared with placebo.
- In Germany, the Commission E supports using galenical preparations of milk thistle to treat dyspeptic complaints. Extracts standardized to contain at least 70% silymarin are recommended for toxic liver damage, as supportive treatment in chronic inflammatory liver disease, and for hepatic cirrhosis.[1]
- Milk thistle is official in the USP24-NF19.

REFERENCES

Except when specifically referenced, the following book was referred to in the compilation of the pharmacologic and clinical information: Mills S, Bone K: *Principles and Practice of Phytotherapy: Modern Herbal Medicine,* Edinburgh, 2000, Churchill Livingstone.

1 Blumenthal M et al, eds: *The complete German Commission E monographs: therapeutic guide to herbal medicines,* Austin, 1998, American Botanical Council.
2 Madaus G: *Lehrbuch der biologischen heilmittel,* Band I, Hildesheim, Germany, 1976, Georg Olms Verlag.
3 Grieve M: *A modern herbal,* New York, 1971, Dover Publications.

MISTLETOE

Other Common Name:	European mistletoe
Botanical Name:	*Viscum album*
Family:	Viscaceae
Plant Part Used:	Aerial parts

PRESCRIBING INFORMATION

Actions
Hypotensive, peripheral vasodilator, mild sedative

Potential Indications
Based on appropriate evaluation of the patient, practitioners should consider prescribing mistletoe in formulations in the context of:
- Hypertension, tachycardia, cardiac hypertrophy, atherosclerosis (5)
- Epilepsy, nervous excitability (6)

Contraindications
None known.

Warnings and Precautions
None required.

Interactions
None known.

Use in Pregnancy and Lactation
No adverse effects expected.

Eclectic practitioners used large and frequent doses of a preparation of the fresh plant to facilitate labor.[1]

Side Effects
None expected if taken within the recommended dose range. A review of data collected from 1985 to 1992 indicated that the accidental ingestion of mistletoe in the United States is not associated with profound toxicity.[2] The only literature referring to side effects is for fresh mistletoe extracts given by injection.

Dosage

*Dose per day**	*Dose per week**
3-6 ml of 1:2 liquid extract	20-40 ml of 1:2 liquid extract

SUPPORTING INFORMATION

Traditional Prescribing
Traditional Western herbal medicine uses include:
- As a gentle hypotensive suitable for long-term use; hypertension, arteriosclerosis, nervous tachycardia, hypertensive headache, chorea[3,4]
- Epilepsy,[5] nervous excitability[6]

Although Eclectic physicians referred to the use of *Viscum album,* whether this species was actually being used is debatable. These physicians were probably using *V. flavescens,* which is botanically distinct from *V. album.*

Mistletoe *continued on page 330*

*This dose range is extrapolated from the British Herbal Pharmacopoeia 1983 and the author's education and experience.

Pharmacologic Research

Dried mistletoe herb contains lectins, proteins, and polypeptides (viscotoxins), as well as polysaccharides, phenylpropanes, and lignans,[7] although the constituents depend on the host tree on which the mistletoe grew, the location, and in which season it was harvested. Mistletoe extracts vary in the constituents they contain depending on the type of extract and the process used in manufacture.[8] Aqueous alcoholic extracts are unlikely to contain the lectins or proteins,[9] and if the viscotoxins are present, they are decomposed in the gut and not absorbed intact. (This action substantially reduces the potential toxicity of mistletoe aqueous alcoholic extracts when taken orally.)[7]

The results of experimental studies into the hypotensive activity of mistletoe are contradictory.[7] Many studies,[10,11] if not all, used administration by injection. Aqueous extracts were the most active, and a comparative study indicated that the highest activity was demonstrated by an extract of mistletoe grown on *Salix* spp. Suggested mechanisms of action involved inhibiting the excitability of the medulla oblongata vasomotor center and cholinomimetic activity. (This study most likely used administration by injection.)[12]

Clinical Studies

Aqueous mistletoe extracts (which contain lectins) have been used clinically by injection for immune stimulation for many years, particularly in Europe. The concept of using fermented mistletoe extracts for cancer therapy was advocated by Rudolf Steiner in 1916. However, because these extracts or their isolated constituents were administered by injection, the results are not relevant to the clinical use of oral aqueous alcoholic extracts of mistletoe and have not been reported here.

REFERENCES

1 Ellingwood F, Lloyd JU: *American materia medica, therapeutics and pharmacognosy,* ed 11, Portland, 1983, Eclectic Medical Publications.
2 Krenzelok EP, Jacobsen TD, Aronis J: *Am J Emerg Med* 15(5):516-520, 1997.
3 Weiss RF: *Herbal medicine,* English ed, Beaconsfield, UK, 1988, Beaconsfield Publishers.
4 British Herbal Medicine Association's Scientific Committee: *British herbal pharmacopoeia,* Bournemouth, 1983, BHMA.
5 Leclerc H: *Precis de phytotherapie,* ed 5, Paris, 1983, Masson.
6 Bartram T: *Encyclopedia of herbal medicine,* ed 1, Dorset, UK, 1995, Grace Publishers.
7 Bisset NG, ed: *Herbal drugs and phytopharmaceuticals,* Stuttgart, 1994, Medpharm Scientific Publishers.
8 Kleijnen J, Knipschild P: *Phytomed* 1(3):255-260, 1994.
9 Pizzorno JE, Murray MT, eds: *A textbook of natural medicine,* ed 2, Edinburgh, 1999, Churchill Livingstone.
10 Fukunaga T et al: *Yakugaku Zasshi* 109(8):600-605, 1989.
11 Becker H: *Dtsch Apoth Ztg* 126:1229, 1986.
12 Petkov V: *Am J Chin Med* 7:197-236, 1979.

MOTHERWORT

Botanical Name: Leonurus cardiaca
Family: Labiatae
Plant Part Used: Aerial parts

PRESCRIBING INFORMATION

Actions

Nervine tonic, cardiotonic, hypotensive, antiarrhythmic, antithyroid, spasmolytic, emmenagogue

Potential Indications

Based on appropriate evaluation of the patient, practitioners should consider prescribing motherwort in formulations in the context of:
- Adjuvant therapy for hyperthyroidism (4,6)
- Nervous cardiac disorders such as palpitations (4,5)
- Coronary heart disease (4)
- Anxiety, neuralgia, chorea (5)
- Amenorrhea, dysmenorrhea, ovarian pain (5)

Contraindications

Pregnancy.[1]

Warnings and Precautions

None required.

Interactions

None known.

Use in Pregnancy and Lactation

Contraindicated in pregnancy.

Side Effects

None expected if taken within the recommended dose range.

Dosage

Dose per day*	Dose per week*
2.0-3.5 ml of 1:2 liquid extract	15-25 ml of 1:2 liquid extract

SUPPORTING INFORMATION

Traditional Prescribing

Traditional Western herbal medicine uses include:
- Heart disease, cardiac debility, tachycardia, effort syndrome[2]
- Female reproductive problems, including amenorrhea, uterine, and period pain[3]
- Nervous conditions, hysteria, chorea (characterized by involuntary, jerky movements), neuralgia, spinal disorders[3]
- Antithyroid activity for mild hyperthyroidism[4]

Motherwort is considered in European herbal medicine as having antithyroid activity. Being less powerful than orthodox drugs, motherwort is used for mild thyroid hyperfunction and can be used for long-term treatment.[4]

Motherwort *continued on page 332*

*This dose range is extrapolated from the British Herbal Pharmacopoeia 1983, the British Herbal Compendium 1992, and the author's education and experience.

331

Pharmacologic Research

- Motherwort extracts demonstrated hypotensive activity when administered by injection in normal and hypertensive experimental models.[5]
- In early research, a mild sedative effect was demonstrated for motherwort extracts. The effect on intestine and uterus was very slight stimulation.[6] Motherwort extract has also demonstrated antispasmodic activity.[7]
- Leonurine, an alkaloid present in motherwort, is described as the uterotonic principle of the Leonurus species used in TCM.[8,9]
- From Chinese research, an undefined species of Leonurus by injection decreased the development of acute ischemic cerebral edema and reduced disorders of monoamine metabolism and mortality in an experimental model.[10]

Clinical Studies

- Motherwort has been used in China in treating coronary heart disease with favorable results. The species of Leonurus and route of administration were undefined.[10]
- In Germany, the Commission E supports using motherwort to treat nervous cardiac disorders and as an adjuvant therapy for thyroid hyperfunction.[11]

REFERENCES

1 British Herbal Medicine Association: *British herbal compendium,* Bournemouth, 1992, BHMA.

2 British Herbal Medicine Association's Scientific Committee: *British herbal pharmacopoeia,* Bournemouth, 1983, BHMA.

3 Felter HW, Lloyd JU: *King's American dispensatory,* ed 18, rev 3, Portland, 1905, reprinted 1983, Eclectic Medical Publications.

4 Weiss RF: *Herbal medicine,* English ed, Beaconsfield, UK, 1988, Beaconsfield Publishers.

5 Arustamova FA: *Izv Akad Nauk Arm SSR Biol Nauki* 16(7):47-52, 1963.

6 Erspamer LV: *Arch Int Pharmacodyn* 76:132-152, 1948.

7 Isaev I, Bojadzieva M: *Nauchni Tr Visshiya Med Inst Sofiya* 37(5):145-152, 1960.

8 Cheng KF et al: *Experientia* 35(5):571-572, 1979.

9 Kong YC et al: *Am J Chin Med* 4(4):373-382, 1976.

10 Kuang PG et al: *J Tradit Chin Med* 8(1):37-40, 1988.

11 Blumenthal M et al, eds: *The complete German Commission E monographs: therapeutic guide to herbal medicines,* Austin, 1998, American Botanical Council.

MULLEIN

Botanical Name: *Verbascum thapsus*
Family: Scrophulariaceae
Plant Part Used: Leaf

PRESCRIBING INFORMATION

Actions

Expectorant, demulcent, anticatarrhal, vulnerary

Potential Indications

Based on appropriate evaluation of the patient, practitioners should consider prescribing mullein in formulations in the context of:
- Acute or chronic bronchitis, tracheitis, the common cold, influenza, respiratory catarrh, tonsillitis (5)
- Gastrointestinal conditions requiring demulcency, such as ulceration, diarrhea, and hemorrhoids (5)

Contraindications

None known.

Warnings and Precautions

None required.

Interactions

None known.

Use in Pregnancy and Lactation

No adverse effects expected.

Side Effects

None expected if taken within the recommended dose range.

Dosage

Dose per day*	**Dose per week***
4.5-8.5 ml of 1:2 liquid extract	30-60 ml of 1:2 liquid extract

SUPPORTING INFORMATION

Traditional Prescribing

Traditional Western herbal medicine uses include:
- Bronchitis, particularly with hard cough; the common cold, influenza, respiratory catarrh, inflammation of the larynx or trachea, tuberculosis[1,2]
- Diarrhea, dysentery, hemorrhoids[2], intestinal bleeding[3]
- As a poultice for sore throat, tonsillitis, mumps[2]; oil infusion topically for inflamed mucosa, hemorrhoids, ulcers[1,2]

Native Americans used mullein leaf mainly in external applications and smoked to relieve asthma and sore throat. Other uses included inhalation of fumes from smoke smudge for catarrh and as a leaf poultice for pain, swelling, sprains, bruises, wounds, and headache. Mullein leaf was official in the NF from 1916 to 1936 and was used as a demulcent and emollient.[4]

Mullein *continued on page 334*

*This dose range is extrapolated from the British Herbal Pharmacopoeia 1983 and the author's education and experience.

Pharmacologic Research

No pharmacologic information has been found for mullein leaf.

Clinical Studies

No clinical studies using mullein leaf have been found.

REFERENCES

1 British Herbal Medicine Association's Scientific Committee: *British herbal pharmacopoeia,* Bournemouth, 1983, BHMA.
2 Felter HW, Lloyd JU: *King's American dispensatory,* ed 18, rev 3, Portland, 1905, reprinted 1983, Eclectic Medical Publications.
3 Grieve M: *A modern herbal,* New York, 1971, Dover Publications.
4 Vogel VJ: *American Indian medicine,* Norman, Okla, 1970, University of Oklahoma Press.

MYRRH

Botanical Names: *Commiphora molmol, Commiphora myrrha*[+]
Other species of Commiphora with comparable chemical composition
may be used.
Family: Burseraceae
Plant Part Used: Resin (oleo-gum resin) obtained from the stem

PRESCRIBING INFORMATION

Actions

Astringent, antimicrobial, antibacterial, antiinflammatory, vulnerary

Potential Indications

Based on appropriate evaluation of the patient, practitioners should
consider prescribing myrrh in formulations in the context of:
- Chronic bronchitis, the common cold, chronic catarrh; inflammation
  of the mouth and throat *(5)*
- Gastritis, dyspepsia; amenorrhea, leukorrhea *(5)*
- Topical treatment for inflammations of the mouth and throat, skin
  inflammations, wounds, abrasions *(4,5)*

Contraindications

Known allergy.

According to TCM, myrrh is contraindicated in pregnancy and in cases
of excessive uterine bleeding.[1]

Warnings and Precautions

Depending on the level of dilution of the tincture, a transient burning
sensation on the skin or mucous membranes may be experienced.
Myrrh should not be ingested for prolonged periods (more than a few
weeks) because of the potential of allergic contact dermatitis.

Interactions

None known.

Use in Pregnancy and Lactation

Contraindicated in pregnancy.

Side Effects

Allergic contact dermatitis has been reported from using myrrh.[2,3] For
this reason, internal use should be restricted to short-term use.

Dosage

Dose per day*	Dose per week*
1.5-4.5 ml of 1:5 tincture	10-30 ml of 1:5 tincture

SUPPORTING INFORMATION

Traditional Prescribing

Traditional Western herbal medicine uses include:
- Mouth ulcers, pharyngitis, gingivitis, laryngitis, respiratory catarrh,
  the common cold, chronic catarrh, bronchitis, excessive mucous
  secretion, boils[4,5]

Myrrh *continued on page 336*

[+]Medicinally interchangeable species.
*This dose range is interpreted from the British Herbal Pharmacopoeia 1983, British Pharmaceutical Codex 1934 and 1973, and the author's education and
experience.

- Chronic gastritis, atonic dyspepsia; amenorrhea, female reproductive tract disorders accompanied by a dragging sensation and leukorrhea[5]
- Topically for damaged gums, wounds, abrasions, poorly healing skin ulcers, and sinusitis[4-6]

Uses and properties from TCM include:
- Invigorating the *blood*, dispersing *congealed blood*, reducing swelling, and alleviating pain; thus used to treat trauma, sores, boils, swelling, abdominal masses or pain, chest pain, amenorrhea[1]
- Topically for chronic poorly healing sores[1]

Traditional Ayurvedic uses include:
- Dyspepsia, chlorosis (hypochromic anemia), amenorrhea, uterine disorders, menstrual disorders in young girls, chronic bronchitis, tuberculosis[7]
- A mouthwash for mouth ulcers and sore throat[7]

Pharmacologic Research

Myrrh oleo-gum resin contains an essential oil containing sesquiterpenes and a resin fraction containing commiphoric acids and esters.[8]
- A sesquiterpene fraction from myrrh (a mixture of furanodiene-6-one and methoxyfuranoguaia-9-ene-8-one) demonstrated local anesthetic activity *in vivo* and showed antibacterial and antifungal activity against standard pathogenic strains of *Escherichia coli*, *Staphylococcus aureus*, *Pseudomonas aeruginosa*, and *Candida albicans*, with minimum inhibitory concentrations ranging from 0.18 to 2.8 μg/ml.[9]
- Myrrh increased glucose tolerance *in vivo* under both normal and diabetic conditions.[10] Two furanosesquiterpenes isolated from myrrh exhibited hypoglycemic activity in an experimental model of diabetes.[11]
- Myrrh exhibited strong antithrombotic activity *in vivo*.[12]
- Pretreatment with an aqueous suspension of myrrh (250 to 1000 mg/ml) protected against the ulcerogenic effects of several necrotizing agents, including ethanol and indomethacin. The protective effect of myrrh was attributed to its effect on mucus production and an increase in nucleic acid and non-protein sulfhydryl concentrations, which appears to be mediated through its free radical–scavenging, thyroid-stimulating, and prostaglandin-inducing properties.[13]
- Petroleum ether extract of myrrh (500 mg/kg, oral route) produced significant antiinflammatory activity in carrageenan-induced inflammation and cotton pellet granuloma models. Antipyretic activity was also observed *in vivo*.[14] Myrrh demonstrated significant antiinflammatory activity in the following experimental models: xylene-induced ear edema (400 mg/kg pretreatment by injection) and cotton pellet granuloma (400 mg/kg, oral).[15]
- An analgesic activity was demonstrated after oral administration of myrrh *in vivo*. The active analgesic compounds were identified as two sesquiterpenes, particularly furanoeudesma-1,3-diene. This compound was shown to bind to opioid receptors in isolated brain membrane.

Myrrh continued on page 337

Naloxone, an opioid antagonist, completely inhibited the analgesic effect of this compound by injection *in vivo*. Furanoeudesma-1,3-diene exhibited structural similarities with two opioid agonists (morphiceptin and DPDPE).[16,17]

- Treatment with myrrh was found to have an anticarcinogenic effect *in vivo* on solid tumors induced by Ehrlich carcinoma cells. The activity was comparable to the standard cytotoxic drug cyclophosphamide and was more pronounced after 25 days compared with 50 days of treatment.[18,19] Another study found that pretreatment with myrrh did not alter the biochemical and cytologic effects of cyclophosphamide and did not show any additive effect.[20]
- Both an extract and a fraction of myrrh stimulated phagocytosis *in vivo* after intraperitoneal injection.[21]

Clinical Studies

No clinical studies using myrrh have been found.
- In Germany, the Commission E supports using myrrh topically to treat mild inflammations of the oral and pharyngeal mucosa.[22]
- ESCOP recommends myrrh for the topical treatment of gingivitis, stomatitis (mouth ulcers), minor skin inflammations, minor wounds, and abrasions and as a supportive treatment for pharyngitis and tonsillitis.[23]

REFERENCES

1 Bensky D, Gamble A: *Chinese herbal medicine materia medica,* Seattle, 1986, Eastland Press.
2 Al-Suwaidan SN et al: *Contact Dermatitis* 39(3):137, 1998.
3 Gallo R et al: *Contact Dermatitis* 41(4):230-231, 1999.
4 British Herbal Medicine Association's Scientific Committee: *British herbal pharmacopoeia,* Bournemouth, 1983, BHMA.
5 Felter HW: *The eclectic materia medica, pharmacology and therapeutics,* Portland, 1922, reprinted 1983, Eclectic Medical Publications.
6 British Herbal Medicine Association: *British herbal compendium,* Bournemouth, 1992, BHMA.
7 Chopra RN et al: *Chopra's indigenous drugs of India,* ed 2, Calcutta, 1958, reprinted 1982, Academic Publishers.
8 Wagner H, Bladt S: *Plant drug analysis: a thin layer chromatography atlas,* ed 2, Berlin, 1996, Springer-Verlag.
9 Dolara P et al: *Planta Med* 66(4):356-358, 2000.
10 Al-Awadi FM, Gumaa KA: *Acta Diabetol Lat* 24(1):37-41, 1987.
11 Ubillas RP et al: *Planta Med* 65(8):778-779, 1999.
12 Olajide OA: *Phytother Res* 13(3):231-232, 1999.
13 al-Harbi MM et al: *J Ethnopharmacol* 55(2):141-150, 1997.
14 Tariq M et al: *Agents Actions* 17(3-4):381-382, 1986.
15 Atta AH, Alkofahi A: *J Ethnopharmacol* 60:117-124, 1998.
16 Dolara P et al: *Nature* 379(6560):29, 1996.
17 Dolara P et al: *Phytother Res* 10(supp 1):S81-S83, 1996.
18 al-Harbi MM et al: *Chemotherapy* 40(5):337-347, 1994.
19 Qureshi S et al: *Cancer Chemother Pharmacol* 33(2):130-138, 1993.
20 al-Harbi MM et al: *Am J Chin Med* 22(1):77-82, 1994.
21 Delaveau P, Lallouette P, Tessier AM: *Planta Med* 40(1):49-54, 1980.
22 Blumenthal M et al, eds: *The complete German Commission E monographs: therapeutic guide to herbal medicines,* Austin, 1998, American Botanical Council.
23 Scientific Committee of the European Scientific Cooperative on Phytotherapy [ESCOP]: *ESCOP monographs: Myrrha.* European Scientific Cooperative on Phytotherapy, ESCOP Secretariat, Argyle House, Gandy Street, Exeter, Devon, EX4 3LS, United Kingdom, October 1999.

NEEM LEAF

Botanical Names: *Azadirachta indica, Melia azadirachta*[#]
                        Note: *Melia azedarach* is not a medicinally interchangeable species.
Family: Meliaceae
Plant Part Used: Leaf

PRESCRIBING INFORMATION

Actions

Antimicrobial, antifungal, antiviral, antipyretic, adaptogenic, antipruritic, antitussive, depurative, antiinflammatory, anxiolytic, emmenagogue, hypoglycemic, immune-enhancing

Potential Indications

Based on appropriate evaluation of the patient, practitioners should consider prescribing neem leaf in formulations in the context of:
- Diabetes mellitus (4)
- Psoriasis, in combination with topical treatment (4)
- Skin conditions, fever, blood disorders (5)
- Allergies, hypertension, gastrointestinal disorders, hepatitis, cancer (6)
- Inflammatory conditions, enhancing immunity (7)
- Topical treatment for scabies, alone and in combination with turmeric (4)
- Topical treatment for eczema and ringworm infection (4,5)
- Topical treatment as a cream or pessary for vaginosis resulting from infections, in combination with saponins from *Sapindus mukorossi* and an aromatic extract called citrata oil (4)
- Topical treatment for ulcers, boils, and other skin conditions (5)

Contraindications

Use during pregnancy and treatments for infertility (of both sexes) is not recommended.

Warnings and Precautions

Extracts of neem leaf should not be taken for prolonged periods at high doses. Toxicology studies of leaf extracts and some isolated constituents (limonoids) show a very low toxicity, especially when taken orally. However, toxic effects have been observed in animals grazing on neem leaf.[1]

Interactions

None known.

Use in Pregnancy and Lactation

Given the uncertain relevancy of the animal experiments, neem leaf is best avoided during pregnancy, especially in the first trimester.

Side Effects

None expected if taken within the recommended dose range.

Dosage

Dose per day*	Dose per week*
1.5-3.5 ml of 1:2 liquid extract	10-25 ml of 1:2 liquid extract

Neem Leaf *continued on page 339*

[#]Alternative name.

*This dose range is extrapolated from traditional Ayurvedic medicine[2] and the author's education and experience.

338

SUPPORTING INFORMATION

Traditional Prescribing

Traditional Ayurvedic uses of neem leaf include:
- As a bitter tonic and for blood purification[3]
- Skin diseases, fevers[3]
- Blood disorders, eye diseases[2]
- Neuromuscular pain, diarrhea, hyperacidity, nausea; hepatitis, enlarged spleen[4]
- As a cough suppressant, tuberculosis; urinary disorders, dysmenorrhea[4]
- As an emmenagogue[5]
- Intestinal worm infestation, including filariasis[4,5]
- Venomous bites[5]
- Diabetes, hypertension, cancer, allergies[4]
- Topically for ulcers, glandular swellings, boils and other skin diseases, such as eczema, scabies, and pemphigus[3,5,6]

Indian monks consumed the juice of fresh green neem leaves to suppress sexual desire.[7] Neem leaf and leaf oil are used traditionally as an insecticide,[5,8] but the main insecticidal activity is found in the seeds.

Traditional Fijian medicine uses include asthma, diabetes, and syphilis.[9]

Pharmacologic Research

Neem leaf contains limonoids (including aradirachtins) and simple terpenoids.[10] Limonoids are modified triterpenes.
- Oral administration of neem leaf extract reduced blood sugar levels in normal and streptozocin-induced diabetic models.[11] The hypoglycemic effect was comparable to glibenclamide (an antidiabetic drug).[12] Pretreatment with neem leaf prevented the rise in blood glucose levels compared with control diabetic animals.[12] Neem leaf extract demonstrated an antihyperglycemic effect against glucose and epinephrine (adrenaline)-induced models of hyperglycemia[13] and blocked the peripheral utilization of glucose and the glycogenolytic effect of epinephrine in normal and diabetic experimental models.[14]
- The anxiolytic activity of neem leaf extract (up to 200 mg/kg) was comparable to that induced by diazepam (1 mg/kg) after oral administration.[15] Neem leaf extract demonstrated analgesic[16] and sedative[17] activity *in vivo* after intraperitoneal administration.
- Aqueous extracts of neem leaf dose-dependently reduced gastric ulcer severity in animals subjected to stress and decreased ethanol-induced gastric mucosal damage. The extract appeared to prevent mast cell degranulation and to increase the amount of adherent gastric mucus in stressed rats.[18]
- An aqueous extract of neem leaf reduced elevations of cholesterol and urea and attenuated gastric ulcerogenesis and suppression of humoral immune response in experimental models of stress.[19]

Neem Leaf continued on page 340

- After oral administration, the water-soluble portion of an alcohol extract of neem leaf exhibited antiinflammatory activity in the cotton pellet granuloma assay.[20] Dose-dependent antiinflammatory activity was also demonstrated in carrageenan-induced acute inflammation (oral[21] and intraperitoneal[22] routes) and formaldehyde-induced subacute inflammation (oral route).[21]

- An aqueous extract of neem leaf augmented both humoral and cell-mediated immune responses after oral administration,[23] enhanced phagocytic activity of macrophages both *in vitro* and *in vivo*, and induced expression of MHC-II antigens on macrophages.[24] Neem leaf (2 g/kg, orally) enhanced antibody titers against Newcastle disease virus antigen in chickens that had survived an outbreak of infectious bursal disease.[25]

- Neem leaf extract demonstrated an inhibitory action against a wide spectrum of microorganisms *in vitro,* including protozoa *(Plasmodium falciparum),*[26,27] viruses,[28-30] bacteria[31] and fungi.[32,33] The *in vivo* activity of neem leaf extract against mouse plasmodia was not convincing.[1]

- Administration of an alcohol extract of neem leaf during the early phase of fever development reduced rectal temperature to near normal values in *Escherichia coli* endotoxin–induced fever. Pretreatment did not significantly reduce fever.[34]

- A methanol extract of neem leaf exhibited direct antimutagenic activity *in vitro*.[35] An aqueous extract inhibited cyclophosphamide- and mitomycin-induced chromosomal aberrations after intraperitoneal administration[36] and inhibited chemically induced oral squamous cell carcinomas after oral administration.[37]

- Histopathologic studies confirm that oral administration of an aqueous extract of neem leaf protected against increases in serum liver enzymes induced by acetominophen (paracetamol).[38,39] This finding demonstrates hepatoprotective activity.

- Oral pretreatment with neem leaf extract decreased the formation of lipid peroxides and enhanced levels of antioxidants and detoxifying enzymes in the stomach, liver, and circulation of rats treated with the carcinogen MNNG.[40]

- Neem leaf extract given orally at the early postimplantation stage terminated pregnancy in rodents and primates.[41] Oral administration of aqueous neem leaf extract demonstrated antifertility activity in male mice.[42] Neem leaf powder by the oral route resulted in reversible atrophic and biochemical changes in male reproductive tissue *in vivo*.[43-45]

- Morphologic changes in spermatozoa have been observed in rats treated with powdered neem leaf, which may be the result of an antiandrogenic effect.[46] Oral administration of a neem leaf aqueous extract decreased serum testosterone but did not affect the fertility index in male rats. After intraperitoneal administration, a neem leaf fraction containing predominately steroidal compounds impaired spermatogenesis and altered the morphology and motility of spermatozoa, leading to a reduced fertility index.[7] However, in another study,

Neem Leaf *continued on page 341*

neem leaf extract was not observed to interfere with spermatogenesis in male rats fed the extract, but antiimplantation and abortifacient effects were observed in females mated by these males.[47]

- Neem leaf alcoholic extract produced a dose-dependent hypotensive effect *in vivo* after intravenous administration.[48,49]

Clinical Studies

- In an uncontrolled trial, patients with diabetes were able to reduce their dose of insulin by up to 30% to 50% (without significant changes in blood glucose) when ingesting neem leaf, which was prescribed either as 5 g of an aqueous leaf paste or the equivalent amount of dried leaf in capsules.[50]
- Oral neem leaf extract in combination with topical coal tar reduced erythema, desquamation, and infiltration of psoriatic lesions in patients with psoriasis in an uncontrolled trial.[51]
- Phase I clinical trials, which have been completed in India, Egypt, and the Dominican Republic, indicate the safety, acceptability, and beneficial action of a topical herbal formulation containing neem leaf, saponins from *Sapindus mukorossi,* and an aromatic extract called citrata oil, in treating infectious vaginosis.[52]
- In a poorly controlled clinical trial, an improvement was observed in 16 cases of acute eczema, ringworm infection, and scabies after several days of topical treatment with a concentrated neem leaf preparation. In the three cases of chronic eczema, response was slow, and improvement occurred after 15 to 20 days. Application of the vehicle solution by one person in each group before neem treatment did not produce any effect.[53]
- Topical treatment with fresh neem leaf (80%) and turmeric (20%) combined in a paste cured 97% of 814 cases of scabies within 3 to 15 days in an uncontrolled study.[54]

REFERENCES

1 van der Nat JM et al: *J Ethnopharmacol* 35(1):1-24, 1991.

2 Kapoor LD: *CRC handbook of Ayurvedic medicinal plants,* Boca Raton, Fla, 1990, CRC Press.

3 Thakur RS, Puri HS, Husain A: *Major medicinal plants of India,* Lucknow, India, 1989, Central Institute of Medicinal and Aromatic Plants.

4 Chaturvedi VS: *Neem in Ayurveda,* Mumbai, India, 1996, Arogya Sansthan.

5 Nadkarni AK: *Dr. K.M. Nadkarni's Indian materia medica,* ed 3, Bombay, 1976, Popular Prakashan.

6 Chopra RN et al: *Chopra's indigenous drugs of India,* ed 2, Calcutta, 1958, reprinted 1982, Academic Publishers.

7 Parshad O et al: *Phytother Res* 11(2):168-170, 1997.

8 Wagner H et al, eds: *Economic and medicinal plant research,* London, 1989, Academic Press.

9 Cambie RC, Ash J: *Fijian medicinal plants,* Melbourne, Victoria, Australia, 1994, CSIRO Publishing.

10 Dai J et al: *J Agric Food Chem* 49(3):1169-1174, 2001.

11 Chattopadhyay RR: *J Ethnopharmacol* 67(3):367-372, 1999.

12 Khosla P et al: *Indian J Physiol Pharmacol* 44(1):69-74, 2000.

13 Chattopadhyay RR et al: *Bull Calcutta Sch Trop Med* 35:29-35, 1992.

14 Chattopadhyay RR: *Gen Pharmacol* 27(3):431-434, 1996.

15 Jaiswal AK, Bhattacharya SK, Acharya SB: *Indian J Exp Biol* 32(7):489-491, 1994.

16 Khanna N et al: *Indian J Exp Biol* 33(11):848-850, 1995.

17 Parshad O, Young LE, Young RE: *Phytother Res* 11(5):398-400, 1997.

18 Garg GP, Nigam SK, Ogle CW: *Planta Med* 59(3):215-217, 1993.

Neem Leaf *continued on page 342*

19 Sen P, Medriatta PK, Ray A: *Indian J Exp Biol* 30(12):1170-1175, 1992.

20 Chattopadhyay RR: *Indian J Exp Biol* 36(4):418-420, 1998.

21 Koley KM, Lal J, Tandan SK: *Fitoterapia* 65(6):524-528, 1994.

22 Chattopadhyay RR et al: *Fitoterapia* 65(2):146-148, 1994.

23 Ray A, Banerjee BD, Sen P: *Indian J Exp Biol* 34(7):698-701, 1996.

24 Upadhyaya S, Dhawan S: *Neem (Azadirachta indica): immunomodulatory properties and therapeutic potential*, Bombay, February 1994, abstract PR 2, Update Ayurveda.

25 Sadekar RD et al: *Indian J Exp Biol* 36(11):1151-1153, 1998.

26 Rochanakij S et al: *Southeast Asian J Trop Med Public Health* 16(1):66-72, 1985.

27 MacKinnon S et al: *J Nat Prod* 60(4):336-341, 1997.

28 Badam L, Joshi SP, Bedekar SS: *J Commun Dis* 31(2):79-90, 1999.

29 Rao AR et al: *Indian J Med Res* 57:495-502, 1969.

30 Rai A, Sethi MS: *Indian J Animal Sci* 42:1066-1070, 1972.

31 Sohni YR, Padmaja K, Bhatt RM: *J Ethnopharmacol* 45(2):141-147, 1995.

32 Bhowmick BN, Choudhary BK: *Indian Bot Report* 1:164-165, 1982.

33 Pant N et al: *Fitoterapia* 57:302-304, 1985.

34 Ashorobi RB: *Phytother Res* 12(1):41-43, 1998.

35 Kusamran WR, Tepsuwan A, Kupradinun P: *Mutat Res* 402(1-2):247-258, 1998.

36 Mukhopadhyay MJ, Mukherjee A: *Phytother Res* 12(6):409-412, 1998.

37 Balasenthil S et al: *J Ethnopharmacol* 67(2):189-195, 1999.

38 Chattopadhyay RR et al: *Indian J Exp Biol* 30(8):738-740, 1992.

39 Bhanwra S et al: *Indian J Physiol Pharmacol* 44(1):64-68, 2000.

40 Arivazhagan S, Balasenthil S, Nagini S: *Cell Biochem Funct* 18(1):17-21, 2000.

41 Talwar GP et al: *Am J Reprod Immunol* 37(6):485-491, 1997.

42 Deshpande VY, Mendulkar KN, Sadre NL: *J Postgrad Med* 26(3):167-170, 1980.

43 Katsutri M et al: *Indian J Physiol Pharmacol* 41(3):234-240, 1997.

44 Katsutri M et al: *Indian J Exp Biol* 33(10):725-729, 1995.

45 Joshi AR et al: *Indian J Exp Biol* 34(11):1091-1094, 1996.

46 Aladakatti RH, Ahamed RN: *Indian J Exp Biol* 37(12):1251-1254, 1999.

47 Choudhary DN et al: *Indian J Exp Biol* 28(8):714-716, 1990.

48 Koley KM, Lal J: *Indian J Physiol Pharmacol* 38(3):223-225, 1994.

49 Chattopadhyay RR: *Gen Pharmacol* 28(3):449-451, 1997.

50 Shukla R, Singh S, Bhandari CR: *Med Surg* 13:11-12, 1973.

51 Pandey SS, Jha AK, Kaur V: *Indian J Dermatol Venereol Leprol* 60:63, 1994.

52 Talwar GP et al: *Immunol Cell Biol* 75(2):190-192, 1997.

53 Singh N et al: *Antiseptic* 70:677-680, 1979.

54 Charles V, Charles SX: *Trop Geogr Med* 44(1-2):178-181, 1992.

NETTLE LEAF

Other Common Name:	Nettles
Botanical Names:	*Urtica dioica, Urtica urens*+
Family:	Urticaceae
Plant Part Used:	Leaf

PRESCRIBING INFORMATION

Actions

Antirheumatic, antiallergic, depurative, styptic (hemostatic)

Potential Indications

Based on appropriate evaluation of the patient, practitioners should consider prescribing nettle leaf in formulations in the context of:
- Allergic *rhinitis (2)*
- Osteoarthritis, rheumatoid arthritis *(4)*
- Chronic skin eruptions, especially eczema *(5)*
- Inflammatory diseases of the lower urinary tract, prevention and treatment of kidney gravel *(4,5)*
- Internal blood loss, including uterine hemorrhage, melena *(5)*
- Topical treatment for nosebleeds, burns, wounds, inflammation of the mouth and throat *(6)*

Contraindications

Patients who are allergic to nettle stings should not apply the fresh or unprocessed dried leaves topically.

Warnings and Precautions

In rare cases, nettle leaf may cause allergic reactions in susceptible patients.

Interactions

None known.

Use in Pregnancy and Lactation

No adverse effects expected.

Side Effects

Hypersensitivity reactions to contact with nettle have been documented. A man who had developed a contact dermatitis after treating his eczema with a poultice of herbs including chamomile also exhibited a diffuse edematous gingivostomatitis; he regularly drank nettle tea. This reaction was believed to be an allergic contact reaction to the chamomile and the nettle (and not an irritant reaction).

Dosage

*Dose per day**	*Dose per week**
2-6 ml of 1:2 liquid extract	15-40 ml of 1:2 liquid extract

SUPPORTING INFORMATION

Traditional Prescribing

Traditional Western herbal medicine uses include:
- Cutaneous eruptions, particularly eczema of a nervous or psychologic origin or those of a chronic nature and especially in children[1,2]

Nettle Leaf *continued on page 344*

+Medicinally interchangeable species.
*This dose range is extrapolated from the British Herbal Pharmacopoeia 1983, the British Herbal Compendium 1992, and the author's education and experience.

343

- Chronic diarrhea, dysentery, disorders of the bowel with secretion of mucus[2]
- Blood loss including uterine hemorrhage, nosebleeds, melena[1]
- Bronchial or asthmatic conditions,[3] bladder disorders, including stones[2]
- Topically (by beating the leaves or as a poultice) for relieving joint pain (including arthritis, rheumatism, gout, and sciatica),[3,4] burns, wounds, and inflammation of the mouth and throat[3]

Pharmacologic Research

- Nettle leaf extract or its constituents have demonstrated antiinflammatory activity *in vitro* by inhibiting cyclooxygenase- and 5-lipoxygenase–derived reactions.
- Nettle hairs and whole plant extract were found to contain high levels of leukotrienes, as well as histamine. Nettle hairs therefore resemble insect venoms and cutaneous mast cells with regard to their spectrum of mediators.
- The solubility of the silicon in nettle leaf was investigated in a Polish study. A 1:100 decoction of the dried leaves simmered for 30 minutes yields approximately 5 mg of soluble silicon for every 1 g of nettle used.[5]

Clinical Studies

- Studies with volunteers suggest the immediate reaction to nettle sting is the result of histamine introduced by the nettle. The persistence of the stinging sensation may be caused by the presence of substances directly toxic to nerves or capable of inducing secondary release of other mediators. Acetylcholine is present in the hairs and contributes to the stinging reaction.
- Lipopolysaccharide (LPS) stimulation of cytokine release from the whole blood of healthy human volunteers was investigated as an experimental model. In this assay system, LPS stimulation causes an increase of TNF-α and interleukin-1β (IL-1β) secretion, which is correlated with the number of monocytes-macrophages in the blood of each volunteer. In confirmation of possible antiinflammatory activity, nettle leaf extract significantly reduced this release of cytokines in a concentration-dependent manner. The nettle leaf extract also independently stimulated the secretion of interleukin-6 (IL-6). Because IL-6 acts antagonistically to IL-1β in decreasing prostaglandin E$_2$ synthesis, and induces inhibitors of proteinases as well, this finding might also reflect a favorable antiinflammatory result. Phenolic acid derivatives and flavonoids showed no activity in this assay, thus the cytokine inhibitory components are currently unknown.
- Twenty healthy volunteers ingested 1.34 g per day of a nettle leaf extract for 21 days. Although the nettle leaf had no effect on basal levels of cytokines, it did significantly decrease the release of TNF-α and IL-1β after LPS stimulation *ex vivo*. However, the increase in IL-6, which was observed *in vitro,* was not observed after oral ingestion, confirming that *in vitro* results are not necessarily translatable into clinical findings. This result is probably because some compounds in the plant exhibit poor bioavailabilties after oral doses.

Nettle Leaf *continued on page 345*

- Sixty nine volunteers completed a randomized, double-blind, placebo-controlled study investigating the effect of a freeze-dried preparation of nettle leaf on allergic rhinitis. Patients were advised to take nettle leaf (600 mg) or placebo at the onset of symptoms. Nettle was rated higher than placebo in the global assessments but was only slightly higher in diary data after 1 week.

- A multicenter, postmarketing surveillance study examined the safety and therapeutic benefit of a nettle leaf preparation (dose unknown) in nearly 9000 patients with osteoarthritis and rheumatoid arthritis. After a 3-week period, 82% of patients believed that the treatment had relieved their symptoms, 38% indicated that they might have their NSAID therapy reduced, and 26% no longer required NSAID therapy.

- Several uncontrolled studies have indicated that using nettle leaf extract in conjunction with standard NSAID therapy may achieve a dose reduction of the latter in treating rheumatic complaints. Doses equivalent to 9.1 g per day of leaf or 50 g per day stewed fresh young leaf were prescribed.

- The sting of nettle leaf has been shown to be beneficial in treating osteoarthritic pain at the base of the thumb or index finger in a randomized, double-blind, controlled, crossover trial. Nettle or placebo leaf was stroked over the painful area daily.[6]

- In Germany, the Commission E supports using nettle leaf as supportive therapy for rheumatic aliments by internal and external application. Nettle leaf is also recommended internally with copious fluid intake for inflammatory diseases of the lower urinary tract and prevention and treatment of kidney gravel.[7]

- ESCOP recommends nettle leaf as an adjuvant therapy for rheumatic conditions and irrigation in inflammatory conditions of the lower urinary tract.[8]

REFERENCES

Except when specifically referenced, the following book was referred to in the compilation of the pharmacologic and clinical information : Mills S, Bone K: *Principles and Practice of Phytotherapy: Modern Herbal Medicine,* Edinburgh, 2000, Churchill Livingstone.

1 British Herbal Medicine Association's Scientific Committee: *British herbal pharmacopoeia,* Bournemouth, 1983, BHMA.

2 Felter HW, Lloyd JU: *King's American dispensatory,* ed 18, rev 3, Portland, 1905, reprinted 1983, Eclectic Medical Publications.

3 Grieve M: *A modern herbal,* New York, 1971, Dover Publications.

4 Sales H: *Culpeper's complete herbal & English physician.* Reproduced from an original edition published in 1826, Bath, UK, 1981, Pitman Press.

5 Piekos R, Paslawska S: *Planta Med* 27(2):145-150, 1975.

6 Randall C et al: *J R Soc Med* 93(6):305-309, 2000.

7 Blumenthal M et al, eds: *The complete German Commission E monographs: therapeutic guide to herbal medicines,* Austin, 1998, American Botanical Council.

8 Scientific Committee of the European Scientific Cooperative on Phytotherapy [ESCOP]: *ESCOP monographs: Urticae folium/herba.* European Scientific Cooperative on Phytotherapy, ESCOP Secretariat, Argyle House, Gandy Street, Exeter, Devon, EX4 3LS, United Kingdom, July 1997.

NETTLE ROOT

Botanical Names: *Urtica dioica, Urtica urens*[+]
Family: Urticaceae
Plant Part Used: Root

PRESCRIBING INFORMATION

Actions

Antiprostatic

Potential Indications

Based on appropriate evaluation of the patient, practitioners should consider prescribing nettle root in formulations in the context of:
- Improving urologic symptoms in benign prostatic hyperplasia *(2,4)*
- Improving urologic symptoms in benign prostatic hyperplasia, in combination with saw palmetto *(2)*

Contraindications

None known.

Warnings and Precautions

The Commission E advises that using nettle root for benign prostatic hyperplasia (BPH) should occur under professional supervision.

Interactions

None known.

Use in Pregnancy and Lactation

No adverse effects expected.

Side Effects

Occasional, mild gastrointestinal discomfort may occur from ingesting nettle root.

Dosage

Dose per day*	*Dose per week**
4.5-8.5 ml of 1:2 liquid extract	30-60 ml of 1:2 liquid extract

SUPPORTING INFORMATION

Traditional Prescribing

Traditional Western herbal medicine uses include:
- Similar uses to those for nettle leaf, including cutaneous skin eruptions, hemorrhages, and particularly bowel disorders[2]
- Asthma[3]

Pharmacologic Research

- Several studies have indicated that the lignans in the root of nettle inhibited the binding activity of human sex hormone binding globulin (SHBG) *in vitro*.
- Five subfractions of an aqueous-methanolic extract of nettle root inhibited cellular proliferation in BPH tissue. A reduction in the cellular proliferation of BPH tissue was observed *ex vivo* after treating patients with an aqueous-methanolic nettle root extract.
- Nettle root extract was shown to be a very weak inhibitor of 5-α-reductase (which converts testosterone into 5-α-DHT) *in vitro*.

Nettle Root *continued on page 347*

[+]Medicinally interchangeable species.
*This dose range is extrapolated from the German Commission E and ESCOP monographs.[1]

A mild inhibition of DHT binding to cytosolic androgen receptors in isolated rat prostate was observed.

- Other *in vitro* studies indicated that nettle root inhibited aromatase (which converts testosterone into estradiol). A pharmacologic effect for nettle root from the lipophilic compounds in nettle might occur in fatty tissues where androgens are aromatized. Nettle root and saw palmetto each inhibit aromatase by a different mechanism.
- Nettle root extract demonstrated a specific and dose-dependent inhibition of human leukocyte elastase (HLE) *in vitro*. (The presence of the proteolytic enzyme HLE in seminal plasma is an important marker in clinically silent genitourinary tract infection or inflammation.)
- Oral administration of five nettle root extracts was tested in experimentally induced BPH. The methanolic extract demonstrated the greatest inhibition of prostate growth compared with controls.
- *Urtica dioica* agglutinin (UDA), a small, single-chain lectin, demonstrated antifungal, antiviral, cytotoxic, immunomodulatory, and anticancer activities, mainly *in vitro* or *in vivo* (by injection). However, such activities are uncertain for normal oral doses of nettle root preparations resulting from the poor bioavailability of UDA. An *in vitro* study has shown that UDA binds to cell membranes of smooth muscle and epithelial cells within BPH tissue.

Clinical Studies

- Morphologic studies of BPH cells were conducted in 31 patients treated with nettle root extract (equivalent to 6 g/day of root) for 20 weeks. The observed changes in the nucleus and cytoplasm of prostate cells may have been the result of inhibition of the binding capacity of SHBG. In a randomized, double-blind, placebo-controlled trial, 3 months' treatment with nettle root produced a significant improvement of International Prostate Symptom Score (IPSS) and a moderate reduction of residual urine volume.[4]
- In a number of uncontrolled clinical trials conducted from 1979 to 1988, nettle root extract (equivalent to 3 to 6 g/day of root) administered for 3 weeks to 20 months demonstrated improvement in urologic symptoms in patients with BPH.
- Long-term treatment over 8 to 10 years of 226 patients with BPH found that therapy with nettle root extract was able to maintain more than 50% of patients without the need for surgery. After long-term treatment, the usual enlargement of the prostate was not evident.
- In a randomized, controlled, open trial, the zinc, calcium, and sodium levels in prostatic secretions from patients with BPH were investigated. The authors concluded that nettle root extract (equivalent 9 g/day of root for 7 days) may alter the zinc-testosterone metabolism and lower zinc secretion in adenomatous tissue.
- Sixty seven patients experienced a reduction of nocturnal micturition frequency after 6 months of treatment with nettle root tincture (equivalent to 1 g/day of root). In patients with a mild condition, symptoms were relieved within approximately 3 weeks.

Nettle Root *continued on page 348*

- Nettle root extract (equivalent to 3 g/day of root for 6 to 9 weeks) improved the symptoms of BPH in two double-blind, placebo-controlled trials.
- In a placebo-controlled, clinical trial, 40 patients with BPH were treated with combined nettle root and saw palmetto extract or placebo over 24 weeks. Significant improvement in symptoms was observed in the herbal treatment group compared with placebo. The daily dose was equivalent to 2.4 g per day of nettle root and 2.9 g per day of saw palmetto berries.
- In a randomized, double-blind, multicenter, clinical trial, the efficacy of combined nettle root and saw palmetto extract was compared with the drug finasteride in treating BPH stages I to II over 48 weeks. Improvements in IPSS and peak urinary flow were observed for both groups. Although no significant difference was demonstrated between the two treatments, fewer adverse events were reported for the herbal combination, especially in terms of diminished ejaculation volume, erectile dysfunction, and headache. The herbal treatment was evaluated as more cost effective. The daily dose was equivalent to 2.4 g per day of nettle root and 2.9 g per day of saw palmetto berries.
- In Germany, the Commission E supports using nettle root for treating difficult urination in BPH stages I and II.[1]
- ESCOP recommends nettle root for the symptomatic treating of micturition disorders (e.g., nocturia, dysuria, urine retention) in BHP stages I and II.[5]

REFERENCES

Except when specifically referenced, the following book was referred to in the compilation of the pharmacologic and clinical information: Mills S, Bone K: *Principles and Practice of Phytotherapy: Modern Herbal Medicine,* Edinburgh, 2000, Churchill Livingstone.

1 Blumenthal M et al, eds: *The complete German Commission E monographs: therapeutic guide to herbal medicines,* Austin, 1998, American Botanical Council.
2 Felter HW, Lloyd JU: *King's American dispensatory,* ed 18, rev 3, Portland, 1905, reprinted 1983, Eclectic Medical Publications.
3 Grieve M: *A modern herbal,* New York, 1971, Dover Publications.
4 Engelmann U, Boos G, Kres H: *Urologe B* 36(4):287-291, 1996.
5 Scientific Committee of the European Scientific Cooperative on Phytotherapy [ESCOP]: *ESCOP monographs: Urticae radix.* European Scientific Cooperative on Phytotherapy, ESCOP Secretariat, Argyle House, Gandy Street, Exeter, Devon, EX4 3LS, United Kingdom, March 1996.

OATS

Botanical Name: Avena sativa
Family: Gramineae
Plant Parts Used: Oats seed: mature seed
Green oats: aerial parts, including seed at the immature, milky stage

PRESCRIBING INFORMATION

Actions	Oats seed: nervine tonic, tonic, thymoleptic
	Green oats: nervine tonic, anxiolytic
Potential Indications	Based on appropriate evaluation of the patient, practitioners should consider prescribing oats seed in formulations in the context of: • Nervous system support during nicotine withdrawal (results are conflicting) (3) • Nervous exhaustion and conditions resulting from nervous exhaustion, such as insomnia, feverish conditions; general debility, convalescence; depression, menopausal neurasthenia (5)
	Based on appropriate evaluation of the patient, practitioners should consider prescribing green oats in formulations in the context of: • Nervous system support during nicotine withdrawal (results are conflicting) (2) • Nervous system support during drug use withdrawal (4) • Nervous exhaustion (5)
Contraindications	None known.
Warnings and Precautions	None required.
Interactions	None known.
Use in Pregnancy and Lactation	No adverse effects expected.
Side Effects	None expected if taken within the recommended dose range.
Dosage	Oats seed:

Oats seed:

Dose per day*	Dose per week*
3-6 ml of 1:1 liquid extract	20-40 ml of 1:1 liquid extract

Green oats:

Dose per day**	Dose per week**
3-6 ml of 1:2 liquid extract	20-40 ml of 1:2 liquid extract

Oats *continued on page 350*

*This dose range is extrapolated from the British Herbal Pharmacopoeia 1983 and the author's education and experience.
**This dose range is extrapolated from King's American Dispensatory 1983 and the author's education and experience.

349

Traditional Prescribing

Traditional Western herbal medicine uses of oats seed include:
- Depression, menopausal neurasthenia, general debility[1]
- Spermatorrhea[2]
- Nervous prostration, nervous exhaustion resulting from typhoid and other fevers, insomnia resulting from nervous exhaustion[2]
- Enfeebled states of the heart muscle, acting as a tonic and improving the energy of the heart[2]

Traditional Western herbal medicine uses of green oats include calming and regenerating the nervous system.[3]

Green oats extract is recorded in *King's American Dispensatory* as having little effect in assisting with opium withdrawal.[2]

Pharmacologic Research

- Fresh green plant tincture administered by stomach tube or intraperitoneal injection antagonized the analgesic effect of morphine in two separate tests. Extracts diluted with water, exposed to light, and allowed to stand for 2 weeks resulted in reduced activity. Extracts of fresh green plant were superior to the seed. Dried brown leaves showed little activity. When morphine and fresh plant tincture were chronically administered together, physical dependence on morphine was reduced. (The green oats tincture was administered by stomach tube.) The pressor response to intravenously administered nicotine in anesthetized rats was antagonized by prior injection of fresh green plant tincture.[4]
- Results from a controlled experimental study suggest that oats extract (chaff) prevented atherosclerosis. Oat chaff extract produced a more favorable blood lipid profile compared with control animals and a reduction in the formation of atherosclerotic plaques.[5]

Clinical Studies

- Treating opium addiction by green oats may have originated from homeopathy.[6]
- In a randomized, placebo-controlled, clinical study involving healthy volunteers and bronchial patients who were habitual smokers, those given green oats extract achieved a significant reduction in tobacco use compared with controls. The reduction was still observed 2 months later. A tincture made from fresh whole oats plant (1:5, 90% ethanol) was prescribed at a dosage of 1 ml four times per day for a period of 28 days.[7] These results were not replicated in a later controlled trial.[8]
- Green oats plant juice in alcohol was ineffective for reducing cigarette cravings in an uncontrolled trial involving 76 patients. The oats extract and dosage were the same as those in the previously noted trial for the first 2 months but were then altered. For the following 2 months, 1 L of plant juice was added to 500 ml of 90%

Oats continued on page 351

ethanol and was not diluted with water until just before administration to the patient. The author noted that oats had been effective in general practice (by minimizing cigarette cravings) on several occasions when patients really wanted to give up smoking, but it was only one feature of the total therapeutic approach used.[9]

- Oats seed extract (15 ml/day of 1:2 extract) containing malic acid (for flavoring) prescribed in apple juice produced a reduction of 66% in daily cigarette consumption compared with no change for those receiving placebo (apple juice alone).[10]

- In a double-blind study involving participants wanting to stop smoking, no significant difference was observed between those treated with green oats extract (equivalent to 1.2 g/day fresh oat plant) compared with a placebo group (approximately 35% stopped smoking in both groups). In both the placebo and oats groups, the light smokers stopped smoking at a higher rate than those with a high consumption of cigarettes.[11] In a single-blind, placebo-controlled study, oats extract did not produce a reduction in tobacco use by smokers who were not attempting to quit. The oats extract (1:5, 90% ethanol) was made from a green plant with full-sized ears and a ripe plant dug up 1 week before harvest (roots included). The dose was 1 ml four times per day.[12]

- In a clinical study conducted in 1968 to 1969, 6 out of 10 chronic opium addicts gave up the drug after treatment with green oats (27 to 45 days). Two addicts reduced their intake. The participant's status was maintained on follow-ups (3 to 19 months later). No serious withdrawal symptoms or side effects were noted.[13] The administered dose was 2 ml three times per day of tincture made from fresh whole plant excluding root (1.5:5, 90% ethanol).

REFERENCES

1 British Herbal Medicine Association's Scientific Committee: *British herbal pharmacopoeia,* Bournemouth, 1983, BHMA.
2 Felter HW, Lloyd JU: *King's American dispensatory,* ed 18, rev 3, Portland, 1905, reprinted 1983, Eclectic Medical Publications.
3 Vogel A: *The nature doctor,* Teufen, Switzerland, 1977, Verlag A. Vogel.
4 Connor J et al: *J Pharm Pharmac* 27(2):92-98, 1975.
5 Juzwiak S et al: *Herba Polonica* 40(1-2):50-58, 1994.
6 Jack RA: *Br Med J* 4(778):48, 1971.
7 Anand CL: *Nature* 233(5320):496, 1971.
8 Geckeler K, Schmidt K, Schmidt F: *Munch Med Wochenschr* 116(11):581-582, 1974.
9 Gabrynowicz JW: *Med J Aust* 2(8):306-307, 1974.
10 Netherlands Patent 7412625, 1976.
11 Schmidt K, Geckeler K: *Int J Clin Pharmacol* 14(3):214-216, 1976.
12 Bye C et al: *Nature* 252(5484):580-581, 1974.
13 Anand CL: *Br Med J* 3(775):640, 1971.

OLIVE LEAF

Botanical Name: *Olea europaea*
Family: Oleaceae
Plant Part Used: Leaf

PRESCRIBING INFORMATION

Actions

Hypotensive, antioxidant, bitter tonic

Potential Indications

Based on appropriate evaluation of the patient, practitioners should consider prescribing olive leaf in formulations in the context of:

- Hypertension *(4,6)*
- Angina pectoris *(6)*
- Possible uses for gout and fluid retention *(4)*

The much-publicized clinical antibacterial and antiviral activities of olive leaf are not supported by a rational analysis of the pharmacologic data. Even if any clinical improvement in infected patients after using olive leaf was definitely established by controlled clinical trials, this would not be proof of antimicrobial activity because other mechanisms of action (such as immune-enhancing activity) might apply.

Contraindications

None known.

Warnings and Precautions

None required.

Interactions

None known.

Use in Pregnancy and Lactation

No adverse effects expected.

Side Effects

Traditional sources indicate that olive leaf may cause gastric upset, thus it should be taken before meals.[1]

Dosage

*Dose per day**	*Dose per week**
3.5-7.0 ml of 1:2 liquid extract	25-50 ml of 1:2 liquid extract

SUPPORTING INFORMATION

Traditional Prescribing

Traditional Western herbal medicine uses include:

- For lowering blood pressure; angina, possibly associated with hypertension[2]
- Cough,[3] obstinate fever,[4] intermittent fever[5]
- As a diuretic, febrifuge, emmenagogue[3]
- As a liver stimulant[6]; for stomachache resulting from acidity[6]
- Topically for snakebite, mouth ulcers[3]

Olive Leaf *continued on page 353*

*This dose range is extrapolated from traditional use.

Traditional South African medicinal uses include:
- As a hypotensive and to enhance renal function[7]
- Scrofula, intermittent fevers[8]

Pharmacologic Research

Key constituents of the olive leaf (dried leaf) include iridoid glycosides (oleuropein 6% to 9%) and flavonoids.[9] In the 1960s, elenolic acid (calcium elenolate) was isolated from aqueous extracts of various parts of olive plant after mild acid hydrolysis. Various agents can hydrolyze oleuropein to produce elenolic acid and hydroxytryrosol. This hydrolysis also occurs over time in herbal liquid extracts. Hydroxytyrosol is an antioxidant constituent of olive fruit and olive oil. Oleuropeoside is also referred to in the literature, and this compound may be identical to oleuropein (this has not been verified).
- Olive leaf extract exhibited antihypertensive activity after oral administration in an experimental model of hypertension.[10] Oleuropein has been shown to reduce blood pressure in both normotensive and hypertensive models after injection.[11]
- A decoction of olive leaf caused relaxation of isolated aorta preparations. Oleuropeoside was shown to be one of the constituents responsible for this vasodilating action.[12]
- Oleuropein increased coronary flow in isolated heart preparations *in vitro*. By injection, oleuropein decreased changes in the electrocardiogram (ECG) resulting from pituitrin-induced coronary spasm, indicating coronary vasodilation. Oleuropein demonstrated antiarrhythmic activity in a number of experimental models after injection.[11]
- An aqueous extract of olive leaf inhibited ACE *in vitro*. A strong ACE inhibitor, oleacein, was isolated from olive leaf.[13]
- Hypoglycemic, hypoinsulinemic, and hypocholesterolemic activities were demonstrated after oral administration of a leaf decoction of *Olea europea* var. *oleaster* to rats prone to develop obesity, insulin-resistance, hyperlipidemia, and diabetes.[14,15] Olive leaf treatment also reduced capillary wall thickening in the skin and pancreas and prevented this event in the kidney.[15] The hypocholesterolemic effect of olive leaf was superior to that of simvastatin (a hypocholesterolemic drug).[14]
- Long-term administration of olive leaf (route unknown) decreased tissue injury, urea, cholesterol, aspartate transaminase, and alanine transaminase levels raised by streptozotocin in an experimental model of diabetes.[16] Olive leaf and oleuropeoside exhibited hypoglycemic and antidiabetic activity *in vivo*.[17]
- An aqueous extract of olive leaf exhibited antiinflammatory activity in carrageenan-induced edema and protected against aspirin-induced gastric ulcers. At low doses, olive leaf stimulated the central nervous system, but at high doses it caused central nervous system depression.[18]
- Topical application of oleuropein inhibited experimentally induced edema. Oleuropein also strongly inhibited the enzyme myeloperoxidase, which is a marker of the accumulation of neutrophils in inflamed tissue.[19]

Olive Leaf *continued on page 354*

- Olive leaf extract and isolated flavonoids inhibited the classical pathway of the complement system *in vitro* but had no effect on the alternative pathway.[20] Oleuropein inhibited leukocyte 5-lipoxygenase *in vitro*.[21]

- Oleuropein dose-dependently enhanced nitrite production in LPS-challenged macrophages. A nitric oxide (NO) synthase inhibitor blocked this effect. Oleuropein also increased expression of NO synthase in macrophages. These results suggest that oleuropein potentiates macrophage response during endotoxin challenge, resulting in higher NO production, which is believed to be beneficial for cellular protection.[22]

- Oleuropein demonstrated antioxidant activity *in vitro*.[23,24] Olive leaf extract was also antioxidant *in vitro* and the activity was attributed to its oleuropein content and to a lesser extent the flavonoid content.[25] Consumption of olive oil containing oleuropein aglycone and hydroxytyrosol resulted in a dose-dependent reduction in the urinary excretion of 8-iso-prostaglandin $F_{2\alpha}$ (a marker of oxidative stress) in volunteers.[26]

- Dietary oleuropein reduced plasma levels of total, free, and ester cholesterol and increased the ability of LDL to resist oxidation in an experimental model.[27]

- Hydroxytyrosol demonstrated broad antimicrobial activity *in vitro* against a range of bacteria known to cause intestinal or respiratory tract infections in humans. Oleuropein inhibited several of these strains but was less active than hydroxytyrosol.[28] In other *in vitro* studies, oleuropein inhibited the growth of a number of pathogenic bacteria,[29-31] the production of *Staphylococcus aureus* enterotoxin B,[31] and the germination and outgrowth of *Bacillus cereus* T spores.[32] Calcium elenolate exhibited virucidal activity against a variety of RNA and DNA viruses *in vitro*,[33-35] including members of most of the groups of influenza and parainfluenza viruses. Virucidal activity and a reduction in viral yield were demonstrated *in vivo* after intranasal administration to animals infected with parainfluenza-3 virus.[36]

- However, no *in vivo* studies or rigorous clinical studies have been found demonstrating antimicrobial activity for oral doses of olive leaf extract or oleuropein. Claims made in the popular media and by certain manufacturers suggesting that olive leaf has extensive antibacterial and antiviral actions, with the ability to treat a wide variety of microbial illnesses are potentially dangerous, unsupported, and represent considerable extrapolations from the previously outlined *in vitro* activity as follows. Such claims are based on extrapolating activity from one virus type to all types of viruses, from *in vitro* activity to *in vivo* activity in humans (with no consideration of dosage issues), and from the activity of calcium elenolate to the activity of olive leaf extracts. The only evidence of activity in humans is from anecdotal reports and a collection of case reports inappropriately presented as a clinical trial (see the "Clinical Studies" section in this monograph).

Olive Leaf continued on page 355

Clinical Studies

- Olive leaf decreased systolic and diastolic blood pressure, glycemia, and calcemia from baseline values in two groups of patients with moderate essential hypertension. On average, total reductions were approximately 18 mm Hg for systolic blood pressures and approximately 10 mm Hg for diastolic blood pressures. One group of patients was presenting for the first time, and the other group was already receiving antihypertensive medication (which was gradually withdrawn 2 weeks before beginning the study). The trial was of single-blind design; for 2 weeks, a placebo was prescribed followed by 3 months' treatment with an aqueous olive leaf extract (1600 mg/day).[37]
- Olive leaf infusion caused marked diuresis in hypertensive patients.[38] Administering olive leaf infusion or decoction for 20 to 25 days to 10 patients increased daily urinary output, but blood potassium, sodium, and chloride remained unchanged in most cases. Blood uric acid was decreased, especially in hyperuricemic cases.[39]
- Olive leaf concentrated extract was claimed to produce beneficial antimicrobial effects in 500 Hungarian patients with respiratory diseases, lung conditions, dental problems, skin conditions of bacterial and viral origin, *Helicobacter pylori* infection, and lowered immunity. No placebo was administered, and dosage and duration of treatment were not indicated. The success of the treatment appears to have been assessed on subjective criteria only. In other case reports, a Bulgarian gynecologist described the reduction of elevated Pap smear category readings for women at high risk of cervical cancer. This reduction is said to have occurred by removing or reducing fungal infection of *Candida guilliermondii* following both oral ingestion and topical application of olive leaf extract. No further details were listed.[40]

REFERENCES

1 Weiss RF: *Herbal medicine*, English ed, Beaconsfield, UK, 1988, Beaconsfield Publishers.

2 Leclerc H: *Précis de phytothérapie*, ed 5, Paris, 1966, Masson.

3 Miller AG, Morris M: *Plants of Dhofar. The southern region of Oman. Traditional, economic and medicinal uses*, Diwan of Royal Court Sultanate of Oman, 1988, The Office of the Adviser for Conservation of the Environment.

4 Grieve M: *A modern herbal*, New York, 1971, Dover Publications.

5 Felter HW, Lloyd JU: *King's American dispensatory*, ed 18, rev 3, Portland, 1905, reprinted 1983, Eclectic Medical Publications.

6 Leporatti ML, Corradi L: *J Ethnopharmacol* 74(1):17-40, 2001.

7 van Wyk B-E, van Oudtshoorn B, Gericke N: *Medicinal plants of South Africa*, Arcadia, Pretoria, South Africa, 1997, Briza Publications.

8 Hutchings A: *Zulu medicinal plants: an inventory*, Pietermaritzburg, South Africa, 1996, University of Natal Press in association with University of Zululand, National Botanical Institute.

9 Wagner H, Bladt S: *Plant drug analysis: a thin layer chromatography atlas*, ed 2, Berlin, 1996, Springer-Verlag.

10 Ribeiro R et al: *J Ethnopharmacol* 15(3):261-269, 1986.

11 Petkov V, Manolov P: *Arzneim Forsch* 22(9):1476-1486, 1972.

12 Zarzuelo A et al: *Planta Med* 57(5):417-419, 1999.

13 Hansen K et al: *Phytomed* 2(4):319-325, 1996.

14 Bennani-Kabchi N et al: *Ann Pharm Fr* 58(4):271-277, 2000.

15 Bennani-Kabchi N et al: *Therapie* 54(6):717-723, 1999.

16 Onderoglu S et al: *J Pharm Pharmacol* 51(11):1305-1312, 1999.

Olive Leaf *continued on page 356*

17 Gonzalez M et al: *Planta Med* 58(6):513-515, 1992.

18 Fehri B et al: *Boll Chim Farm* 135:42-49, 1996.

19 de la Peurto R, Martinez-Dominguez E, Ruiz-Gutierrez V: *Z Naturforsch [C]* 55(9-10):814-819, 2000.

20 Pieroni A et al: *Pharmazie* 51(10):765-768, 1996.

21 de la Puerta, Ruiz-Gutierrez V, Hoult JR: *Biochem Pharmacol* 57(4):445-449, 1999.

22 Visioli F, Bellosta S, Galli C: *Life Sci* 62(6):541-546, 1998.

23 Benavente-Garcia O et al: *Food Chem* 68(4):457-462, 2000.

24 Speroni E et al: *Phytother Res* 12(suppl 1):S98-S100, 1998.

25 le Tutour B, Didier G: *Phytochem* 31(4):1173-1178, 1992.

26 Visioli F et al: *Biochem Biophys Res Commun* 278(3):797-799, 2000.

27 Coni E et al: *Lipids* 35(1):45-54, 2000.

28 Bisignano G et al: *J Pharm Pharmacol* 51(8):971-974, 1999.

29 Aziz NH et al: *Microbios* 93(374):43-55, 1998.

30 Tassou CC, Nychas GJ: *Lett Appl Microbiol* 20(2):120-124, 1995.

31 Tranter HS, Tassou SC, Nychas GJ: *J Appl Bacteriol* 74(3):253-259, 1993.

32 Tassou CC, Nychas GJ, Board RG: *Biotechnol Appl Biochem* 13(2):231-237, 1991.

33 Renis HE: *Antimicrob Agents Chemother* 9:167-172, 1969.

34 Hirschman SZ: *Nat New Biol* 238(87):277-279, 1972.

35 Renis HE: *Antimicrob Agents Chemother* 8(2):194-199, 1975.

36 Soret MG: *Antimicrob Agents Chemother* 9:160-166, 1969.

37 Cherif S et al: *J Pharm Belg* 51(2):69-71, 1996.

38 Balansard J, Dephaut J: *Acta Phytother* 17:197, 1953.

39 Capretti G, Bonaconza E: *Giorn Clin Med* 30:630-642, 1949.

40 Walker M: *Townsend Letter for Doctors and Patients* 204:92-96, 2000.

OREGON GRAPE

Botanical Names: *Berberis aquifolium, Mahonia aquifolium*[#][^]
Family: Berberidaceae
Plant Part Used: Root and rhizome

PRESCRIBING INFORMATION

Actions — Antipsoriatic, antiinflammatory, depurative, antimicrobial

Potential Indications — Based on appropriate evaluation of the patient, practitioners should consider prescribing Oregon grape in formulations in the context of:
- Chronic skin diseases, psoriasis, acne, eczema *(5)*
- Anorexia *(6)*
- Topical treatment for psoriasis* *(2)*
- Topical treatment for acne vulgaris* *(3)*

Contraindications — Berberine-containing herbs are contraindicated in pregnancy[2,3] and for jaundiced neonates.[3]

Warnings and Precautions — None required.

Interactions — None known.

Use in Pregnancy and Lactation — Contraindicated in pregnancy.

Side Effects — None expected when taken within the recommended dose range.

Dosage

Dose per day**	Dose per week**
3.5-7.0 ml of 1:2 liquid extract	25-50 ml of 1:2 liquid extract

SUPPORTING INFORMATION

Traditional Prescribing — Traditional Western herbal medicine uses include:
- Chronic skin disease, including psoriasis, eczema, syphilitic dyscrasia, pimples, acne; dyspepsia, gastritis, cholecystitis, liver disorders[4-6]
- Constitutional syphilis, leukorrhea[4,5]

Native Americans used Oregon grape as a bitter tonic for appetite loss and general debility. Other possible native uses included biliousness and topically for ulcerated gums or sore throats. Oregon grape was official in the USP from 1905 to 1916 and NF from 1916 to 1947 and was listed as a bitter tonic.[7]

Oregon Grape *continued on page 358*

[#]Alternative name.
[^]Adopted by the American Herbal Products Association as the new botanical name.[1]
* Trials were conducted using Oregon grape stem bark, although given the similar alkaloid profile, extracts of Oregon grape root could not be expected to provide similar effects.
**Higher doses may be necessary in acute conditions for which the effect of berberine is required. In fact, barberry is a better choice for such applications. This dose range is extrapolated from the British Herbal Pharmacopoeia 1983 and the author's education and experience.

Pharmacologic Research

The following alkaloids have been isolated from Oregon grape root: magnoflorine, berberine, palmatine, jatrorrhizine, columbamine, oxyacanthine, berbamine, aromoline, baluchistine, and aquifoline.[8-11] Oregon grape root is, however, not as rich a source of berberine as barberry (*Berberis vulgaris*) and golden seal (*Hydrastis canadensis*). Oregon grape stem bark, which has been used traditionally[7] and features in most of the pharmacologic and clinical studies conducted on Oregon grape, contains the following major alkaloids: berberine, magnoflorine, palmatine, jatrorrhizine, and minor alkaloids (e.g., berbamine, oxyacanthine, columbamine).[12] Oregon grape root may contain a larger alkaloid content than stem bark.[13]

- Berberine demonstrated antimicrobial activity *in vivo*[14] and was found to synergistically enhance the antibacterial activity of previously inactive plant constituents isolated from Oregon grape leaf *in vitro*.[15]
- Lipogenesis in hamster sebaceous glands was suppressed 63% by berberine *in vitro*, indicating that Oregon grape may be of benefit for the topical treatment of acne vulgaris.[16]
- Oregon grape stem bark extracts have demonstrated antiinflammatory, antioxidant, and antifungal activities *in vitro*.[12,17] Methanol extract of Oregon grape root demonstrated antifungal activity *in vitro*.[18]
- Oregon grape stem bark extract exhibited immunostimulating activity in two phagocytosis assays.[12]
- Oregon grape bark extract and several of the main alkaloids inhibited human keratinocyte growth *in vitro*. This antiproliferative activity is relevant to treating psoriasis.[19] A possible mechanism of action involves the interference of DNA synthesis by berberine.[20]

Clinical Studies

In the clinical trials listed in this section, the ointment or cream contained 10% Oregon grape mother tincture prepared according to the HAB from stem bark.

- Oregon grape extract demonstrated a beneficial effect in a prospective case report study and a small placebo-controlled clinical trial investigating the treatment of acne. Treatment produced good results, with a reduction in oiliness of the skin. In the clinical trial, nine male and female patients with mild or moderate acne applied either Oregon grape cream or the corresponding placebo base twice per day for 8 weeks. Both groups showed a decrease in the number of inflamed lesions, but only a tendency was shown to diminished sebum levels in the Oregon grape group.[21,22] Stronger preparations may be necessary to show a significant activity.
- Topical ointments containing Oregon grape stem bark extract are marketed in Europe for psoriasis. Several clinical studies have confirmed their activity. In one open trial, the ointment was used for 12 weeks, with a large proportion of patients continuing treatment for 1 year or until their skin cleared.[23,24] Oregon grape ointment improved cellular cutaneous immune mechanisms and reduced the hyperproliferation of keratinocytes in a comparative trial with

Oregon Grape *continued on page 359*

dithranol conducted over 4 weeks.[25] In a placebo-controlled, intra-individual trial, Oregon grape ointment produced a benefit according to patients' assessment. Improvement was greater in more severe cases.[26]

REFERENCES

1 McGuffin M, ed: *Herbs of commerce*, ed 2 [draft 3.3], Bethesda, Md, 1998, American Herbal Products Association.
2 De Smet PAGM et al, eds: *Adverse effects of herbal drugs*, Berlin, 1992, Springer-Verlag.
3 Chan E: *Biol Neonate* 63(4):201-208, 1993.
4 British Herbal Medicine Association's Scientific Committee: *British herbal pharmacopoeia*, Bournemouth, 1983, BHMA.
5 Felter HW, Lloyd JU: *King's American dispensatory*, ed 18, rev 3, Portland, 1905, reprinted 1983, Eclectic Medical Publications.
6 Ellingwood F, Lloyd JU: *American materia medica, therapeutics and pharmacognosy*, ed 11, Portland, 1983, Eclectic Medical Publications.
7 Vogel VJ: *American Indian medicine*, Norman, Okla, 1970, University of Oklahoma Press.
8 Kostalova D, Brazdovicova B, Tomko J: *Chem Zvesti* 35(2):279-283, 1981.
9 Schwabe W: *Dtsch Apoth Ztg* 54:326-327, 1939.
10 Kostalova D, Hrochova V, Tomko J: *Chem Pap* 40(3):389-394, 1986.
11 Kostalova D et al: *Collect Czech Chem Commun* 52(1):242-246, 1987.
12 Galle K et al: *Phytomed* 1(1):59-62, 1994.
13 Neugebauer H, Brunner K: *Pharm Zentralhalle* 80:241-245, 1939.
14 Mills S, Bone K: *Principles and practice of phytotherapy: modern herbal medicine*, Edinburgh, 2000, Churchill Livingstone.
15 Stermitz FR et al: International Conference: 2000 Years of Natural Product Research—Past, Present and Future, Amsterdam, July 26-30, 1999, abstract L 29.
16 Seki T, Morohashi M: *Skin Pharmacol* 6(1):56-60, 1993.
17 Lampert ML, Andenmatten C, Schaffner W: *Z Phytother* 19(2):107-118, 1998.
18 McCutcheon AR et al: *J Ethnopharmacol* 44(3):157-169, 1994.
19 Muller K, Ziereis K, Gawlik I: *Planta Med* 61(1):74-75, 1995.
20 Creasey WA: *Biochem Pharmacol* 28(7):1081-1084, 1979.
21 Lampert ML, Rufli TH, Schaffner W: 2nd International Congress on Phytomedicine, Munich, September 11-14, 1996, abstract P-71.
22 Mennet-von Eiff M, Meier B: *Ars Medici* 85(4):255-259, 1995.
23 Gieler U, von der Weth A, Heger M: *Ars Medici* 85(14):1018-1019, 1995.
24 Gieler U, von der Weth A, Heger M: *J Dermatol Treat* 6(1):31-34, 1995.
25 Augustin M et al: *Forsch Komplementarmed* 6(suppl 2):19-21, 1999.
26 Wiesenauer M, Ludtke R: *Phytomed* 3(3):231-235, 1996.

PASQUE FLOWER

Other Common Name:	Pulsatilla
Botanical Names:	*Anemone pulsatilla, Pulsatilla vulgaris*[#]
Family:	Ranunculaceae
Plant Part Used:	Dried* aerial parts

PRESCRIBING INFORMATION

Actions

Spasmolytic, analgesic

Potential Indications

Based on appropriate evaluation of the patient, practitioners should consider prescribing pasque flower in formulations in the context of:
- Painful or inflammatory conditions of the male or female reproductive tract, including dysmenorrhea, ovarian pain, orchitis, and epididymitis *(5)*
- Hyperactivity, insomnia, tension headache *(5)*

Contraindications

Pregnancy and lactation.[1]

Warnings and Precautions

The recommended dose range must not be exceeded.

Interactions

None known.

Use in Pregnancy and Lactation

Contraindicated in pregnancy and lactation.

Side Effects

None expected if taken within the recommended dose range. Excessive (undefined) doses can cause violent gastritis.[1]

Dosage

*Dose per day***	*Dose per week***
0.4-1.5 ml of 1:2 liquid extract	3-10 ml of 1:2 liquid extract

SUPPORTING INFORMATION

Traditional Prescribing

Traditional Western herbal medicine uses include:
- Painful or inflammatory conditions of the male or female reproductive system, such as dysmenorrhea, orchitis, ovarian pain, and epididymitis[2]
- Hyperactivity, insomnia, tension headache, asthma[2]
- Skin eruptions and boils[2]

Eclectic physicians used only fresh plant preparations but at lower doses[3] to those that British herbalists advocated, who were mainly advocating dried plant preparations.[2]

Pasque Flower *continued on page 361*

[#]Alternative name.

*The fresh plant should not be used because it contains a constituent (protoanemonin) that causes irritant side effects.[1]

**This dose range is extrapolated from the British Herbal Pharmacopoeia 1983, the British Herbal Compendium 1992, and the author's education and experience.

Pharmacologic Research

No pharmacologic information relevant to the current use of pasque flower has been found.

Clinical Studies

No clinical studies have been conducted using liquid extract of pasque flower.

REFERENCES

1 British Herbal Medicine Association: *British herbal compendium,* Bournemouth, 1992, BHMA.
2 British Herbal Medicine Association's Scientific Committee: *British herbal pharmacopoeia,* Bournemouth, 1983, BHMA.
3 Ellingwood F, Lloyd JU: *American materia medica, therapeutics and pharmacognosy,* ed 11, Portland, 1983, Eclectic Medical Publications.

PASSION FLOWER

Other Common Name:	Passiflora
Botanical Name:	*Passiflora incarnata*
Family:	Passifloraceae
Plant Part Used:	Aerial parts

PRESCRIBING INFORMATION

Actions

Anxiolytic, spasmolytic, mild sedative, hypnotic

Potential Indications

Based on appropriate evaluation of the patient, practitioners should consider prescribing passion flower in formulations in the context of:
- Anxiety *(2,4,5)*
- Achieving mild sedation in healthy individuals *(2)*
- Adjuvant therapy for opiate withdrawal *(2)*
- Insomnia, in combination with valerian *(3)*
- Restlessness and irritability with difficulty in falling asleep *(4,5)*
- Cardiac insufficiency (NHYA functional class II) for anxiolytic effects, in combination with hawthorn leaf and flower *(2)*
- Nervous tachycardia, nervous headache *(5)*
- Nervous symptoms resulting from menstrual disturbances *(5)*
- Spasmodic conditions, including dysmenorrhea, asthma, whooping cough, and epilepsy *(5)*
- Neuralgic pain, including facial, rectal, and cardiac pain *(5)*

Contraindications

None known.

Warnings and Precautions

None required.

Interactions

None known.

Use in Pregnancy and Lactation

No adverse effects expected.

Side Effects

None expected if taken within the recommended dose range.

Dosage

*Dose per day**	*Dose per week**
3-6 ml of 1:2 liquid extract	20-40 ml of 1:2 liquid extract

SUPPORTING INFORMATION

Traditional Prescribing

Traditional Western herbal medicine uses include:
- Restlessness, wakefulness, nervous irritability, especially when resulting from exhaustion or prolonged illness[1]
- Hysteria, nervous tachycardia[1,2]
- Insomnia in infants and older adults or resulting from mental worry or overwork[1,2]

Passion Flower *continued on page 363*

*This dose range is extrapolated from the British Herbal Pharmacopoeia 1983, the British Herbal Compendium 1992, and the author's education and experience.

- Spasmodic conditions, including tetanus, chorea, and whooping cough[1]
- Generalized seizures,[2] epilepsy[1]
- Spasmodic asthma,[2] oppressed breathing[1]
- Neuralgic pain,[2] including facial, rectal, and cardiac pain[1]
- Nervous headache[1]
- Nervous symptoms resulting from menstrual disturbances, spasmodic dysmenorrhea[1]
- Topically for burns, scalds, hemorrhoids, painful ulcers, and toothache[1]

Native Americans used passion flower topically for ringworm, swellings, and sore eyes. Passion flower was official in the NF from 1916 to 1936 and was recommended as an antispasmodic and sedative.[3]

Passion flower has also been used traditionally in Brazil for treating insomnia.[4]

Pharmacologic Research

The main documented constituents of dried aerial parts of *Passiflora incarnata* are flavonoids (up to 1.2%), especially flavone-C-glycosides, including isovitexin.[5] The presence of trace amounts of the harmane alkaloids appears to depend on the stage of development of the plant, and in many samples, they are absent.[6] The German Commission E recommends that passion flower not contain more than 0.01% of harmane alkaloids.

- Experimental studies have investigated the sedative and anxiolytic activity of passion flower constituents in an attempt to find the active components. An experimental study conducted in 1976 found sedative activity for maltol after high doses by injection.[7] Maltol is an artifact and is present only in passion flower preparations at low concentrations.[8] A recent study, which found sedative and anxiolytic activity for an aqueous extract and aqueous alcohol extract, respectively, found no activity for several combinations of constituents (maltol + harmane alkaloids, maltol + flavonoids, or maltol alone) at low or high concentrations.[9] (All preparations were administered by injection.) This finding suggests that as yet unidentified compounds are responsible for the activity of passion flower.
- Aqueous and ethanolic extracts of passion flower demonstrated sedative activity after oral and intraperitoneal administration in experimental models.[9-14] The sedation index was comparable to meprobamate (250 mg/kg) and higher than that of diazepam (10 mg/kg) and chlordiazepoxide (10 mg/kg).[12]
- Oral administration of a passion flower extract exhibited anxiolytic activity *in vivo*,[15] and analgesic activity was demonstrated *in vivo* after oral administration of an aqueous extract of passion flower.[10] After oral administration, passion flower extract demonstrated antiinflammatory activity in three experimental models.[16]
- Passion flower extract did not interact with benzodiazepine, dopaminergic, or histaminergic receptors *in vitro*.[17]

Passion Flower *continued on page 364*

- Inhaling the essential oil of passion flower, or of its volatile constituents (maltol, 2-phenylethanol), did not decrease the motility of mice under normal conditions. Motility was decreased after caffeine-induced overagitation.[18]

Clinical Studies

- A randomized, double-blind, controlled, 14-day trial compared clonidine (an alpha-2 adrenergic agonist, maximum dose 0.8 mg/day) plus passion flower extract against clonidine plus placebo in the outpatient detoxification of opiate addicts. Both treatments were equally efficacious in treating the physical symptoms of withdrawal, but the group receiving passion flower showed superiority over clonidine alone in terms of managing mental symptoms. The dosage of the undefined passion flower extract was 60 drops per day.[19]
- In a pilot, randomized, double-blind, controlled trial, passion flower extract was as efficacious as oxazepam (a benzodiazepine drug) for managing generalized anxiety disorder. However, passion flower treatment resulted in a lower incidence of impairment of job performance. The daily dose of the undefined passion flower extract was 45 drops.[20]
- A passion flower and valerian combination improved symptoms of insomnia in uncontrolled trials.[21,22] Side effects characteristic of benzodiazepine tranquilizers were not observed.[22] In a controlled trial with comparison against chlorpromazine (an antipsychotic drug), EEG recordings showed sedative activity after 6 weeks' treatment with the herbal combination.[21] The dosage administered in one of these trials was 1.0 to 2.5 dessert-spoonfuls per day of syrup (100 g of which contained 25 g of passion flower extract 1:1 and 12.5 g of valerian extract 1:1).[22]
- In a randomized, double-blind, placebo-controlled study, a single dose of passion flower extract (equivalent to 7 g of dried herb) demonstrated a sedative effect when compared with baseline values in healthy female volunteers as assessed by a self-rating scale for alertness.[23]
- In a randomized, double-blind trial, hawthorn (leaf and flower) combined with passion flower reduced heart rate at rest, diastolic blood pressure during exercise, plasma cholesterol and increased exercise capacity compared with placebo in NHYA stage II heart failure patients.[24]
- In Germany, the Commission E supports using passion flower to treat nervous restlessness.[25]
- ESCOP recommends passion flower for treating nervous tension, restlessness, and irritability with difficulty in falling asleep.[26]

REFERENCES

1 Felter HW, Lloyd JU: *King's American dispensatory,* ed 18, rev 3, Portland, 1905, reprinted 1983, Eclectic Medical Publications.
2 British Herbal Medicine Association's Scientific Committee: *British herbal pharmacopoeia,* Bournemouth, 1983, BHMA.
3 Vogel VJ: *American Indian medicine,* Norman, Okla, 1970, University of Oklahoma Press.
4 Bernardes A: *A pocket book of Brazilian herbs: forklore, history, uses,* Rio de Janeiro, Brazil, 1983, Shogun Arte.

Passion Flower *continued on page 365*

5 Wagner H, Bladt S: *Plant drug analysis: a thin layer chromatography atlas,* ed 2, Berlin, 1996, Springer-Verlag.

6 British Herbal Medicine Association: *British herbal compendium,* Bournemouth, 1992, BHMA.

7 Aoyagi N, Kimura R, Murata T: *Chem Pharm Bull* 22(5):1008-1013, 1974.

8 Meier B: *Z Phytother* 16(2):115-126, 1995.

9 Soulimani R et al: *J Ethnopharmacol* 57(1):11-20, 1997.

10 Speroni E, Minghetti A: *Planta Med* 54(6):488-491, 1988.

11 Sopranzi N et al: *Clin Ter* 132(5):329-333, 1990.

12 Galliano G, Foussard-Blanpin O, Bretaudeau J: *Phytotherapy* (40/41):18-22, 1994.

13 Capasso A, Pinto A: *Acta Ther* 21(2):127-140, 1995.

14 Speroni E et al: *Phytother Res* 10(suppl 1):S92-S94, 1996.

15 Della Loggia R, Tubaro A, Redaelli C: *Riv Neurol* 51(5):297-310, 1981.

16 Borrelli F et al: *Phytother Res* 10(suppl 1):S104-S106, 1996.

17 Burkard W et al: *Pharm Pharmacol Lett* 7(1):25-26, 1997.

18 Buchbauer G, Jirovetz L, Jager W: *Arch Pharm* 325(4):247-248, 1992.

19 Akhondzadeh S et al: *J Clin Pharm Ther* 26(5):369-373, 2001.

20 Akhondzadeh S et al: *J Clin Pharm Ther* 26(5):363-367, 2001.

21 Kammerer E, Wegener T: *Natura Med* 10(2):1-8, 1995.

22 Mollenhauer C: *Z Phytother Abstractband* 22, 1995.

23 Schulz H, Jobert M, Hubner WD: *Phytomed* 5(6):449-458, 1998.

24 von Eiff M et al: *Acta Ther* 20:47-66, 1994.

25 Blumenthal M et al, eds: *The complete German Commission E monographs: therapeutic guide to herbal medicines,* Austin, 1998, American Botanical Council.

26 Scientific Committee of the European Scientific Cooperative on Phytotherapy [ESCOP]: *ESCOP monographs: Passiflorae herba.* European Scientific Cooperative on Phytotherapy, ESCOP Secretariat, Argyle House, Gandy Street, Exeter, Devon, EX4 3LS, United Kingdom, July 1997.

PAU D'ARCO

Other Common Name:	Lapacho
Botanical Names:	*Tabebuia avellanedae, Tabebuia impetiginosa,*# *Tabebuia ipe*+
Family:	Bignoniaceae
Plant Part Used:	Bark

PRESCRIBING INFORMATION

Actions

Immune-enhancing, antitumor, antibacterial, antifungal, antiparasitic, depurative

Potential Indications

Based on appropriate evaluation of the patient, practitioners should consider prescribing pau d'arco in formulations in the context of:
- Adjuvant therapy for cancer *(4a,6)*
- Adjuvant therapy for protozoal infections *(7)*
- Topical treatment for skin diseases, fungal infections, skin cancer, varicose ulcers *(6)*

Contraindications

Patients on anticoagulant therapy should not be prescribed pau d'arco because of the potential warfarinlike action of naphthoquinones at high doses.

Warnings and Precautions

Although pau d'arco contains potentially toxic active constituents that can generate free radicals and interfere with mitochondrial respiration and blood coagulation, no evidence has been found that the long-term use of pau d'arco is unsafe, provided certain precautions are observed: the dose should not be too high, and patients on anticoagulant therapy should not take pau d'arco. The therapeutic effects of pau d'arco are likely to be mild, and it should not be trusted as a sole treatment for cancer or infections.

Interactions

Prescribing pau d'arco with anticoagulants is contraindicated.

Use in Pregnancy and Lactation

Caution in pregnancy resulting from possible abortive and teratogenic actions.

Side Effects

Adverse effects have been recorded during clinical trials using lapachol, but no evidence has been found to suggest that pau d'arco would cause similar effects. No adverse effects are expected when consumed within the recommended dosage.

Dosage

Dose per day*	Dose per week*
3-7 ml of 1:2 liquid extract	20-50 ml of 1:2 liquid extract

Pau d'arco *continued on page 367*

#Alternative name.

+Medicinally interchangeable species.

*This dose range is adapted from dried plant dosages administered by decoction in traditional South American medicine.[1] The author's experience and the fact that ethanol-water is a more effective solvent than water for many phytochemicals are taken into account.

SUPPORTING INFORMATION

Traditional Prescribing

Traditional South American medicine uses of pau d'arco include:
- As a depurative and tonic[1,2]
- Dysentery, fever, sore throat, wounds, snakebites, intestinal inflammation, inflamed joints, circulatory and degenerative disorders, carcinomas[2]
- Topically for treating skin diseases, such as eczema, psoriasis, fungal infections, and skin cancers[2]

Traditional use of the bark of other species of Tabebuia include:[3]
- Stomach ulcers *(T. insignis var. monophylla)*
- Malaria, chronic anemia, ulcer pains *(T. neochrysantha)*
- Rheumatic conditions *(T. obscura)*

In the mid-1960s, a Brazilian news magazine printed reports of the "miracle cures" of cases of terminal leukemia and cancer following the use of pau d'arco tea. The bark was dispensed from hospitals in São Paulo for treating leukemia, diabetes, ulcers, rheumatism, and cancer. Other instances were reported of topical use of the decoction successfully treating skin cancer and chronic varicose ulcers.[1]

Pharmacologic Research

The most widely used species of pau d'arco in Western counties are *Tabebuia impetiginosa (T. avellanedae)* and *T. ipe.* Other species used include *Tabebuia rosea (T. pentaphylla), T. chrysantha, T. cassinoides,* and *T. serratifolia.*

Key constituents of *Tabebuia impetiginosa* bark include naphthoquinones of the 1,4 type (especially lapachol) and furanonaphthoquinones. Although much of the active component research has concentrated on lapachol, other naphthoquinones and their furano derivatives are likely to contribute significantly to the therapeutic activity of pau d'arco.
- Lapachol, other naphthoquinones, and furanonaphthoquinones have inhibited growth of cultured tumor cells. Lapachol has demonstrated significant antitumor activity *in vitro* and *in vivo.* Oral administration of lapachol resulted in inhibition of tumor growth in several carcinosarcoma models, particularly Walker 256 carcinosarcoma. Statistical analysis revealed a link between the redox potentials of various compounds in pau d'arco and their antitumor activity. The oxidative stress theory, in which quinones are reduced to oxygen-radical-activating compounds, is one explanation for their cytotoxic activity.
- Pau d'arco extracts and other components have also demonstrated *in vivo* antitumor effects in skin carcinogenesis and leukemia P-388 models.
- *In vitro* investigations of compounds isolated from *T. impetiginosa* confirmed dose-dependent, immune-enhancing effects on human granulocytes and lymphocytes.

Pau d'arco *continued on page 368*

- Pau d'arco, and some of its constituents, including lapachol, were found to be active against various tropical parasites *in vitro*. Studies at Harvard Medical School confirmed these results.
- Naphthoquinones tested against drug-resistant strains of *Plasmodium falciparum* were superior to the controls chloroquine and quinine. Lapachol has been used as a chemoprophylactic against *Schistosoma mansoni* penetration and infection *in vivo*. Lapachol and its derivatives were also shown to work by topical applications.
- Pau d'arco extracts and isolated constituents demonstrated antibacterial and antifungal activity *in vitro*. *T. impetiginosa* extract inhibited a penicillin-resistant strain of *Staphylococcus aureus*.
- Antiviral activity was demonstrated *in vitro* for lapachol against a number of viruses, including herpes and retroviruses. Extracts of the inner bark of *T. avellanedae* were found to inhibit induction of Epstein-Barr virus (EBV)–associated early antigen in EBV genome–carrying human lymphoblastic cell lines. The antiviral activity of lapachol may involve redox reactions, stimulation of interferon production, or enzyme inhibition.
- Lapachol and related naphthoquinones are known anticoagulants. Some authors link this anticoagulant activity to the anticancer applications of pau d'arco.
- Oral administration of aqueous extract of *Tabebuia avellandae* inner bark demonstrated antiinflammatory activity in rat paw edema and analgesic activity in an experimental pain model.[4]

Clinical Studies

- A phase I clinical trial using lapachol was initiated in 1967 at the Baltimore Cancer Research Center. The trial involved 21 patients with leukemia, each of whom was initially given capsules containing 0.25 or 0.5 g lapachol and later switched to a syrup formulation. The trial was stopped prematurely because prolonged prothrombin times were observed at the high oral doses required to test for antitumor activity. These doses also resulted in nausea and vomiting, and measurements of plasma lapachol showed that intestinal absorption of lapachol was considerably less than previously determined in rats. However, lapachol may be much better absorbed from its natural plant matrix.
- Prescription of lapachol (20 to 30 mg/kg/day) caused shrinkage of tumors and reduction in pain for nine patients with cancer who were participating in a small clinical trial. Three patients ceased the treatment because of nausea and vomiting; the other patients had no significant side effects. Three patients experienced complete remissions.

REFERENCES

Except when specifically referenced, the following book was referred to in the compilation of the pharmacologic and clinical information: Mills S, Bone K: *Principles and Practice of Phytotherapy: Modern Herbal Medicine,* Edinburgh, 2000, Churchill Livingstone.

1 Jones K: *Pau d'arco: immune power from the rain forest,* Rochester, Vt, 1995, Healing Arts Press.

2 Oswald EH: *Br J Phytother* 3(3):112-117, 1993-1994.

3 Evans Schultes R, Raffauf RF: *The healing forest: medicinal and toxic plants of the Northwest Amazonia,* Portland, 1990, Dioscorides Press.

4 Goncalves de Miranda FG et al: *BMC Pharmacology* 1:6, 2001.

PEPPERMINT

Botanical Name: Mentha piperita
Family: Labiatae
Plant Part Used: Leaf

PRESCRIBING INFORMATION

Actions

Spasmolytic, carminative, cholagogue, antiemetic, antitussive, antimicrobial (internally and topically), mild sedative, diaphoretic, analgesic (topically), antipruritic (topically)

Potential Indications

Based on appropriate evaluation of the patient, practitioners should consider prescribing peppermint in formulations in the context of:
- Nonulcer dyspepsia,* in combination with fennel, caraway, and wormwood (2)
- Chronic digestive problems, bloating, flatulence,* in combination with fennel, caraway, and gentian (2)
- Spastic complaints of the gastrointestinal tract, gallbladder, and bile ducts (4,5)
- Gastritis, enteritis (4)
- Respiratory tract catarrh, cough, the common cold (5)
- Nausea, vomiting, morning sickness (5)
- Nervous conditions, dysmenorrhea (5)
- Topical treatment for headaches (5)

Contraindications

Because of its ability to lower esophageal sphincter pressure, peppermint is contraindicated in patients with esophageal reflux.

Warnings and Precautions

Peppermint should be used with care in patients with salicylate sensitivity and aspirin-induced asthma, as well as those with gallstones.

Interactions

Peppermint tea reduced the absorption of iron by 84% from a bread meal (compared with a water control) in adult volunteers. The inhibition was dose-dependent and related to its tannin content. Inhibition by black tea was 79% to 94%.[1] This finding indicates a potential interaction for concomitant administration of peppermint during iron intake. In anemia and cases for which iron supplementation is required, peppermint should not be taken simultaneously with meals or iron supplements.

Use in Pregnancy and Lactation

No adverse effects expected.

Side Effects

None known for peppermint leaf. Allergic reactions to peppermint appear to be rare or of a relatively minor nature.

Peppermint *continued on page 370*

*Peppermint has also been used in traditional herbal medicine for treating dyspepsia and flatulence and is recommended for this use by both the Commission E and ESCOP. (4,5)

Skin rashes, headache, bradycardia, muscle tremor, heartburn, and ataxia are rarely reported side effects associated with using enteric-coated capsules of peppermint oil. Fibrillation has been associated with the excessive consumption of peppermint-flavored confectionery. Gastrointestinal irritation or aggravation of gastrointestinal complaints, including stomatitis, severe esophagitis, gastritis, unexplained diarrhea, and pancreatitis, have been associated with using peppermint preparations, including confectionery.

Dosage

Dose per day**	Dose per week**
1.5-4.5 ml of 1:2 liquid extract	10-30 ml of 1:2 liquid extract

SUPPORTING INFORMATION

Traditional Prescribing

Traditional Western herbal medicine uses include:
- Spasm or cramps of the stomach,[2] gastrointestinal pain, flatulent dyspepsia,[3] gallbladder disorders[4]
- Nausea, vomiting,[2] morning sickness[3]
- The common cold[3]
- Dysmenorrhea,[3] hysteria[2]
- To disguise the unpleasant taste of other medicines and to allay the painful effect of cathartic remedies[2]
- As a poultice for upset stomach and headaches[2]

Peppermint oil solution has been traditionally used as an inhalation for bronchitic cough and pneumonia.[2]

Pharmacologic Research

Key constituents of peppermint leaves include phenolic acids, tannins, and an essential oil (0.5% to 4.0%) consisting mostly of menthol (35% to 45%).
- Peppermint extract produced analgesic activity in two experimental models, indicating central and peripheral effects (400 mg/kg pretreatment by injection and 200 to 400 mg/kg oral pretreatment, respectively). Peppermint exhibited antiinflammatory activity in acute (200 mg/kg, pretreatment by injection) and chronic inflammation (400 mg/kg, oral).[5]
- Peppermint extract and essential oil markedly reduced experimentally induced contractile responses in isolated gastrointestinal smooth muscle preparations.
- Oral administration of a fraction obtained from an aqueous ethanolic extract of peppermint inhibited nasal symptoms, sneezing, and nasal rubbing in an experimental model of allergic rhinitis.[6]
- Peppermint oil inhibited gastrointestinal enterocyte glucose uptake via a direct action at the brush border membrane *in vitro*.
- Peppermint oil has exhibited significant antibacterial and antifungal activity *in vitro*.

Peppermint continued on page 371

**This dose range is extrapolatd from the British Herbal Compendium 1992 and the author's education and experience.

- Single oral doses of menthol or cineole inhibited 3-hydroxy-3-methyl-glutaryl coenzyme A (HMG CoA) reductase activity in experimental models by up to 70%.
- Menthol inhalation significantly reduced cough frequency and increased cough latency in experimental models of chemically induced cough.
- Acetylcholine-induced bronchospasm decreased by 50% in experimental models when an ointment containing menthol, camphor, and essential oils was insufflated through the respiratory tract. Topical application produced only slight reduction.
- Dietary menthol and limonene significantly inhibited experimentally induced mammary tumors in experimental models.
- Menthol has calcium ion–channel blocking activity and a pharmacologic profile similar to that of calcium antagonists.

Clinical Studies

- A liquid herbal formula containing peppermint, fennel, caraway *(Carum carvi)*, and wormwood was significantly superior to metoclopramide (a spasmolytic drug) in terms of relieving symptoms in a randomized, double-blind, controlled trial involving patients with dyspepsia. A trial of similar design demonstrated a significant improvement in the gastrointestinal complaint scores and a reduction in intestinal gas in patients with chronic digestive problems, such as flatulence or bloating, treated with a tablet formula containing these ingredients (but with gentian instead of wormwood).
- Pain intensity was significantly decreased in two randomized trials,[7,8] and pain intensity and global clinical impression were significantly improved in a double-blind, placebo-controlled, multicenter trial involving patients with nonulcer dyspepsia. Doses of 180 to 270 mg/day of peppermint oil and 100 to 150 mg/day of caraway oil were prescribed for 4 weeks. No significant difference was observed between the peppermint-caraway combination and the drug cisapride (a motility drug; 30 mg/day) in terms of clinical outcome.[7]
- A meta-analysis of five randomized, double-blind, placebo-controlled trials found that peppermint oil (0.6 to 1.2 ml/day for 2 to 4 weeks) might be efficacious for symptom relief in irritable bowel syndrome but was unable to provide a definitive judgment because of methodologic flaws associated with most studies.[9] Enteric-coated capsules were used to prevent the gastric reflux, which such high doses will inevitably cause. In a randomized, double-blind, multicenter, placebo-controlled trial published since the meta-analysis, 75% of children with irritable bowel syndrome who received peppermint oil experienced reduced severity of pain after 2 weeks of treatment.[10]
- Gynecologic patients experienced a significant reduction in postoperative nausea after inhaling peppermint oil in a placebo-controlled trial. Patients were provided with 5 ml of oil but used no more than a total of 1 ml.
- Peppermint oil solution administered (dose unknown) via the biopsy channel of the colonoscope relieved colonic spasm within 30 seconds

Peppermint continued on page 372

in an uncontrolled study, allowing easier passage of the instrument. A more recent placebo-controlled trial confirmed that a spasmolytic effect was seen in 89% of patients undergoing colonoscopy after intracolonic administration of approximately 200 ml of a 0.8% peppermint oil solution (compared with 33% in the control group). In patients with irritable bowel syndrome, efficacy was significantly lower.[11]

- Topical application of a solution of 10% peppermint oil in ethanol significantly reduced headache sensitivity and intensity, comparable to acetaminophen (paracetamol, 1 g), in a randomized, double-blind, placebo-controlled, crossover trial.

- Patients with cholesterol gallstones were treated with either ursodeoxycholic acid (UDCA, 11.1 mg/kg/day) or a combination of UDCA (4.75 mg/kg/day) and menthol (4.75 mg/kg/day) in a double-blind trial. After 15.0 to 16.9 months, complete dissolution of stones was achieved in 53% of patients treated with the combination and 38% of patients treated with the higher dose of UDCA alone. The response rate (complete + partial dissolution) was 76% in the combination group and 75% in the UDCA alone group. One case of stone calcification occurred in the UDCA alone group, whereas no cases occurred in the combination treatment group.

- Long-term inhalation of menthol (20 mg/day for 4 weeks via a nebulizer) significantly decreased airway hyperresponsiveness in patients with asthma in a placebo-controlled trial.

- Administration of menthol (11 mg) as a lozenge decreased the sensation of nasal congestion in patients with the common cold in an uncontrolled trial.

- In Germany, the Commission E supports using peppermint leaf to treat spastic complaints of the gastrointestinal tract, gallbladder, and bile ducts. Peppermint oil can be used to treat discomfort of the upper gastrointestinal tract and bile ducts, irritable colon, catarrh of the respiratory tract, and inflammation of the oral mucosa.[12]

- ESCOP recommends peppermint leaf for the symptomatic treatment of digestive disorders, such as dyspepsia, flatulence, gastritis, and enteritis, and peppermint oil for irritable bowel syndrome and the symptomatic treatment of digestive disorders, coughs, and the common cold.[13]

- Peppermint has remained official in the USP since the first entry in 1820 and is currently official in the USP24-NF19.

REFERENCES

Except when specifically referenced, the following book was referred to in the compilation of the pharmacologic and clinical information: Mills S, Bone K: *Principles and Practice of Phytotherapy: Modern Herbal Medicine,* Edinburgh, 2000, Churchill Livingstone.

1 Hurrell RF, Reddy M, Cook JD: *Br J Nutr* 81(4):289-295, 1999.
2 Felter HW, Lloyd JU: *King's American dispensatory,* ed 18, rev 3, Portland, 1905, reprinted 1983, Eclectic Medical Publications.
3 British Herbal Medicine Association's Scientific Committee: *British herbal pharmacopoeia,* Bournemouth, 1983, BHMA.

Peppermint *continued on page 373*

4 British Herbal Medicine Association: *British herbal compendium,* Bournemouth, 1992, BHMA.

5 Atta AH, Alkofahi A: *J Ethnopharmacol* 60(2):117-124, 1998.

6 Inoue T et al: *Biol Pharm Bull* 24(1):92-95, 2001.

7 Madisch A et al: *Arzneim Forsch* 49(11):925-932, 1999.

8 Freise J, Kohler S: *Pharmazie* 54(3):210-215, 1999.

9 Pittler MH, Ernst E: *Am J Gastroenterol* 93(7):1131-1135, 1998.

10 Kline RM et al: *J Pediatr* 138(1):125-128, 2001.

11 Asao T et al: *Gastrointest Endosc* 53(2):172-177, 2001.

12 Blumenthal M et al, eds: *The complete German Commission E monographs: therapeutic guide to herbal medicines,* Austin, 1998, American Botanical Council.

13 Scientific Committee of the European Scientific Cooperative on Phytotherapy [ESCOP]: *ESCOP monographs: Menthae piperitae folium/aetheroleum.* European Scientific Cooperative on Phytotherapy, ESCOP Secretariat, Argyle House, Gandy Street, Exeter, Devon, EX4 3LS, United Kingdom, July 1997.

PLEURISY ROOT

Botanical Name: *Asclepias tuberosa*
Family: Asclepiadaceae
Plant Part Used: Root

PRESCRIBING INFORMATION

Actions

Diaphoretic, expectorant

Potential Indications

Based on appropriate evaluation of the patient, practitioners should consider prescribing pleurisy root in formulations in the context of:
- Respiratory disorders, especially of a catarrhal, chronic, or inflammatory nature, including the common cold, influenza, pneumonia, pleurisy, bronchitis, and fevers *(5)*
- Other conditions for which diaphoresis is of benefit, such as arthritic and rheumatic conditions *(5)*

Contraindications

None known.

Warnings and Precautions

None required.

Interactions

None known.

Use in Pregnancy and Lactation

No adverse effects expected.

Side Effects

None expected if taken within the recommended dose range. Very large (undefined) doses are said to cause diarrhea and vomiting.[1]

Dosage

*Dose per day**	*Dose per week**
1.5-3.0 ml of 1:2 liquid extract	10-20 ml of 1:2 liquid extract

SUPPORTING INFORMATION

Traditional Prescribing

Traditional Western herbal medicine uses include:
- Bronchitis, pneumonitis, pleurisy, influenza, pulmonary congestion, tuberculosis, dry asthma with fever; the common cold, particularly in children[1,2]
- Diarrhea, dysentery, flatulent colic; rheumatism, neuralgia, dry skin conditions[2]

Pleurisy root was regarded as a lung tonic[3] and the best diaphoretic in the *Eclectic Materia Medica*.[2]

Native Americans used pleurisy root both internally and externally for bronchial and pulmonary disorders, including pneumonia and fever, and for dysentery. Pleurisy root was used externally for wounds, sores,

Pleurisy Root *continued on page 375*

*This dose range is extrapolated from the British Herbal Pharmacopoeia 1983 and the author's education and experience.

and bruises. Pleurisy root was official in the USP from 1820 to 1905 and the NF from 1916 to 1936 and was used as a diaphoretic and expectorant and in large doses as an emetic and purgative.[4]

Pharmacologic Research

No pharmacologic information relevant to the current use of pleurisy root has been found.

Clinical Studies

No clinical studies using pleurisy root have been found.

REFERENCES

1 British Herbal Medicine Association's Scientific Committee: *British herbal pharmacopoeia*, Bournemouth, 1983, BHMA.
2 Felter HW, Lloyd JU: *King's American dispensatory*, ed 18, rev 3, Portland, 1905, reprinted 1983, Eclectic Medical Publications.
3 Grieve M: *A modern herbal*, New York, 1971, Dover Publications.
4 Vogel VJ: *American Indian medicine*, Norman, Okla, 1970, University of Oklahoma Press.

POKE ROOT

Botanical Names: *Phytolacca decandra, P. americana*[#]
Family: Phytolaccaceae
Plant Part Used: Root

PRESCRIBING INFORMATION

Actions

Antiinflammatory, lymphatic, depurative, immune-enhancing

Potential Indications

Based on appropriate evaluation of the patient, practitioners should consider prescribing poke root in formulations in the context of:
- Skin conditions, as a depurative acting primarily via the lymphatic system (5)
- Treating inflammatory conditions or infections, especially of the respiratory tract and reproductive systems (5)
- Mastitis, mammary abscess (5)
- Possible treatment for uterine and breast cancers (6)
- Topical treatment of skin irritation, infection, or infestation (5)

Contraindications

Poke root is contraindicated in:
- Pregnancy, lactation (because of its potential toxicity)
- Lymphocytic leukemia (resulting from increased lymphocyte count in a woman consuming the fresh root and the lymphocyte-stimulating activity of the lectins *in vitro*)
- Gastrointestinal irritation (resulting from the emetic activity and saponin content)

Warnings and Precautions

The recommended dosage of poke root has been exceeded in some cases (see the "Side Effects" section in this monograph) because of variation in the potency of the root with resultant side effects. Fresh plant tinctures should be used with extreme caution, if at all. Accurate measurement of dried plant tincture volumes is vital to ensure that the safe dosage is not exceeded, because toxic effects are possible from overdose. Topical application of poke root should be restricted to dried plant tinctures and contact with the eyes should be avoided.

Interactions

Concurrent use with immunosuppressive drugs should be avoided.

Use in Pregnancy and Lactation

Contraindicated in pregnancy and lactation.

Side Effects

Poisonings occurred in North America during the nineteenth century following overdose of dried plant tinctures and ingestion of berries or roots mistaken for other vegetables. More recently, poisoning has occurred from inappropriate use of the root, such as

Poke Root continued on page 377

[#]Alternative name.

ingesting the fresh root without boiling first and ingesting decocted powdered root. Adverse events have occurred in Australia resulting from excessive intake: in some cases hospitalization was required, and in one case, a shock reaction with pronounced hypotension and tachycardia occurred. Topical application of preparations derived from the green plant and root has produced inflammation of the skin.

Dosage

Dose per day*	Dose per week*
0.15-0.7 ml of 1:5 tincture	1-5 ml of 1:5 tincture

Using liquid extracts and fresh plant tinctures should be avoided because of potential toxic effects.

SUPPORTING INFORMATION

Traditional Prescribing

Traditional Western herbal medicine uses include:
- Action on the skin and the glandular structures, particularly of the mouth, throat, or reproductive tract (tonsillitis, laryngitis, lymphadenitis, mumps, ovaritis, glandular swellings) and marked action on the mammary glands[1,2]
- Breast cancer[3]
- Chronic rheumatism[1]
- Topically for treating skin and glandular disorders, including scabies, tinea, acne, mastitis, and mammary abscess[1]
- Uterine cancer[3]

Native Americans used poke root as a poultice, and the root was applied to the hands and feet of individuals afflicted with fever. Poke root was official in the USP from 1820 to 1916, the NF from 1916 to 1947, and was used for emetic and purgative purposes, as a depurative, in skin diseases, and for relief of pain and inflammation.[4]

Pharmacologic Research

- The immunologic activity of poke root may be caused by the presence of traces of mitogenic lectins, which may interact with gut-associated lymphoid tissue and may even be absorbed in small quantities. These lectins are used pharmacologically to agglutinate some erythrocytes, stimulate mitosis and antibody synthesis in lymphocytes, and induce activation of plasma cells.
- The crude saponins from poke root exhibited antiinflammatory activity by injection in experimental models.

Clinical Studies

No clinical studies using poke root have been found.

Poke Root *continued on page 378*

*This dose range is extrapolated from the British Pharmaceutical Codex 1923, the British Herbal Pharmacopoeia 1983, and the author's education and experience.

REFERENCES

Except where specifically referenced, the following book was referred to in the compilation of the pharmacologic information: Mills S, Bone K: *Principles and Practice of Phytotherapy: Modern Herbal Medicine,* Edinburgh, 2000, Churchill Livingstone.

1 British Herbal Medicine Association's Scientific Committee: *British herbal pharmacopoeia,* Bournemouth, 1983, BHMA.
2 Felter HW, Lloyd JU: *King's American dispensatory,* ed 18, rev 3, Portland, 1905, reprinted 1983, Eclectic Medical Publications.
3 Grieve M: *A modern herbal,* New York, 1971, Dover Publications.
4 Vogel VJ: *American Indian medicine,* Norman, Okla, 1970, University of Oklahoma Press.

PRICKLY ASH

Botanical Names: *Zanthoxylum clava-herculis, Zanthoxylum americanum,*[+]
                       Xanthoxylum americanum[#]
Family: Rutaceae
Plant Part Used: Bark

PRESCRIBING INFORMATION

Actions

Circulatory stimulant, diaphoretic, antirheumatic, sialogogue

Potential Indications

Based on appropriate evaluation of the patient, practitioners should consider prescribing prickly ash in formulations in the context of:
- Hemorrhoids and varicose veins *(2)*
- Conditions requiring circulatory stimulation, including peripheral circulatory insufficiency, intermittent claudication, and Raynaud's syndrome *(5)*
- Cramps, chronic rheumatic conditions, neuralgia *(5)*
- Osteoarthritis *(6)*

Contraindications

None known.

Warnings and Precautions

None required.

Interactions

None known.

Use in Pregnancy and Lactation

No adverse effects expected.

Side Effects

None expected if taken within the recommended dose range.

Dosage

Dose per day*	Dose per week*
1.5-4.5 ml of 1:2 liquid extract	10-30 ml of 1:2 liquid extract

SUPPORTING INFORMATION

Traditional Prescribing

Traditional Western herbal medicine uses include:
- Conditions of sluggish circulation, peripheral circulatory insufficiency, intermittent claudication, Raynaud's syndrome,[1] cold hands and feet, and complaints arising from bad circulation[2]
- Chronic rheumatic conditions,[1] arthritic tendency[3]
- Cramps, neuralgia[1,4]
- Conditions of mucous membranes such as pharyngitis and postnasal catarrh[4]
- As a gastrointestinal tonic for atonic dyspepsia, constipation[4]

Prickly Ash *continued on page 380*

[+]Medicinally interchangeable species.
[#]Alternative name.
*This dose range is extrapolated from the British Herbal Pharmacopoeia 1983, the British Herbal Compendium 1992, and the author's education and experience.

Pharmacologic Research

Aqueous extract of prickly ash inhibited swelling and improved vascular permeability in experimental models of hemorrhoids and varicose veins.[5]

Clinical Studies

A high dose of prickly ash extract (standardized for total alkaloids and magnoflorine) demonstrated symptom improvement in treating hemorrhoids and varicose veins in two randomized, double-blind, placebo-controlled trials. Venous circulation was improved in varicose veins patients.[5]

REFERENCES

1 British Herbal Medicine Association's Scientific Committee: *British herbal pharmacopoeia,* Bournemouth, 1983, BHMA.

2 Grieve M: *A modern herbal,* New York, 1971, Dover Publications.

3 Bartram T: *Encyclopedia of herbal medicine,* ed 1, Dorset, UK, 1995, Grace Publishers.

4 Felter HW, Lloyd JU: *King's American dispensatory,* ed 18, rev 3, Portland, 1905, reprinted 1983, Eclectic Medical Publications.

5 Jia Q et al: *Phytomed* 7(supp 2):46, 2000.

RASPBERRY LEAF

Other Common Name:	Red raspberry leaf
Botanical Name:	*Rubus idaeus*
Family:	Rosaceae
Plant Part Used:	Leaf

PRESCRIBING INFORMATION

Actions

Astringent, partus preparator, parturifacient, antidiarrheal

Potential Indications

Based on appropriate evaluation of the patient, practitioners should consider prescribing raspberry leaf in formulations in the context of:
- Ensuring healthy uterine function at childbirth (when taken during pregnancy) *(4,5)*
- Abnormal bleeding from the uterus, stomach, or bowels *(5)*
- Mouth ulcers, diarrhea *(5)*
- Dysmenorrhea *(6)*
- Topical treatment for tonsillitis, conjunctivitis, sore throat *(5,6)*

Contraindications

None known.

Warnings and Precautions

None required.

Interactions

None known.

Use in Pregnancy and Lactation

No adverse effects expected in pregnancy or lactation, but confining use to the second and third trimesters is more appropriate.

Side Effects

None expected if taken within the recommended dosage.

Dosage

Dose per day*	Dose per week*
4.5-14 ml of 1:2 liquid extract	30-100 ml of 1:2 liquid extract

SUPPORTING INFORMATION

Traditional Prescribing

Traditional Western herbal medicine uses include:
- Diarrhea, dysentery, cholera[1,2]
- During pregnancy and to facilitate delivery,[1,2] dysmenorrhea[3]
- Stomatitis;[1] hemorrhage from the stomach, bowel, or uterus; prolapsed uterus[2]
- Topically for tonsillitis and conjunctivitis,[1] as a gargle for sore throats[4]
- Stomach complaints of children, topically for wounds and ulcers[4]

Pharmacologic Research

The leaves of raspberry contain flavonoids, gallotannins, and ellagitannins.[5]

Raspberry Leaf *continued on page 382*

*This dose range is extrapolated from the British Herbal Pharmacopoeia 1983 and the author's education and experience.

- Aqueous extract of raspberry leaf (1 g/15 ml) had little or no effect on isolated uteri from nonpregnant rats but inhibited contractions of those from pregnant rats. A variable response was obtained from uteri in induced estrus. Inhibition lasted 3 to 4 minutes, and intrinsic contractions were resumed. Epinephrine (adrenaline)-like resistance did not develop and the inhibitory effect was not prevented by propranolol. The extract contracted strips of human uterus at 10 to 16 weeks of pregnancy. For pregnant human and rat uteri, the intrinsic rhythm (over a 20-minute period while the extract remained in contact with the tissue) appeared to become more regular in most cases, and contractions were less frequent.[6]
- Aqueous extract of raspberry leaf stimulated isolated smooth muscle, particularly the uterus. When the tannins were removed from this extract, spasmolytic activity was exhibited. Both stimulant and relaxant components were present in the extract, with a weak anticholinesterase component demonstrating stimulation.[7]
- Raspberry leaf extracts relaxed isolated intestinal smooth muscle.[8]
- A concentrate of raspberry leaf infusion relaxed the uterus and intestine *in situ* (by intravenous injection), provided the tone of the organs was normal. For the uterus, the relaxation was occasionally followed by contraction and further relaxation. The degree of relaxation increased with successive doses. Secondary contractions were eliminated, and those that occurred were evenly spaced. The experimental model included mainly nonpregnant uteri and one animal in late pregnancy. Relaxation was also promoted in tonically contracted isolated (presumably nonpregnant) uteri, but if allowed to relax, raspberry leaf caused the organ to contract. When little tone was present in isolated uterus, raspberry leaf caused stimulation, but when the uterus was toned, raspberry leaf induced relaxation.[9] This finding implies a regulatory action on uterine tone.

Clinical Studies

- A retrospective, observational, controlled study involving 108 women found that women can consume raspberry leaf during their pregnancy to shorten labor, with no side effects identified for the women or their babies. Ingesting raspberry leaf may also decrease the likelihood of preterm and postterm labor, evidenced by a smaller spread of the gestation period among the raspberry leaf group. An unexpected finding of the study was that women who ingest raspberry leaf might be less likely to require artificial rupture of their membranes, cesarean section, forceps, or vacuum birth. Treatment began as early as 8 weeks' gestation, with the majority commencing at 30 to 34 weeks. The daily dose ranged from 1 to 6 cups of tea or 1 to 8 tablets, with 6 cups or tablets per day being the most popular intake. The weight of the tablets was not defined.[10]
- A follow-up trial of randomized, double-blind, placebo-controlled design was conducted by the same authors and involved 192 women who were followed from 32 weeks of pregnancy to labor. The women in the treatment group received 1.2 g of raspberry leaf twice a day.

Raspberry Leaf *continued on page 383*

No adverse effects were observed, but also, no effect on shortening the first stage of labor was indicated. A shortening of the second stage of labor occurred (a difference of 9.6 minutes) and a lower rate of forceps deliveries was noted for the raspberry leaf group compared with the control group (19.3% and 30.4%, respectively). The authors suggested that earlier intervention and a higher dose should be studied.[11]

- A pharmacologic study conducted in the 1940s observed that uterine contractions decreased in frequency and strength in three pregnant women administered a raspberry leaf extract. Secondary contractions were also eliminated. A very slight fall in the systolic blood pressure was noticeable. The authors noted that raspberry leaf may be useful for treating irregular uterine action during labor and menstruation. The dose was recorded as 20 to 40 grains (approximately 1.3 to 2.6 g) of crude extract of dried raspberry leaves, containing fragarine. "Fragarine" is the term the authors proposed for the active principle of this crude extract of raspberry leaves.[3] This term has been used in popular and scientific literature ever since, but no evidence has been found to verify the existence of fragarine, let alone its chemical structure.

REFERENCES

1 British Herbal Medicine Association's Scientific Committee: *British herbal pharmacopoeia,* Bournemouth, 1983, BHMA.
2 Felter HW, Lloyd JU: *King's American dispensatory,* ed 18, rev 3, Portland, 1905, reprinted 1983, Eclectic Medical Publications.
3 Whitehouse B: *Br Med J* 2:370-371, 1941.
4 Grieve M: *A modern herbal,* New York, 1971, Dover Publications.
5 Wagner H, Bladt S: *Plant drug analysis: a thin layer chromatography atlas,* ed 2, Berlin, 1996, Springer-Verlag.
6 Bamford DS, Percival RC, Tothill AU: *Br J Pharmacol* 40(1):161P-162P, 1970.
7 Beckett AH et al: *J Pharm Pharmacol* 6:785-796, 1954.
8 Patel AV et al: *J Pharm Pharmacol* 47(12B):1129, 1990.
9 Burn JH, Withell ER: *Lancet* 2(6149):1-3, 1941.
10 Parsons M, Simpson M, Ponton T: *J Aust Coll Midwives* 12(3):20-25, 1999.
11 Simpson M et al: *J Midwifery Womens Health* 46(2):51-59, 2001.

RED CLOVER

Botanical Name: *Trifolium pratense*
Family: Leguminosae
Plant Part Used: Flower

PRESCRIBING INFORMATION

Actions

Depurative, antitumor (traditional use)

Potential Indications

Based on appropriate evaluation of the patient, practitioners should consider prescribing red clover in formulations in the context of:
- Skin disorders, including eczema, psoriasis, and ulcers (5)
- Respiratory conditions, especially with spasmodic cough, including bronchitis (5)

Contraindications

None known.

Warnings and Precautions

None required.

Interactions

None known.

Use in Pregnancy and Lactation

No adverse effects expected.

Side Effects

None expected if taken within the recommended dose range.

Dosage

Dose per day*	Dose per week*
1.5-6.0 ml of 1:2 liquid extract	10-40 ml of 1:2 liquid extract

SUPPORTING INFORMATION

Traditional Prescribing

Traditional Western herbal medicine uses include:
- Chronic skin disease, including eczema, psoriasis, leg ulcers, and burns[1,2]
- Bronchitis, whooping cough, laryngitis[1,2]
- Cancer[2]

Pharmacologic Research

Red clover flowers contain isoflavones, including biochanin A, formononetin, and genistein.[3] Isoflavones have demonstrated weak estrogenic activity and under certain circumstances exert an antiestrogenic competitive activity.[4] However, in 25% aqueous ethanolic extracts of red clover flowers, these constituents are present in low quantities.[3]

Clinical Studies

Trials using concentrated extracts of red clover leaf and flower, standardized for isoflavone content have been conducted. However, given that traditional liquid extracts are low in isoflavones, this information has not been reviewed here.

Red Clover *continued on page 385*

*This dose range is extrapolated from the British Herbal Pharmacopoeia 1983, the British Herbal Compendium 1992, and the author's education and experience.

REFERENCES

1 British Herbal Medicine Association's Scientific Committee: *British herbal pharmacopoeia*, Bournemouth, 1983, BHMA.

2 Felter HW, Lloyd JU: *King's American dispensatory*, ed 18, rev 3, Portland, 1905, reprinted 1983, Eclectic Medical Publications.

3 Lehmann R, Penman K: Technical Report. MediHerb Pty Ltd, PO Box 713, Warwick, Queensland 4370, Australia.

4 Messina MJ: *Am J Clin Nutr* 70(suppl 3):439S-450S, 1999.

REHMANNIA

Botanical Name: Rehmannia glutinosa
Family: Gesneriaceae
Plant Part Used: Root

PRESCRIBING INFORMATION

Actions

Antipyretic, adrenal tonic, antihemorrhagic, antiinflammatory

Potential Indications

Based on appropriate evaluation of the patient, practitioners should consider prescribing Rehmannia in formulations in the context of:
- Rheumatoid arthritis, asthma, urticaria (4)
- Chronic nephritis, in combination with other traditional Chinese herbs, including Astragalus (4)
- Fevers, hemorrhage, skin rashes, diabetes, insomnia, constipation (5)
- Benefit in supporting adrenal function, particularly if hypertension is present (Unlike licorice, Rehmannia is not contraindicated in hypertension.) (5,7)
- Preventing the suppressive effects of corticosteroid drugs on endogenous levels of corticosteroids (7)

Contraindications

None known.

Warnings and Precautions

None required.

Interactions

None known.

Use in Pregnancy and Lactation

No adverse effects expected.

Side Effects

In a small, open trial involving patients with rheumatoid arthritis, intermittent treatment with Rehmannia decoction elicited mild edema in a minority of patients. Excessive doses can cause diarrhea.

Dosage

Dose per day*	Dose per week*
4.5-8.5 ml of 1:2 liquid extract	30-60 ml of 1:2 liquid extract

SUPPORTING INFORMATION

Traditional Prescribing

In TCM, Rehmannia in its uncured form is the dried root of *Rehmannia glutinosa*. The cured form consists of the clean, fresh root stewed in wine. In this process, the root is washed in wine, steamed, dried, then resteamed, and dried several times. Unless stated otherwise, liquid extracts of Rehmannia usually consist of the uncured form.

Rehmannia *continued on page 387*

*This dose range is adapted from dried plant dosages administered by decoction in TCM.[1] The author's experience and the fact that ethanol-water is a more effective solvent than water for many phytochemicals are taken into account.

TCM uses for uncured Rehmannia include:
- Febrile diseases with reddened tongue and thirst[1,2]
- Hemorrhage[2]
- Spitting of blood, skin eruptions[1]
- Diabetes caused by *internal heat*[1]
- Conditions caused by *heart fire:* mouth sores, insomnia, low-grade fevers, constipation[2]
- Conditions of *yin deficiency* with *internal heat*[1]

TCM uses for cured Rehmannia include:
- To regulate menstruation, to promote blood production and tone the kidneys[3]
- Anemia, dizziness, weakness, tinnitus[1]
- Amenorrhea, metrorrhagia[3]
- Night sweats[1]

Pharmacologic Research

Pharmacologic research conducted using polysaccharides from Rehmannia *in vitro* and by injection has not been listed, because this activity is probably not relevant to the oral use of Rehmannia liquids prepared with ethanol.

Rehmannia root contains a number of constituents, including iridoid glycosides and other glycosides.
- Uncured Rehmannia inhibited the metabolism of cortisol by hepatocytes *in vitro*. Oral administration in a model of adrenal cortex depletion (induced by chronic treatment with glucocorticoids) resulted in raised serum corticosterone levels. Rehmannia treatment also prevented or reversed morphologic changes in the pituitary and adrenal cortex, appearing to antagonize the suppressive effect of glucocorticoids on the hypothalamic-pituitary-adrenal axis.
- Cured Rehmannia abolished the suppressive effects of cyclophosphamide and dexamethasone on immune function and demonstrated protective effects on disturbances in hematopoiesis, immunity, and heart, liver, and kidney functions during chemotherapy in various experimental models.
- An *in vitro* study found that three compounds from Rehmannia demonstrated aldose reductase inhibitory activity.
- Orally administered uncured Rehmannia improved hemorrheology in experimental models of arthritis and thrombosis.

Clinical Studies

- Uncontrolled trials using uncured Rehmannia produced therapeutic effects in patients with rheumatoid arthritis, asthma, and urticaria.
- Oral administration of an herbal preparation that included Rehmannia and Astragalus demonstrated therapeutic effects in patients with chronic nephritis. Significant improvement was observed for 91% of the treatment group compared with 67% of the control group.

Rehmannia continued on page 388

The preparation also demonstrated antiallergic effects and promotion and modulation of immune function. The design of this clinical research was not rigorous and its results should be interpreted with caution.

REFERENCES

The following book was referred to in the compilation of the pharmacologic and clinical information: Mills S, Bone K: *Principles and Practice of Phytotherapy: Modern Herbal Medicine,* Edinburgh, 2000, Churchill Livingstone.

1 Pharmacopoeia Commission of the People's Republic of China: *Pharmacopoeia of the People's Republic of China,* English ed, Beijing, 1997, Chemical Industry Press.
2 Bensky D, Gamble A: *Chinese herbal medicine materia medica,* Seattle, 1986, Eastland Press.
3 Chang HM, But PP: *Pharmacology and applications of Chinese materia medica,* Singapore, 1987, World Scientific.

ROSEMARY

Botanical Name: *Rosmarinus officinalis*
Family: Labiatae
Plant Part Used: Leaf

PRESCRIBING INFORMATION

Actions

Carminative, spasmolytic, antioxidant, antimicrobial, circulatory stimulant, hepatoprotective

Potential Indications

Based on appropriate evaluation of the patient, practitioners should consider prescribing rosemary in formulations in the context of:

- Increasing mental alertness and memory *(6)*
- Enhancing phase I and II detoxification by the liver *(7)*
- Achieving antioxidant and hepatoprotective effects, preventing atherosclerosis *(7)*
- Circulatory weakness, including hypotension *(5,6)*
- Dyspeptic conditions and particularly for improvement of hepatic and biliary function *(4)*
- Headache, depression, debility *(5)*
- Topical treatment for promoting wound healing, as a mild antiseptic, for alleviating symptoms of rheumatic diseases and circulatory problems *(4)*
- Topical treatment for myalgia, sciatica, and intercostal neuralgia *(5)*

Contraindications

No known contraindications have been found for rosemary, although caution may be warranted in women wishing to conceive, based on the cineole content in its essential oil. In an embryotoxic study involving rats, rosemary aqueous extract did not cause significant changes in postimplantation loss or in the number of malformation of fetuses. Preimplantation loss increased in the treated group, although the difference was not significant compared with the control.[1]

Warnings and Precautions

None required.

Interactions

Nonheme iron absorption was significantly decreased in female volunteers who consumed a phenolic-rich extract of rosemary (8.2% by weight of polyphenols, including carnosic acid, carnosol, and rosmarinic acid). The extract was administered via the meat component of a test meal and compared with a control meal over a total of 4 days.[2] This finding indicates a potential interaction for concomitant administration of rosemary during iron intake. In anemia and cases for which iron supplementation is required, rosemary should not be taken simultaneously with meals or iron supplements.

Use in Pregnancy and Lactation

No adverse effects expected. (See also the "Contraindications" section in this monograph.)

Rosemary *continued on page 390*

Side Effects

None expected if taken within the recommended dose range. Contact allergy has been reported for rosemary and may be the result of the constituent carnosol.[3]

Dosage

*Dose per day**	*Dose per week**
2.0-4.5 ml of 1:2 liquid extract	15-30 ml of 1:2 liquid extract

SUPPORTING INFORMATION

Traditional Prescribing

Traditional Western herbal medicine uses include:
- To stimulate the mind, memory, and the senses[4,5]
- Flatulent dyspepsia associated with psychogenic tension[6]
- Migrainous or hypertensive headaches[6]
- Depressive states with general debility and indications of cardiovascular weakness[6]
- All states of chronic circulatory weakness, including hypotension; debility; anorexia and poor digestion, particularly in older adults[7]
- Topically for myalgia, sciatica, and intercostal neuralgia[6]

Pharmacologic Research

Rosemary leaf contains an essential oil (1% to 2%), consisting of 1,8-cineole, borneol, bornyl acetate, α-pinene, and camphene; phenolic diterpenes, including carnosol and carnosic acid; rosmarinic acid; flavonoids; and triterpenoids.[8,9] (Carnosic acid is also known as carnosolic acid or salvin.)
- Rosemary is a strong antioxidant. The antioxidant activity is attributed to the phenolic diterpenes (particularly carnosic acid and carnosol), as well as rosmarinic acid. These components have inhibited lipid peroxidation, are good scavengers of free radicals, and protect red blood cells against oxidative hemolysis *in vitro*.[10,11] Rosemary extract has inhibited oxidative alterations to skin surface lipids *in vitro* and *in vivo*.[12]
- Because of its strong antioxidant activity, rosemary is used in the food industry as a preservative, particularly for meat products.[13] An *in vitro* comparison with 15 other herbs found that rosemary exhibited the highest antioxidant index in all the tested fats, particularly in animal fats.[14] (Carnosol and carnosic acid are fat-soluble.) Rosmarinic acid is also a potent antioxidant, but its solubility in fat is low, thus it acts best in aqueous systems. The strong antioxidant activity toward saturated fats is unusual, given that most antioxidant plant extracts and phytochemicals demonstrate activity only in aqueous systems. This action may indicate a valuable role in treating and preventing pathologic processes that involve lipid peroxidation, such as the development of atherosclerosis.
- Experimental studies indicated that oral administration of rosemary leaf is hepatoprotective, which has been attributed to the antioxidant phenolic compounds.[15] Oral administration of a methanolic extract of

Rosemary *continued on page 391*

*This dose range is extrapolated from the British Herbal Pharmacopoeia 1983 and the author's education and experience.

rosemary enhanced liver microsomal metabolism of endogenous estrogens. Rosemary also inhibited the uterotropic action of estradiol and estrone.[16]

- Oral intake of rosemary extract reduced the development of mammary carcinoma *in vivo*.[17] Rosemary extract may assist in reversing multidrug resistance in mammary tumors, as indicated by its ability to inhibit the transmembrane transport pump activity in isolated breast cancer cells.[18]

- Rosemary extract, or its components, carnosol or carnosic acid, are potent inhibitors of DNA adduct formation induced by benzo(a)pyrene or aflatoxin B1 *in vitro*.[19] These substances act by inhibiting cytochrome P-450 activity (phase I enzymes) and inducing glutathione S-transferase (phase II).[20] Oral administration of rosemary extract (0.25% to 1.0%) in the diet of rats increased the activity of the phase II enzymes glutathione S-transferase and NADPH-quinone reductase.[21] Water-soluble extract of rosemary induced phase I and II enzymes *in vivo* (by oral route). This activity was attributed to flavones, monoterpenes, or an additive effect of all components but not to rosmarinic acid alone.[22] A further *in vivo* study using oral doses indicated that the fraction containing the diterpenes induced phase II enzymes.[23]

- Rosemary extract demonstrated *in vitro* antimicrobial activity toward food-borne microorganisms,[24] *Leishmania mexicana* (80% ethanol extract),[25] *Yersinia enterocolitica* (ethanol extract),[26] and HSV type 2.[27]

- Rosemary oil also demonstrated antimicrobial activity *in vitro* toward *Candida albicans*[28] and a number of bacteria that cause respiratory and gastrointestinal disorders (e.g., *Pseudomonas aeruginosa, Escherichia coli, Aspergillus fumigatus*) by gaseous contact. Rosemary oil also delayed sporulation of several filamentous fungi.[29]

- Normal and diabetic mice with unlimited access to a rosemary infusion for 3 months had lower blood glucose levels compared with controls.[30]

- Aqueous-alcoholic extract of rosemary (1 g/kg, orally) inhibited experimentally induced gastric lesions. This activity may be the result of enhanced mucosal defense.[31]

- Oral administration of rosemary infusion demonstrated diuretic activity *in vivo*.[32]

- Rosemary oil produced a relaxant effect on experimentally induced contractions in isolated tracheal smooth muscle,[33] aortic segments,[34] and intestine.[35] Rosemary extract demonstrated spasmolytic activity on experimentally contracted isolated ileum.[36]

- Topical application of a chloroform extract of rosemary demonstrated a dose-dependent antiinflammatory activity in the croton oil–induced ear edema model.[37] Rosmarinic acid inhibited experimentally induced anaphylaxis (by oral route). Further tests indicated a selectivity of this compound for complement-dependent (inflammatory) processes.[38]

- Injection of freeze-dried rosemary extract (flowering stems) produced an increase in bile flow from both the liver and gallbladder *in vivo*.[39]

Rosemary continued on page 392

- Both inhalation and oral administration of rosemary oil stimulated locomotor activity in an experimental model.[40]

Clinical Studies

No clinical studies using rosemary leaf have been found. However, some clinical studies have used rosemary essential oil.

- Inhaling rosemary leaf oil for 3 minutes by volunteers produced decreased frontal alpha and beta power (measured from electro-encephalographic [EEG] recordings), suggesting increased alertness. Anxiety scores were lowered. Volunteers reported feeling more relaxed and alert and were faster (but not more accurate) at mathematical computations compared with baseline values. The trial was randomized and controlled.[41]
- In an uncontrolled trial, an aqueous emulsion of rosemary oil (1:10) inhibited the growth of Candida albicans when applied to the mouths (five times per day) of 12 patients with cancer, pneumonia, and oral candidiasis, which was unresponsive to nystatin.[42]
- In Germany, the Commission E supports using rosemary leaf to treat dyspeptic conditions. Externally, rosemary leaf can be used as supportive therapy for rheumatic diseases and circulatory problems.[43]
- ESCOP recommends rosemary leaf and flower for improving hepatic and biliary function and in dyspeptic conditions. In addition to the recommendations previously listed for topical use, which are also listed by the Commission E, rosemary can be used externally for the promotion of wound healing and as a mild antiseptic.[44]

REFERENCES

1 Lemonica IP, Damasceno DC, di-Stasi LC: *Braz J Med Biol Res* 29(2):223-227, 1996.
2 Samman S et al: *Am J Clin Nutr* 73(3):607-612, 2001.
3 Hjorther AB et al: *Contact Dermatitis* 37(3):99-100, 1997.
4 Gerard J, Woodward M: *Gerard's herbal: the essence thereof distilled by Marcus Woodward from the edition of Th. Johnson, 1636,* London, 1985, Bracken Books.
5 Culpeper N: *Culpeper's complete herbal, and English physician,* Manchester, 1826, J. Gleave & Son, reprinted Bath, 1981, Harvey Sales.
6 British Herbal Medicine Association's Scientific Committee: *British herbal pharmacopoeia,* Bournemouth, 1983, BHMA.
7 Weiss RF: *Herbal medicine,* English ed, Beaconsfield, UK, 1988, Beaconsfield Publishers.
8 Wagner H, Bladt S: *Plant drug analysis: a thin layer chromatography atlas,* ed 2, Berlin, 1996, Springer-Verlag.
9 Bisset NG, ed: *Herbal drugs and phytopharmaceuticals,* Stuttgart, 1994, Medpharm Scientific Publishers.
10 Haraguchi H et al: *Planta Med* 61(4):333-336, 1995.
11 Aruoma OI et al: *Xenobiotica* 22(2):257-268, 1992.
12 Calabrese V et al: *Int J Tissue React* 22(1):5-13, 2000.
13 Schwarz K, Ternes W: *Z Lebensm Unters Forsch* 195(2):95-98, 1992.
14 Halliwell B et al: *Food Chem Toxicol* 33(7):601-617, 1995.
15 Fahim FA et al: *Int J Food Sci Nutr* 50(6):413-427, 1999.
16 Zhu BT et al: *Carcinogenesis* 19(10):1821-1827, 1998.
17 Singletary KW, Nelshoppen JM: *Cancer Lett* 60(2):169-175, 1991.
18 Plouzek CA et al: *Eur J Cancer* 35(10):1541-1545, 1999.
19 Offord EA et al: *Cancer Lett* 114(1-2):275-281, 1997.
20 Mace K et al: *Arch Toxicol Suppl* 20:227-236, 1998.
21 Singletary K, Gutierrez E: *FASEB J* 7(4):A866, 1993.
22 Debersac P et al: *Food Chem Toxicol* 39(2):109-117, 2001.

Rosemary *continued on page 393*

23 Debersac P et al: *Food Chem Toxicol* 39(9):907-918, 2001.

24 Del Campo J, Amiot MJ, Nguyen-The C: *J Food Prot* 63(10):1359-1368, 2000.

25 Schnitzler AC, Nolan LL, Shetty K: *Acta Hort* 426:235-241, 1996.

26 Bara MTF, Vanetti MCD: *J Herbs Spices Med Plant* 3(4):51-58, 1995.

27 Romero E, Tateo F, Debiaggi M: *Mitt Gebiete Lebensm Hyg* 80:113-119, 1989.

28 Steinmetz MD, Moulin-Traffort J, Regli P: *Mycoses* 31(1):40-51, 1988.

29 Larrondo JV, Agut M, Calvo-Torras MA: *Microbios* 82(332):171-172, 1995.

30 Erenmemisoglu A, Saraymen R, Ustun S: *Pharmazie* 52(8):645-646, 1997.

31 Dias PC et al: *J Ethnopharmacol* 69(1):57-62, 2000.

32 Haloui M et al: *J Ethnopharmacol* 71(3):465-472, 2000.

33 Aqel MB: *J Ethnopharmacol* 33(1-2):57-62, 1991.

34 Aqel MB: *Int J Pharmacogn* 30(4):281-288, 1992.

35 Hof S, Gropper B, Ammon HPT: *Arch Pharm* 321:702, 1988.

36 Forster HB, Niklas H, Lutz S: *Planta Med* 40(4):309-319, 1980.

37 Brkic D et al: International Congress and 48th Annual Meeting of the Society for Medicinal Plant Research and the 6th International Congress on Ethnopharmacology of the International Society for Ethnopharmacology, Zurich, September 3-7, 2000, abstract P2A/1.

38 Englberger W et al: *Int J Immunopharmacol* 10(6):729-737, 1988.

39 Mongold JJ et al: *Plant Med Phytother* 25(1):6-11, 1991.

40 Kovar KA et al: *Planta Med* 53(4):315-318, 1987.

41 Diego MA et al: *Int J Neurosci* 96(3-4):217-224, 1998.

42 Durakovic Z, Durakovic S: *J Indian Med Assoc* 72(7):175-176, 1979.

43 Blumenthal M et al, eds: *The complete German Commission E monographs: therapeutic guide to herbal medicines*, Austin, 1998, American Botanical Council.

44 Scientific Committee of the European Scientific Cooperative on Phytotherapy [ESCOP]: *ESCOP monographs: Rosmarinus folium cum flore*. European Scientific Cooperative on Phytotherapy, ESCOP Secretariat, Argyle House, Gandy Street, Exeter, Devon, EX4 3LS, United Kingdom, July 1997.

SAGE

Botanical Name: Salvia officinalis
Family: Labiatae
Plant Part Used: Aerial parts

PRESCRIBING INFORMATION

Actions

Spasmolytic, antioxidant, astringent, antihyperhidrotic, antimicrobial

Potential Indications

Based on appropriate evaluation of the patient, practitioners should consider prescribing sage in formulations in the context of:
- Inflammations and infections of the mouth and throat (4,5)
- Dyspepsia (4,5)
- Excessive sweating (4,5)
- Menopausal hot flashes* and night sweating, in combination with Medicago sativa (4)
- Reducing or stopping lactation (5)
- Febrile conditions (5)
- Nervous debility, nervous exhaustion (6)
- Topical treatment for inflammations of the mucous membranes of the nose (4)
- Topical treatment to stop the flow of milk (5)

Contraindications

Pregnancy and lactation.[1] (See also the "Use in Pregnancy and Lactation" section in this monograph.)

Warnings and Precautions

The recommended dose must not be exceeded. Caution should be taken with long-term use.[1] (These cautions are made because of the presence of the potentially toxic component thujone in the essential oil of sage leaf.)

Interactions

None known.

Use in Pregnancy and Lactation

Contraindicated in pregnancy and lactation. However, sage has been used traditionally to stop milk flow.

Side Effects

None expected if taken within the recommended dose range.

Dosage

Dose per day**	Dose per week**
2.0-4.5 ml of 1:2 liquid extract	15-30 ml of 1:2 liquid extract

SUPPORTING INFORMATION

Traditional Prescribing

Traditional Western herbal medicine uses include:
- Inflammation of the mouth, tongue, or throat and topically for these conditions[2]

Sage continued on page 395

*Sage has also been used in traditional herbal medicine for treating hot flashes. (6)
**This dose range is extrapolated from the British Herbal Pharmacopoeia 1983 and the author's education and experience.

- Flatulent dyspepsia, debilitated digestion,[2,3] bilious and kidney disorders[4]
- Excessive sweating,[2,3] hot flashes of menopause[5]
- Nervous exhaustion, debility of the nervous system, joint pain, tension headache[4]
- To improve the memory and stimulate the senses[6]
- To stop the flow of milk, both oral[2] and topical use[3]

Pharmacologic Research

The aerial parts of sage contain 1.5% to 2.5% essential oil, the composition of which varies depending on its origin. The essential oil contains monoterpenes, including approximately 30% thujone in some varieties. High doses of thujone may cause neurotoxicity. Other constituents of sage include flavonoids, rosmarinic acid, and phenolic diterpenes, including carnosol and carnosic acid.[7,8] (Carnosic acid is also known as carnosolic acid or salvin.)

- Sage extract caused inhibition of lipid peroxidation *in vitro*.[9] Isolated constituents of sage found to have *in vitro* antioxidant activity include the phenolic diterpenes carnosol, rosmanol, and carnosic acid.[10]
- Sage extract administered by injection demonstrated hypotensive and spasmolytic activity in experimental models.[11]
- Sage extract and sage oil inhibited acetylcholinesterase in a concentration-dependent manner in human brain tissue *in vitro*.[12] Diterpenes isolated from sage were found to interact with the GABA-benzodiazepine receptor.[13]
- Aqueous extract of sage demonstrated moderate antibacterial activity *in vitro*.[14]
- Topical application of a chloroform extract of sage demonstrated dose-dependent antiinflammatory activity in the croton oil–induced ear edema model.[15]

Clinical Studies

- In a number of open studies, sage has reduced sweat production in patients with hyperhidrosis (excessive sweating). Daily dose ranged from the equivalent of 2.6 to 4.5 g of leaf.[1]
- A product containing sage and alfalfa *(Medicago sativa)* extracts produced improvement in the menopausal symptoms of hot flashes and night sweats in an open trial conducted for 3 months. The product appeared to produce a slight central antidopaminergic activity.[16]
- In Germany, the Commission E supports using sage to treat dyspeptic symptoms, excessive perspiration, and externally for inflammations of the mucous membranes of the nose and throat.[17]
- ESCOP recommends sage leaf for treating inflammations and infections of the mouth and throat, such as stomatitis, gingivitis, and pharyngitis, as well as hyperhidrosis.[1]

REFERENCES

1 Scientific Committee of the European Scientific Cooperative on Phytotherapy [ESCOP]: *ESCOP monographs: Salviae folium.* European Scientific Cooperative on Phytotherapy, ESCOP Secretariat, Argyle House, Gandy Street, Exeter, Devon, EX4 3LS, United Kingdom, March 1996.
2 British Herbal Medicine Association's Scientific Committee: *British herbal pharmacopoeia,* Bournemouth, 1983, BHMA.

Sage continued on page 396

3 Felter HW, Lloyd JU: *King's American dispensatory*, ed 18, rev 3, Portland, 1905, reprinted 1983, Eclectic Medical Publications.

4 Grieve M: *A modern herbal*, New York, 1971, Dover Publications.

5 Bartram T: *Encyclopedia of herbal medicine*, ed 1, Dorset, UK, 1995, Grace Publishers.

6 Culpeper N: *Culpeper's complete herbal, and English physician*, Manchester, 1826, J. Gleave & Son, reprinted Bath, 1981, Harvey Sales.

7 Wagner H, Bladt S: *Plant drug analysis: a thin layer chromatography atlas*, ed 2, Berlin, 1996, Springer-Verlag.

8 Bisset NG, ed: *Herbal drugs and phytopharmaceuticals*, Stuttgart, 1994, Medpharm Scientific Publishers.

9 Hohmann J et al: *Planta Med* 65(6):576-578, 1999.

10 Wang M et al: *J Nat Prod* 62(3):454-456, 1999.

11 Todorov S et al: *Acta Physiol Pharmacol Bulg* 10(2):13-20, 1984.

12 Perry N et al: *Int J Geriatr Psychiatry* 11(12):1063-1069, 1996.

13 Rutherford DM et al: *Neurosci Lett* 135(2):224-226, 1992.

14 Brantner A, Grein E: *J Ethnopharmacol* 44(1):35-40, 1994.

15 Brkic D et al: International Congress and 48th Annual Meeting of the Society for Medicinal Plant Research and the 6th International Congress on Ethnopharmacology of the International Society for Ethnopharmacology, Zurich, September 3-7, 2000, abstract P2A/1.

16 De Leo V et al: *Minerva Ginecol* 50(5):207-211, 1998.

17 Blumenthal M et al, eds: *The complete German Commission E monographs: therapeutic guide to herbal medicines*, Austin, 1998, American Botanical Council.

SARSAPARILLA

Common Name:	Sarsaparilla
Botanical Names:	Smilax ornata, Smilax regelii,[+] Smilax febrifuga,[+] Smilax medica[+]
	Note: Other species have also been listed in traditional texts, although they were less favored (e.g., S. officinalis). Smilax aristolochiifolia is a botanical synonym of S. medica and therefore is also a medicinally interchangeable species for Smilax ornata.
Family:	Smilacaceae
Plant Part Used:	Root and rhizome

PRESCRIBING INFORMATION

Actions

Antirheumatic, depurative, antiinflammatory

Potential Indications

Based on appropriate evaluation of the patient, practitioners should consider prescribing sarsaparilla in formulations in the context of:
- Psoriasis *(4a,4,5)*
- Chronic skin disorders *(5)*
- Rheumatoid arthritis *(5)*
- Providing general tonic effects *(6)*

Contraindications

None known.

Warnings and Precautions

The German Commission E advises that taking sarsaparilla preparations leads to gastric irritation and temporary kidney impairment (diuresis). The absorption of simultaneously administered substances (such as digitalis glycosides or bismuth) is increased. The elimination of other substances (e.g., hypnotics) is accelerated. This action can cause an uncontrolled condition of increased or decreased action of treatments taken simultaneously.[1] However, these concerns are theoretical and not based on animal experiments or clinical case reports, and they would apply for any herb containing saponins. Such concerns would be alleviated by not taking sarsaparilla simultaneously with drug medication.

Interactions

None known.

Use in Pregnancy and Lactation

No adverse effects expected.

Side Effects

None expected if taken within the recommended dose range.

Dosage

*Dose per day**	*Dose per week**
3-6 ml of 1:2 liquid extract	20-40 ml of 1:2 liquid extract

Although these doses reflect recent modern use, nineteenth century clinicians used substantially higher doses, possibly because of the

Sarsaparilla *continued on page 398*

[+]Medicinally interchangeable species.
*This dose range is extrapolated from the British Herbal Pharmacopoeia 1983.

antisyphilitic application. For example, the *British Pharmacopoeia* 1898 recommended 8 to 15 ml three times per day of a 1:1 extract.

The clinical trial with psoriasis patients (see later discussion) used 15 g per day by decoction, but water does not effectively extract saponins. Hence lower doses of ethanol-water extracts may still be as effective. Nonetheless, a case may be made for increasing the sarsaparilla dose if the patient's condition does not respond to treatment.

SUPPORTING INFORMATION

Traditional Prescribing

Traditional Western herbal medicine uses include:
- Chronic skin conditions, especially psoriasis[2,3]
- Rheumatoid arthritis, syphilis, dropsy[2,3]
- Adjuvant therapy for leprosy[2]

Smilax regelii root has also been used traditionally in Guatemala for treating skin diseases, including abscess, boils, and acne, as well as urinary tract infections.[4,5] Species of Smilax ("zarzaparrilla" [*S. aristolochiaefolia* and other species] and "cuculmeca" [*Smilax* spp.])[6] have been used traditionally in Central America for blood and skin disorders, snakebite, and as a tonic to enhance vigor and treat weakness.[7]

Sarsaparilla, which was introduced into North America from Spanish America, is listed in Spanish pharmacopoeias from 1739 to 1954, with the major actions being sudorific (inducing sweating, similar to a diaphoretic), antivenereal, and antirheumatic. Sarsaparilla was used extensively in the sixteenth and seventeenth centuries for treating syphilis.[8]

Sarsaparilla from several species of Smilax (not to be confused with the American or wild sarsaparilla, *Aralia nudicaulis*) was official in the USP from 1820 to 1955 and the NF from 1955 to 1965 and was used as a tonic and flavoring agent. Native Americans used sarsaparilla to treat many diverse diseases.[9]

Natives of the Amazon have used the root *(Smilax officinalis)* to reestablish virility in men and to treat symptoms of menopause.[10] Such applications might well be anticipated, given the steroidal saponin content of the plant.

Pharmacologic Research

Species of sarsaparilla contain steroidal saponins for which sarsasapogenin and smilagenin have been identified as aglycones.[11]
- Aqueous extract of *Smilax regelii* root inhibited the following dermatophytes *in vitro: Epidermophyton floccosum, Microsporum canis,* and *Trichophyton mentagrophytes.*[4]
- Oral pretreatment of rats with *Smilax regelii* extract inhibited carbon tetrachloride—induced hepatocellular metabolic changes.[12]

Sarsaparilla *continued on page 399*

- Sarsaparilla products have been popular among athletes and body-builders for testosterone supplementation. Despite this traditional use, sarsaparilla does not contain testosterone, and the steroidal saponins do not behave as anabolic steroids. A study reviewing all clinical trials published between 1966 and 1992 found no documented evidence to substantiate claims that diosgenin, smilagenin, and hecogenin increase growth hormone release in the body.[13]

Clinical Studies

- Oral administration of sarsaparilla improved psoriasis in over 50% of patients treated in open, uncontrolled trials.[14-18] The daily dose provided for one of these trials was a sarsaparilla root decoction (15 g in 1 L).[15] In many of these trials, a low-fat diet and ointments were also used, and long-term use of sarsaparilla (2 to 3 months) was required. Saponins from sarsaparilla produced greater improvement in psoriasis patients compared with controls. Sarsaparilla saponins were more beneficial for chronic plaque psoriasis. The average period of treatment was 4 months, with a range of 4 weeks to 7 months.[19]
- *Smilax ornata* extract (equivalent to 30 g root/day) taken for several months was superior to sulfones in treating leprosy.[20] Favorable results were obtained in a later uncontrolled trial using a combination of sarsaparilla and sulfones for leprosy treatment.[21]
- Sarsaparilla root extract (2.4 g/day) produced a decrease in serum urea in both healthy volunteers and patients with nephritis. According to the authors, this finding may have been the result of increased urinary excretion. Symptoms of acute uremia (e.g., headaches, appetite loss) were relieved with the reduction in serum urea.[22]

REFERENCES

1 Blumenthal M et al, eds: *The complete German Commission E monographs: therapeutic guide to herbal medicines,* Austin, 1998, American Botanical Council.
2 British Herbal Medicine Association's Scientific Committee: *British herbal pharmacopoeia,* Bournemouth, 1983, BHMA.
3 Felter HW, Lloyd JU: *King's American dispensatory,* ed 18, rev 3, Portland, 1905, reprinted 1983, Eclectic Medical Publications.
4 Caceres A et al: *J Ethnopharmacol* 31(3):263-276, 1991.
5 Caceres A et al: *J Ethnopharmacol* 20(3):223-237, 1987.
6 Hersch-Martinez P: *Econ Bot* 51(2):107-120, 1997.
7 Villalobos R: *Rev Forest Centroam* 32:39-42, 2000.
8 Fernandez Negri MA, Lopez Andujar G: *Ars Pharm* 31(3-4):223-231, 1990.
9 Vogel VJ: *American Indian medicine,* Norman, Okla, 1970, University of Oklahoma Press.
10 Evans Schultes R, Raffauf RF: *The healing forest: medicinal and toxic plants of the Northwest Amazonia,* Portland, 1990, Dioscorides Press.
11 Hostettmann K, Marston A: *Chemistry & pharmacology of natural products: saponins,* Cambridge, 1995, Cambridge University Press.
12 Rafatullah S et al: *Int J Pharmacogn* 29(4):296-301, 1991.
13 Barron RL, Vanscoy GJ: *Ann Pharmacother* 27(5):607-615, 1993.
14 Deneke T: *Dtsch Med Wochenschr* 62:337-341, 1936.
15 Philippsohn A: *Dermatol Wochenschr* 93:1220-1223, 1931.
16 Ritter H: *Dtsch Med Wochenschr* 62:1629-1631, 1936.
17 Zaun H: *Dtsch Med Wochenschr* 64:1073, 1938.
18 Baird PC Jr: *N Engl J Med* 220:794-801, 1939.
19 Thurman FM: *N Engl J Med* 227:128-133, 1942.
20 Rollier R et al: *Maroc Med* 30:776-780, 1951.
21 Rollier R: *Int J Leprosy* 27:328-340, 1959.
22 Rittmann R, Schneider F: *Klin Wochschr* 9:401-408, 1930.

SAW PALMETTO

Botanical Names: *Serenoa serrulata, Serenoa repens,# Sabal serrulata#*
Family: Palmae
Plant Part Used: Fruit

PRESCRIBING INFORMATION

Actions	Antiinflammatory, male tonic, antiprostatic, spasmolytic, possibly antiandrogenic
Potential Indications	Based on appropriate evaluation of the patient, practitioners should consider prescribing saw palmetto in formulations in the context of: • Mild to moderate BPH *(4,5)* • Inflammation of the genitourinary tract, especially cystitis, atrophy of sexual tissues; as an aphrodisiac; sex hormone deficiency *(5)* • Noninfectious prostatitis *(7)*
Contraindications	None known.
Warnings and Precautions	None required.
Interactions	None known.
Use in Pregnancy and Lactation	No adverse effects expected.
Side Effects	Saw palmetto is well tolerated by most patients and causes relatively few side effects. Most side effects are minor gastrointestinal problems, such as nausea, which are usually resolved when the herb is taken with meals. One case of hemorrhage during surgery, which was associated with intake of saw palmetto extract, has been reported.[1]

Dosage

Dose per day*	**Dose per week***
2.0-4.5 ml of 1:2 liquid extract	15-30 ml of 1:2 liquid extract

Capsules containing 160 mg of the liposterolic extract (LESP) are usually recommended at two capsules per day.** This extract is an 8:1 to 10:1 concentrate of the original dried berries (i.e., approximately 2.88 g/day of saw palmetto berries). Hence using LESP reflects a higher dosing strategy than that stated here.

Saw Palmetto *continued on page 401*

#Alternative name.

*This dose range is extrapolated from the British Pharmaceutical Codex 1934, the British Herbal Pharmacopoeia 1983, and the German Commission E.
**This dose range is extrapolated from clinical trials and the German Commission E.

Traditional Prescribing

Traditional Western herbal medicine uses include:

- Prostatic hypertrophy, inflammation of the genitourinary tract (especially cystitis), genitourinary tract discharge, atrophy of sexual tissues, sex hormone disorders; as an aphrodisiac[2,3]; enlarged ovaries, undeveloped mammary glands[4]
- Irritative cough, chronic bronchial coughs, whooping cough, laryngitis, acute catarrh, asthma[3]
- To improve digestion; as a tonic for the nervous system[4]

Native Americans ate saw palmetto berries. Saw palmetto was official in the USP from 1906 to 1916 and the NF from 1926 to 1950 and was used as a diuretic, sedative, and anticatarrhal.[5]

Pharmacologic Research

Saw palmetto berries contain free fatty acids, triglycerides, phytosterols (mainly β-sitosterol), fatty alcohols, flavonoids, and polysaccharides.

LESP is a specially prepared extraction of dried saw palmetto berries using hexane, 90% ethanol, or supercritical carbon dioxide. The liposterolic extract contains 85% to 95% fatty acids (mostly as triglycerides) and 0.2% to 0.4% total sterols (with 0.1% to 0.3% β-sitosterol). Flavonoids are unlikely to be present, except in the extract prepared using 90% ethanol.

- Androgen deprivation can decrease the obstructive symptoms of BPH. *In vitro* studies confirm that the lipid component of LESP weakly inhibits 5α-reductase (an enzyme that converts testosterone to its more potent form: DHT), but saw palmetto probably does not possess clinically significant activity as a 5α-reductase inhibitor.
- *In vitro* research found that LESP inhibited testosterone and DHT binding in several tissue specimens, including vaginal skin and prepuce. Another study found that LESP did not inhibit binding of DHT to prostatic androgen receptor in an experimental model.
- LESP had a proliferative effect on androgen-responsive prostate cancer cells at low concentrations and a cytotoxic effect at higher concentrations. In cells unresponsive to androgen stimulation, LESP exerted a concentration-dependent, antiproliferative action. This antiandrogenic activity was confirmed for LESP in several animal models.
- LESP inhibited the effects of prolactin on hamster ovary cells, suggesting that the extract may inhibit prolactin-induced prostate growth.
- Dynamically caused urinary outlet obstruction is associated with increased smooth muscle tone. Saponifiable and ethanolic liposterolic extracts of saw palmetto produced a spasmolytic effect on isolated uterus, bladder, and aorta.
- BPH is associated with congestion and a noninfectious prostatitis, which is evidenced by white cell infiltration of the prostate.

Saw Palmetto continued on page 402

Agents with antiinflammatory and edema-protective activities may improve the clinical picture. LESP was found, *in vitro*, to be a dual inhibitor of cyclooxygenase and 5-lipoxygenase. The activity was found to reside in the acidic lipophilic fraction.

- A pronounced antiedematous effect was observed for oral doses of an alcohol extract of saw palmetto in carrageenan-induced edema of rat paw. LESP demonstrated antiedematous activity in a number of experimental models, with an antagonistic effect observed against histamine-induced edema but not in relation to serotonin- or bradykinin-induced weals. The participation of glucocorticoids in this antiinflammatory activity was excluded.

- In experimental models of BPH, high oral doses of LESP inhibited prostatic growth in castrated mice given testosterone. A moderate dose achieved a similar outcome in a rat model. A model of BPH that uses transplants of human prostrate tissue into hairless mice found high oral doses of LESP reversed the hormonal stimulation (by DHT and estradiol) of prostate growth.

Clinical Studies

Except when specified, all of the clinical studies listed here used 320 mg/day of LESP, which is equivalent to an average daily dose of 2.88 g of saw palmetto berries. Saw palmetto liquid extracts will also provide such therapeutic benefits, provided similar dosage considerations are observed.

- A systematic review of randomized clinical trials found that LESP improved urologic symptoms and flow measures compared with placebo. LESP produced similar improvement in urinary symptoms and flow compared with finasteride and is associated with fewer adverse reactions.[6] The trials outlined in this section were covered in this review.

- Several randomized, double-blind, placebo-controlled trials demonstrated that treatment with LESP for 28 to 90 days significantly reduced symptoms and nocturnal frequency and increased peak urinary flow rates and postvoid residual (PVR) in patients with BPH. One randomized, double-blind, placebo-controlled trial found that although LESP treatment improved BPH symptoms, equal improvement was observed in the placebo group.

- One hundred and seventy six (176) nonresponders to placebo were selected for a double-blind, placebo-controlled, multicenter study investigating BPH. LESP treatment significantly improved dysuria, significantly increased peak urinary flow rate, and decreased daytime and nocturnal urinary frequency compared with a placebo. This trial had a relatively short assessment period (30 days).

- A number of double-blind, comparative studies involving LESP have been completed. No significant differences were observed between LESP and finasteride (5 mg/day) for improving quality of life and IPSS, but finasteride did significantly increase peak flow rate over LESP in a large-scale, randomized trial. This trial was 26 weeks in duration, and finasteride can show increasing efficacy up to 1 year

Saw Palmetto continued on page 403

after initiation of therapy. Mean PVR and peak urinary flow outcomes were not significantly different between LESP and alfuzosin (7.5 mg/day), but the Boyarsky and obstructive scores were significantly better for alfuzosin in a 3-week trial. (Alfuzosin is a fast-acting drug.) LESP compared favorably with mepartricin (100,000 international units/day) for nocturnal frequency, dysuria, and PVR and with prazosin (4 mg/day for 12 weeks) for urinary frequency, mean urinary flow rate, and PVR.

- Results from several uncontrolled clinical trials demonstrated significant therapeutic effects for LESP in patients with BPH over the long term (3 years in one study), with good to excellent tolerability.
- Double-blind, controlled trials of combination therapy with LESP and other phytotherapeutic agents have been undertaken. Urinary flow, micturition time, residual urine, frequency of micturition, and a subjective assessment of the effect of treatment were all significantly improved over placebo for LESP and pumpkin seed extract (480 mg/day of extract) combination therapy. When LESP was combined with nettle root (equivalent to 2.4 g/day of root) and compared with placebo over 24 weeks, significant improvements were seen in IPSS and peak flow but not PVR. When the LESP-nettle root combination was compared with finasteride (5 mg/day) over 48 weeks, both treatments significantly improved urinary flow and IPSS, and no significant differences were observed between the two treatments. The herbal combination had better tolerability than finasteride. A subsequent analysis of a subgroup of patients from this trial indicated that efficacy was unrelated to prostate volume.[7] A randomized, placebo-controlled trial published in 2000 indicated that a blend of LESP, nettle root, pumpkin seed oil, and lemon flavonoid extract improved clinical parameters in symptomatic BPH slightly more than placebo. The blend was associated with significant epithelial contraction, especially in the transition zone, indicating a possible mechanism of action for the clinical effect.[8] This blend also induced suppression of prostatic tissue DHT levels in a randomized clinical trial involving patients with BPH.[9]
- In Germany, the Commission E supports using saw palmetto to treat urination problems in BPH stages I and II.[10]
- Saw palmetto has been reinstated to the USP and is official in the USP24-NF19.

REFERENCES

Except when specifically referenced, the following book was referred to in the compilation of the pharmacologic and clinical information: Mills S, Bone K: *Principles and Practice of Phytotherapy: Modern Herbal Medicine*, Edinburgh, 2000, Churchill Livingstone.

1 Cheema P, El-Mefty O, Jazieh AR: *J Intern Med* 250(2):167, 2001.
2 British Herbal Medicine Association's Scientific Committee: *British herbal pharmacopoeia*, Bournemouth, 1983, BHMA.
3 Felter HW, Lloyd JU: *King's American dispensatory*, ed 18, rev 3, Portland, 1905, reprinted 1983, Eclectic Medical Publications.

Saw Palmetto continued on page 404

4 Ellingwood F, Lloyd JU: *American materia medica, therapeutics and pharmacognosy,* ed 11, Portland, 1983, Eclectic Medical Publications.

5 Vogel VJ: *American Indian medicine,* Norman, Okla, 1970, University of Oklahoma Press.

6 Wilt TJ et al: *JAMA* 280(18):1604-1609, 1998; *Cochrane Database Syst Rev* (2):CD001423, 2000.

7 Sokeland J: *BJU Int* 86(4):439-442, 2000.

8 Marks LS et al: *J Urol* 163(5):1451-1456, 2000.

9 Marks LS et al: *Urology* 57(5):999-1005, 2001.

10 Blumenthal M et al, eds: *The complete German Commission E monographs: therapeutic guide to herbal medicines,* Austin, 1998, American Botanical Council.

SCHISANDRA

Other Common Name: Schizandra
Botanical Names: *Schisandra chinensis, Schizandra chinensis*[#]
Family: Schisandraceae
Plant Part Used: Fruit

PRESCRIBING INFORMATION

Actions	Hepatoprotective, antioxidant, adaptogenic, nervine tonic, antitussive, oxytocic, mild antidepressant
Potential Indications	Based on appropriate evaluation of the patient, practitioners should consider prescribing Schisandra in formulations in the context of: • Acute or chronic liver diseases, including hepatitis *(3)* • Improving the detoxifying capacity of the liver *(7)* • Improving physical performance, endurance, and resistance to the effects of stress *(3)* • Improving mental performance *(4)* • Chemical liver damage, poor liver function *(7)* • Chronic cough, asthma *(5)* • Spontaneous or night sweating, nocturnal emission, spermatorrhea, enuresis, frequent urination *(5)*
Contraindications	In TCM, Schisandra is contraindicated in the early stages of cough or rash and in excess heat patterns.[1] Schisandra is contraindicated in pregnancy, except at birth.
Warnings and Precautions	None required.
Interactions	None known.
Use in Pregnancy and Lactation	Contraindicated in pregnancy, except to assist childbirth.
Side Effects	Mild gastrointestinal symptoms (e.g., heartburn, indigestion, nausea) and headache have been reported. In one trial, 4 out of the 107 patients treated with the equivalent of 1.5 g per day of dried fruit developed mild and transient nausea, headache, and stomachache.[2,3]

	Dose per day*	**Dose per week***
Dosage	3.5-8.5 ml of 1:2 liquid extract	25-60 ml of 1:2 liquid extract

SUPPORTING INFORMATION

Traditional Prescribing	Uses and properties from TCM include: • Chronic cough, asthma[1,4]

Schisandra *continued on page 406*

[#]Alternative name.
*This dose range is adapted from dried plant dosages administered by decoction in TCM.[4] The author's experience and the fact that ethanol-water is a more effective solvent than water for many phytochemicals are taken into account.

- Nocturnal emission, spermatorrhea, leukorrhea, enuresis, frequent urination[1,4]
- Protracted diarrhea[1,4]
- Spontaneous or night sweating, impairment of body fluid with thirst[1,4]
- Shortness of breath and feeble pulse, diabetes caused by *internal heat*, palpitation, amnesia, and insomnia[1,4]

Pharmacologic Research

Dibenzocyclooctene lignans (such as schisandrin) are key constituents of Schisandra fruit.

- Numerous studies, *in vitro*[5,6] and *in vivo* after oral administration,[7-14] have demonstrated the hepatoprotective activity of Schisandra and its constituents in response to toxic challenge.
- Schisandra and its constituents have shown antioxidant activity *in vitro*[7,15] and *in vivo* via oral administration.[13,15,16]
- The mechanism of action of the hepatoprotective activity of Schisandra is likely to include:
  - Antioxidant activity within the liver[8,17]
  - Facilitation of glutathione regeneration via the glutathione reductase–catalyzed and NADPH-mediated pathways[13]
  - Inhibition of the activation of the hepatotoxin[8] and the binding of its resultant metabolites to liver microsomes[18]
- Despite being a postulated powerful inducer of phase I enzymes, Schisandra does not increase harmful bioactivation (the production of a more toxic compound) *in vivo* (e.g., after coadministration of acetaminophen) and *in vitro* studies have indicated that constituents of Schisandra decrease the mutagenicity of benzo(a)pyrene by favorably influencing hepatic metabolism.[19,20]
- Schisandra was shown to have adaptogenic and tonic effects in several experimental models. Renal and gonadal RNA, glycogen, and enzyme levels were increased in mature animals compared with those in younger rabbits. Reproductive cell numbers were increased in both sexes[21] and working capacity was increased *in vivo*, all by oral administration.[22]
- Schisandra treatment reduced heart rate, respiratory frequency, and lactate levels and increased plasma glucose and performance in a randomized, double-blind, placebo-controlled, crossover study involving race and show-jump horses.[23]
- In a placebo-controlled trial, significant reductions in serum levels of glutamic pyruvic transaminase (GPT), glutamic oxaloacetic transaminase (GOT), and creatine kinase were observed after oral administration of standardized Schisandra extracts to poorly performing horses with persistently high enzyme levels.[24]
- Intraperitoneal injection of Schisandra significantly reduced sleeping time induced by phenobarbital, ethanol, and ether *in vivo*. This finding suggests antidepressant activity.[25]
- Schisandra preparations strengthened the rhythmic contractions of nonpregnant, pregnant, and postpartum uteri in isolated tissue and *in vivo*.[2]

Schisandra *continued on page 407*

Clinical Studies

- Schisandra extract (equivalent to 1.5 g dried fruit/day) was shown to be superior to combined liver extract and vitamin E in treating patients with chronic viral hepatitis in an open, controlled trial. Serum GPT levels normalized at a much faster rate and remained normal after the withdrawal of Schisandra. Schisandra was also more effective at relieving symptoms of sleeplessness, fatigue, abdominal tension, and diarrhea.[3]
- Early uncontrolled trials in Russia reported that Schisandra increased endurance and physical efficiency in humans and decreased sickness in factory workers and children.[26,27] Flight attendants working on nonstop 7- to 9-hour flights treated with Schisandra did not display the increase in heart rate and blood pressure that was experienced by controls not receiving treatment. In a placebo-controlled trial, physical work capacity increased in athletes treated with Schisandra.[28]
- Standardized Schisandra extract significantly increased basal levels of salivary NO in a randomized, double-blind, placebo-controlled study on athletes. NO is thought to be a marker for adaptation to heavy exercise and is likely to have a role in nonspecific immunity. A daily dose containing 12.4 mg of schisandrins was administered.[29]
- Uncontrolled trials indicate that Schisandra might increase mental efficiency in humans.[26] Schisandrin (5 to 10 mg) improved concentration, fine coordination, and endurance in healthy young male adults.[2] Schisandra is reported to improve vision and hearing, enlarge the visual field, improve adaptation to the dark, and increase the discrimination of skin receptors.[2]
- Schisandra liquid extract successfully induced labor in 72 of 80 women with prolonged labor. The dose administered was 20 to 25 drops per hour for 3 hours of 1:3 extract for 3 consecutive days.[30] Schisandra tincture (1:10, 30 to 40 drops, three times/day) improved cardiovascular symptoms in hypotensive pregnant women. The Schisandra-treated group experienced fewer birth complications than the untreated women. No effects were observed on contraction or on labor.[31]

REFERENCES

1 Bensky D, Gamble A: Chinese herbal medicine materia medica, Seattle, 1986, Eastland Press.

2 Chang HM, But PP: Pharmacology and applications of Chinese materia medica, Singapore, 1987, World Scientific.

3 Wagner H, Hikino H, Farnsworth NR, eds: Economic and medicinal plant research, London, 1988, Academic Press.

4 Pharmacopoeia Commission of the People's Republic of China: Pharmacopoeia of the People's Republic of China, English ed, Beijing, 1997, Chemical Industry Press.

5 Hikino H et al: Planta Med 50(3):213-218, 1984.

6 Jiaxiang N et al: J Appl Toxicol 13(6):385-388, 1993.

7 Mak DH et al: Mol Cell Biochem 165(2):161-165, 1996.

8 Ip SP, Ko KM: Biochem Pharmacol 52(11):1687-1693, 1996.

9 Ip SP et al: Biochem Pharmacol 54(2):317-319, 1997.

10 Ip SP, Che CT, Ko KM: Chung Kuo Yao Li Hsueh Pao 19(4):313-316, 1998.

11 Pao TT et al: Chung Hua I Hsueh Tsa Chih 54:275-278, 1974.

12 Zhu M et al: J Ethnopharmacol 67:61-68, 1999.

13 Ko KM et al: Planta Med 61(2):134-137, 1995.

Schisandra continued on page 408

14 Chang HM et al, eds: *Advances in Chinese medicinal materials research,* Singapore, 1985, World Scientific.

15 Lu H, Liu GT: *Chung Kuo Yao Li Hsueh Pao* 11(4):331-335, 1990.

16 Lu H, Liu GT: *Chem Biol Interact* 78(1):77-84, 1991.

17 Ip SP et al: *Free Radic Biol Med* 21(5):709-712, 1996.

18 Liu KT, Lesca P: *Chem Biol Interact* 41(1):39-47, 1982.

19 Liu KT et al: *Chem Biol Interact* 39(3):315-330, 1982.

20 Liu KT, Lesca P: *Chem Biol Interact* 39(3):301-314, 1982.

21 Peng GR et al: *Shanghai J Trad Chin Med* 2:43-45, 1989.

22 Azizov AP, Seifulla RD: *Eksp Klin Farmakol* 61(3):61-63, 1998.

23 Hancke J et al: *Fitoterapia* 65(2):113-118, 1994.

24 Hancke J et al: *Phytomed* 3(3):237-240, 1996.

25 Hancke JL, Wikman G, Hernandez DE: *Planta Med* 52:542-543, 1986.

26 Brekhman I, Dardymov IV: *Annu Rev Pharmacol* 9:419-430, 1969.

27 Fulder S: *The root of being: ginseng and the pharmacology of harmony,* London, 1980, Hutchinson.

28 Lupandin AV: *Fiziol Cheloveka* 16(3):114-119, 1990.

29 Panossian AG et al: *Phytomed* 6(1):17-26, 1999.

30 Trifonova AT: *Akush Ginekol* 4:19-22, 1954.

31 Gaistruk AN, Taranovskij KL: *Urg Probl Obstet Gynecol L'vov* 1:183-186, 1968.

SHATAVARI

Botanical Names: *Asparagus racemosus, Protasparagus racemosus#*
Family: Asparagaceae (broadly, Liliaceae)
Plant Part Used: Root

PRESCRIBING INFORMATION

Actions

Tonic, galactagogue, sexual tonic, adaptogenic, spasmolytic, antidiarrheal, diuretic

Potential Indications

Based on appropriate evaluation of the patient, practitioners should consider prescribing shatavari in formulations in the context of:
- Promoting conception and for sexual debility in both sexes (5)
- A female reproductive tonic and aphrodisiac (6)
- Infertility in both sexes, impotence (6)
- Promoting lactation, menopause (6)
- Promoting appetite in children (6)
- Infections, immunosuppression (7)
- Diarrhea (5)

Contraindications

None known.

Warnings and Precautions

None required.

Interactions

None known.

Use in Pregnancy and Lactation

No adverse effects expected.

Side Effects

None expected if taken within the recommended dosage.

Dosage

*Dose per day**	*Dose per week**
4.5-8.5 ml of 1:2 liquid extract	30-60 ml of 1:2 liquid extract

SUPPORTING INFORMATION

Traditional Prescribing

Traditional Ayurvedic uses include:
- As a tonic and for rejuvenative action on the female reproductive organs, which is said "to give the capacity to have a hundred husbands"[2]
- As a nutritive tonic[3]
- To promote conception (treating both sexes);[2] sexual debility in both sexes[3]
- Menopause[2]
- Leukorrhea,[3] gonorrhea,[1] herpes[2]
- As a galactagogue[4]
- Dyspepsia, dysentery,[1] diarrhea,[1,3] stomach ulcers, hyperacidity[2]

Shatavari *continued on page 410*

#Alternative name.
*This dose range is extrapolated from traditional Ayurvedic medicine[1] and the author's education and experience.

- Biliousness, liver complaints[1]
- Lung abscesses, hematemesis, cough, convalescence, dehydration[2]
- Inflammation, rheumatism[1]
- Tumors, diseases of the blood,[1] chronic fevers[2]

Preparations based on shatavari are often recommended for threatened miscarriage.[5]

Shatavari is regarded as a remedy from the *rasayana* group. *Rasayana* literally means that path that *rasa* or the primordial tissue takes. A remedy that improves the quality of *rasa* should strengthen or promote the health of all tissues of the body.[6] Shatavari is used in Southeast Asia for promoting appetite and providing nourishment to children.[7]

Aboriginal Australians used shatavari topically. A decoction of the young root with the bark removed was used traditionally as a wash for scabies, infected or ulcerating skin lesions, and chickenpox. The crushed young root (bark and cortex removed) was applied as a paste for breast lumps and breast swelling.[8]

Pharmacologic Research

Steroidal saponins, including shatavarin I[9]; alkaloids, including the pyrrolizidine alkaloid asparagamine A[10]; and mucilage[11] are key constituents of shatavari root. (Based on its chemical structure, asparagamine A would not be expected to be toxic.) The presence of steroidal saponins in shatavari suggests its activity on the female reproductive system may be the result of subtle estrogen modulating activity.

When referred here, shatavari suspension is the dried, powdered root of shatavari boiled in water without separating the insoluble part, as prescribed in Ayurveda.
- Oral administration of shatavari increased the weight of mammary lobulo-alveolar tissue[12] and corrected irregular, low milk yields[13] in experimental models. The authors suggested that shatavari may act directly on the mammary gland or via the pituitary and adrenal glands.[12]
- Shatavarin-I inhibited experimentally induced contractions in isolated uterine tissue and *in vivo* (administered by injection).[14,15] Antioxytocic activity was demonstrated for the alkaloid asparagamine A in later work.[10]
- Oral pretreatment with shatavari suspension had the following adaptogenic effects in experimental models. Shatavari:
  - Reduced mortality from intra-abdominal sepsis[16-18]; one model used concurrent immunosuppression[18]
  - Protected against neutropenia and leukopenia from immunosuppression[18-20] with results comparable to two known immunomodulators (glucan and lithium carbonate)[20]
  - Increased both the phagocytic and killing capacity of macrophages[18,21] and possibly neutrophils[22]

Shatavari *continued on page 411*

- Produced leukocytosis with predominant neutrophilia[16,18,20]
- Enhanced humoral and cell-mediated immunity[23]
- Stimulated granulocyte-macrophage colony formation, indicating the presence of the cytokine that stimulates the growth of this colony[22]
- Reduced bleomycin-induced fibrosis of the lung[6]
- Enhanced the clearance of injected colloidal carbon, indicating enhancement of the activity of the reticulo-endothelial system (a major component of the immune system)[24]
- Reduced stress-induced gastric damage, plasma steroid increase, and macrophage function suppression[25]
- Decreased ethanol-induced gastric ulceration and cisplatin-induced gastroparesis[6]

- Shatavari extract showed considerable antibacterial activity against a variety of bacteria *in vitro* and was comparable to chloramphenicol (an antibiotic) in its activity.[26]
- Shatavari decreased adhesion scores and increased peritoneal macrophage activity in an experimental model investigating intraperitoneal adhesions.[27]
- Oral dosing with an ethanolic extract of shatavari inhibited ochratoxin A (carcinogen)–induced suppression of both chemotactic activity and production of IL-1 and TNF by macrophages. Moreover, shatavari induced excess production of TNF-α when compared with controls.[28] In an earlier study, ingestion of shatavari powder before exposure to the carcinogen DMBA reduced the incidence of mammary tumors in rats.[29]
- Shatavari extract demonstrated antitussive activity against sulfur dioxide–induced cough after oral administration. Results were comparable to those for codeine (a proven antitussive).[30] Hepatoprotective activity was also demonstrated for pretreatment with a shatavari extract.[23]
- Oral administration of shatavari suspension increased weight gain, lung weight, and adrenal gland ascorbic acid content and decreased body temperature, adrenal gland weight, and plasma cortisol levels in young rats. Shatavari did not increase weight gain in adult rats. This finding indicates a mild growth promoting activity, which was milder than that obtained from treatment with ashwaganda.[31]
- An extract of shatavari inhibited carrageenan- and serotonin-induced edema, indicating antiinflammatory activity.[32]
- Shatavari extract exhibited potent antioxidant activity in isolated liver mitochondrial membranes subjected to gamma-radiation.[33]
- Shatavari fresh root juice protected against experimental models of gastric and duodenal ulceration when administered orally.[34]

Clinical Studies

- In a multicenter, randomized, double-blind, placebo-controlled trial, a formulation of herbs containing 68% shatavari was not found to be superior to placebo in promoting lactation in mothers with lactational inadequacy.[35]

Shatavari *continued on page 412*

- Shatavari prevented the presence in gastric aspirates of hemoglobin and reduced the DNA content and the rise in pepsin caused by aspirin ingestion in healthy volunteers. Two doses of shatavari were administered (1.5 g/day and 3 g/day), both of which produced these results.[36]
- Shatavari reduced gastric emptying time from baseline values and had similar activity to metoclopramide (an antiemetic drug) in a small, controlled trial involving healthy male volunteers. Two grams of shatavari powdered root were administered for 2 days between baseline and test readings.[37]

REFERENCES

1 Kapoor LD: *CRC handbook of Ayurvedic medicinal plants,* Boca Raton, Fla, 1990, CRC Press.

2 Frawley D, Lad V: *The yoga of herbs: an Ayurvedic guide to herbal medicine,* ed 2, Santa Fe, 1988, Lotus Press.

3 Thakur RS, Puri HS, Husain A: *Major medicinal plants of India,* Lucknow, India, 1989, Central Institute of Medicinal and Aromatic Plants.

4 Nadkarni AK: *Dr. K.M. Nadkarni's Indian materia medica,* ed 3, Bombay, 1976, Popular Prakashan.

5 Dev S: *Environ Health Perspect* 107(10):783-789, 1999.

6 Rege NN, Thatte UM, Dahanukar SA: *Phytother Res* 13(4):275-291, 1999.

7 World Health Organization: *The use of traditional medicine in primary health care: a manual for health workers in Southeast Asia,* New Delhi, 1990, WHO Regional Office for Southeast Asia.

8 Aboriginal Communities of the Northern Territory of Australia, Conservation Commission of the Northern Territory: *Traditional aboriginal medicines in the Northern Territory of Australia,* Darwin, 1993, Conservation Commission of the Northern Territory of Australia.

9 Hostettmann K, Marston A: *Chemistry & pharmacology of natural products: saponins,* Cambridge, 1995, Cambridge University Press.

10 Sekine T et al: *Perkin Transactions* 1(4):391-393, 1995.

11 Bharatiya Vidya Bhavan's Swami Prakashananda Ayurveda Research Centre: *Selected medicinal plants of India,* Bombay, 1992, Chemexcil.

12 Sabnis PB, Gaitonde BB, Jetmalani M: *Indian J Exp Biol* 6(1):55-57, 1968.

13 Patel AB, Kanitkar UK: *Indian Vet J* 46(8):718-721, 1969.

14 Gaitonde BB, Jetmalani MH: *Arch Int Pharmacodyn Ther* 179(1):121-129, 1969.

15 Joshi J, Dev S: *Indian J Chem* 27B:12-16, 1988.

16 Thatte UM et al: *Indian Drugs* 25(3):95-97, 1987.

17 Dahanukar SA et al: *Indian Drugs* 24:125, 1986.

18 Thatte UM, Dahanukar SA: *Phytother Res* 3(2):43-49, 1989.

19 Thatte UM et al: *J Postgrad Med* 33(4):185-188, 1987.

20 Thatte UM, Dahanukar SA: *Methods Find Exp Clin Pharmacol* 10(10):639-644, 1988.

21 Rege NN, Dahanukar SA: *J Postgrad Med* 39(1):22-25, 1993.

22 Thatte UM et al: International Symposium of Immunological Adjuvants and Modulators of Nonspecific Resistance to Microbial Infections, Columbia, Md, June 30-July3, 1986, abstract 53.

23 Muruganandan S et al: *J Med Arom Plant Sci* 22-23(4A-1A):49-52, 2000-2001.

24 Dahanukar SA, Thatte UM: *Phytomed* 4:297-306, 1997.

25 Dahanukar SA, Thatte UM: *Indian Pract* 41(4):245-252, 1988.

26 Mandal SC et al: *Phytother Res* 14(2):118-119, 2000.

27 Rege NN et al: *J Postgrad Med* 35(4):199-203, 1989.

28 Dhuley JN: *J Ethnopharmacol* 58(1):15-20, 1997.

29 Rao AR: *Int J Cancer* 28(5):607-610, 1981.

30 Mandal SC et al: *Fitoterapia* 71(6):686-689, 2000.

31 Sharma S, Dahanukar S, Karandikar SM: *Indian Drugs* 23(3):133-139, 1985.

32 Mandal SC et al: *Nat Prod Sci* 4(4):230-233, 1998.

33 Kamat JP et al: *J Ethnopharmacol* 71(3):425-435, 2000.

34 Bipul D et al: *Indian J Exp Biol* 35(10):1084-1087, 1997.

35 Sharma S et al: *Indian Pediatr* 33(8): 675-677, 1996.

36 Thatte UM: In Pushpangadan P et al, eds: *Glimpses of Indian ethnopharmacology,* Kerala, India, 1995, Tropical Botanic Garden and Research Institute.

37 Dalvi SS, Nadkarni PM, Gupta KC: *J Postgrad Med* 36(2):91-94, 1990.

SHEPHERD'S PURSE

Botanical Name: *Capsella bursa-pastoris*
Family: Cruciferae
Plant Part Used: Aerial parts

PRESCRIBING INFORMATION

Actions

Antihemorrhagic, urinary antiseptic

Potential Indications

Based on appropriate evaluation of the patient, practitioners should consider prescribing shepherd's purse in formulations in the context of:
- Excessive or irregular menstrual bleeding *(4,5)*
- Hematemesis, hematuria, hemorrhoids, diarrhea *(5)*
- Topical treatment for nosebleed *(4)*

Contraindications

None known.

Warnings and Precautions

None required.

Interactions

None known.

Use in Pregnancy and Lactation

No adverse effects expected.

Side Effects

None expected if taken within the recommended dose range.

Dosage

Dose per day*	*Dose per week**
3-6 ml of 1:2 liquid extract	20-40 ml of 1:2 liquid extract

SUPPORTING INFORMATION

Traditional Prescribing

Traditional Western herbal medicine uses include:
- Menorrhagia, uterine hemorrhage, hematemesis, hematuria, hemorrhoids[1,2]
- Diarrhea, atopic dyspepsia[1,2]

Pharmacologic Research

- *Ex vivo* tests indicated shepherd's purse extracts accelerated coagulation of blood.[3] However, an *in vivo* experiment conducted in 1969 found no hemostatic activity.[4] Injection of extract fractions mildly increased peripheral blood flow. Contractile activity was demonstrated on isolated smooth muscle.[5]
- *In vivo* studies indicate diuretic, antiinflammatory, and antiulcer activities for shepherd's purse extracts. The extract was administered by injection in the majority of these studies.[6]
- Injection of shepherd's purse extract caused inhibition of solid tumor growth in an experimental model.[7] In another model, oral administration inhibited hepatoma induction. The active constituent was believed to be fumaric acid.[8]

Shepherd's Purse *continued on page 414*

---

*This dose range is extrapolated from the British Herbal Pharmacopoeia 1983 and the author's education and experience.

Clinical Studies

No clinical studies using shepherd's purse have been found.

In Germany, the Commission E supports using shepherd's purse for symptomatic treatment of mild menorrhagia and metrorrhagia and topical application for nosebleeds.[9]

REFERENCES

1 British Herbal Medicine Association's Scientific Committee: *British herbal pharmacopoeia,* Bournemouth, 1983, BHMA.

2 Felter HW, Lloyd JU: *King's American dispensatory,* ed 18, rev 3, Portland, 1905, reprinted 1983, Eclectic Medical Publications.

3 Vermathen M, Glasl H: *Planta Med* 59(suppl 1):A670, 1993.

4 Kuroda K, Kaku T: *Life Sci* 8(1):151-155, 1969.

5 Kuroda K, Takagi K: *Arch Int Pharmacodyn* 178:382-391, 1969.

6 Kuroda K, Takagi K: *Arch Int Pharmacodyn* 178:392-399, 1969.

7 Kuroda K et al: *Cancer Res* 36(6):1900-1903, 1976.

8 Kuroda K et al: *Gann* 65(4):317-321, 1974.

9 Blumenthal M et al, eds: *The complete German Commission E monographs: therapeutic guide to herbal medicines,* Austin, 1998, American Botanical Council.

SKULLCAP

Botanical Name: *Scutellaria lateriflora*
Family: Labiatae
Plant Part Used: Aerial parts

Actions

Nervine tonic, spasmolytic, mild sedative

Potential Indications

Based on appropriate evaluation of the patient, practitioners should consider prescribing skullcap in formulations in the context of:
- Nervous excitability, restlessness, wakefulness, anxiety (5)
- Physical or mental tiredness (5)
- Headache, depression (6)
- Epilepsy, neuralgia, tremor (5)

Contraindications

None known.

Warnings and Precautions

None required.

Interactions

None known.

Use in Pregnancy and Lactation

No adverse effects expected.

Side Effects

None expected if taken within the recommended dose range.

Dosage

Dose per day*	Dose per week*
2.0-4.5 ml of 1:2 liquid extract	15-30 ml of 1:2 liquid extract

Traditional Prescribing

Traditional Western herbal medicine uses include:
- Epilepsy, particularly grand mal and other nervous system disorders, such as hysteria, chorea (characterized by involuntary, jerky movements), nervous tension, tremors, neuralgia, and delirium tremens[1,2]
- As a calmative to the nervous system and for nervous excitability, restlessness, wakefulness, and disorders arising from physical or mental overwork[2]
- Functional cardiac disorders that resulted from nervous causes, particularly with intermittent pulse[2]
- As an infusion for children with teething pain[2]
- Headache, particularly arising from incessant coughing and pain[3]
- Depression[4]

Skullcap *continued on page 416*

---

*This dose range is extrapolated from the British Herbal Pharmacopoeia 1983 and the author's education and experience.

Pharmacologic Research

No pharmacologic information relevant to the current usage of skullcap has been found.

Clinical Studies

No clinical studies using skullcap have been found.

REFERENCES

1 British Herbal Medicine Association's Scientific Committee: *British herbal pharmacopoeia,* Bournemouth, 1983, BHMA.
2 Felter HW, Lloyd JU: *King's American dispensatory,* ed 18, rev 3, Portland, 1905, reprinted 1983, Eclectic Medical Publications.
3 Grieve M: *A modern herbal,* New York, 1971, Dover Publications.
4 Bartram T: *Encyclopedia of herbal medicine,* ed 1, Dorset, UK, 1995, Grace Publishers.

SPINY JUJUBE

Other Common Names:	Zizyphus, sour Chinese date seed
Botanical Names:	*Zizyphus jujuba* var. *spinosa*, *Zizyphus spinosa*,[#] *Ziziphus spinosa*[#]
Family:	Rhamnaceae
Plant Part Used:	Seed

PRESCRIBING INFORMATION

Actions

Hypnotic, mild sedative, hypotensive, anxiolytic

Potential Indications

Based on appropriate evaluation of the patient, practitioners should consider prescribing spiny jujube in formulations in the context of:

- Anxiety,* insomnia,* in combination with hoelen, Cnidium, Anemarrhena, and licorice (3)
- Irritability, palpitations, excessive sweating resulting from debility, night sweats (5)

Contraindications

None known.

Warnings and Precautions

None required.

Interactions

None known.

Use in Pregnancy and Lactation

No adverse effects expected.

Side Effects

A 30-year-old woman experienced chills, fever, and joint pain that were attributed to taking *Zizyphus spinosa* seeds (dose not defined).[1]

Dosage

Dose per day**	**Dose per week****
6.0-11.5 ml of 1:2 liquid extract	40-80 ml of 1:2 liquid extract

SUPPORTING INFORMATION

Traditional Prescribing

Uses and properties from TCM include:

- To nourish the *liver*[2,3] and *heart* and calm the *spirit*[3]
- Dream-disturbed sleep,[2] insomnia[2,3]
- Irritability, palpitations with anxiety[3]
- Excessive sweating resulting from debility,[2,3] night sweats[3]

Note: *Zizyphus jujuba* is a different species that is used for different therapeutic purposes in TCM. The part used of this species is the date-like fruit.

Spiny Jujube *continued on page 418*

[#]Alternative name.

*Spiny jujube has also been used in TCM for treating anxiety and insomnia. (5)

**This dose range is adapted from dried plant dosages administered by decoction in TCM.[2] The author's experience and the fact that ethanol-water is a more effective solvent than water for many phytochemicals are taken into account.

Pharmacologic Research

The active constituents of *Zizyphus spinosa* seed include dammarane-type saponins called jujubosides A and B and a flavone C-glycoside called spinosin.[4]

- Oral administration of spiny jujube seed demonstrated sedative activity in experimental models:
  - Inhibiting spontaneous activity[5,6]
  - Prolonging pentobarbital sodium-induced sleep[5]
  - Reducing the response to sound stimulus[6]
  - Inhibiting the convulsive effect of pentylenetetrazole[6]
- Spiny jujube demonstrated immunopotentiating activity *in vivo*. Oral administration of the seed extract increased the lymphocyte transformation rate, hemolysin formation, and clearance of carbon particles. Spiny jujube treatment also enhanced the delayed hypersensitivity reaction to sheep erythrocytes in both normal and cyclophosamide-treated mice.[7]
- Jujubosides inhibited histamine release from peritoneal exudate cells induced by antigen-antibody reaction[8] and exhibited potent immunologic adjuvant activity *in vivo* (route unknown).[9] (An immune adjuvant enhances or modulates immune response.)
- Spiny jujube is also anticonvulsant, hypotensive, and prolongs survival after burns. The herb has very low toxicity, and it improved hypoxia tolerance in rats.[5]

Clinical Studies

Suanzaorentang is a TCM formula containing *Zizyphus spinosa* (45.5%), hoelen (*Poria cocos*, 23%), Cnidium (*Cnidium monnieri*, 13.5%), Anemarrhena (*Amenarrhena asphodeloides*, 13.5%), and licorice (*Glycyrrhiza uralensis*, 4.5%).

- Suanzaorentang (750 mg/day) demonstrated almost the same anxiolytic effect as diazepam (6 mg/day) in a short-term, double-blind trial. Suanzaorentang, but not diazepam, improved psychomotor performance during the daytime. Mood was improved and sympathetic nervous system symptoms decreased. No significant subjective side effects were observed during treatment. Laboratory tests of the major systems were normal after 1 week of administration.[10]
- Significant improvements in all ratings of sleep quality and well being were observed in patients with sleep disorders during suanzaorentang treatment compared with the baseline and placebo periods. Patients ingested capsules containing 1 g of suanzaorentang each night (30 minutes before bedtime) for 2 weeks.[11] In patients with anxiety and cardiac symptoms, treatment with suanzaorentang also demonstrated an anxiolytic effect.[12]

REFERENCES

1 Zhang L, Wang H: *China J Chin Materia Med* 14(2):116, 1989.

2 Pharmacopoeia Commission of the People's Republic of China: *Pharmacopoeia of the People's Republic of China*, English ed, Beijing, 1997, Chemical Industry Press.

3 Bensky D, Gamble A: *Chinese herbal medicine materia medica*, Seattle, 1986, Eastland Press.

4 Tang W, Eisenbrand G: *Chinese drugs of plant origin*, Berlin, 1992, Springer-Verlag.

Spiny Jujube *continued on page 419*

5 Chang HM, But PP: *Pharmacology and applications of Chinese materia medica,* Singapore, 1987, World Scientific.

6 Lou SN, Feng BL, Xia LY: *Zhongchengyao Yanjiu* (2):18-19, 1987.

7 Lang X et al: *Bull Chin Materia Medica* 13(11):683-685, 1988.

8 Yoshikawa M et al: *Chem Pharm Bull* 45(7):1186-1192, 1997.

9 Matsuda H et al: *Chem Pharm Bull* 47(12):1744-1748, 1999.

10 Chen HC, Hsieh MT, Shibuya TK: *Int J Clin Pharmacol Ther Toxicol* 24(12):646-650, 1986.

11 Chen HC, Hsieh MT: *Clin Ther* 7(3):334-337, 1985.

12 Hsieh MT, Chen HC: *Eur J Clin Pharmacol* 30(4):481-484, 1986.

ST. JOHN'S WORT

Other Common Name:	Hypericum
Botanical Name:	*Hypericum perforatum*
Family:	Guttiferae
Plant Part Used:	Aerial parts, harvested during the early flowering period

PRESCRIBING INFORMATION

Actions

Antidepressant, nervine tonic, antiviral, vulnerary, antimicrobial (topically)

Potential Indications

Based on appropriate evaluation of the patient, practitioners should consider prescribing St. John's wort in formulations in the context of:
- Mild to moderate depression *(1,4,5)*
- Depressive symptoms in patients addicted to alcohol *(2)*
- Recurrent orofacial herpes, genital herpes *(2)*
- Anxiety, nervousness, restlessness *(4,5)*
- Obsessive-compulsive disorder, mild psychosomatic and somatoformic disorders *(4)*
- Seasonal affective disorder *(4)*
- Seasonal affective disorder, in combination with light therapy *(3)*
- Psychologic symptoms of menopause *(4,5)*
- Enhancing mood in stressed individuals, such as athletes *(3)*
- Enhancing aerobic endurance capacity in athletes, in combination with vitamin E *(2)*
- PMS *(4)*
- Conditions requiring increased nocturnal melatonin plasma levels, such as circadian rhythm–associated sleep disorders *(4)*
- Afflictions of the nervous system, such as spinal injuries, neuralgia, and sciatica *(5)*
- Treating and preventing acute and chronic infections caused by enveloped viruses (e.g., cold sores, herpes genitalis, chickenpox, shingles) *(7)*

Contraindications

Despite the contraindication given in the *British Herbal Pharmacopoeia* 1983, clinical trials have shown that St. John's wort is efficacious for treating depression.

Concurrent administration of high doses of St. John's wort is contraindicated with the following drugs: warfarin, digoxin, and cyclosporine, as well as indinavir and related anti-HIV drugs.

Warnings and Precautions

Not suited to treating serious depression with psychotic symptoms or suicidal risk.

St. John's wort is not advisable in cases of known photosensitivity. Patients taking higher doses should avoid excessive exposure to sunlight and UV radiation.

St. John's Wort *continued on page 421*

Interactions

St. John's wort may interact with a number of drugs, possibly via cytochrome P-450 induction. Practitioners should avoid prescribing St. John's wort if patients are taking the following drugs: immune suppressants (cyclosporin), cardiac glycosides (digoxin), HIV nonnucleoside reverse transcriptase inhibitors (nevirapine)[1] and other HIV protease inhibitors (indinavir), the chemotherapeutic drug irinotecan (Camptosar)[2], and the anticoagulants warfarin and phenprocoumon. Caution should be exercised when prescribing St. John's wort to patients taking selective serotonin reuptake inhibitors (SSRIs) because of potential effects on serotonin levels and the risk of subsequent serotonin syndrome (confusion, fever, shivering, sweating, diarrhea, and muscle spasm). Several reports indicate breakthrough bleeding occurring in women taking St. John's wort while on the oral contraceptive pill (OCP) and recent reports from Sweden and Britain of unwanted pregnancies. Practitioners should exercise caution with women who are taking a very low dose OCP. No interaction was observed between St. John's wort and alcohol in terms of cognitive capabilities in a clinical trial. Concerns have also been raised about concurrent administration of St. John's wort with theophylline (a bronchorelaxant) and phenytoin (an anticonvulsant). A case was reported in which St. John's wort reduced serum levels of theophylline.[3] However, no clinical adverse effects have been reported for phenytoin or any other anticonvulsant drugs. In fact, an open trial demonstrated that St. John's wort extract had no effect on carbamazepine pharmacokinetics in eight healthy volunteers.[4]

A randomized, double-blind, placebo-controlled study investigating the pharmacokinetic interaction between St. John's wort preparations and digoxin in healthy volunteers found that the interaction was dose-related and not inherent to the standardized extract. Doses equivalent to 1 g per day of St. John's wort herb produced no differences in pharmacokinetic parameters compared with placebo.[5]

Use in Pregnancy and Lactation

No adverse effects expected.

Side Effects

In patients who are HIV-positive receiving oral St. John's wort, mild, reversible elevations of serum liver enzymes were observed.

A postmarketing surveillance study of 3250 depressed patients reported that 2.4% experienced side effects that were mainly mild gastrointestinal complaints and allergic reactions, such as pruritis.

A case of adynamic ileus associated with the use of St. John's wort by a 67-year-old woman has been reported.

No reliable evidence of phototoxicity in humans has been found. Investigations involving volunteers found that the threshold daily dose for a mild increase in photosensitization was approximately 2 to 4 g of commercial extract (containing 5 to 10 mg of hypericin).[6]

St. John's Wort continued on page 422

Reversible photosensitivity has been observed in patients receiving oral doses of isolated hypericin (0.05 to 0.10 mg/kg of body weight/day).[7] Avoiding excessive exposure to sunlight or artificial UVA light is advisable for patients taking high doses, and St. John's wort should be used cautiously in patients with known photosensitivity.

Several cases of hypomania were reported for individuals with no history of bipolar disorder after taking St. John's wort.[8,9] Episodes of mania were also reported for two people with a history of bipolar depression[10] and in one depressed patient concurrently taking sertraline.[11] In the last case, the adverse reaction may have been the result of the drug alone. A psychotic episode associated with using St. John's wort was reported for a woman who was later diagnosed as having Alzheimer's disease.[12]

Some reports indicate a phenomenon that appears to be a sensory nerve hypersensitivity. The evidence suggests that the St. John's wort preparations were manufactured from late harvested herb containing high levels of resinous compounds that appeared as sediment in the liquids. The problem can be avoided by not dispensing the sediment and by using St. John's wort harvested at the onset of full flowering.

Dosage

Dose per day*	Dose per week*
2-6 ml of 1:2 liquid extract	15-40 ml of 1:2 liquid extract
2-6 ml of 1:2 high hypericin liquid extract	15-40 ml of 1:2 high hypericin liquid extract

Extracts providing quantified levels of total hypericins are recommended. Ideally, aqueous ethanol extracts should contain not less than 0.2 mg/ml hypericins, and high hypericin extracts should contain not less than 0.4 mg/ml hypericins.

SUPPORTING INFORMATION

Traditional Prescribing

Traditional Western herbal medicine uses include:
- Excitability, hysteria, nervous conditions with depression, menopausal neurosis[13,14]
- Neuralgia, fibrositis, sciatica, spinal injuries or irritations, shock, concussion, throbbing of the body without fever[13,14]
- Hemorrhage, menorrhagia, diarrhea, jaundice, chronic urinary conditions[14]
- Internally and topically for wounds[13,14]
- Externally as an oil maceration for wounds, ulcers, and swellings[14]

The Eclectic physicians regarded St. John's wort as having "undoubted power over the nervous system, and particularly the spinal cord."[14]

St. John's Wort *continued on page 423*

*This dose range is extrapolated from the British Herbal Pharmacopoeia 1983 and the author's education and experience.

Pharmacologic Research

Key constituents of the aerial parts of St. John's wort include the naphthodianthrones hypericin and pseudohypericin (collectively referred to as total hypericin [TH]), flavonoids, and phenolic compounds such as hyperforin.

- Experimental studies suggest that St. John's wort is the only antidepressant agent capable of inhibiting the reuptake of serotonin, norepinephrine (noradrenaline), and dopamine with similar potencies.[15] St. John's wort extracts may have a similar mechanism of action to SSRIs but probably to a lesser extent.[16]
- Many compounds in St. John's wort, including the hypericins, hyperforin, and flavonoids, appear to contribute to the antidepressant activity.[17]
- Hypericin and pseudohypericin demonstrated activity against several enveloped viruses in vitro and against several retroviruses in vitro and in vivo (by oral administration or injection). Both antiviral and antiretroviral activity was enhanced by exposure to light.
- Hypericin produced a potent antitumor activity in vitro against several tumor cells, but did not show any toxic effects toward normal cells at higher concentrations. Antitumor activity in vivo was also demonstrated after intraperitoneal injection. An antimutagenic activity was demonstrated for St. John's wort extract in terms of DNA repair in Escherichia coli.
- St. John's wort extract demonstrated bactericidal activity in vitro against a number of gram-positive and gram-negative bacteria, including Staphylococcus aureus, Proteus vulgaris, Escherichia coli, and Pseudomonas aeruginosa.
- In an experimental model, oral administration of an extract of St. John's wort (26.5 mg/kg) induced a sedation similar to that produced by diazepam (2 mg, orally). None of the isolated fractions from this extract exhibited the same sedative activity as the whole extract. The previously described dose of concentrated St. John's wort extract was equivalent to 125 mg/kg of dried, powdered herb. This amount is only slightly higher than normal therapeutic doses of the standardized extract but is lower than doses typically used for liquids.
- Oral administration of St. John's wort extracts dose-dependently and significantly reduced alcohol intake in two genetic animal models of human alcoholism.
- Oral administration of St. John's wort tincture demonstrated improved wound healing in experimental models. In a controlled in vivo test, oily extract of St. John's wort demonstrated a significant antiirritant effect against croton oil applied to the skin.

Clinical Studies

- Meta-analysis and systematic reviews, including the Cochrane review, published from 1996 to 2000 concluded that St. John's wort extracts are more efficacious than placebo for treating mild to moderate depression. More data is required to assess its efficacy compared with other antidepressant medication. Fewer side effects were, however, reported for St. John's wort extracts compared with

St. John's Wort continued on page 424

standard antidepressants.[18-20] For the trials considered in one of the previously listed reviews[20] and based on recent formulation specifications, the most common daily dose of extract prescribed corresponded to approximately 5 g of dried herb, containing 2.7 mg of TH. One trial investigated the efficacy of a high daily dose (twice this dose).

- Since the publication of these reviews, further trials have been published. Two randomized, double-blind, multicenter studies found St. John's wort extract to be more efficacious than placebo and at least as beneficial as imipramine (a tricyclic antidepressant) in treating mild to moderate depression.[21,22] St. John's wort extract (equivalent to 6 g/day of dried herb and containing 2.6 mg/day of TH and 26 mg of hyperforin) was compared against 100 mg/day imipramine or placebo for 8 weeks.[21] The other trial compared the effects of St. John's wort extract containing 1 mg per day hypericin with 150 mg per day of imipramine over a 6-week period.[22] Side effects were less common in patients taking the St. John's wort extract in both studies. The design of these studies has been questioned,[23-26] notably the use of imipramine as a comparison instead of a more modern antidepressant, the short duration of treatment, and the absence of a placebo group (in the case of one trial).

- A number of trials found that standardized St. John's wort extracts compared favorably with the SSRI fluoxetine,[27-30] particularly for treating depressed patients with anxiety symptoms.[30] The dose of St. John's wort used was equivalent to 4.8 g per day of dried herb in one of these trials[27] and was standardized to contain 1 mg per day hypericin in two others.[28,29] Duration of treatment was typically 6 weeks. A review of controlled trials found St. John's wort as efficacious as fluoxetine for mild depression.[31] St. John's wort compared favorably with the SSRI sertraline for treating mild to moderate depression in a randomized, placebo-controlled pilot trial involving a small group of outpatients.[32]

- A randomized, double-blind, placebo-controlled, multicenter trial published in 2001 concluded that standardized St. John's wort extract administered for 8 weeks was not an effective treatment for severe depression compared with placebo. Although St. John's wort was found to be safe and well tolerated, no significant benefits above placebo were observed for the Hamilton Depression Scale (HAM-D) or other measures of anxiety or depression. However, the number of patients reaching remission of their illness was significantly higher in the St. John's wort group compared with placebo (based on intention-to-treat analysis). This effect was not regarded as clinically significant by the authors. The daily doses corresponded to approximately 5 to 7 g of original dried herb.[33] A number of letters were published criticizing the design of this trial (see letters published in *JAMA* 286(1):42, 2001). Of relevance is that a trial included in one of the systematic reviews found similar efficacy for St. John's wort compared with imipramine (150 mg/day) in treating severe depression. The response rates were low for both groups, but fewer side effects were

St. John's Wort continued on page 425

recorded in the herbal treatment group. The daily dose of St. John's wort extract corresponded to approximately 8 g of original dried herb and provided 5.4 mg of TH.

- A randomized, double-blind, placebo-controlled trial involving mild to moderately depressed patients (International Classification of Diseases [ICD]-10 categories F32.0, F32.1, F33.0, F33.1**) and patients with dysthymia (ICD-10 category F34.1**) found a large discrepancy in response between dysthymic and nondysthymic patients, the latter being more sensitive to St. John's wort therapy.[34]

- The results of a postmarketing surveillance study suggest that St. John's wort is beneficial for treating mild to moderate depression in children under 12 years of age. The 76 children who completed the study were treated with a St. John's wort extract, the majority of patients receiving daily doses corresponding to approximately 1.7 to 3.3 g of original dried herb (containing 0.9 to 1.8 mg of TH) for 4 to 6 weeks. No adverse events were reported.[35]

- St. John's wort extract reduced depressive symptoms in patients addicted to alcohol and was well tolerated in a randomized, double-blind, placebo-controlled trial involving 119 male and female patients. The daily dose corresponded to 2.7 mg of TH.[36]

- St. John's wort extract for 4 weeks (containing 2.7 mg/day TH) significantly reduced HAM-D scores in patients with seasonal affective disorder (SAD) when combined with either bright or dim light therapy in a single-blind trial. In an uncontrolled trial, survey results showed a significant improvement from baseline values for anxiety, loss of libido, and insomnia in patients with SAD treated with St. John's wort alone and in those treated with both St. John's wort and light therapy. No significant between-group differences were observed, except that improvement in sleep was greater in the combined treatment group.[37] New findings suggest that the photodynamic impact of St. John's wort increases the effect of normal light, as if the patient were subject to continuous light therapy.[38]

- In an open, pilot trial, administering St. John's wort extract (standardized to 2.7 mg/day hypericin for 12 weeks) produced promising results in treating obsessive-compulsive disorder.[39]

- Oral treatment with St. John's wort extract reduced the number of patients experiencing herpetic episodes and the total symptom score compared with placebo in two double-blind, randomized trials lasting 90 days. The trials included 94 patients with recurrent orofacial herpes and 110 patients with genital herpes.[40]

- In a randomized, double-blind trial, St. John's wort extract (0.9 mg/day TH) did not demonstrate a significant effect over placebo for treating painful polyneuropathy.[41] However, a tendency to improvement was observed, which did not achieve statistical significance, possibly because of the low patient numbers involved.

St. John's Wort continued on page 426

**International Classification of Diseases*, rev 10, Chapter V (F), World Health Organization, 1991. (Categories F32.0, F32.1, F33.0, F33.1 refer to mild to moderate depression; F34.1 refers to dysthymia [chronic mood disorder].)

- In an open, observational study, improvement in symptoms was observed in premenopausal and postmenopausal women after 12 weeks of treatment with St. John's wort (standardized to 0.9 mg/day TH). Climacteric complaints such as irritability and outbreaks of sweating decreased or disappeared in the majority of women. Sexual well being also improved.[42] A St. John's wort and black cohosh combination significantly reduced menopausal symptoms compared with placebo in a randomized, double-blind trial involving 179 women. The daily dose of herbal treatment corresponded to 0.5 mg of TH and 2 mg of 27-deoxyactein (a marker compound in black cohosh).[43]

- An uncontrolled, pilot study with St. John's wort found improvement in PMS scores and a decrease in symptom severity when the herb was administered for two menstrual cycles. The daily dose of extract contained 0.9 mg TH.[44]

- In an uncontrolled trial, St. John's wort extract (standardized to deliver 0.5 mg/day TH) for 3 weeks produced a significant increase in nocturnal melatonin plasma concentration in healthy volunteers.

- A placebo-controlled, crossover study found that 6 weeks of treatment with St. John's wort extract (equivalent to 2 g/day of dried herb) significantly improved vigor while reducing anger, fatigue, confusion, and mood disturbance in athletes.[45] In a double-blind, placebo-controlled trial, athletes were randomized into three groups: St. John's wort plus vitamin E, vitamin E, and placebo. The St. John's wort plus vitamin E group demonstrated a significantly better aerobic endurance capacity compared with the other groups. The daily dose of St. John's wort used was approximately 170 mg of standardized extract, probably corresponding to approximately 1 g of dried herb.

- In Germany, the Commission E supports using St. John's wort internally to treat anxiety-related symptoms and depressive moods, as well as anxiety, nervous unrest, or both. Oily St. John's wort preparations are recommended internally for dyspeptic complaints and externally for treatment and posttherapy of acute and contused injuries, myalgia, and first-degree burns.[46]

- ESCOP recommends St. John's wort for treating mild to moderate depressive states (ICD-10 categories F32.0, F32.1**) and somatoformic disturbances, including symptoms such as restlessness, anxiety, and irritability.[47]

- St. John's wort has been reinstated to the USP and is official in the USP24-NF19.

REFERENCES

Except when specifically referenced, the following book was referred to in the compilation of the pharmacologic and clinical information: Mills S, Bone K: *Principles and Practice of Phytotherapy: Modern Herbal Medicine,* Edinburgh, 2000, Churchill Livingstone.

St. John's Wort *continued on page 427*

**International Classification of Diseases,* rev 10, Chapter V (F), World Health Organization, 1991. (Categories F32.0, F32.1, F33.0, F33.1 refer to mild to moderate depression; F34.1 refers to dysthymia [chronic mood disorder].)

1 [No authors listed]: *Treatment Update* 12(11):6, 2001.

2 Mathijssen HJ et al: Annual Meeting of the American Association for Cancer Research, San Francisco, April 6-10, 2002, abstract 2443.

3 Nebel A et al: *Ann Pharmacother* 33:502, 1999.

4 Burstein AH et al: *Clin Pharmacol Ther* 68(6):605-612, 2000.

5 Uehleke B et al: *Phytomed* 7(supp 2):20, 2000.

6 Schulz V: *Schweiz Rundsch Med Prax* 89(50):2131-2140, 2000.

7 [No authors listed]: *Treatment Update* 12(11):4-5, 2001.

8 Schneck C: *J Clin Psychiatry* 59(12):689, 1998.

9 O'Breasail AM, Argouarch S: *Can J Psychiatry* 43(7):746-747, 1998.

10 Nierenberg AA et al: *Biol Psychiatry* 46(12):1707-1708, 1999.

11 Barbenel DM et al: *J Psychopharmacol* 14(1):84-86, 2000.

12 Laird RD, Webb M: *J Herb Pharmacother* 1(2):87, 2001.

13 British Herbal Medicine Association's Scientific Committee: *British herbal pharmacopoeia,* Bournemouth, 1983, BHMA.

14 Felter HW, Lloyd JU: *King's American dispensatory,* ed 18, rev 3, Portland, 1905, reprinted 1983, Eclectic Medical Publications.

15 Nathan P: *Mol Psychiatry* 4(4):333-338, 1999.

16 Kasper S, Schulz V: *Wien Med Wochenschr* 149(8-10):191-196, 1999.

17 International Conference: 2000 Years of Natural Product Research—Past, Present and Future, Amsterdam, July 26-30, 1999.

18 Stevinson C, Ernst E: *Eur Neuropsychopharmacol* 9(6):501-505, 1999.

19 Linde K, Mulrow CD: *Cochrane Database Syst Rev* (2):CD000448, 2000.

20 Gaster B, Holroyd J: *Arch Intern Med* 160(2):152-156, 2000.

21 Woelk H: *BMJ* 321(7260):536-539, 2000.

22 Philipp M, Kohnen R, Hiller KO: *BMJ* 319:1534-1539, 1999.

23 Cornwall PL: *BMJ* 322(7284):493, 2001.

24 Spira JL: *BMJ* 322(7284):493, 2001.

25 Alkhenizan A: *BMJ* 322(7284):493, 2001.

26 Volp A: *BMJ* 322(7284):493-494, 2001.

27 Harrer G et al: *Arzneim Forsch* 49(1):289-296, 1999.

28 Schrader E: *Int Clin Psychopharmacol* 15(2):61-68, 2000.

29 Hasler A, Brattstrom A, Meier B: International Conference: 2000 Years of Natural Product Research, Amsterdam, July 26-30, 1999, abstract 413.

30 Friede M, Henneicki-von Zepelin H-H, Freudenstein J: *Phytomed* 7(supp 2):18-19, 2000.

31 Volz HP, Laux P: *Compr Psychiatry* 41(2, suppl 1):133-137, 2000.

32 Brenner R et al: *Clin Ther* 22(4):411-419, 2000.

33 Shelton RC et al: *JAMA* 285(15):1978-1986, 2001.

34 Randlov C et al: *Altern Ther Health Med* 7(3):108-109, 2001.

35 Hubner WD, Kirste T: *Phytother Res* 15(4):367-370, 2001.

36 Winkel R et al: *Phytomed* 7(supp 2):19, 2000.

37 Wheatley D: *Curr Med Res Opin* 15(1):33-37, 1999.

38 Harrer G: *Schweiz Rundsch Med Prax* 89(50):2123-2129, 2000.

39 Taylor LH, Kobak KA: *J Clin Psychiatry* 61(8):575-578, 2000.

40 Mannel M, Koytchev R, Dundarov S: *Phytomed* 7(supp 2):17, 2000.

41 Sindrup SH et al: *Pain* 91(3):361-365, 2001.

42 Grube B, Walper A, Wheatley D: *Adv Ther* 16(4):177-186, 1999.

43 Boblitz N et al: *Focus Alternat Complement Ther* 5(1):85-86, 2000.

44 Stevinson C, Ernst E: *BJOG* 107(7):870-876, 2000.

45 Chapman M: *Australian Doctor,* October 6, 2000.

46 Blumenthal M et al, eds: *The complete German Commission E monographs: therapeutic guide to herbal medicines,* Austin, 1998, American Botanical Council.

47 Scientific Committee of the European Scientific Cooperative on Phytotherapy [ESCOP]: *ESCOP monographs: Hyperici herba.* European Scientific Cooperative on Phytotherapy, ESCOP Secretariat, Argyle House, Gandy Street, Exeter, Devon, EX4 3LS, United Kingdom, March 1996.

THUJA

Other Common Names: Arbor-vitae, tree of life, white cedar (American)
Botanical Name: *Thuja occidentalis*
Family: Cupressaceae
Plant Part Used: Leaf

PRESCRIBING INFORMATION

Actions

Antimicrobial, depurative, antiviral, antifungal

Potential Indications

Based on appropriate evaluation of the patient, practitioners should consider prescribing Thuja in formulations in the context of:
- Infections from wart viruses, oral and topical use *(5,7)*
- Treating and preventing nonspecific URTIs, in combination with *Echinacea* spp. root and Baptisia *(2)*
- Sinusitis, in combination with *Echinacea* spp. root and Baptisia *(3)*
- Topical application for wart infection of the foot *(2)*
- Topical application for fungal infections of the skin *(5)*

Contraindications

Pregnancy[1] and lactation (resulting from the presence of the potentially toxic component thujone in the essential oil of Thuja leaf).

Warnings and Precautions

Thuja should not be taken in high doses over a prolonged period. Caution is advised in epilepsy because of the thujone content in the essential oil.[2]

Interactions

None known.

Use in Pregnancy and Lactation

Contraindicated in pregnancy and lactation.

Side Effects

None expected if taken within the recommended dose range.

High doses of thujone (obtained from ingesting the essential oil) have caused convulsions and neurotoxicity in animals and humans.[2] High doses of Thuja may cause headaches attributed to the thujone content. The addictive syndrome known as absinthism (from the liqueur absinthe) has been attributed to the toxic effects of thujone.

Dosage

Dose per day*	Dose per week*
1.5-3.0 ml of 1:5 tincture	10-20 ml of 1:5 tincture

SUPPORTING INFORMATION

Traditional Prescribing

Traditional Western herbal medicine uses include:
- Bronchial catarrh, bronchitis with cardiac weakness, intermittent fever[1]
- Warts (oral and topical use)[1]

Thuja *continued on page 429*

*This dose range is extrapolated from the British Herbal Pharmacopoeia 1983 and the author's education and experience.

- Enuresis, cystitis,[1] urinary incontinence, bedwetting, urethritis[3]
- Psoriasis, rheumatism[1]
- Amenorrhea, uterine carcinoma[1]
- Enlarged prostate[3]
- Disorders of the blood and glands[3]
- To counter the ill effects of smallpox vaccination[1]
- Topically for wounds, skin ulcers, bedsores, fungal infections of the skin, carcinomatous ulcerations, trachoma, rheumatism, leukorrhea; to stop hemorrhage caused by uterine tumor[3]

Native Americans used Thuja for a wide variety of reasons: as a remedy for cough and headache, as a diaphoretic and to treat intermittent fevers, as a blood purifier, and to flavor other medicines. A poultice of Thuja leaves was used for swollen hands and feet and for heart pain. Thuja was official in the USP from 1882 to 1894 and the NF from 1942 to 1950. Thuja was used as a stimulant to heart and uterine muscle and as a stimulant, irritant, and antiseptic.[4]

Pharmacologic Research

An important component of Thuja leaf is the essential oil, which contains monoterpenes (especially terpenic ketones, including thujone) and other terpenes.[5]

Pharmacologic research conducted using (TPS, a high molecular weight polysaccharide fraction isolated from Thuja, is not listed here. The quantity of polysaccharides present in Thuja preparations containing 50% ethanol or more (such as Thuja tincture) would be negligible.

- Constituents of Thuja have shown anticarcinogenic activity *in vitro*. The concentration of tumor-promoted ornithine decarboxylase was inhibited.[6]
- Phagocytosis of erythrocytes by Kupffer cells *in vitro* was significantly improved by a formulation containing Thuja, Baptisia, *Echinacea angustifolia*, and *E. purpurea* roots combined with homeopathic remedies. Single herbal extracts also demonstrated activity, with Thuja extract having a prominent effect on the first phase of phagocytosis.[7]
- Antiviral activity was observed using Thuja extracts against HSV *in vitro*. Using highly purified fractions of Thuja, the minimal antiviral dose was lower than 50 µg/ml, and the 50% cytotoxic dose was 400 µg/ml.[8] A 70% ethanolic extract of Thuja also inhibited HSV *in vitro*. Using activity-guided fractionation, the main active component was found to be deoxypodophyllotoxin, a known antiviral agent. Commercial tinctures of Thuja were found to contain approximately 0.3 mg/ml of this component.[9] Deoxypodophyllotoxin is also known to be active against the wart virus.
- Thuja essential oil demonstrated fungicidal activity against the ringworm fungi *Microsporum audouinii in vitro*.[10]

Clinical Studies

- Herbal formulations containing Thuja have been used successfully for treating and preventing nonspecific URTI in randomized, double-blind,

Thuja *continued on page 430*

placebo-controlled trials.[11,12] These formulations consisted of Thuja, Baptisia, and *Echinacea* spp. root or these herbs combined with homeopathic remedies. In trials, the daily dose of herbs was well below the normal therapeutic limit (more similar to a homeopathic protocol).

- A controlled trial found combined use of Thuja, Baptisia, and *Echinacea* spp. root with the antibiotic doxycycline had better success than doxycycline alone in treating acute sinusitis.[13]
- Thuja extract applied topically for 3 weeks demonstrated benefit for treating foot warts in a randomized, double-blind, placebo-controlled clinical trial involving children and adults.[14]

REFERENCES

1 British Herbal Medicine Association's Scientific Committee: *British herbal pharmacopoeia,* Bournemouth, 1983, BHMA.
2 Millet Y et al: *Clin Toxicol* 18(12):1485-1498, 1981.
3 Felter HW, Lloyd JU: *King's American dispensatory,* ed 18, rev 3, Portland, 1905, reprinted 1983, Eclectic Medical Publications.
4 Vogel VJ: *American Indian medicine,* Norman, Okla, 1970, University of Oklahoma Press.
5 Leung AY, Foster S: *Encyclopedia of common natural ingredients used in food, drugs and cosmetics,* ed 2, New York-Chichester, 1996, John Wiley.
6 Chang LC et al: *J Nat Prod* 63(9):1235-1238, 2000.
7 Vomel T: *Arzneim Forsch* 35(9):1437-1439, 1985.
8 Beuscher N, Kopanski L: *Planta Med* 52:555-556, 1986.
9 4th International Congress on Phytotherapy, Munich, September 10-13, 1992.
10 Yadav P, Dubey NK: *Indian J Pharm Sci* 56(6):227-231, 1994.
11 Barrett B, Vohman M, Calabrese C: *J Fam Prac* 48(8):628-635, 1999.
12 Henneicke-von Zepelin HH et al: *Curr Med Res Opin* 15(3):214-227, 1999.
13 Zimmer M: *Therapiewoche* 35:4024-4028, 1985.
14 Khan MT et al: *J Eur Acad Dermatol Venereol* 12(suppl 2):S251-S252, 1999.

THYME

Botanical Name: *Thymus vulgaris*
Family: Labiatae
Plant Part Used: Leaf

PRESCRIBING INFORMATION

Actions

Expectorant, spasmolytic, antibacterial, antifungal, antioxidant, rubefacient (topically), antimicrobial

Potential Indications

Based on appropriate evaluation of the patient, practitioners should consider prescribing thyme in formulations in the context of:
- Productive cough *(2,5)*
- Bronchitis, whooping cough, catarrh of the upper respiratory tract *(4,5)*
- Stomatitis and halitosis *(4)*
- Laryngitis, sore throat, fever in the common cold *(5)*
- Dyspepsia, chronic gastritis, colic, flatulence, diarrhea *(5)*
- Tonsillitis, as a gargle *(5)*

Contraindications

None known.

Warnings and Precautions

None required.

Interactions

None known.

Use in Pregnancy and Lactation

No adverse effects expected.

Side Effects

In a group of 100 patients with leg ulcers, 5% responded with a positive reaction to patch testing with thyme oil. Allergic contact dermatitis caused by thymol has been reported for a proprietary antiseptic mouthwash used for treating paronychia. Thyme inhaled as dust can cause occupational asthma, which has been confirmed by inhalation challenges.

Dosage

Dose per day*	Dose per week*
2-6 ml of 1:2 liquid extract	15-40 ml of 1:2 liquid extract

SUPPORTING INFORMATION

Traditional Prescribing

Traditional Western herbal medicine uses include:
- Dyspepsia, chronic gastritis, colic, flatulence, diarrhea[1,2]
- Bronchitis, asthma, whooping cough, laryngitis, sore throat, catarrh, fever in the common cold[1,2]
- Hysteria, dysmenorrhea, bedwetting[1,2]

Thyme *continued on page 432*

*This dose range is extrapolated from the British Pharmaceutical Codex 1949, the British Herbal Pharmacopoeia 1983, and the author's education and experience.

- As a stimulating tonic in convalescence after exhausting illness[2]
- Topically for tonsillitis[1]

Pharmacologic Research

- Thyme extracts exhibited a spasmolytic effect on isolated smooth muscle and inhibited agents that stimulate smooth muscle. The relaxing effect of bradykinin was potentiated.
- The antibacterial and antifungal activity of thymol is well recognized. Essential oil of thyme demonstrated antimicrobial and fungicidal activity *in vitro* in several studies.
- Components of thyme oil inhibited the growth of seven standard strains of gram-positive and gram-negative bacteria *in vitro*. A broad spectrum of activity was observed for thymol and carvacrol against bacteria involved in URTIs. Aqueous and ethanolic extracts of thyme demonstrated significant inhibition of *Helicobacter pylori in vitro*.
- Thyme extracts have exhibited antioxidant activity *in vitro*.

Clinical Studies

- Oral treatment with large doses of thymol resolved Kaposi's sarcoma, dermatomyositis, and progressive scleroderma in separate case studies. The thymol was administered at a dose of 1 to 4 g per day in two cycles of 64 and 169 days, with a 35-day interval with no treatment.
- In conjunction with maintaining a continuous state of dryness, topical thymol was successfully used in treating paronychia and onycholysis.
- In a randomized, double-blind study, 60 patients with productive cough received either syrup of thyme or bromhexine for a period of 5 days. No significant difference was observed between the two groups, based on self-reported symptom relief. Both groups made similar gains. A nonstatistically significant improvement was observed in the recovery rate of nonsmokers compared with smokers in both groups.
- Vulval lichen sclerosis in two patients was successfully treated with a cream containing thyme extract. No side effects were reported.
- In Germany, the Commission E supports using thyme to treat symptoms of bronchitis and whooping cough and catarrh of the upper respiratory tract.[3]
- ESCOP recommends thyme for treating catarrh of the upper respiratory tract, bronchial catarrh, pertussis, stomatitis, and halitosis.[4]

REFERENCES

The following book was referred to in the compilation of the pharmacologic and clinical information: Mills S, Bone K: *Principles and Practice of Phytotherapy: Modern Herbal Medicine,* Edinburgh, 2000, Churchill Livingstone.

1 British Herbal Medicine Association's Scientific Committee: *British herbal pharmacopoeia,* Bournemouth, 1983, BHMA.
2 Felter HW, Lloyd JU: *King's American dispensatory,* ed 18, rev 3, Portland, 1905, reprinted 1983, Eclectic Medical Publications.
3 Blumenthal M et al, eds: *The complete German Commission E monographs: therapeutic guide to herbal medicines,* Austin, 1998, American Botanical Council.
4 Scientific Committee of the European Scientific Cooperative on Phytotherapy [ESCOP]: *ESCOP monographs: Thymi herba.* European Scientific Cooperative on Phytotherapy, ESCOP Secretariat, Argyle House, Gandy Street, Exeter, Devon, EX4 3LS, United Kingdom, March 1996.

TIENCHI GINSENG

Botanical Name: *Panax notoginseng*
Family: Araliaceae
Plant Part Used: Root

PRESCRIBING INFORMATION

Actions

Antihemorrhagic, cardioprotective, antiinflammatory, antiarrhythmic, hypocholesterolemic

Potential Indications

Based on appropriate evaluation of the patient, practitioners should consider prescribing Tienchi ginseng in formulations in the context of:

- Hemoptysis, hematuria *(4,5)*
- Angina pectoris, high blood cholesterol *(4)*
- Hemorrhage, hematemesis, melena, abnormal uterine bleeding *(5)*
- Injury from trauma, especially with hematoma, swelling, and bruising *(5)*

Contraindications

Pregnancy, according to TCM.[1]

Warnings and Precautions

None required.

Interactions

None known.

Use in Pregnancy and Lactation

Contraindicated in pregnancy.

Side Effects

None expected if taken within the recommended dose range.

Dosage

*Dose per day**	*Dose per week**
3.5-8.5 ml of 1:2 liquid extract	25-60 ml of 1:2 liquid extract

Higher doses may be required for trauma and severe hemorrhage.[3]

SUPPORTING INFORMATION

Traditional Prescribing

Uses from TCM include:

- Hemorrhage, nosebleed, hemoptysis, hematemesis, metrorrhagia, hematoma, melena, sharp pain of chest and abdomen[2,3]
- Swelling and pain caused by trauma[2]

Pharmacologic Research

The main active constituents of Tienchi ginseng are saponins, including ginsenosides and notoginsenosides.[4]

- Tienchi ginseng increased coronary blood flow in isolated heart tissue and *in vivo* (by injection),[3,5] decreased myocardial oxygen

Tienchi Ginseng *continued on page 434*

*This dose range is adapted from dried plant dosages administered by decoction in TCM.[2] The author's experience and the fact that ethanol-water is a more effective solvent than water for many phytochemicals are taken into account.

consumption, and prolonged the survival time from anoxia (by injection).[3] Total saponins protected against myocardial ischemia and ischemia-reperfusion damage *in vivo* (route unknown).[6]

- A diluted root extract increased cardiac function in an isolated heart preparation. A hypotensive effect was demonstrated for root and total saponins in an experimental model (by injection).[3] Injection of Tienchi ginseng saponins protected against experimentally induced hemorrhagic shock, which was attributed to the improvement in heart function.[7]

- Aqueous extract of Tienchi ginseng lowered systemic blood pressure *in vivo,* an effect that was not blocked or reversed by multiple antagonists.[5] *In vitro* studies indicated that Tienchi ginseng had a selective blocking effect on calcium channels.[8,9]

- Panaxatriol saponins exerted an antiarrhythmic effect *in vivo* (route unknown). A significant protective effect was observed toward atrial fibrillation.[10]

- Tienchi ginseng saponins dilated coronary blood vessels *in vivo* (by injection).[11] An antiatherosclerotic effect was demonstrated experimentally for oral application of the total saponins of Tienchi ginseng.[12] Injection of Tienchi ginseng saponins inhibited experimentally induced abnormal increases in platelet aggregation and platelet adhesiveness.[13]

- The saponin fraction of Tienchi ginseng demonstrated antiinflammatory, analgesic, and immunomodulatory actions in experimental models (by injection).[14] Antiinflammatory activity was not observed in the adjuvant-induced inflammation model after injection of Tienchi ginseng decoction.[15]

- Tienchi ginseng total saponins decreased total cholesterol and triglycerides *in vivo* after oral administration.[16]

- Ginsenoside Rg_1 isolated from Tienchi ginseng lowered hyperglycemia and acted synergistically with insulin *in vivo* (route unknown). The uptake of glucose by hepatocytes was increased *in vitro*.[17]

- Oral doses of Tienchi ginseng improved experimentally induced learning and memory deficit[18] and increased spontaneous locomotor activity *in vivo.* Treated animals showed less anxious behavior than controls.[19]

Clinical Studies

- In uncontrolled trials in China, Tienchi ginseng has satisfactorily treated heart disease, especially angina pectoris. A typical dose is 1 g of powder taken three times per day.[3]

- A hemostatic effect was achieved for hemoptysis in an uncontrolled trial involving 10 patients. Tienchi ginseng powder (6 to 9 g, two to three times/day) was administered. In another uncontrolled trial, success was noted in hematuria by the third day of treatment (0.9 to 1.5 g every 6 to 8 hours).[3]

- In a trial involving 57 patients, Tienchi ginseng demonstrated similar hypocholesterolemic activity to clofibrate. The clinical hypocholesterolemic activity of Tienchi ginseng has, however, been disputed.[3]

Tienchi Ginseng continued on page 435

REFERENCES

1 Bensky D, Gamble A: *Chinese herbal medicine materia medica,* Seattle, 1986, Eastland Press.
2 Pharmacopoeia Commission of the People's Republic of China: *Pharmacopoeia of the People's Republic of China,* English ed, Beijing, 1997, Chemical Industry Press.
3 Chang HM, But PP: *Pharmacology and applications of Chinese materia medica,* Singapore, 1987, World Scientific.
4 Tang W, Eisenbrand G: *Chinese drugs of plant origin,* Berlin, 1992, Springer-Verlag.
5 Lei XL, Chiou GC: *Am J Chin Med* 14(3-4):145-152, 1986.
6 Li X, Chen JX, Sun JJ: *Chung Kuo Yao Li Hsueh Pao* 11(1):26-29, 1990.
7 Li LX et al: *Chung Kuo Yao Li Hsueh Pao* 9(1):52-55, 1988.
8 Xiong ZG, Chen JX, Sun JJ: *Chung Kuo Yao Li Hsueh Pao* 10(2):122-125, 1989.
9 Kwan CY: *Clin Exp Pharmacol Physiol* 22 (suppl 1):S297-299, 1995.
10 Gao BY et al: *Yao Hsueh Hsueh Pao* 27(9):641-644, 1992.
11 Wu JX, Sun JJ: *Chung Kuo Yao Li Hsueh Pao* 13(6):520-523, 1992.
12 Shi L et al: *Chung Kuo Yao Li Hsueh Pao* 11(1):29-32, 1990.
13 Ma LY, Xiao PG: *Phytother Res* 12:138-140, 1998.
14 Wang YL, Chen D, Wu JL: *Chung Kuo Chung Hsi I Chieh Ho Tsa Chih* 14(1):5, 35-36, 1994.
15 Wei F et al: *J Altern Complement Med* 5(5):429-436, 1999.
16 Xu Q, Zhao Y, Cheng GR: *Chung Kuo Chung Yao Tsa Chih* 18(6):367-368, 383, 1993.
17 Gong YH et al: *Yao Hsueh Hsueh Pao* 26(2):81-85, 1991.
18 Hsieh MT et al: *Phytother Res* 14(5):375-377, 2000.
19 Cicero AF, Bandieri E, Arletti R: *J Ethnopharmacol* 73(3):387-391, 2000.

TURMERIC

Botanical Name: *Curcuma longa*
Family: Zingiberaceae
Plant Part Used: Rhizome

PRESCRIBING INFORMATION

Actions

Antiinflammatory, antiplatelet, antioxidant, hypolipidemic, choleretic, antimicrobial, carminative, depurative

Potential Indications

Based on appropriate evaluation of the patient, practitioners should consider prescribing turmeric in formulations in the context of:
- Dyspepsia (2,4,5)
- Stomach ulcer (3,6)
- Adjuvant therapy for precancerous conditions (3)
- Osteoarthritis, in combination with ashwaganda, *Boswellia serrata,* and zinc (3)
- Rheumatoid arthritis (5)
- Antioxidant activity (4)
- Liver dysfunction (5,7)
- Hypercholesterolemia (7)

Contraindications

According to the Commission E, turmeric is contraindicated when obstruction of the biliary tract is present and should be used only after seeking professional advice if gallstones are present.

Warnings and Precautions

High doses should not be given to patients taking antiplatelet or anticoagulant drugs. Care should be exercised with women wishing to conceive and patients complaining of hair loss. Patients applying topical doses should not be exposed to excessive sunlight.

Interactions

High doses of turmeric (greater than 15 g/day) should not be given to patients taking antiplatelet or anticoagulant drugs.

Use in Pregnancy and Lactation

No adverse effects expected.

Side Effects

None expected if taken within the recommended dose range.

Dosage

Dose per day*	Dose per week*
5-14 ml of 1:1 liquid extract	35-100 ml of 1:1 liquid extract

SUPPORTING INFORMATION

Traditional Prescribing

Traditional Ayurvedic uses include:
- Liver disorders, poor digestion,[1,2] diarrhea, vomiting of pregnancy[1]
- Fevers, the common cold, catarrhal cough[1,2]
- Leprosy, snakebite[1]

Turmeric *continued on page 437*

*This dose range is adapted from doses used in clinical trials.

- Externally for conjunctivitis, ophthalmia,[1] skin infections, ulcers, wounds, arthritis, and eczema[1,2]

Uses from TCM include:
- Amenorrhea, dysmenorrhea[3,4]
- Chest and abdominal pain and abdominal distention[3,4]
- Jaundice with dark urine[3]
- Impairment of consciousness in febrile diseases, epilepsy, mania[3]
- Traumatic injury, swelling, and pain[3]

Traditional Thai medicinal uses include:
- Intestinal ulcer, peptic ulcer[5]
- Promoting health, preventing gonorrhea, the common cold, dizziness[5]
- Anal hemorrhage, hemorrhage in women, uremia[5]
- Topically for skin diseases, ringworm, wounds, insect bites, to strengthen teeth[5]

Traditional Western herbal medicine uses include:
- Jaundice[6]
- As a mild, aromatic stimulant (Eclectic physicians)[7]

Pharmacologic Research

Key constituents of turmeric rhizome include an essential oil (containing sesquiterpene ketones) and yellow pigments known as diarylheptanoids, including curcumin.
- Oral doses of curcumin have displayed significant antiinflammatory activity in both acute and chronic experimental models. Curcumin is a dual inhibitor of arachidonic acid metabolism, inhibiting both the enzymes 5-lipoxygenase and cyclooxygenase in vitro.
- The antiplatelet activity of curcumin is supported by a number of in vitro and ex vivo studies, suggesting that curcumin inhibits thromboxane production from platelets. A recent study found that curcumin inhibited platelet aggregation induced by arachidonate, epinephrine (adrenaline), and collagen in vitro.
- The antioxidant activity of curcumin and extracts of turmeric are consistently supported by in vitro and oral in vivo studies.
- Dietary levels of curcumin as low as 0.1% significantly reduced the rises in serum and liver cholesterol in an experimental model of hypercholesterolemia. A subsequent study verified that turmeric increased the ratio of HDL cholesterol to total cholesterol.
- Early studies indicated that injection of turmeric essential oil or curcumin increased bile synthesis. Oral administration of curcumin caused regression of gallstones in an experimental model with preestablished cholesterol gallstones.
- Oral doses of turmeric extract produced significant protection against gastric ulceration in a number of experimental models. Turmeric extract increased gastric wall mucus production and enhanced its cytoprotective quality.

Turmeric continued on page 438

- Hepatoprotective activity for turmeric extract against carbon tetrachloride–induced hepatotoxicity has been demonstrated *in vivo*.
- Numerous *in vitro* and *in vivo* (oral route) studies show that turmeric and curcumin possess antimutagenic and antipromotion activity, which is probably related to the antioxidant and antiinflammatory activities of curcumin. Oral administration of curcumin significantly inhibited the tumor incidence and tumor burden of both invasive and noninvasive tumors in various experimental models of cancer.
- Turmeric, its essential oil, and curcumin inhibited the growth of gram-positive bacteria *in vitro*. The essential oil of turmeric displayed significant antifungal activity *in vitro*. Low concentrations of curcumin have shown significant phototoxicity toward Salmonella *in vitro*.

Clinical Studies

- In a randomized, double-blind, placebo-controlled trial, treatment with turmeric (2 g/day for 7 days) was significantly better than placebo for patients with dyspepsia.
- In a small, uncontrolled trial, turmeric (2 g/day) produced favorable results for treating stomach ulcer after 4 to 12 weeks.[8] In a controlled trial, 88% of participants treated with turmeric (4 g/day) showed improvement in abdominal pain caused by gastric ulceration compared with 40% in the group receiving magnesium silicate and aluminum hydroxide.[9]
- In a randomized, double-blind, placebo-controlled, crossover trial, patients with osteoarthritis received a preparation containing turmeric, ashwaganda, *Boswellia serrata* resin, and a zinc complex or placebo for 3 months. Treatment with the herbal-mineral preparation produced a significant drop in severity of pain and disability.
- In uncontrolled trials, turmeric extract (equivalent to approximately 50 g/day dried root for 12 weeks) dramatically decreased blood lipid peroxide levels in healthy males and lowered plasma cholesterol and triglycerides. The therapeutic effect was at least equivalent to clofibrate.
- Turmeric given to chronic smokers (1.5 g/day for 30 days) significantly reduced urinary mutagens in a placebo-controlled study.
- Patients with submucosal fibrosis (a precancerous condition) treated orally with turmeric preparations for 3 months experienced a normalization in the number of micronucleated cells, both in exfoliated oral mucosal cells and in circulating lymphocytes. Results were compared with healthy volunteers who served as a control group. The dose for the treatment group was turmeric extract 3 g per day given alone or mixed with either turmeric essential oil 600 mg per day or turmeric oleoresin 600 mg per day.
- In Germany, the Commission E supports using turmeric to treat dyspeptic conditions.[10]

REFERENCES

Except when specifically referenced, the following book was referred to in the compilation of the pharmacologic and clinical information: Mills S, Bone K: *Principles and Practice of Phytotherapy: Modern Herbal Medicine,* Edinburgh, 2000, Churchill Livingstone.

Turmeric *continued on page 439*

1 Chopra RN et al: *Chopra's indigenous drugs of India,* ed 2, Calcutta, 1958, reprinted 1982, Academic Publishers.
2 Kapoor LD: *CRC handbook of Ayurvedic medicinal plants,* Boca Raton, Fla, 1990, CRC Press.
3 Pharmacopoeia Commission of the People's Republic of China: *Pharmacopoeia of the People's Republic of China,* English ed, Beijing, 1997, Chemical Industry Press.
4 Bensky D, Gamble A: *Chinese herbal medicine materia medica,* Seattle, 1986, Eastland Press.
5 Farnsworth NR, Bunyapraphatsara N, eds: *Thai medicinal plants,* Bangkok, 1992, Medicinal Plant Information Center.
6 Grieve M: *A modern herbal,* New York, 1971, Dover Publications.
7 Felter HW, Lloyd JU: *King's American dispensatory,* ed 18, rev 3, Portland, 1905, reprinted 1983, Eclectic Medical Publications.
8 Prucksunand C et al: *Thai J Pharmacol* 8(3):139-151, 1986.
9 Intanonta A et al: Report submitted to Primary Health Care Office, Ministry of Public Health, Thailand, 1986.
10 Blumenthal M et al, eds: *The complete German Commission E monographs: therapeutic guide to herbal medicines,* Austin, 1998, American Botanical Council.

TYLOPHORA

Other Common Names: Indian ipecac, Indian lobelia
Botanical Names: *Tylophora indica, Tylophora asthmatica*#
Family: Asclepiadaceae
Plant Part Used: Leaf

PRESCRIBING INFORMATION

Actions

Antiasthmatic, antiinflammatory, immune depressant, antiallergic, emetic

Potential Indications

Based on appropriate evaluation of the patient, practitioners should consider prescribing Tylophora in formulations in the context of:
- Asthma *(2,6)*
- Allergic rhinitis *(4)*
- Autoimmune and chronic immune-mediated inflammatory diseases *(7)*
- Providing protection against inhaled allergen challenge *(3)*

Contraindications

Because of the strong pharmacologic activity of Tylophora, it is contraindicated in pregnancy and lactation and should not be used long term.

Warnings and Precautions

Tylophora is best taken short term and intermittently, rather than continuously. The recommended dosage must not be exceeded.

Interactions

None known.

Use in Pregnancy and Lactation

Contraindicated in pregnancy and lactation.

Side Effects

Nausea and vomiting may occur, even at a low dose, especially in sensitive individuals. Sore mouth and loss of taste for salt have also been reported in a clinical trial after patients swallowed one chopped fresh leaf per day for 6 days.[1] The frequency and severity of side effects were less in a subsequent trial conducted by the same research group, for which an undefined dried ethanolic extract of Tylophora leaf (40 mg/day for 6 days) was used instead of the fresh leaf.[2]

Dosage

Tylophora should be used only for short-term intermittent treatment, up to 4 weeks at a time. The best way to prescribe Tylophora is to recommend between 20 to 50 drops per day of a 1:5 tincture (the highest dose in that range that does not cause nausea for that particular batch in that particular patient) for the first 10 to 14 days of each calendar month.*

Tylophora *continued on page 441*

#Alternative name.
*This dose range is extrapolated from clinical trial data.

SUPPORTING INFORMATION

Traditional Prescribing

Traditional Ayurvedic uses include:
- Bronchial asthma,[3] chronic bronchitis, catarrh, dysentery[4]
- As an emetic, diaphoretic and expectorant; as a substitute for Ipecacuanha[4]
- Snakebite (in large doses)[5]

Pharmacologic Research

The leaves of Tylophora contain several alkaloids, including tylophorine and tylophorinine.[6]
- Tylophora has short-lived bronchodilator activity *in vitro,* but this is probably not the basis of its effects in asthma.[7]
- Studies show that the antiasthma effects are more likely to be mediated through depression of some aspects of cell-mediated immunity. Tylophora extract reduced total leukocyte count *in vivo* (by injection); and 21 days after administration, eosinophils and lymphocytes were still reduced.[7] Oral administration of Tylophora demonstrated a pronounced inhibition of the cell-mediated immune response in experimental models, as evidenced by the increased survival time of skin grafts.[8]
- Tylophorine enhanced adenylate cyclase activity in intact leukocytes taken from children with asthma but had no effect in cells from children without asthma. The authors suggested that tylophorine acts by stimulating beta-adrenergic receptor activity in patients with bronchial asthma, possibly in a manner similar to that of hydrocortisone.[9]
- Pretreatment with Tylophora significantly increased lung flow rates in antigen-sensitized animals, demonstrating an antiallergic activity. Tylophora was administered as an aqueous extract by injection before sensitization and challenge or directly by perfusion before challenge but after sensitization. Tylophora demonstrated similar antiallergic activity to the preventative drug disodium cromoglycate. Tylophora also increased flow rates in normal animals, which possibly indicates a bronchodilating activity. In sensitized animals, the effect of Tylophora was greater, possibly because of an immunosuppressive action.[10]
- Pretreatment with tylophorine injection (25 mg/kg) inhibited systemic anaphylaxis induced by sensitization with egg albumen. The protection afforded by tylophorine exceeded that of dexamethasone. When sheep red blood cells were added to a sensitized lymphoid cell suspension from animals treated with tylophorine, immunocyto-adherence was only 15% (compared with 40% in the absence of tylophorine). Tylophorine did not prevent the mast cell–degranulating effect of agents that act on the surface membrane but did inhibit mast cell rupture induced by diazoxide (which causes cell degranulation by reducing intracellular levels of cAMP).[11]
- Injection of tylophorine exhibited pronounced antiinflammatory activity compared with placebo, dexamethasone, and phenylbutazone (antiinflammatory drugs) in experimental models of acute and chronic inflammation.[12]

Tylophora continued on page 442

- Primary and secondary responses of adjuvant-induced arthritis were significantly inhibited by injecting tylophorine.[11]
- Extracts of Tylophora have been shown to stimulate the adrenal cortex, increase plasma steroid levels, and antagonize steroid-induced suppression of adrenal activity via intraperitoneal injection.[13] This activity might be the basis of its antiinflammatory effects.
- Tylophorine caused central nervous system depression (100 to 300 mg/kg), potentiated phenobarbital-induced sleeping time (100 mg/kg), and potentiated the analgesic effect of subanalgesic doses of morphine (50 to 100 mg/kg). The tylophorine was administered by injection.[12]

Clinical Studies

- In an open, preliminary trial conducted in the 1960s, chewing one leaf of Tylophora daily for 6 days produced relief of symptoms in many of the patients with asthma and allergic rhinitis.[14] In a randomized, double-blind trial, Tylophora (one fresh leaf/day) or placebo was administered for 6 days to patients with asthma. At the end of the first week, 62% of patients in the active group had moderate to complete relief of symptoms compared with 28% in the placebo group. By the end of the 12-week follow-up period, 16% of the treated group had still maintained complete to moderate relief compared with 0% in the placebo group. After the 12-week period, the crossover (and double-blind) phase of the trial was initiated. Patients on placebo were given Tylophora and vice-versa. One week after crossover, 50% of the Tylophora group had complete to moderate relief compared with 11% of the placebo group.[1]
- In another randomized, double-blind, placebo-controlled trial involving patients with asthma, at the end of the 6-day treatment period, 56.3% of the Tylophora group had complete to moderate symptom improvement compared with 31.6% in the placebo group. At the end of the 12-week follow-up period, 14.8% of the Tylophora group and 7.2% of the placebo group still had complete to moderate relief. The efficacy of Tylophora was verified in a subgroup of patients who were crossed over. Patients in the treatment group received 40 mg per day of an undefined dried ethanolic extract of Tylophora leaf.[2]
- Tylophora (one dry leaf/day for 6 days) provided protection from inhaled allergen challenge (administered 55 hours after the treatment period) in patients with asthma who were symptom free and who had demonstrated positive bronchial sensitivity. No protection was available in the control group for which no treatment was received. A subgroup of these patients was challenged further, and the duration of the protection was found to last for 7 to 9 days after the Tylophora treatment had ceased.[15]
- Tylophora (350 mg dried leaf/day for 7 days) demonstrated greater symptomatic improvement in patients with bronchial asthma than placebo and no significant difference when compared with a standard antiasthmatic drug (containing mainly theophylline), in randomized, double-blind, crossover trials. Tylophora had a more gradual and long-lasting effect than the drug treatment.[16]

Tylophora continued on page 443

- In a placebo-controlled trial that investigated the treatment of asthma, results were not significant, but they did show a tendency to improvement for Tylophora treatment. However, the "placebo" consisted partly of Ipecacuanha, an herb that is not devoid of bronchial activity.[17]
- In an open, controlled study, Tylophora leaf (200 mg/day for 6 days) depressed absolute eosinophil count and increased urine levels of 17-ketosteroid in both healthy volunteers and patients with asthma. The authors postulated that increased release of steroid hormones from the adrenal gland may reduce the development of sensitivity to foreign antigen, thus giving relief to patients with asthma. Lung function tests were significantly improved compared with baseline in both healthy volunteers and patients with asthma when tested on the seventh day after administering Tylophora. The improvement in lung function was superior to that produced by isoprenaline (a bronchodilator).[18]

REFERENCES

1 Shivpuri DN, Menon MPS, Prakash D: *J Allergy* 43(3):145-150, 1969.
2 Shivpuri DN, Singhal SC, Parkash D: *Ann Allergy* 30(7):407-412, 1972.
3 Nadkarni AK: *Dr. K.M. Nadkarni's Indian materia medica,* ed 3, Bombay, 1976, Popular Prakashan.
4 Chopra RN et al: *Chopra's indigenous drugs of India,* ed 2, Calcutta, 1958, reprinted 1982, Academic Publishers.
5 Nyman P et al: *Glimpses of Indian ethnopharmacology,* Kerala, India, 1995, Tropical Botanic Garden and Research Institute.
6 Karnick CR: *Planta Med* 27(4):333-336, 1975.
7 Haranath PSRK, Shyamalakumari S: *Indian J Med Res* 63(5):661-669, 1975.
8 Atal CK et al: *J Ethnopharmacol* 18(2):133-141, 1986.
9 Raina V, Raina S: *Biochem Biophys Res Comm* 94(4):1074-1077, 1980.
10 Nayampalli SS, Sheth UK: *Indian J Pharmacol* 11(3):229-232, 1979.
11 Gopalakrishnan C et al: *Indian J Med Res* 71:940-948, 1980.
12 Gopalakrishnan C et al: *Indian J Med Res* 69:513-520, 1979.
13 Udupa AL, Udupa SL, Guruswamy MN: *Planta Med* 57(5):409-413, 1991.
14 Shivpuri DN, Menon MPS, Parkash D: *J Assoc Physicians India* 16(1):9-15, 1968.
15 Shivpuri DN, Agarwal MK: *Ann Allergy* 31(2):87-94, 1973.
16 Thiruvengadam KV et al: *J Indian Med Assoc* 71(7):172-176, 1978.
17 Gupta S et al: *Indian J Med Res* 69:981-989, 1979.
18 Gore KV, Rao AK, Guruswamy MN: *Indian J Med Res* 71:144-148, 1980.

UVA URSI

Other Common Name: Bearberry
Botanical Name: *Arctostaphylos uva-ursi*
Family: Ericaceae
Plant Part Used: Leaf

PRESCRIBING INFORMATION

Actions

Urinary antiseptic, astringent, antiinflammatory

Potential Indications

Based on appropriate evaluation of the patient, practitioners should consider prescribing uva ursi in formulations in the context of:
• Inflammatory or infectious conditions of the lower urinary tract, particularly cystitis *(4,5)*
• Cystitis, in combination with dandelion leaf and root *(2)*
• Urinary stones *(5)*

Contraindications

According to the *British Herbal Compendium*, uva ursi is contraindicated in kidney disorders, but data to support this is minimal.

According to the Commission E, uva ursi is contraindicated in pregnancy and lactation and for children under 12 years of age.

Warnings and Precautions

Uva ursi is not suitable for prolonged use.

Interactions

Uva ursi should not be given with treatments that will lead to the production of acidic urine, because this will reduce the antibacterial effect. Uva ursi will work best when urine has an alkaline pH.

The high tannin levels will interfere with the absorption of various nutrients.

Use in Pregnancy and Lactation

Contraindicated in pregnancy and lactation.

Side Effects

Because of the high tannin content, internal use of uva ursi may cause cramping, nausea, vomiting, and constipation.

Dosage

Dose per day*	Dose per week*
4.5-8.5 ml of 1:2 liquid extract	30-60 ml of 1:2 liquid extract

SUPPORTING INFORMATION

Traditional Prescribing

Traditional Western herbal medicine uses include:
• Inflammatory diseases of the bladder and kidneys, including cystitis, urethritis, and pyelitis; dysuria, chronic irritation of the bladder, enuresis, excessive mucus and bloody discharges in the urine, strangury, urinary stones, chronic gonorrhea[1,2]

Uva Ursi *continued on page 445*

*This dose range is extrapolated from the *British Herbal Compendium* 1992 and the author's education and experience.

- Specifically indicated for lack of tone, feeble circulation, and lack of innervation in the urinary tract[2]
- Chronic diarrhea, dysentery, menorrhagia, leukorrhea, diabetes[2]

Pharmacologic Research

Uva ursi leaves contain hydroquinone glycosides (including arbutin) and tannins.

- Uva ursi extracts have shown antimicrobial activity *in vitro* against *Escherichia coli, Proteus vulgaris, Enterobacter aerogenes, Streptococcus fecalis, Staphylococcus aureus, Salmonella typhi,* and *Candida albicans.*
- Although the bactericidal activity of uva ursi decoction was relatively low, it markedly increased the hydrophobicity of the microbial species tested, which included *E. coli.* Uva ursi may therefore influence the microbe's surface characteristics.[3]
- Uva ursi extract is most effective against bacterial infection in an alkaline environment. Alkaline urine indicates the presence of certain microorganisms that are capable of urea splitting, such as *Proteus* spp., *Klebsiella* spp., some *Citrobacter* spp., some *Hemophilus* spp., *Bilophila wadsworthia,* the yeast *Cryptococcus neoformans,* and several other bacteria and fungi. Based on the research highlighted here, infection with these organisms should be susceptible to treatment with uva ursi. Alkalinization of the urine with buffering agents containing sodium bicarbonate, sodium citrate, citric acid, and tartaric acid in conjunction with uva ursi intake is desirable in these circumstances.
- Arbutin, in conjunction with antiinflammatory drugs, showed an inhibitory effect on swelling in a delayed-type hypersensitivity model. The effect was superior to the drugs used alone. Arbutin may therefore have a synergistic antiinflammatory activity on type IV reaction–induced inflammation.

Clinical Studies

- In a double-blind, placebo-controlled, randomized, clinical trial, 57 women with recurrent cystitis received either herbal treatment (standardized uva ursi extract and dandelion leaf and root extract) or placebo. Treatment for 1 month significantly reduced the recurrence of cystitis during the 1-year follow-up period, with no incidence of cystitis in the herbal group and a 23% occurrence in the placebo group. No side effects were reported. The dose of the individual herbs was not specified.
- In Germany, the Commission E supports using uva ursi to treat inflammatory disorders of the efferent (descending) urinary tract.[4]
- ESCOP recommends uva ursi for treating uncomplicated infections of the lower urinary tract, such as cystitis, when antibiotic treatment is not considered essential.[5]

REFERENCES

Except when specifically referenced, the following book was referred to in the compilation of the pharmacologic and clinical information: Mills S, Bone K: *Principles and Practice of Phytotherapy: Modern Herbal Medicine,* Edinburgh, 2000, Churchill Livingstone.

Uva Ursi *continued on page 446*

1 Felter HW, Lloyd JU: *King's American dispensatory,* ed 18, rev 3, Portland, 1905, reprinted 1983, Eclectic Medical Publications.

2 British Herbal Medicine Association's Scientific Committee: *British herbal pharmacopoeia,* Bournemouth, 1983, BHMA.

3 Turi M et al: *Acta Pathol Microbiol Immunol Scand* 105(12):956-962, 1997.

4 Blumenthal M et al, eds: *The complete German Commission E monographs: therapeutic guide to herbal medicines,* Austin, 1998, American Botanical Council.

5 Scientific Committee of the European Scientific Cooperative on Phytotherapy [ESCOP]: *ESCOP monographs: Uvae ursi folium.* European Scientific Cooperative on Phytotherapy, ESCOP Secretariat, Argyle House, Gandy Street, Exeter, Devon, EX4 3LS, United Kingdom, June 1997.

VALERIAN

Common Name:	Valerian
Botanical Name:	*Valeriana officinalis*
Family:	Valerianaceae
Plant Part Used:	Root and rhizome

Common Name:	Mexican valerian
Botanical Name:	*Valeriana edulis*
Family:	Valerianaceae
Plant Part Used:	Root and rhizome

PRESCRIBING INFORMATION

Actions

Valerian and Mexican valerian: anxiolytic, mild sedative, hypnotic, spasmolytic

Potential Indications

Based on appropriate evaluation of the patient, practitioners should consider prescribing valerian in formulations in the context of:
- Insomnia *(2,4,5)*
- Insomnia, in combination with lemon balm or hops *(2)*
- Depression, in combination with St. John's wort *(2)*
- Stress *(3)*
- Anxiety, in combination with St. John's wort *(3)*
- Restlessness, nervous tension *(4,5)*
- Depression, anxiety, migraine, nervous headache, cramps, intestinal colic, dysmenorrhea, rheumatic pains, chorea, mild spasmodic movements, epilepsy *(5)*

Based on appropriate evaluation of the patient, practitioners should consider prescribing Mexican valerian in formulations in the context of:
- Anxiety *(4a,6)*
- Insomnia *(2,6)*

Contraindications

None known.

Warnings and Precautions

None required.

Interactions

Although no reports to date have been presented, valerian may increase the effects of central nervous system depressants or alcohol when taken together, according to the *U.S. Pharmacopeia.* Despite this warning, early animal studies indicated that valepotriates do not add to the depressant effect of alcohol. A human study confirmed that simultaneous intake of alcohol with a valerian and St. John's wort combination did not increase the effects of the herbal product, and a mixture of valepotriates (valtrate, acevaltrate, and didrovaltrate [200 to 400 mg]) combined with ethanol did not cause a reduction of efficiency.

Valerian root extract may attenuate some symptoms of benzodiazepine withdrawal, based on animal models.[1]

Valerian *continued on page 448*

Use in Pregnancy and Lactation

No adverse effects expected.

Side Effects

In some individuals, valerian can aggravate a sensation of tiredness or drowsiness, particularly in higher doses, but this is usually more a case of an increased awareness of the body's needs rather than a negative depressant effect. A few individuals find valerian stimulating and should avoid its use. Headaches have been reported after overdose with valerian.

A male patient taking multiple medications experienced serious cardiac complications and delirium following a surgical procedure.[2] The man had self-medicated for "many years" with valerian root extract (530 mg to 2 g/dose, five times daily). However, given the person's multiple medications, valerian cannot be causally linked to his symptoms. These other factors may have increased the risk of a withdrawal reaction.

Dosage

Valerian:

Dose per day*	Dose per week*
2-6 ml of 1:2 liquid extract	15-40 ml of 1:2 liquid extract

Mexican valerian:

Dose per day**	Dose per week**
1.5-4.5 ml of 1:2 liquid extract	10-30 ml of 1:2 liquid extract

SUPPORTING INFORMATION

Traditional Prescribing

Traditional Western herbal medicine uses of valerian include:
- Insomnia, hysterical states, excitability, hypochondria, nervousness; migraine, nervous headache, depressive states, reduced cerebral circulation[3,4]
- Cramps, intestinal colic, dysmenorrhea, rheumatic pains, chorea, mild spasmodic movements, epilepsy[3,4]

Mexican valerian is used traditionally in Mexico for its tranquilizing and sedative effects.[5] Native Americans used Mexican valerian internally for hemorrhages and tapeworm infestation and topically for rheumatism, swollen and bruised parts, wounds, and to draw out boils.[6-8]

Pharmacologic Research

Valerian root contains iridoids (known as valepotriates), essential oil, and cyclopentane sesquiterpenes (e.g., valerenic acid). Mexican valerian root has a higher percentage of valepotriates (and a larger valtrate-isovaltrate content) than valerian; it does not contain valerenic acid.

Valerian *continued on page 449*

*This dosage is extrapolated from the British Pharmaceutical Codex 1949, the British Herbal Pharmacopoeia 1983, the British Herbal Compendium 1992, and the author's education and experience.
**This dose range is extrapolated from the pharmacologic and clinical information available on valepotriates.

Valepotriates are unstable compounds; they decompose under acid or alkaline conditions or in alcoholic solutions (such as liquid extracts). However, the initial decomposition products of valepotriates are active as sedatives and are probably among the active products in the human system after ingestion of valerian.

- Aqueous extract of valerian induced the release of GABA from brain tissue. Many *in vitro* studies have investigated the interaction of valerian or its components with receptors mediating sedation, such as GABA, adenosine, and 5-hydroxytryptamine (5-HT$_{1A}$, serotonin) receptors.
- The sedative effect of the valepotriates has been demonstrated in several experimental models. Oral valepotriates improved coordination, and (by unknown dose route) valepotriates decreased anxiety and aggression. In an experimental model, intraperitoneal administration of valerenic acid demonstrated sedative activity resembling central nervous system depression, rather than muscle relaxation or a neuroleptic effect.
- Antispasmodic effects on smooth muscle tissue (ileum) were observed for valepotriates and an essential oil component of valerian *in vitro* and *in vivo* (by injection).[9]

Clinical Studies

- The sedative effects of valepotriates on humans was confirmed a number of times in German research conducted in the late 1960s.
- A randomized, placebo-controlled, double-blind trial demonstrated single or repeated administrations of valerian did not have a negative impact on reaction time, alertness, and concentration the morning after intake. The dose used was equivalent to 3 g per day of root and was prescribed for 2 weeks.[10]
- In a randomized, double-blind trial, valerian tablets demonstrated similar efficacy to oxazepam (10 mg/day) for treating insomnia. The daily dose of valerian corresponded to approximately 3 g of original root.[11]
- A randomized, double-blind, placebo-controlled, crossover study using valerian extract (equivalent to 3 g/day of root for 14 days) confirmed positive effects on sleep structure and sleep perception in patients with mild psychophysiologic insomnia.[12] The effect of Mexican valerian (MV) and valerian (V) extracts were investigated using polysomnographic recordings in a double-blind, crossover trial involving 20 patients with insomnia. Patients received a single dose of extract in tablet form: the MV extract dose contained 2.4 mg valepotriates; the V extract dose contained 0.3 mg valerenic acid. The following results were obtained:[13]
  - Decrease in waking episodes (MV only)
  - Increase in REM sleep (both extracts, but V better)
  - Increase in sleep efficiency index (compared with baseline; V better)
  - Decreased time for stages 1 and 2 in non-REM sleep and an increase in delta sleep (MV better)
  - Decrease in morning sleepiness (V better)
  - No residual hypnotic effect (MV better)

Valerian *continued on page 450*

- In a large, uncontrolled, multicenter trial involving over 11,000 patients, treatment with aqueous valerian extract (equivalent to 0.25 g/day dried root) was rated as successful in treating difficulty in falling asleep (72%), discontinuous sleep (76%), and restlessness and tension (72%).
- In a double-blind, placebo-controlled, crossover trial, a combination of valerian (equivalent to 400 mg of root) with hops and lemon balm demonstrated a significant subjective effect on poor sleep compared with placebo (which also contained hops and lemon balm) over 2 consecutive nights. Good sleep was reported in 44% and 89% of patients reported improved sleep.
- A Swiss study found that a freeze-dried aqueous valerian extract improved sleep latency and sleep quality without increasing sleepiness the next morning, compared with placebo. The group of participants who rated themselves as good sleepers were largely unaffected by valerian, but the poor or irregular sleepers reported a significant improvement. Valerian did not increase the frequency of "more sleepy than usual (the next morning)" responses. A dosage of approximately 1.2 g of valerian root per day was given over 3 nonconsecutive nights.
- A randomized, double-blind study was conducted on patients with diagnosed insomnia. Practitioners rated sleep improvement higher following valerian therapy than they did after placebo. Patients preferred valerian, with significant improvements being noted in sleep quality and the feeling of being rested after sleep. The dose was equivalent to approximately 2.4 g of dried root per day and administered for 4 weeks.
- Two randomized, double-blind, placebo-controlled trials compared a number of herbal extracts, including dried ethanolic extract of valerian (equivalent to 6 g of root), in sleep-disturbed volunteers. In contrast to diazepam (10 mg), valerian displayed an increase in delta and theta frequencies and a decrease in beta frequency on electro-encephalographic recordings. In contrast to placebo, most of the herbal extracts (as with diazepam) induced an increase in subjectively evaluated sleepiness.
- A double-blind, placebo-controlled crossover trial on healthy volunteers showed valerian tended to normalize the sleep profile, lower periods of wakefulness, and increase the efficiency of the sleep period. Valerian was administered as a single dose (equivalent to 6 g) and as a repeated dose (equivalent to 3 g/day for 14 days).
- A combination of valerian and hops extracts reduced the noise-induced disturbance of sleep stage patterns (slow-wave sleep and REM) in sleep-disturbed volunteers. The combination (equivalent to 1 g/day of valerian root and 2 g/day of hops) was given to volunteers during the second or third of 3 consecutive nights disturbed by heavy traffic noise. A randomized, double-blind, controlled trial demonstrated equivalent efficacy and tolerability for a hops-valerian preparation when compared against a benzodiazepine drug in patients with temporary sleep-onset and sleep-interruption disorders.[14]

Valerian continued on page 451

- A randomized, double-blind, placebo-controlled, multicenter trial investigated the use of a combination of dried aqueous ethanol extracts of valerian and lemon balm in ambulatory patients with light insomnia. Improvements in sleep quality, daily condition, time to fall asleep, total duration of sleep, concentration, and ability to perform occurred with no hangover, withdrawal, or rebound phenomena in the treated group. Doses equivalent to 2.9 g per day of valerian root and 1.7 g per day of lemon balm herb were given for 3 weeks.
- In a randomized, controlled, double-blind study, a combination of valerian and St. John's wort extracts (containing 0.45 to 0.9 mg/day of TH) was shown to have comparable benefits to the antidepressant amitriptyline (75 to 150 mg/day) in treating depression over 6 weeks. Compared with an improvement rate of 77% in the amitriptyline group, benefit was observed for 82% of patients in the herbal group, without the high frequency of side effects of amitriptyline such as dry mouth and lethargy.
- In a pilot study, patients with stress-induced insomnia were treated with kava, then valerian, then a combination of kava and valerian, with washout periods in between each treatment. Total stress severity was significantly relieved by kava and valerian single treatments. Stress was measured in the areas of social, personal, and life events. The combination of kava and valerian significantly relieved insomnia.[15]
- In a double-blind, multicenter trial, a valerian-St. John's wort combination demonstrated a comparable reduction in symptoms of fear and depressive mood compared with amitriptyline (75 to 125 mg). The daily dose was 3 to 6 capsules. Each capsule contained valerian extract corresponding to approximately 0.3 g of dried root and St. John's wort extract containing 0.15 mg of TH. In another double-blind trial, the same combination demonstrated significant improvement compared with the antidepressant desipramine.
- A double-blind study found that 2 weeks of daily treatment with a valerian-St. John's wort combination (containing approximately 0.2 g of valerian root and 0.3 to 0.6 mg/day of TH) was more effective than diazepam (2 mg) in patients with moderate anxiety. Fewer side effects were observed in the herbal treatment group (4%) compared with diazepam treatment (14%).
- A double-blind, placebo-controlled technique examining activation, performance, and mood in healthy volunteers showed that valerian extract influenced subjective feelings of somatic arousal, despite high physiologic activation. No sedative effects were demonstrated, and suggestions were that valerian has thymoleptic activity.
- A double-blind, placebo-controlled, three-way crossover trial investigated the effect of a valerian and St. John's wort extract combination on safety-related performance in 12 volunteers. The herbal product was shown to be comparable to placebo with respect to safety in terms of performance and well being. The effects when taken with alcohol were not greater than those of alcohol alone.

Valerian *continued on page 452*

- In Germany, the Commission E supports using valerian to treat restlessness and sleeping disorders based on nervous conditions.[16]
- ESCOP recommends valerian root for treating tenseness, restlessness, and irritability with difficulty in falling asleep.[17]
- Valerian has been reinstated to the USP and is official in the USP24-NF19.

REFERENCES

Except when specifically referenced, the following book was referred to in the compilation of the pharmacologic and clinical information: Mills S, Bone K: *Principles and Practice of Phytotherapy: Modern Herbal Medicine,* Edinburgh, 2000, Churchill Livingstone.

1 Andreatini R, Loire JR: *Eur J Pharmacol* 260:233-235, 1994.
2 Garges HP, Varia I, Doraiswamy PM: *JAMA* 280(18):1566-1567, 1998.
3 British Herbal Medicine Association's Scientific Committee: *British herbal pharmacopoeia,* Bournemouth, 1983, BHMA.
4 Felter HW, Lloyd JU: *King's American dispensatory,* ed 18, rev 3, Portland, 1905, reprinted 1983, Eclectic Medical Publications.
5 *Valeriana edulis,* Secretaria de Medio Ambiente, Recursos Naturales y Pesca (SEMARNAP, a Mexican government environmental department). Information available via URL: http:www.semarnap.gob.mx/
6 Chamberlin RV: *Mem Am Anthropol Assoc* 2(5):331-405, 1911.
7 Smith HH: *Bull Public Mus City Milw* 4:1-174, 1923.
8 Smith HH: *Bull Public Mus City Milw* 4:175-326, 1928.
9 Hazelhoff B, Malingre TM, Meijer DK: *Arch Int Pharmacodyn Ther* 257(2):274-287, 1982.
10 Kuhlmann J et al: *Pharmacopsychiatry* 32(6):235-241, 1999.
11 Dorn M: *Forsch Komplementarmed Klass Naturheilkd* 7(2):79-84, 2000.
12 Donath F et al: *Pharmacopsychiatry* 33(2):47-53, 2000.
13 Herrera-Arellano A et al: *Planta Med* 67(8):695-699, 2001.
14 Schmitz M, Jackel M: *Wien Med Wochenschr* 148(13):291-298, 1998.
15 Wheatley D: *Phytother Res* 15(6):549-551, 2001.
16 Blumenthal M et al, eds: *The complete German Commission E monographs: therapeutic guide to herbal medicines,* Austin, 1998, American Botanical Council.
17 Scientific Committee of the European Scientific Cooperative on Phytotherapy [ESCOP]: *ESCOP monographs: Valerianae radix.* European Scientific Cooperative on Phytotherapy, ESCOP Secretariat, Argyle House, Gandy Street, Exeter, Devon, EX4 3LS, United Kingdom, July 1997.

VERVAIN

Botanical Name: *Verbena officinalis*
Family: Verbenaceae
Plant Part Used: Aerial parts

PRESCRIBING INFORMATION

Actions

Nervine tonic, mild antidepressant, mild diaphoretic, astringent

Potential Indications

Based on appropriate evaluation of the patient, practitioners should consider prescribing vervain in formulations in the context of:
- Infantile colic, in combination with lemon balm, chamomile, licorice, and fennel *(3)*
- Anorexia, gastrointestinal irritation, jaundice *(5)*
- Depression, nervous breakdown, epilepsy *(5)*
- Feverish conditions including influenza, debility following illnesses or fever *(5)*
- Promotion of lactation *(5)*

Contraindications

Vervain is sometimes recommended as contraindicated during pregnancy, resulting from *in vitro* Chinese research conducted in 1975 and earlier *in vivo* studies using one of its constituents (verbenalin). This contraindication is not carried in most traditional Western herbal medicine texts, TCM texts, or the German Commission E monographs.

Warnings and Precautions

None required.

Interactions

Vervain tea reduced the absorption of iron by 59% from a bread meal (compared with a water control) in adult volunteers. The inhibition was dose-dependent and related to its polyphenol content (phenolic acids, monomeric flavonoids, polymerized polyphenols). Inhibition by black tea was 79% to 94%.[1] This finding indicates a potential interaction for concomitant administration of vervain during iron intake. In anemia and cases for which iron supplementation is required, vervain should not be taken simultaneously with meals or iron supplements.

Use in Pregnancy and Lactation

No adverse effects expected.

Side Effects

None expected if taken within the recommended dose range.

Dosage

Dose per day*	Dose per week*
3-6 ml of 1:2 liquid extract	20-40 ml of 1:2 liquid extract

Vervain *continued on page 454*

*This dose range is extrapolated from the British Herbal Pharmacopoeia 1983 and the author's education and experience.

SUPPORTING INFORMATION

Traditional Prescribing

Traditional Western herbal medicine uses include:
- Depression, nervous breakdown, epilepsy[2]
- As a galactagogue,[2] amenorrhea[3]
- Feverish conditions, debility following acute conditions, especially influenza[2,3]
- Anorexia, intestinal colic,[4] gallbladder pain, jaundice[2]
- As a poultice for headache, earache, rheumatism, hemorrhoids[4]

Uses from TCM include amenorrhea and dysmenorrhea, as well as malaria, abdominal masses, inflammation of the throat, boils, acute infections of the urinary tract, and edema.[5]

The Eclectics regarded *Verbena hastata*, a species of Verbena, as having similar properties to *V. officinalis*. *Verbena hastata* was official in the NF from 1916 to 1926 and was used as a diaphoretic and expectorant. Native Americans used *Verbena hastata* to treat stomachache and as a beverage.[6]

Pharmacologic Research

The aerial parts of vervain contain a number of constituents, including iridoid glycosides (e.g., verbenalin) and caffeic acid derivatives.[7]
- Synergistic effects were observed on contraction of isolated uterus by the combination of vervain with either prostaglandin E_2 or prostaglandin $F_{2\alpha}$. The Chinese researchers suggested using vervain preparations with prostaglandin E_2 for inducing abortion.[8] Verbenalin has been reported to exhibit uterine stimulation-contraction *in vivo* (route unknown).[9,10]
- Vervain extracts were active against the following viruses *in vitro*: influenza A, parainfluenza type 1, and respiratory syncytial virus. Stimulation of phagocytosis and increased secretion of IL-6 was also observed.[11] However, this observed activity might be caused by the polyphenols and may not translate to *in vivo* activity.
- Verbenalin by oral administration demonstrated hepatoprotective activity in acute carbon tetrachloride–induced liver injury.[12]
- Antiinflammatory activity was observed for vervain extract in experimental models after topical and oral administration (in high doses).[13]

Clinical Studies

- A double-blind study on babies with colic investigated the effect of an instant herb tea preparation containing vervain, lemon balm, chamomile, licorice, and fennel. After 7 days, the colic improvement scores were significantly better in the herbal tea group, and more babies in the treatment group had their colic eliminated. The tea preparation was offered with every episode of colic, up to 150 ml per dose, but not more than three times per day. The exact composition of the preparation was not defined.[14]
- In an uncontrolled trial conducted in China, a high dose of vervain decoction (60 g/day) was successful in treating malaria.[15]

Vervain *continued on page 455*

REFERENCES

1 Hurrell RF, Reddy M, Cook JD: *Br J Nutr* 81(4):289-295, 1999.
2 British Herbal Medicine Association's Scientific Committee: *British herbal pharmacopoeia,* Bournemouth, 1983, BHMA.
3 Felter HW, Lloyd JU: *King's American dispensatory,* ed 18, rev 3, Portland, 1905, reprinted 1983, Eclectic Medical Publications.
4 Grieve M: *A modern herbal,* New York, 1971, Dover Publications.
5 Pharmacopoeia Commission of the People's Republic of China: *Pharmacopoeia of the People's Republic of China,* English ed, Beijing, 1997, Chemical Industry Press.
6 Vogel VJ: *American Indian medicine,* Norman, Okla, 1970, University of Oklahoma Press.
7 Bisset NG, ed: *Herbal drugs and phytopharmaceuticals,* Stuttgart, 1994, Medpharm Scientific Publishers.
8 Research Group on Reproductive Physiology, Peking Medical College: *Tung Wu Hseuh Pao* 20(4):340-345, 1974.
9 Zufall CJ, Richtmann WO: *Pharm Arch* 14:65-93, 1943.
10 Farnsworth NR et al: *J.Pharm Sci* 64(4):535-598, 1975.
11 Mende-Weber R et al: 2nd International Congress on Phytomedicine, Munich, September 11-14, 1996, abstract SL-118.
12 Singh B et al: *Fitoterapia* 69(2):135-140, 1998.
13 Calvo MI et al: *Phytomed* 5(6):465-467, 1998.
14 Weizman Z et al: *J Pediatrics* 122(4):650-652, 1993.
15 Huang KC: *The pharmacology of Chinese herbs,* Boca Raton, Fla, 1993, CRC Press.

WHITE HOREHOUND

Botanical Name: *Marrubium vulgare*
Family: Labiatae
Plant Part Used: Aerial parts

PRESCRIBING INFORMATION

Actions

Expectorant, spasmolytic, bitter tonic

Potential Indications

Based on appropriate evaluation of the patient, practitioners should consider prescribing white horehound in formulations in the context of:
- Acute or chronic bronchitis, nonproductive cough, the common cold, asthma *(5)*
- Dyspepsia *(4,5)*
- Loss of appetite, bloating, flatulence *(4)*

Contraindications

None known.

Warnings and Precautions

None required.

Interactions

None known.

Use in Pregnancy and Lactation

No adverse effects expected.

Side Effects

None expected if taken within the recommended dose range.

Dosage

Dose per day*	Dose per week*
2-6 ml of 1:2 liquid extract	15-40 ml of 1:2 liquid extract

SUPPORTING INFORMATION

Traditional Prescribing

Traditional Western herbal medicine uses include:
- Acute or chronic bronchitis, whooping cough, respiratory conditions with nonproductive cough, the common cold, asthma[1,2]
- As a warm infusion for diaphoresis, jaundice, hoarseness, amenorrhea, excitability, and asthma[2]
- Dyspepsia, intestinal worms[2]

Pharmacologic Research

The aerial parts of white horehound contain bitter principles, including the diterpene marrubiin.[3]
- Experimental studies indicate that white horehound has an expectorant action (route unknown), which was attributed to marrubiin and the volatile oil.[4]

White Horehound *continued on page 457*

*This dose range is extrapolated from the British Herbal Pharmacopoeia 1983, the British Herbal Compendium 1992, and the author's education and experience.

- Extract of leaves, stems, and roots demonstrated antispasmodic activity in several isolated smooth muscle preparations by inhibiting the action of some neurotransmitters.[5]
- Marrubiin, by injection, exhibited potent analgesic effects in two experimental models. The findings suggest marrubiin and the whole plant extract do not interact with opioid systems.[6]

Clinical Studies

No clinical studies using white horehound have been found.
- In Germany, the Commission E supports using white horehound to treat loss of appetite and dyspepsia, including bloating and flatulence.[7]

REFERENCES

1 British Herbal Medicine Association's Scientific Committee: *British herbal pharmacopoeia,* Bournemouth, 1983, BHMA.

2 Felter HW, Lloyd JU: *King's American dispensatory,* ed 18, rev 3, Portland, 1905, reprinted 1983, Eclectic Medica Publications.

3 Bisset NG, ed: *Herbal drugs and phytopharmaceuticals,* Stuttgart, 1994, Medpharm Scientific Publishers.

4 British Herbal Medicine Association: *British herbal compendium,* Bournemouth, 1992, BHMA.

5 Schlemper V et al: *Phytomed* 3(2):211-216, 1996.

6 de Jesus RA et al: *Phytomed* 7(2):111-115, 2000.

7 Blumenthal M et al, eds: *The complete German Commission E monographs: therapeutic guide to herbal medicines,* Austin, 1998, American Botanical Council.

WHITE PEONY

Other Common Name:	Paeonia
Botanical Name:	*Paeonia lactiflora*
Family:	Paeoniaceae
Plant Part Used:	Root

PRESCRIBING INFORMATION

Actions

Spasmolytic, mild skeletal muscle relaxant, anticonvulsant, antiinflammatory, cognition-enhancing

Potential Indications

Based on appropriate evaluation of the patient, practitioners should consider prescribing white peony in formulations in the context of:

- Polycystic ovary syndrome, infertility, dysmenorrhea,* in combination with licorice (4)
- Skeletal muscle cramps and spasm, in combination with licorice (3)
- Fibroids, in combination with *Paeonia suffruticosa, Poria cocos, Cinnamomum cassia,* and *Prunus persica (4)*
- Angina, in combination with *Stevia rebaudiana* and ginsenosides (4)
- Epilepsy, in combination with licorice and fossilized mammalian tooth (4)
- Rheumatoid arthritis (4a)
- Menstrual dysfunction (5)
- Assisting memory and learning (7)

Contraindications

None known.

Warnings and Precautions

Because of the anticoagulant findings in experimental models, caution should be exercised in patients taking warfarin and other anticoagulant medication.

Interactions

None known.

Use in Pregnancy and Lactation

No adverse effects expected.

Side Effects

None expected if taken within the recommended dose range.

Dosage

Dose per day*	**Dose per week***
4.5-8.5 ml of 1:2 liquid extract	30-60 ml of 1:2 liquid extract

SUPPORTING INFORMATION

Traditional Prescribing

Uses and properties from TCM include:
- To *invigorate* and *cool* the *blood,* dispel *congealed blood,* and clear *heat* and *liver fire*[2]

White Peony *continued on page 459*

---

*White peony has also been used in TCM for treating dysmenorrhea. (5)

**This dose range is adapted from dried plant dosages administered by decoction in TCM.[1] The author's experience and the fact that ethanol-water is a more effective solvent than water for many phytochemicals are taken into account.

- Dysmenorrhea, amenorrhea, gynecological problems from *hot blood*; abdominal pain or immobile masses, chest pain[2]
- Swellings, trauma, abscess, boils; swollen painful eyes[1,2]
- Nosebleed, hematemesis[1]

Pharmacologic Research

White peony root contains the unusual constituent paeoniflorin, which is a glucoside with a cagelike monoterpene structure.[3]

- The results of *in vitro* studies suggest that paeoniflorin inhibits testosterone synthesis in ovaries but does not affect estradiol synthesis. Binding to glucocorticoid receptors was moderate, but binding was absent for progesterone receptors.[4,5] White peony reduces testosterone production from ovaries but not from adrenal glands.[6,7] Oral administration of a white peony and licorice combination resulted in a lower incidence of experimental uterine adenomyosis compared with controls.[8] In an ovariectomized model, this combination increased DHEA and brought about an increase in serum estrogen concentration.[9]
- White peony has exhibited smooth muscle relaxant activity in isolated tissue (ileum and uterus) from several animal species.[10] Paeoniflorin and related compounds inhibited twitch responses of skeletal muscle in response to direct and indirect stimulation.[10] This effect was potentiated by GL from licorice and was confirmed *in vivo*.[10]
- Intragastric administration of white peony decoction exhibited antiinflammatory activity in the adjuvant-induced arthritis model.[11]
- Oral administration of white peony decoction or paeoniflorin attenuated the performance deficit produced by scopolamine,[12] and paeoniflorin reduced learning impairment[13] in experimental models.
- Aqueous extract of white peony inhibited the convulsant activity of the drug pentylenetetrazol in isolated neuronal tissue. The most active constituents were albiflorin and the gallotannin fraction.[14] White peony showed a clear inhibitory effect on the bursting activity of neurons induced by pentylenetetrazol *in vitro*.[15]
- An aqueous methanol extract of white peony demonstrated anticholinergic activity *in vivo*. Paeoniflorin was one of the active constituents *in vivo* but had no effect on isolated tissue,[16] probably because the active form is a metabolite of paeoniflorin.
- White peony and licorice decoction demonstrated antidiarrheal activity in cisplatin-induced diarrhea.[17]
- White peony, which was found to inhibit nine types of common pathogenic bacteria, also enhanced the phagocytic activity of macrophages and increased T lymphocytes.[18]
- White peony inhibited platelet aggregation, increased fibrinolytic activity, and prolonged prothrombin time *in vitro*.[19] Anticoagulant activity was demonstrated *in vivo* for paeoniflorin.[20]
- An antiatherogenic activity was demonstrated after oral administration of white peony in an experimental model of hypercholesterolemia.[21]

White Peony continued on page 460

- Oral administration of Shimotsu-to, an herbal formula containing equal amounts of white peony, Rehmannia root, *Angelica acutiloba* root, and *Cnidium officinale* rhizome prevented the development of brain infarction and rarefaction induced by chronic brain ischemia in an animal model.[22]

Clinical Studies

The white peony and licorice combination (TJ-68, Shakuyaku-kanzo-to [Japanese]; Shaoyao Gancao Tang [Chinese]) referred to here is approved for use in clinical practice in Japan and has been used to treat pain accompanying acute muscle spasms, including dysmenorrhea. TJ-68 is a granular extract, 7.5 g of which contains a dried concentrate made from 6 g of dried white peony root and 6 g of dried licorice root.

- Eight infertile, hyperandrogenic, and oligomenorrheic women were investigated for the lowering of serum testosterone levels and inducing regular ovulation by treatment with TJ-68 (5 to 10 g/day for 2 to 8 weeks).[23] After the treatment period, serum testosterone levels had normalized in seven patients, and six patients were ovulating regularly. Two of these six patients subsequently became pregnant.
- The effect of white peony and licorice combination (TJ-68, 7.5 g/day for 24 weeks) in patients with polycystic ovary syndrome (PCOS) was studied over a 24-week period. Serum testosterone and free testosterone levels were significantly decreased after 4 weeks. However, testosterone levels after 12 weeks were lower only in the patients who became pregnant. After 24 weeks, the LH/FSH ratio was significantly lower in the treated group. In an earlier uncontrolled trial, the effect of treatment with the same herbal combination varied according to the type of PCOS treated. Plasma testosterone tended to remain higher in PCOS of the general cystic type than in the peripheral cystic type, and the pregnancy rate in individuals with the general cystic type was lower.[24,25]
- In an uncontrolled study, 110 premenopausal patients with fibroids were treated with a traditional Chinese formula containing white peony, *Paeonia suffruticosa, Poria cocos, Cinnamomum cassia,* and *Prunus persica.* Clinical symptoms were improved in 90% of cases, and the fibroids shrunk in approximately 60% of cases.[26]
- TJ-68 has shown benefit in clinical trials for treating muscle spasm. In a multicenter, double-blind, placebo-controlled trial, treatment with the combination (7.5 g/day for 2 weeks) resulted in significantly greater improvement in muscle spasm (mainly of the calf muscle) than placebo treatment for patients with liver cirrhosis.[27]
- White peony combined with licorice and fossilized mammalian tooth provided benefit for almost one half of 43 cases of epilepsy.[28]
- The total glucosides of white peony (TGP) have been used clinically for treating rheumatoid arthritis.[29] This use of TGP capsules was approved in China in 1995.[30]
- Tablets containing mainly white peony, *Stevia rebaudiana,* and ginsenosides were used to treat patients with angina, with a 93% success

White Peony *continued on page 461*

rate in symptoms and improvement in ECG in 53%. Microcirculation was also significantly improved.[31] (Ginsenosides are present in *Panax ginseng*.)

- In case observation studies, TJ-68 was effective in treating the following cases without side effects: neuroleptic-induced hyperprolactinemia, reduced sexual desire in male schizophrenic patients, and risperidone-induced amenorrhea in a schizophrenic woman (7.5 g/day).[32]

REFERENCES

1. Pharmacopoeia Commission of the People's Republic of China: *Pharmacopoeia of the People's Republic of China*, English ed, Beijing, 1997, Chemical Industry Press.
2. Bensky D, Gamble A: *Chinese herbal medicine materia medica*, Seattle, 1986, Eastland Press.
3. Tang W, Eisenbrand G: *Chinese drugs of plant origin*, Berlin, 1992, Springer-Verlag.
4. Takeuchi T et al: *Am J Chin Med* 19(1):73-78, 1991.
5. Tamaya T, Sato S, Okada H: *Acta Obstet Gynecol Scand* 65(8):839-842, 1986.
6. Takeuchi T: *Nippon Naibunpi Gakkai Zasshi* 64(11):1124-1139, 1988.
7. Takeuchi T et al: *Am J Chin Med* 19(1):73-78, 1991.
8. Mori T et al: *Am J Chin Med* 21(3-4):263-268, 1993.
9. Kato T, Okamoto R: *Nippon Sanka Fujinka Gakkai Zasshi* 44(4):433-439, 1992.
10. Hikino H: *Oriental medicinal plants*. In Farnsworth NR et al, eds: *Economic and medicinal plant research*, London, 1985, Academic Press.
11. Cho S et al: *Shoyakugaku Zasshi* 36:78-81, 1982.
12. Ohta H et al: *Pharmacol Biochem Behav* 45(3):719-723, 1993.
13. Ohta H et al: *Pharmacol Biochem Behav* 49(1):213-217, 1994.
14. Sugaya A et al: *J Ethnopharmacol* 33(1-2):159-167, 1991.
15. Sugaya A et al: *Planta Med* 51(1):60-61, 1985.
16. Kobayashi M et al: *Yakugaku Zasshi* 110(12):964-968, 1990.
17. Xu JD, Liu ZH, Chen SZ: *Chung Kuo Chung Hsi I Chieh Ho Tsa Chih* 14(11):673-674, 1994.
18. Liang MR et al: *New J Trad Chin Med* 21(3):51, 1989. Cited in *Abst Chin Med* 3(3):274, 1989.
19. Wang Y, Ma R: *Chung Hsi I Chieh Ho Tsa Chih* 10(2):101, 70, 1990.
20. Ishida H et al: *Chem Pharm Bull* 35(2):849-852, 1987.
21. Zhang YZ, Yan XF: *Chung Hsi I Chieh Ho Tsa Chih* 10(11):669, 645, 1990.
22. Watanabe H, Shibuya T, eds: *Pharmacologic research on traditional herbal medicines*, Amsterdam, 1999, Harwood Academic Publishers.
23. Yaginuma T et al: *Nippon Sanka Fujinka Gakkai Zasshi* 34(7):939-944, 1982.
24. Takahashi K, Kitao M: *Int J Fertility Menopausal Stud* 39(2):69-76, 1994.
25. Takahashi K et al: *Nippon Sanka Fujinka Gakkai Zasshi* 40(6):789-792, 1988.
26. Sakamoto S et al: *Am J Chin Med* 20(3-4):313-317, 1992.
27. Kumada T et al: *J Clin Therapeut Med (Jpn)* 15:499-523, 1999.
28. Lin WB: *Hunan Zhongyizazhi* (3):6, 1986. Cited in *Abst Chin Med* 1(3):417, 1987.
29. Lao ZY et al: *Hsin Yao Yu Lin Ch'uang* 14:193-197, 1995.
30. Prendergast HDV, ed: *Plants for food and medicine*, Kew, UK, 1998, Royal Botanic Gardens.
31. Hu JX, Huang GM: *Chin J Integr Trad West Med* 8(7):427, 1988.
32. Yamada K et al: *J Clin Psychopharmacol* 19(4):380-381, 1999.

WILD CHERRY

Botanical Name: *Prunus serotina*
Family: Rosaceae
Plant Part Used: Bark

PRESCRIBING INFORMATION

Actions	Antitussive, mild sedative, astringent
Potential Indications	Based on appropriate evaluation of the patient, practitioners should consider prescribing wild cherry in formulations in the context of: • Respiratory conditions, especially cough, bronchitis, pleurisy, and pneumonia (5) • Tracheitis is said to be a specific indication (5) • The common cold (6)
Contraindications	None known.
Warnings and Precautions	None required.
Interactions	None known.
Use in Pregnancy and Lactation	No adverse effects expected.
Side Effects	None expected if taken within the recommended dose range.

Dosage

Dose per day*	Dose per week*
2.0-4.5 ml of 1:2 liquid extract	15-30 ml of 1:2 liquid extract

SUPPORTING INFORMATION

Traditional Prescribing	Traditional Western herbal medicine uses include: • Persistent cough, whooping cough, bronchitis, pleurisy, pneumonia, tracheitis, tuberculosis[1,2] • Loss of appetite, nervous dyspepsia[1,2] Native Americans used infusion of wild cherry bark to relieve pains and soreness in the chest, as well as for coughs and the common cold.[3]
Pharmacologic Research	Wild cherry bark contains the cyanogenic glycoside prunasin, which is believed to confer the antitussive activity.[4]
Clinical Studies	No clinical studies using wild cherry have been found.

Wild Cherry *continued on page 463*

*This dose range is extrapolated from the British Pharmaceutical Codex 1934 and the author's education and experience.

REFERENCES

1 British Herbal Medicine Association's Scientific Committee: *British herbal pharmacopoeia*, Bournemouth, 1983, BHMA.

2 Felter HW, Lloyd JU: *King's American dispensatory*, ed 18, rev 3, Portland, 1905, reprinted 1983, Eclectic Medical Publications.

3 Vogel VJ: *American Indian medicine*, Norman, Okla, 1970, University of Oklahoma Press.

4 Leung AY, Foster S: *Encyclopedia of common natural ingredients used in food, drugs and cosmetics*, ed 2, New York-Chichester, 1996, John Wiley.

WILD YAM

Other Common Names: Colic root, rheumatism root
Botanical Name: *Dioscorea villosa*
Family: Dioscoreaceae
Plant Part Used: Root and rhizome

PRESCRIBING INFORMATION

Actions

Spasmolytic, antiinflammatory, antirheumatic, estrogen-modulating

Potential Indications

Based on appropriate evaluation of the patient, practitioners should consider prescribing wild yam in formulations in the context of:
- Any conditions of gastrointestinal spasm or irritation, including intestinal colic, diverticulitis, cholecystitis *(5)*
- Uterine or ovarian cramping, including dysmenorrhea *(5)*
- Alleviation of menopausal symptoms *(6, oral use only)*
- Rheumatoid arthritis *(5)*

Contraindications

None known.

Warnings and Precautions

None required.

Interactions

None known.

Use in Pregnancy and Lactation

No adverse effects expected.

Side Effects

As with all saponin-containing herbs, oral use may cause irritation of the gastric mucous membranes and reflux.

Dosage

Dose per day*	Dose per week*
3-6 ml of 1:2 liquid extract	20-40 ml of 1:2 liquid extract

Extracts providing quantified levels of steroidal saponins as dioscin are recommended. Ideally, aqueous ethanol extracts should contain not less than 15 mg/ml of these steroidal saponins.

SUPPORTING INFORMATION

Traditional Prescribing

Traditional Western herbal medicine uses include:
- All forms of colic, gastrointestinal irritation, and spasm (in men as well), including diverticulitis, cholecystitis[1,2]
- Dysmenorrhea, ovarian, and uterine pain,[2] nausea of pregnant women; uterine pain in the latter stages of pregnancy, false labor pains, postpartum pain[3]
- Neuralgic affections and asthma[1]
- Rheumatoid arthritis (particularly in the acute phase) and muscular rheumatism[2]

Wild Yam *continued on page 465*

*This dose range is extrapolated from the British Herbal Pharmacopoeia 1983 and the author's education and experience.

Native Americans used wild yam for colic and to relieve the pain of childbirth. Wild yam was official in the NF from 1916 to 1942 and was used as a diaphoretic and expectorant.[4]

A more recent Western traditional use of wild yam includes the hormonal imbalance associated with menopause.[5]

In traditional Japanese medicine (Kampo), mixtures containing *Dioscorea japonica* have been used for centuries to treat infertility.[6] High doses of yams can cause infertility, but this is consistent with an estrogenic effect. Lower doses can have the opposite effect (see later discussion) consistent with this traditional use.

Pharmacologic Research

Wild yam root contains steroidal saponins with diosgenin as the aglycone. Many species of Dioscorea have been cultivated for the industrial manufacture of steroidal hormones. The aglycone diosgenin is manufactured from dioscin and then undergoes a series of reactions to produce progesterone, hydrocortisone, and so on.[7] Despite this well-known industrial process, no evidence has been found to suggest that diosgenin is metabolized in the body to produce these steroidal hormones, particularly progesterone. Additionally, diosgenin does not normally occur in untreated wild yam rhizome, although it is probably formed as a result of bowel flora metabolism after ingestion.

Steroidal saponins or their metabolites may exert estrogenic effects by binding with estrogen receptors of the hypothalamus, which are part of the negative-feedback mechanism of estrogen control. In the premenopausal woman, interaction of these compounds with receptors in the hypothalamus or pituitary displaces estrogen from receptors and blocks estrogen feedback. The body thinks that estrogen levels are lower than what they really are and responds by increasing FSH and hence estrogen. In the low estrogen environment of peri- and postmenopause, wild yam may alleviate symptoms of estrogen withdrawal through the binding of its steroidal compounds to vacant receptors in the hypothalamus. Because some menopausal symptoms (e.g., hot flashes) are thought to be initiated via the hypothalamus, this selective binding might be sufficient to reduce such symptoms by convincing the body that more estrogen is present in the bloodstream than what actually is. (Negative-feedback mechanisms would not come into play because ovarian function is minimal around menopause.)

- Estrogenic activity for wild yam has been demonstrated *in vitro*. Wild yam extract enhanced estradiol binding to estrogen receptors and enhanced estrogen receptor–mediated gene expression in estrogen-responsive cells alone and in the presence of estradiol.[8] In an experimental model, subcutaneous administration of diosgenin (20 to 40 mg/kg) demonstrated estrogenic properties and lacked progesteronic effects.[9] Wild yam products were found to be inactive in a progesterone receptor assay.[10]

Wild Yam continued on page 466

- Oral administration of diosgenin:
  - Reduced the acute cholestatic effect induced by estradiol in rats[11]
  - Reduced intestinal inflammation and normalized bile secretion in an experimental model (dose: 80 mg/kg)[12]
  - To cholesterol-fed rats, resulted in increased fecal excretion of cholesterol (neutral sterols) without affecting the excretion of bile acids[13]
  - Decreased plasma cholesterol levels in experimentally induced hypercholesterolemia[14]

Clinical Studies

Claims have arisen in the popular literature that the female body can manufacture progesterone from diosgenin, particularly if a wild yam cream is applied to the skin. No information is currently available about the dermal absorption of dioscin. Convincing evidence published in a peer review journal for a progesterogenic effect of wild yam in postmenopausal women is yet to be provided.

- Analysis of saliva samples from women who were using wild yam cream or tablets indicated that their progesterone levels, DHEA levels, and total progestin activities were no different from those of untreated women. The women tested were taking products that did not contain added hormones, and for the most part, specimens were collected within 12 to 24 hours of product use.[10] In another study by the same research group, the saliva of women who reported consuming herbal products containing yam species was found to contain very low levels of progesterone. Women taking the synthetic progestin MPA also had very low levels of progesterone in their saliva, and the authors suggested that the diosgenin and MPA appeared to suppress progesterone synthesis. Further *in vitro* testing indicated that the saliva from women reporting consumption of yam products did not possess any progesterone bioactivity despite the occurrence of high levels of progesterone receptor–binding components in some samples (20% to 30%). The researchers concluded that, "diosgenin is not converted to progesterone in the human body."[15]
- A trial published in 2001 has found a wild yam cream to have little effect on menopausal symptoms. Twenty three women completed treatment in this randomized, double-blind, placebo-controlled, crossover trial. After a 4-week baseline period, each woman was given the treatment cream and matching placebo for 3 months each. Salivary progesterone levels did not on any occasion exceed the detection limit of the assay. In nearly all the parameters that registered a significant difference from baseline values, the results of the placebo cream exceeded that of the wild yam cream, and no statistical difference was observed between the results for placebo and herbal treatment. One gram of the active cream was said to contain *Dioscorea villosa* extract (100 mg), linseed oil (2 g), geranium oil (100 mg), sage oil (100 mg), and vitamin E (10 mg). The matched placebo was not defined.[16] The possibility exists that if the placebo cream contained the essential oils present in the wild yam cream, this trial recorded effects that were caused by the essential oils.

Wild Yam continued on page 467

- A clinical trial involving seven healthy volunteers (six women, one man) investigated the effect of Mexican yam (*Dioscorea composite,* which contains dioscin) and DHEA administration on serum lipoproteins and DHEA-sulfate (DHEA-S). Participants received placebo for 3 weeks, followed by 3 weeks of Mexican yam (dosage [undefined] doubling each week), followed by another week of placebo. DHEA was then taken in the last week. No rise in DHEA-S values was recorded after the Mexican yam treatment. (An increase was observed during DHEA administration.) Both yam and DHEA significantly reduced serum lipid peroxidation and serum triglyceride and increased HDL cholesterol levels. No changes in total cholesterol or LDL cholesterol were observed for either treatment.[17]
- An uncontrolled study conducted in China supported the hypocholesterolemic activity of Dioscorea saponins given by mouth as tablets (0.2 to 2.0 g/day).[18]

REFERENCES

1 Felter HW, Lloyd JU: *King's American dispensatory,* ed 18, rev 3, Portland, 1905, reprinted 1983, Eclectic Medical Publications.

2 British Herbal Medicine Association's Scientific Committee: *British herbal pharmacopoeia,* Bournemouth, 1983, BHMA.

3 Cook WH: *The Physio-medical dispensatory.* First published in 1869, reprinted by Eclectic Medical Publications, Portland, 1985.

4 Vogel VJ: *American Indian medicine,* Norman, Okla, 1970, University of Oklahoma Press.

5 Bartram T: *Encyclopedia of herbal medicine,* ed 1, Dorset, UK, 1995, Grace Publishers.

6 Hosoyo E, Yamamura Y, eds: *Recent advances in the pharmacology of Kampo medicines,* Tokyo, 1988, Excerpta Medica.

7 Bruneton J: *Pharmacognosy, phytochemistry, medicinal plants,* Paris, 1995, Lavoisier Publishing.

8 Eagon PK et al: 91st Annual Meeting of the American Association for Cancer Research, San Francisco, April 1-5, 2000, abstract 893.

9 Aradhana, Rao AR, Kale RK: *Indian J Exp Biol* 30(5):367-370, 1992.

10 Dollbaum C: *Townsend Letter for Doctors and Patients* 159:104, 1996.

11 Accatino L et al: *Hepatology* 28(1):129-140, 1998.

12 Yamada T et al: *Am J Physiol* 273(2, pt 1):G355-G364, 1997.

13 Cayen MN, Dvornik D: *J Lipid Res* 20:162, 1979.

14 Juarez-Oropeza MA, Diaz-Zagoya JC, Rabinowitz JL: *Int J Biochem* 19(8):679-683, 1987.

15 Zava DT, Dollbaum CM, Blen M: *Proc Soc Exp Biol Med* 217(3):369-378, 1998.

16 Komesaroff PA et al: *Climacteric* 4(2):144-150, 2001.

17 Araghiniknam M et al: *Life Sci* 59(11):147-157, 1996.

18 Chang HM, But PP: *Pharmacology and applications of Chinese materia medica,* Singapore, 1987, World Scientific.

WILLOW HERB

Other Common Names: Epilobium, small-flowered willow herb
Botanical Names: *Epilobium parviflorum, Epilobium montanum,*[+] *Epilobium collinum,*[+] *Epilobium roseum*[+]
Family: Onagraceae
Plant Part Used: Aerial parts

PRESCRIBING INFORMATION

Actions
Antiprostatic

Potential Indications
Based on appropriate evaluation of the patient, practitioners should consider prescribing willow herb in formulations in the context of prostate disorders. (6)

Contraindications
None known.

Warnings and Precautions
None required.

Interactions
None known.

Use in Pregnancy and Lactation
No adverse effects expected.

Side Effects
None expected if taken within the recommended dose range.

Dosage

Dose per day*	Dose per week*
3-6 ml of 1:2 liquid extract	20-40 ml of 1:2 liquid extract

SUPPORTING INFORMATION

Traditional Prescribing
Willow herb was used in European herbal medicine in the mid-twentieth century following its popularization by the traditional Austrian herbalist Maria Treben.[1] Willow herb was recommended for prostatism (chronic disorders of the prostate, especially obstruction to urination by prostatic enlargement).[2]

Pharmacologic Research
Of several extracts of *Epilobium parviflorum* tested *in vitro*, only the aqueous extract showed significant inhibition of 5α-reductase (the enzyme responsible for the biosynthesis of DHT from testosterone).[3]

Clinical Studies
No clinical studies using willow herb have been found.

REFERENCES

1 Treben M: *Health through God's pharmacy,* ed 13, Steyr, Austria, 1989, Wilhelm Ennsthaler.
2 Weiss RF: *Herbal medicine,* English ed, Beaconsfield, UK, 1988, Beaconsfield Publishers.
3 Lesuisse D et al: *J Nat Prod* 59(5):490-492, 1996.

[+]Medicinally interchangeable species.
*This dose range is extrapolated from traditional use of willow herb tea.

WORMWOOD

Botanical Name: *Artemisia absinthium*
Family: Compositae
Plant Part Used: Aerial parts

PRESCRIBING INFORMATION

Actions

Bitter tonic, anthelmintic, antiparasitic

Potential Indications

Based on appropriate evaluation of the patient, practitioners should consider prescribing wormwood in formulations in the context of:
- Anorexia, dyspepsia *(4,5)*
- Conditions involving insufficient flow of gastric or pancreatic enzymes and bile *(4)*
- Worm infestation *(5)*

Contraindications

Pregnancy and lactation, hyperacidity.[1]

Warnings and Precautions

The recommended dose range must not be exceeded.

People with known sensitivity to wormwood or other members of the Compositae family (e.g., ragweed, daisies, chrysanthemums) should avoid using wormwood.

Interactions

None known.

Use in Pregnancy and Lactation

Contraindicated in pregnancy and lactation.

Side Effects

None expected if taken within the recommended dose range. Overdose of wormwood has been reported.[1]

Dosage

Dose per day*	Dose per week*
0.7-3.0 ml of 1:5 tincture	5-20 ml of 1:5 tincture

The low end of the dose range should be used for the bitter effect. Doses at the high end of the dose range are for short-term use only.

SUPPORTING INFORMATION

Traditional Prescribing

Traditional Western herbal medicine uses include:
- Nematode infestation[2,3]
- Anorexia, atonic dyspepsia,[2] flatulent dyspepsia, diarrhea,[3] debility[4]
- Amenorrhea and leukorrhea when resulting from debility[3]

Pharmacologic Research

Constituents of the aerial parts of wormwood include bitter substances (sesquiterpene lactones, particularly absinthin) and an essential oil that contains thujone. High doses of thujone may cause neurotoxicity.[5]

Wormwood *continued on page 470*

*This dose range is extrapolated from the British Herbal Pharmacopoeia 1983 and the author's education and experience.

Bitters are substances capable of strongly stimulating the bitter receptors in the taste buds at the back of the tongue. Bitters applied to the mouth (tasted) before a meal have a priming effect on upper digestive function, which is probably mediated by a nerve reflex from the bitter taste buds and involves an increase in vagal stimulation. This vagal stimulation means bitters might have a promoting effect on all components of upper digestive function, namely the stomach, liver, and pancreas.[6]

- Increased gastric secretory activity and increased stomach acidity was demonstrated after oral doses of isolated absinthin in an experimental model. Wormwood decoction administered by intravenous injection demonstrated a choleretic effect.[1]
- Wormwood decoction demonstrated anthelmintic activity toward the nematode *Trichostrongylus colubriformis in vitro.*[7]

Clinical Studies

- Wormwood given to human volunteers 5 minutes before a meal stimulated gastric secretion.[8]
- Another study found that oral doses of liquid wormwood caused a dramatic increase in duodenal levels of pancreatic enzymes and bile.[9]
- In Germany, the Commission E supports using wormwood to treat loss of appetite, dyspepsia, and biliary dyskinesia[10]
- ESCOP recommends wormwood for treating anorexia and dyspepsia.[1]

REFERENCES

1 Scientific Committee of the European Scientific Cooperative on Phytotherapy [ESCOP]: *ESCOP monographs: Absinthii herba.* European Scientific Cooperative on Phytotherapy, ESCOP Secretariat, Argyle House, Gandy Street, Exeter, Devon, EX4 3LS, United Kindom, July 1997.

2 British Herbal Medicine Association's Scientific Committee: *British herbal pharmacopoeia,* Bournemouth, 1983, BHMA.

3 Felter HW, Lloyd JU: *King's American dispensatory,* ed 18, rev 3, Portland, 1905, reprinted 1983, Eclectic Medical Publications.

4 Grieve M: *A modern herbal,* New York, 1971, Dover Publications.

5 Bisset NG, ed: *Herbal drugs and phytopharmaceuticals,* Stuttgart, 1994, Medpharm Scientific Publishers.

6 Mills S, Bone K: *Principles and practice of phytotherapy: modern herbal medicine,* Edinburgh, 2000, Churchill Livingstone.

7 Bara S, Zaragoza C, Valderrabano J: SEMh Congreso 1999: Sociedad Espanola de Malherbología, Longrono, Spain, November 23-25, 1999.

8 Glatzel H, Hackenberg K: *Planta Med* 3:223-232, 1967.

9 Baumann IC, Glatzel H, Muth HW: *Z Allgemeinmed* 51(17):784-791, 1975.

10 Blumenthal M et al, eds: *The complete German Commission E monographs: therapeutic guide to herbal medicines,* Austin, 1998, American Botanical Council.

YARROW

Other Common Name: Achillea
Botanical Name: *Achillea millefolium*
Family: Compositae
Plant Part Used: Aerial parts

PRESCRIBING INFORMATION

Actions	Diaphoretic, antipyretic, peripheral vasodilator, antiinflammatory, spasmolytic, bitter tonic, styptic (hemostatic), antimicrobial, anti-hemorrhagic, vulnerary
Potential Indications	Based on appropriate evaluation of the patient, practitioners should consider prescribing yarrow in formulations in the context of:

- Loss of appetite, dyspepsia, gastrointestinal spasm *(4)*
- Amenorrhea, menorrhagia *(5)*
- Other conditions involving bleeding, such as hemorrhoids, melena, and hemoptysis *(5)*
- Fevers and conditions in which fever is present, such as the common cold *(5)*
- Conditions of disordered circulation (e.g., hemorrhoids, thrombosis), hypertension *(5)*
- Diarrhea, dysentery *(5)*
- A sitz bath for painful cramping of female reproductive tract *(4)*
- Topical treatment for slow-healing wounds and skin conditions *(5)*

Contraindications	Known allergy.
Warnings and Precautions	Sesquiterpenes are responsible for the allergic contact dermatitis caused by yarrow.[1] People with known sensitivity to other members of the Compositae family (e.g., ragweed, daisies, chrysanthemums) should avoid using yarrow.
Interactions	None known.
Use in Pregnancy and Lactation	No adverse effects expected. However, thujone-containing varieties should be avoided.
Side Effects	None expected if taken within the recommended dose range.

Dosage

Dose per day*	Dose per week*
2-6 ml of 1:2 liquid extract	15-40 ml of 1:2 liquid extract

Yarrow *continued on page 472*

*This dose range is extrapolated from the British Herbal Pharmacopoeia 1983, the British Herbal Compendium 1992, and the author's education and experience.

SUPPORTING INFORMATION

Traditional Prescribing

Traditional Western herbal medicine uses include:
- Fevers, feverish conditions, the common cold, essential hypertension, thrombotic conditions, amenorrhea, dysentery, diarrhea[2,3]
- As an infusion for diuretic action in chronic diseases of the urinary tract and urinary incontinence[4]
- Hemorrhage in which the bleeding is small in amount[4]
- As a tonic for the venous system and mucous membranes and used for treating sore throat, hemorrhoids, dysentery[4]
- Atonic amenorrhea, menorrhagia; flatulence[4]
- Topically for slow-healing wounds and skin conditions[3]

Native Americans used yarrow extensively; it was applied topically for wounds, bruises, swellings, aches, eczema, rash, and earache. Yarrow infusion was taken internally for weak and disordered digestion, general sickness, and as a fever medicine. Yarrow flowers were burnt and inhaled to break fevers. Yarrow leaf and flowering tops were official in the USP from 1863 to 1882 and were used for tonic, stimulant, and emmenagogue purposes. Some Eclectics considered the leaves to be superior to the flowers.[5]

Pharmacologic Research

Using a reliable source of yarrow is important, because many varieties and subspecies of *A. millefolium* that contain varying amounts of phytochemical constituents are available.[6]
- Yarrow aqueous alcohol extract demonstrated *in vitro* antimicrobial activity toward *Staphylococcus aureus* but was inactive against *S. aureus* strains isolated from patients.[7] An ethanol extract demonstrated moderate activity against the following species *in vitro*: *Staph. aureus, Bacillus subtillus, Mycobacterium smegmatis, Escherichia coli, Shigella sonnei,* and *Shigella flexneri*.[8]
- Yarrow showed mild antipyretic activity *in vivo* in early research.[9]
- Aqueous extract of yarrow flower demonstrated antiinflammatory activity both topically (skin irritation test) and systemically (subcutaneous administration, mouse paw edema test). The active fraction was found to be a mixture of protein-carbohydrate complexes.[10]
- Yarrow extracts demonstrated spasmolytic activity on isolated rabbit small intestine. The methanol extract had greater activity than the aqueous extract. Isolated flavonoids were also active.[11]
- Oral administration of yarrow methanolic extract did not demonstrate analgesic activity in an experimental model.[12]
- Yarrow extracts demonstrated hepatoprotective activity in carbon tetrachloride and acetaminophen (paracetamol) liver toxicity models when administered by injection.[13]
- Sesquiterpenes isolated from yarrow were active against experimental leukemia *in vivo*.[14]
- Yarrow flower extracts (ethanolic extract, by injection; aqueous alcohol extract, orally) demonstrated antispermatogenic effects in mice.[15]

Yarrow continued on page 473

Clinical Studies

- In a randomized, double-blind, crossover trial, an herbal preparation effected a similar reduction in subjective symptoms of osteoarthrosis compared with the NSAID ibuprofen but with a lower side effect incidence. The herbal tablet contained feverfew (110 mg), American aspen (*Populus tremuloides*, 90 mg), and yarrow (60 mg). Three tablets were taken daily.[16]
- In Germany, the Commission E supports internal use of yarrow to treat loss of appetite and dyspeptic disorders, such as mild, spastic discomfort of the gastrointestinal tract. As a sitz bath, yarrow is recommended for painful, cramplike conditions of psychosomatic origin in the lower part of the female pelvis.[17]

REFERENCES

1 Rucker G, Manns D, Breuer J: *Arch Pharm* 324(12):979-981, 1991.
2 British Herbal Medicine Association's Scientific Committee: *British herbal pharmacopoeia*, Bournemouth, 1983, BHMA.
3 British Herbal Medicine Association: *British herbal compendium*, Bournemouth, 1992, BHMA.
4 Felter HW, Lloyd JU: *King's American dispensatory*, ed 18, rev 3, Portland, 1905, reprinted 1983, Eclectic Medical Publications.
5 Vogel VJ: *American Indian medicine*, Norman, Okla, 1970, University of Oklahoma Press.
6 Bisset NG, ed: *Herbal drugs and phytopharmaceuticals*, Stuttgart, 1994, Medpharm Scientific Publishers.
7 Molochko VA et al: *Vestn Dermatol Venerol* (8):54-56, 1990.
8 Moskalenko SA: *J Ethnopharmacol* 15(3):231-259, 1986.
9 Nikonorow M: *Acta Polon Pharm* 3:23-56, 1939.
10 Goldberg AS et al: *J Pharm Sci* 58(8):938-941, 1969.
11 Hoerhammer L: Congr Sci Farm Conf Comun 21st [report of the International Congress of the Pharmaceutical Science], Pisa, September 4-8, 1961, abstract S578-588.
12 Ahmad F, Khan RA, Rashid S: *Med J Islam Repub Iran* 10(2):149-152, 1996.
13 Gadgoli C, Mishra SH: *Fitoterapia* 66(4):319-323, 1995.
14 Tozyo T et al: *Chem Pharm Bull* 42(5):1096-1100, 1994.
15 Montanari T, de Carvalho JE, Dolder H: *Contraception* 58(5):309-313, 1998.
16 Ryttig K et al: *Ugeskr Laeger* 153(33):2298-2299, 1991.
17 Blumenthal M et al, eds: *The complete German Commission E monographs: therapeutic guide to herbal medicines*, Austin, 1998, American Botanical Council.

YELLOW DOCK

Other Common Name:	Curled dock
Botanical Name:	*Rumex crispus*
Family:	Polygonaceae
Plant Part Used:	Root

PRESCRIBING INFORMATION

Actions

Mild laxative, cholagogue, depurative

Potential Indications

Based on appropriate evaluation of the patient, practitioners should consider prescribing yellow dock in formulations in the context of:
- Chronic skin disorders (5)
- Constipation, bowel sluggishness, indigestion (5)
- Rheumatism (6)

Yellow dock has been traditionally used as a mild laxative and depurative and might also be used to treat other health problems that may be caused or exacerbated by constipation, including headaches and period pain. Depurative herbs have been traditionally prescribed for chronic rheumatic conditions. (5)

Contraindications

None known.

Warnings and Precautions

Yellow dock should be used with caution during pregnancy because it contains anthraquinone glycosides.

Laxative remedies should not be regarded as a long-term solution to digestive problems. Prolonged use is undesirable. However, the laxative action of yellow dock is very mild.

Interactions

None known.

Use in Pregnancy and Lactation

Yellow dock should be used with caution during pregnancy.

Side Effects

None expected if taken within the recommended dose range.

Dosage

Dose per day*	Dose per week*
2.0-4.5 ml of 1:2 liquid extract	15-30 ml of 1:2 liquid extract

SUPPORTING INFORMATION

Traditional Prescribing

Traditional Western herbal medicine uses include:
- Constipation,[1] dyspepsia, particularly with fullness, pain, and flatulence; painless diarrhea,[2] diphtheria[3]
- Jaundice,[1] bilious complaints[3]

Yellow Dock *continued on page 475*

*This dose range is extrapolated from the British Herbal Pharmacopoeia 1983 and the author's education and experience.

- Chronic skin disorders,[1] chronic lymphatic enlargements, topically for skin disorders[2]
- Rheumatism, disorders of the spleen[4]
- Debilitating conditions, including cancer[3]

Native Americans used Rumex species as a poison antidote and blood purifier. Listed in the USP and NF in the late 1800s and early 1900s, *R. crispus* and *R. obtusifolius* were used for treating skin diseases and for depurative purposes. Later, these herbs were used as laxatives and tonics.[5]

Pharmacologic Research

Yellow dock root contains anthraquinone glycosides, which have demonstrated laxative activity.[6]

Clinical Studies

No clinical studies using yellow dock have been found.

REFERENCES

1 British Herbal Medicine Association's Scientific Committee: *British herbal pharmacopoeia,* Bournemouth, 1983, BHMA.

2 Felter HW, Lloyd JU: *King's American dispensatory,* ed 18, rev 3, Portland, 1905, reprinted 1983, Eclectic Medical Publications.

3 Grieve M: *A modern herbal,* New York, 1971, Dover Publications.

4 Bartram T: *Encyclopedia of herbal medicine,* ed 1, Dorset, UK, 1995, Grace Publishers.

5 Vogel VJ: *American Indian medicine,* Norman, Okla, 1970, University of Oklahoma Press.

6 de Smet PAGM et al, eds: *Adverse effects of herbal drugs,* Berlin, 1993, Springer-Verlag.

APPENDIX A

Dosage **Summary Chart**

Common Name	Botanical Name	Plant Part	Ethanol Content (%)	Extract Strength	Dosage Minimum (ml/day)	Dosage Maximum (ml/day)	Dosage Minimum (ml/wk)	Dosage Maximum (ml/wk)
Albizia	Albizia lebbeck	Stem bark	25	1:2	3.5	8.5	25	60
Aloe vera	Aloe spp.	Juice from the leaf	Negligible	Approx. 4.5:1	25	100	175	700
Andrographis	Andrographis paniculata	Aerial parts	45	1:2	3	6	20	40
Arnica	Arnica montana	Flower	45	1:5	Not taken internally	Not taken internally	Not taken internally	Not taken internally
Ashwaganda	Withania somnifera	Root	45	1:2	5	13	35	90
Astragalus	Astragalus membranaceus	Root	25	1:2	4.5	8.5	30	60
Bacopa	Bacopa monnieri	Aerial parts	25	1:2	5	13	35	90
Baical skullcap	Scutellaria baicalensis	Root	60	1:2	4.5	8.5	30	60
Baptisia	Baptisia tinctoria	Root	60	1:2	2	6	15	40
Bearberry	See Uva ursi							
Barberry	Berberis vulgaris	Root, stem bark	45	1:2	3	6	20	40
Bilberry	Vaccinium myrtillus	Fruit	25	1:1	3	6	20	40
Black cohosh	Cimicifuga racemosa	Root, rhizome	60	1:2	1.5	3	10	20
Black haw	Viburnum prunifolium	Bark	30	1:2	1.5	4.5	10	30
Bladderwrack	Fucus vesiculosus	Thallus	25	1:1	4.5	8.5	30	60
Blue cohosh	Caulophyllum thalictroides	Root	70	1:2	1.5	3	10	20
Blue flag	Iris versicolor	Root	60	1:2	3	6	20	40
Buchu	Agathosma betulina	Leaf	60	1:2	2	4.5	15	30
Bugleweed	Lycopus virginicus	Aerial parts	25	1:2	2	6	15	40
Bupleurum	Bupleurum falcatum	Root	45	1:2	3.5	8.5	25	60
Burdock	Arctium lappa	Root	25	1:2	1.5	3.5	10	25
Calendula	Calendula officinalis	Flower	90	1:2	1.5	4.5	10	30
California poppy	Eschscholzia californica	Aerial parts	45	1:2	3	6	20	40
Cascara	Rhamnus purshiana	Bark	25	1:2	3	8	20	55
Cat's claw	Uncaria tomentosa	Stem bark	60	1:2	4.5	11	30	75
Celery seed	Apium graveolens	Fruit	60	1:2	4.5	8.5	30	60
Chamomile (high grade)	Matricaria recutita	Flower	60	1:2	3	6	20	40

Common name	Botanical name	Part						
Chaste tree	Vitex agnus-castus	Fruit	45	1:2	1	2.5	6	18
Chickweed (fresh plant succus)	Stellaria media	Aerial parts	25	Not applicable	3	6	20	40
Cinnamon	Cinnamomum zeylanicum	Bark	70	1:2	3	6	20	40
Cleavers	Galium aparine	Aerial parts	25	1:2	3.5	7	25	50
Clivers	See Cleavers							
Codonopsis	Codonopsis pilosula	Root	45	1:2	4.5	8.5	30	60
Coleus	Coleus forskohlii	Root	50	1:1	6	13	40	90
Corn silk	Zea mays	Style, stigma	25	1:1	2	6	15	40
Couch grass	Agropyron repens	Rhizome	25	1:1	3	6	20	40
Cramp bark	Viburnum opulus	Bark	30	1:2	3	4.5	15	30
Cranesbill	Geranium maculatum	Root	45	1:2	2	5	15	35
Crataeva	Crataeva nurvala	Bark	25	1:2	6	14	40	100
Damiana	Turnera diffusa	Leaf	60	1:2	3	6	20	40
Dandelion leaf	Taraxacum officinale	Leaf	25	1:1	6	11.5	40	80
Dandelion root	Taraxacum officinale	Root	25	1:2	3	6	20	40
Devil's claw	Harpagophytum procumbens	Root	25	1:2	6	11.5	40	80
Dong quai	Angelica sinensis	Root	45	1:2	4.5	8.5	30	60
Echinacea angustifolia	Echinacea angustifolia	Root	60	1:2	3	6	20	40
Echinacea root blend	Echinacea purpurea and Echinacea angustifolia blend	Root	60	1:2	3	6	20	40
Echinacea purpurea	Echinacea purpurea	Root	60	1:2	3	6	20	40
Echinacea purpurea glycetract	Echinacea purpurea	Root	Not applicable	1:3	4.5	8.5	30	60
Elder flower	Sambucus nigra	Flower	25	1:2	2	6	15	40
Elecampane	Inula helenium	Root	60	1:2	3	6	20	40
Eleutherococcus	Eleutherococcus senticosus	Root	25	1:2	2	8	15	55
Euphorbia	Euphorbia hirta	Aerial parts	60	1:2	0.7	2	5	12
Eyebright	Euphrasia officinalis	Aerial parts	45	1:2	2	4.5	15	30
False unicorn root	Chamaelirium luteum	Root	45	1:2	2	6	15	40
Fennel	Foeniculum vulgare	Fruit	60	1:2	3	6	20	40

Dosage Summary Chart—cont'd

Common Name	Botanical Name	Plant Part	Ethanol Content (%)	Extract Strength	Dosage Minimum (ml/day)	Dosage Maximum (ml/day)	Dosage Minimum (ml/wk)	Dosage Maximum (ml/wk)
Fenugreek	Trigonella foenum-graecum	Seed	45	1:2	2	4.5	15	30
Feverfew	Tanacetum parthenium	Leaf	60	1:5	1	3	7	20
Fringe tree	Chionanthus virginicus	Root bark	45	1:2	3	6	20	40
Gentian	Gentiana lutea	Root	45	1:2	0.7	2	5	15
Ginger	Zingiber officinale	Rhizome	90	1:2	0.7	2	5	15
Ginkgo (standardized extract)	Ginkgo biloba	Leaf	50	2:1	3	4	21	28
Globe artichoke	Cynara scolymus	Leaf	60	1:2	3	8	20	55
Goat's rue	Galega officinalis	Aerial parts	25	1:2	4.5	8.5	30	60
Golden rod	Solidago virgaurea	Aerial parts	45	1:2	3	6	20	40
Golden seal	Hydrastis canadensis	Root, rhizome	45	1:3	2	4.5	15	30
Gotu kola	Centella asiatica	Aerial parts	45	1:2	3	6	20	40
Greater celandine	Chelidonium majus	Aerial parts	45	1:2	1	2	7	15
Green oats	Avena sativa	Aerial parts, including seed at the immature, milky stage	25	1:2	3	6	20	40
Grindelia	Grindelia camporum	Aerial parts	60	1:2	1.5	3	10	20
Gymnema	Gymnema sylvestre	Leaf	25	1:1	3.5	11	25	75
Hawthorn berry	Crataegus monogyna	Berry	45	1:2	3	7	20	50
Hawthorn leaf	Crataegus spp.	Leaf	45	1:2	3	6	20	40
Hemidesmus	Hemidesmus indicus	Root	45	1:2	3.5	8.5	25	60
Hops	Humulus lupulus	Strobile	60	1:2	1.5	3	10	20
Horsechestnut	Aesculus hippocastanum	Seed	35	1:2	2	5	15	35
Horsetail	Equisetum arvense	Aerial parts	25	1:2	2	6	15	40
Hydrangea	Hydrangea arborescens	Root	45	1:2	2	7	15	50
Indian barberry	Berberis aristata	Root, stem bark	45	1:1	2	4.5	15	30
Jamaica dogwood	Piscidia erythrina	Root bark	60	1:2	3	6	20	40
Kava	Piper methysticum	Root	60	1:2	3	8.5	20	60
Korean ginseng	Panax ginseng	Root	60	1:2	1.5	6	10	40
Lavender	Lavandula officinalis	Flower	60	1:2	2	4.5	15	30
Lemon balm	Melissa officinalis	Aerial parts	45	1:2	3	6	20	40

Common name	Botanical name	Part		Ratio				
Licorice	Glycyrrhiza glabra	Root, stolon	20	1:1	2	6	15	40
Licorice (high grade)	Glycyrrhiza glabra	Root, stolon	20	1:1	1.5	4.5	10	30
Lime flowers	Tilia spp	Flower	45	1:2	2	4.5	15	30
Marshmallow leaf	Althaea officinalis	Leaf	25	1:2	3	6	20	40
Marshmallow root	Althaea officinalis	Root	25	1:5	3	6	20	40
Marshmallow root glycetract	Althaea officinalis	Root	Not applicable	1:5	3	6	20	40
Meadowsweet	Filipendula ulmaria	Aerial parts	60	1:2	3	6	20	40
Mexican valerian	Valeriana edulis	Root, rhizome	45	1:2	1.5	4.5	10	30
Milk thistle	Silybum marianum	Fruit	60	1:1	4.5	8.5	30	60
Milk thistle glycetract	Silybum marianum	Fruit	Not applicable	1:1	4.5	8.5	30	60
Mistletoe	Viscum album	Aerial parts	45	1:2	3	6	20	40
Motherwort	Leonurus cardiaca	Aerial parts	25	1:2	2	3.5	15	25
Mullein	Verbascum thapsus	Leaf	25	1:2	4.5	8.5	30	60
Myrrh	Commiphora mol-mol	Resin	90	1:5	1.5	4.5	10	30
Neem leaf	Azadirachta indica	Leaf	45	1:2	1.5	3.5	10	25
Nettle leaf	Urtica dioica	Leaf	25	1:2	2	6	15	40
Nettle root	Urtica dioica	Root	25	1:2	4.5	8.5	30	60
Oats, seed	Avena sativa	Mature seed	25	1:1	3	6	20	40
Oats, green	See Green oats							
Olive leaf	Olea europaea	Leaf	45	1:2	3.5	7	25	50
Oregon grape	Berberis aquifolium	Root, rhizome	25	1:2	3.5	7	25	50
Paeonia	See White peony							
Pasque flower	Anemone pulsatilla	Aerial parts (dried only)	25	1:2	0.4	1.5	3	10
Passion flower	Passiflora incarnata	Aerial parts	45	1:2	3	6	20	40
Pau d'arco	Tabebuia avellanedae	Bark	45	1:2	3	7	20	50
Peppermint	Mentha piperita	Leaf	45	1:2	1.5	4.5	10	30
Pleurisy root	Asclepias tuberosa	Root	45	1:2	1.5	3	10	20
Poke root	Phytolacca decandra	Root	45	1:5	0.15	0.7	1	5
Prickly ash	Zanthoxylum clava-herculis	Bark	45	1:5	1.5	4.5	10	30
Raspberry leaf	Rubus idaeus	Leaf	25	1:2	4.5	14	30	100
Red clover	Trifolium pratense	Flower	25	1:2	1.5	6	10	40
Rehmannia	Rehmannia glutinosa	Root	25	1:2	4.5	8.5	30	60
Rosemary	Rosmarinus officinalis	Leaf	60	1:2	2	4.5	15	30
Sage	Salvia officinalis	Aerial parts	60	1:2	2	4.5	15	30

Continued

Dosage Summary Chart—cont'd

Common Name	Botanical Name	Plant Part	Ethanol Content (%)	Extract Strength	Dosage Minimum (ml/day)	Dosage Maximum (ml/day)	Dosage Minimum (ml/wk)	Dosage Maximum (ml/wk)
Sarsaparilla	Smilax ornata	Root, rhizome	45	1:2	3	6	20	40
Saw palmetto	Serenoa serrulata	Fruit	45	1:2	2	4.5	15	30
Schisandra	Schisandra chinensis	Fruit	45	1:2	3.5	8.5	25	60
Shatavari	Asparagus racemosus	Root	45	1:2	4.5	8.5	30	60
Shepherd's purse	Capsella bursa-pastoris	Aerial parts	25	1:2	3	6	20	40
Siberian ginseng	See Eleutherococcus							
Skullcap	Scutellaria lateriflora	Aerial parts	45	1:2	2	4.5	15	30
Spiny jujube	Zizyphus spinosa	Seed	25	1:2	6	11.5	40	80
St. John's wort	Hypericum perforatum	Aerial parts	45	1:2	2	6	15	40
St. John's wort (high hypericin)	Hypericum perforatum	Aerial parts, harvested during the early flowering period	60	1:2	2	6	15	40
St. Mary's thistle	See Milk thistle							
Thuja	Thuja occidentalis	Leaf	60	1:5	1.5	3	10	20
Thyme	Thymus vulgaris	Leaf	60	1:2	2	6	15	40
Tienchi ginseng	Panax notoginseng	Root	45	1:2	3.5	8.5	25	60
Turmeric	Curcuma longa	Rhizome	45	1:1	5	14	35	100
Tylophora	Tylophora indica	Leaf	45	1:5	1	2	7	14
Uva ursi	Arctostaphylos uva-ursi	Leaf	45	1:2	4.5	8.5	30	60
Valerian	Valeriana officinalis	Root, rhizome	45	1:2	2	6	15	40
Vervain	Verbena officinalis	Aerial parts	25	1:2	3	6	20	40
White horehound	Marrubium vulgare	Aerial parts	25	1:2	2	6	15	40
White peony	Paeonia lactiflora	Root	45	1:2	4.5	8.5	30	60
Wild cherry	Prunus serotina	Bark	25	1:2	2	4.5	15	30
Wild yam	Dioscorea villosa	Root, rhizome	60	1:2	3	6	20	40
Willow herb	Epilobium parviflorum	Aerial parts	25	1:2	3	6	20	40
Withania	See Ashwaganda							
Wormwood	Artemisia absinthium	Aerial parts	45	1:5	0.7	3	5	20
Yarrow	Achillea millefolium	Aerial parts	45	1:2	2	6	15	40
Yellow dock	Rumex crispus	Root	25	1:2	2	4.5	15	30
Zizyphus	See Spiny jujube							

APPENDIX B

Glossary of Herbal Actions

Adaptogenic	A substance that increases the body's resistance to physical, environmental, emotional, or biologic stressors and promotes normal physiologic function
Adrenal tonic	A substance that improves the tone, histology, and function of the adrenal glands (especially the cortex)
Alterative	See Depurative
Analgesic	A substance that relieves pain
Anodyne	See Analgesic
Antacid	A substance that counteracts or neutralizes acidity in the gastrointestinal tract
Anthelmintic	A substance that kills or assists in the expulsion of intestinal worms
Antiallergic	A substance that tones down the allergic response, often by stabilizing mast cells
Antiandrogenic	A substance that inhibits or modifies the action of androgens (male sex hormones)
Antianemic	A substance that prevents or corrects anemia, which is a reduction in the number of circulating red blood cells or in the quantity of hemoglobin
Antiarrhythmic	A substance that prevents or is effective against arrhythmias, which are any variation from the normal rhythm or rate of the heart beat
Antiasthmatic	A substance that prevents or relieves asthma attacks
Antibacterial	A substance that inhibits the growth of bacteria (bacteriostatic) or destroys bacteria (bactericidal)
Anticariogenic	A substance that reduces the incidence of dental caries (tooth decay)
Anticatarrhal	A substance that reduces the formation of catarrh or phlegm (pathologic mucus secretion)
Anticonvulsant	A substance that tends to prevent or arrest seizures (convulsions)
Antidepressant	A substance that alleviates depression
Antidiabetic (see also Hypoglycemic)	A substance that alleviates diabetes or the effects of diabetes
Antidiarrheal	A substance that alleviates diarrhea
Antiecchymotic	A substance that prevents or alleviates bruising
Antiedematous	A substance that prevents or alleviates edema (fluid retention)
Antiemetic	A substance that reduces nausea and vomiting
Antifungal	A substance that inhibits the growth of or destroys fungi
Antihemorrhagic	A substance that reduces or stops bleeding when taken internally
Antihyperhidrotic	A substance that reduces excessive sweating
Antiinflammatory (see also Antiallergic, Antirheumatic, Antiedematous, Immune depressant)	A substance that reduces inflammation
Antilithic	A substance that reduces the formation of calculi (stones) in the urinary tract
Antimicrobial (see also Antibacterial, Antifungal, Antiparasitic, Antiviral)	A substance that inhibits the growth of or destroys microorganisms
Antioxidant	A substance that protects against oxidation and free radical damage
Anti-PAF	A substance that inhibits the activity of PAF (PAF is a potent platelet aggregating agent and inducer of systemic anaphylactic symptoms.)
Antiparasitic	A substance that inhibits the activity of or kills parasites
Antiplatelet	A substance that reduces platelet aggregation (and hence prolongs bleeding time and may prevent thrombus formation)

Continued

Glossary of Herbal Actions—cont'd

Antiprostatic	A substance that reduces symptoms from the prostate gland
Antiprotozoal	A substance that kills protozoa or inhibits their growth and activity
Antipruritic	A substance that relieves or prevents itching
Antipsoriatic	A substance that tends to relieve the symptoms of psoriasis
Antipyretic	A substance that reduces or prevents fever
Antirheumatic	A substance that prevents or relieves rheumatism
Antiseptic	*See Antimicrobial*
Antispasmodic	*See Spasmolytic*
Antithyroid	A substance that reduces the activity of the thyroid gland
Antitumor	A substance that has activity against a malignant tumor
Antitussive	A substance that reduces the amount or severity of coughing
Antiulcer	A substance that prevents or relieves ulceration (usually in the gastrointestinal tract)
Antiviral	A substance that inhibits the growth of or destroys viruses
Anxiolytic	A substance that alleviates anxiety
Aperient	*See Cathartic*
Aphrodisiac	A substance that stimulates sexual desire
Appetite stimulating	A substance that stimulates appetite
Aromatic digestive	A substance that is generally pleasant tasting, smelling, or both that assists digestion (These tonics are warming to the body and are also known as warming digestive tonics.)
Astringent	A substance that causes constriction of mucous membranes and exposed tissues, usually by precipitating proteins (This action has the effect of producing a barrier on the mucus or exposed surfaces.)
Bitter tonic *(also known as a Bitter; see also Digestive stimulant, Gastric stimulant)*	A substance that is bitter tasting and stimulates the upper gastrointestinal tract via the bitter-sensitive taste buds of the mouth, by direct interaction with gastrointestinal tissue, or both (Bitters have a promoting effect on all components of upper digestive function, namely the stomach, liver and pancreas. In addition to appetite and digestion they improve general health and immune function.)
Bladder tonic	A substance that improves the tone and function of the bladder
Bronchospasmolytic	A substance that reduces spasm in the lower respiratory tract
Cancer preventative *(see also Antitumor)*	A substance that prevents the incidence of cancer
Cardioprotective	A substance that protects cardiac tissue against hypoxia (oxygen deficiency) and decreases the risk of heart damage
Cardiotonic	A substance that improves the force of contraction of the heart
Carminative	A substance that relieves flatulence and soothes intestinal spasm and pain, usually by relaxing intestinal muscle and sphincters (These substances are added to herbal formulations to ease the intestinal spasm or pain that may be caused by laxative herbs.)
Cathartic	A substance that assists or induces evacuation of the bowel (i.e., having a strong laxative action) (These substances are also known as purgatives.)
Cholagogue	A substance that increases the release of stored bile from the gallbladder
Choleretic	A substance that increases the production of bile by the liver
Circulatory stimulant	A substance that improves blood flow through body tissues (Circulatory stimulants are warming, and they support vitality in the body tissues.)
Cognition enhancing	A substance that facilitates learning or memory
Collagen stabilizing	A substance that stabilizes collagen (e.g., protects collagen from degradation) (Connective tissue tone is thereby improved.)

Glossary of Herbal Actions—cont'd

Counterirritant	A substance that produces a superficial inflammation of the skin so as to relieve a deeper inflammation (e.g., in muscles, joints, and ligaments)
Demulcent	A substance that has a soothing effect on mucous membranes (e.g., within the respiratory, digestive, and urinary tracts)
Depurative	A substance that improves detoxification and aids elimination to reduce the accumulation of metabolic waste products within the body (These substances were formerly known as alteratives or blood purifiers and are largely used to treat chronic skin and musculoskeletal disorders.)
Diaphoretic	A substance that promotes sweating and thereby controls a fever (also known as sudorifics)
Digestive stimulant (see also *Gastric stimulant* and *Bitter tonic*)	A substance that stimulates the function of the gastrointestinal organs involved with digestion
Diuretic	A substance that increases urinary output
Dopaminergic agonist	A substance that binds to and activates dopamine receptors
Emetic	A substance that causes vomiting
Emmenagogue	A substance that initiates and promotes the menstrual flow (Several of these herbs are also regarded as abortifacients.)
Emollient	A substance used to soothe, soften, or protect skin
Estrogen modulating	In the context of use of herbs, a substance that acts by subtle, poorly understood mechanisms to promote estrogen production and effects in the body (The activity may involve interaction with secondary estrogen receptors such as those in the hypothalamus.)
Expectorant	A substance that improves the clearing of excess mucus from the lungs by either altering the viscosity of mucus or improving the cough reflex
Febrifuge	*See Antipyretic*
Female tonic	A substance that improves the tone, vigor, and function of the female reproductive system
Galactagogue	A substance that increases breast milk production
Gastric stimulant (see also *Bitter tonic* and *Digestive stimulant*)	A substance that stimulates the function of the stomach
General body tonic	*See Tonic*
Hemostatic	*See Styptic*
Hepatic (*Hepatic tonic*)	A substance that improves the tone, vigor, and function of the liver
Hepatoprotective	A substance that protects the hepatocytes (liver cells) against toxic damage
Hepatotrophorestorative	A substance that restores the integrity of liver tissue
Hypnotic	A substance that induces drowsiness and sleep (also known as soporifics)
Hypocholesterolemic (see also *Hypolipidemic*)	A substance that reduces the level of cholesterol in the blood
Hypoglycemic	A substance that reduces the level of glucose in the blood
Hypolipidemic	A substance that reduces the lipid level (cholesterol and triglycerides) of blood
Hypotensive (see also *Peripheral vasodilator*)	A substance that reduces blood pressure
Immune depressant	A substance that reduces immune function and is used particularly when part of the immune system is overactive

Continued

Glossary of Herbal Actions—cont'd

Immune enhancing	A substance that enhances immune function
Immune modulating	A substance that modulates and balances the activity of the immune system
Laxative	A substance that facilitates evacuation of the bowel
Local anesthetic	A substance that removes sensation or pain when applied locally
Lymphatic	A substance that assists detoxification by its effect on lymphatic tissue and often also improves immune function
Male tonic	A substance that improves the tone, vigor, and function of the male reproductive system
Mucolytic	A substance that helps break up and disperse sticky mucus in the respiratory tract
Mucoprotective	A substance that protects the mucous membranes, especially in the context of the gastric lining
Mucous membrane tonic	A substance that improves the tone, vigor, and function of the mucous membranes (particularly of the respiratory tract)
Mucous membrane trophorestorative	A substance that restores the integrity of mucous membranes (e.g., in the respiratory and digestive tracts)
Nervine tonic (*Nervine*)	A substance that improves the tone, vigor, and function of the nervous system (Nervine tonics relax and energize the nervous system).
Neuroprotective	A substance that helps prevent damage to the brain or spinal cord from ischemia, stroke, convulsions, or trauma
Nootropic	*See Cognition enhancing*
Ovarian tonic	A substance that improves the tone, vigor, and function of the ovaries
Oxytocic	A substance that causes contraction of the uterine muscle in association with giving birth
Parturifacient	A substance that induces labor and assists in the efficient delivery of the fetus and placenta
Partus preparator	A substance taken in preparation for labor and childbirth (Treatment usually begins in the second trimester.)
Peripheral vasodilator	A substance that dilates or widens the peripheral blood vessels and thereby improves circulation to peripheral tissues and may assist in reducing blood pressure
Progesterogenic	A substance that promotes the effect or production of progesterone
Prolactin inhibitor	A substance that inhibits the secretion of prolactin
Pungent	A hot-tasting substance that acts on a common group of nerve cell receptors having the effect of warming the body and improving digestion and circulation
Purgative	*See Cathartic*
Refrigerant	A substance that has cooling properties, particularly when applied to the skin
Rubefacient	*See Counterirritant*
Sedative (mild)	A substance that reduces activity, particularly in the nervous system and decreases nervous tension (A sedative may alleviate pain and spasm and induce sleep.)
Sexual tonic	A substance that improves the tone, vigor, and function of the sexual organs
Sialagogue	A substance that increases the secretion of the salivary glands
Skeletal muscle relaxant	A substance that relaxes skeletal muscle tone
Spasmolytic	A substance that reduces or relieves smooth muscle spasm (involuntary contractions)
Stimulant	A substance that heightens the function of an organ or system (e.g., a central nervous system stimulant increases the activity of the central nervous system, particularly behavioral alertness, agitation, or excitation). (The term has a second, more subtle meaning derived from the Thomsonian system [an early branch of herbal therapy in the United States: a substance capable of increasing the action or energy of the living body].)
Stomachic	*See Gastric stimulant*

Glossary of Herbal Actions—cont'd

Styptic	A substance that stops bleeding when applied locally
Thymoleptic *(see also Antidepressant)*	A substance that elevates mood
Thyroid stimulant	A substance that enhances the activity of the thyroid gland
Tissue perfusion enhancing	A substance that enhances the flow of nutrients into a tissue
Tonic *(also known as General body tonic; see also other specific body tonics)*	A substance that improves the tone, vigor, and function of the whole body
Trophorestorative	A substance that has a healing and restorative action on a specific organ or tissue
TSH antagonist	A substance that blocks the activity of TSH
Urinary antiseptic	A substance that inhibits the growth of or destroys microorganisms within the urinary tract
Urinary demulcent	A substance that has a soothing effect on mucous membranes of the urinary tract
Uterine sedative	A substance that reduces the activity of the uterus
Uterine tonic	A substance that increases the tone of the uterine muscle
Vasoconstrictor	A substance that constricts or narrows the blood vessels
Vasodilator	A substance that dilates or widens the blood vessels
Vasoprotective	A substance that protects the integrity of the blood vessels
Venotonic	A substance that improves the tone and function of the veins
Vulnerary *(see also Antiulcer, Astringent, Demulcent)*	A substance that promotes the healing of wounds when applied locally
Weight reducing	A substance that assists in the reduction of body weight

PAF, Platelet-activating factor; *TSH*, thyroid stimulating hormone.

APPENDIX **C**

Glossary of Clinical Trial Terms

Case-control study	Usually in case-control studies, volunteers with existing diagnosed disease (the cases) are enrolled in a study and are matched by identifiable characteristics (e.g., age, race, gender) to disease-free volunteers (the controls). The cases and controls are usually identified without knowledge of an individual's exposure or nonexposure to the factors being investigated. These factors are determined from existing information. Case-control studies usually begin after individuals have already developed or failed to develop the disease being investigated. Hence case-control studies are usually retrospective, although in some circumstances, they can also be prospective.
	Case-control studies are less reliable than either cohort studies or randomized, controlled trials. Often the first type of study to suggest a new medical conclusion, case-control studies may be designed to investigate a hypothesis suggested by a series of case reports.
Cohort study	The terminology surrounding cohort studies has been somewhat confused in the medical literature. A recent definition is: a cohort study compares the experience of a group of people exposed to some factor with another group not exposed to the same factor. If the exposed group has a higher or lower frequency of an outcome (e.g., a disease) than the unexposed group, then an association between exposure and outcome is evident.
	If the exposure occurred in the past and the outcome is investigated in the present, it is termed retrospective. If the exposure occurs in the present and the outcome will be monitored in the future, it is a prospective or concurrent cohort study.
	Cohort studies of disease differ from case-control studies in that cohort studies begin by identifying individuals for study and control groups before the investigator is aware of whether they have or will develop the disease (i.e., exposure → disease). (Case-control studies generally identify individuals with and without the disease and later look at the exposure status of the groups [i.e., disease → exposure].)
Control group	A group of people tested in comparison with a treatment-study group. The control group should be identical to the study group except that it has not been exposed to the treatment under investigation.
Crossover study	A study design in which the same individual receives both treatment and control therapies at different times, and an outcome is assessed for each therapy. A suitable washout period is required between each treatment phase.
Double-blind	When both the investigator and participants do not know who has been assigned to the treatment-study group or to the control group.
Effectiveness	The extent to which a treatment produces a beneficial effect when implemented under the usual conditions of clinical care.
	Both the efficacy of an intervention and its acceptance by those to whom it is offered is considered. A study of effectiveness asks, "Does the medicine help the patient?"
Efficacy	The extent to which a treatment produces a beneficial effect when assessed under the ideal conditions of an investigation (e.g., in a well-designed clinical trial).
	An efficacy study asks, "Does the medicine work?"
Epidemiologic study	A study designed to examine associations between defined parameters and a disease in a relatively large population. Such a study is usually concerned with identifying or measuring the effects of risk factors or exposures. Epidemiologic studies can include case-control studies, cohort studies, and cross-sectional studies (studied at one point in time).

Glossary of Clinical Trial Terms—cont'd

Meta-analysis	A series of methods for systematically combining information from more than one clinical trial so as to draw a stronger conclusion than one drawn solely on the basis of each single trial. Meta-analysis is more quantitative than the systematic review (see later).
Open (unblinded) study	A clinical study that may or may not have been controlled but was conducted without any blinding.
Phase I trial	A clinical trial in which researchers test a new drug or treatment in a small group of healthy people (20-80) for the first time to evaluate its safety, determine a safe dose range, and identify side effects.
Phase II trial	A small-scale, controlled or uncontrolled trial (involving 100-300 people) conducted to determine if a drug or treatment is effective and to further evaluate its safety.
Phase III trial	Usually a randomized, controlled trial involving large groups of people (1000-3000) that is conducted to understand the safety and efficacy of a drug or treatment.
Phase IV study	An uncontrolled study conducted after the drug or treatment has been marketed. Information is gathered in various populations and any side effects associated with long-term use are recorded.
Pilot trial	A small-scale trial often conducted before a large-scale trial.
Placebo	A preparation that has no specific pharmacologic activity against a targeted condition. In clinical trials, placebos, either as dummy treatments or procedures, are administered to control groups to provide results for comparison with the test treatment.
Postmarketing study	An uncontrolled study conducted after the release of a product onto the market to survey the effectiveness and tolerability of the preparation (similar to a phase IV study).
Prospective study	A prospective study is concerned with future information and outcomes. The information characterizing each individual is recorded before the onset of disease. The information obtained relates to the volunteers at the time the study is started and they are then followed throughout the time period of the study. The term may be applied to cohort, case-control, and postmarketing studies.
Randomization	A method of assignment in which individuals have a known, but not necessarily equal, probability of being assigned to a treatment group or control group. As distinguished from random sampling, the individuals being randomized may or may not be representative of a large population.
Retrospective study	A retrospective study looks back on past information. A retrospective study gathers information about individuals who had exposure to a factor under investigation, and the data is analyzed as or after the outcomes have occurred. The term may be applied to cohort and case-control studies.
Single-blind	When the patient is unaware, but the investigator is aware, of which therapy (treatment or control) is being received.
Systematic review	For the purposes of assigning levels of evidence, a review of randomized, controlled trials of a treatment that qualitatively assesses the quality of the trials and the efficacy of the treatment is conducted. (This review is in comparison to a meta-analysis, which makes a quantitative assessment).
Uncontrolled study	A clinical study that tests the therapy on all participants in the study without a control group.

For more information, refer to the following:

- Riegelman RK, Hirsch RP: *Studying a study and testing a test: how to read the health science literature,* ed 3, Boston, 1996, Little Brown.
- Doll R: Cohort studies: history of the method. I. Prospective cohort studies, *Soz Praventivmed* 46(2):75-86, 2001.
- Grimes DA, Schulz KF: Cohort studies: marching towards outcomes, Lancet 359(9303):341-345, 2002.
- Greenhalgh T: *How to read a paper: the basics of evidence based medicine,* ed 2, London, 2001, BMJ Books.

APPENDIX D

Herb Listing by Actions

Action	Herbs
Adaptogenic	ashwaganda, Astragalus, Bacopa (possibly), Eleutherococcus, gotu kola, Korean ginseng, neem leaf, Schisandra, shatavari
Adrenal tonic	licorice, Rehmannia
Analgesic	Arnica (topically only), California poppy, devil's claw, Jamaica dogwood, kava (mild), pasque flower, peppermint (topically)
Antacid	meadowsweet
Anthelmintic	Andrographis, feverfew, wormwood
Antiallergic	Albizia, Baical skullcap, feverfew, nettle leaf, Tylophora
Antiandrogenic	saw palmetto (possibly)
Antianemic	ashwaganda, dong quai
Antiarrhythmic	dong quai, hawthorn (leaf & berry), motherwort, Tienchi ginseng
Antiasthmatic	black haw, Tylophora
Antibacterial	Baical skullcap, barberry, elecampane, golden seal, Indian barberry, myrrh, pau d'arco, thyme
Anticariogenic	licorice
Anticatarrhal	elder flower, eyebright, golden rod, golden seal, mullein
Anticonvulsant	Bacopa (mild), kava, white peony
Antidepressant	lavender, Schisandra (mild), St. John's wort, vervain (mild)
Antidiabetic (see also Hypoglycemic)	goat's rue, Gymnema
Antidiarrheal	cranesbill root, raspberry leaf, shatavari
Antiecchymotic	Arnica (topical only), horsechestnut
Antiedematous	bilberry, horsechestnut
Antiemetic	barberry, fringe tree, ginger, globe artichoke, Indian barberry, peppermint
Antifungal	Calendula (topical), neem leaf, pau d'arco, Thuja, thyme,
Antihemorrhagic	cranesbill root, golden seal, Rehmannia, shepherd's purse, Tienchi ginseng, yarrow
Antihyperhidrotic	sage
Antiinflammatory (see also Antiallergic, Antirheumatic, Antiedematous, Immune depressant)	Aloe juice concentrate, Andrographis, Arnica (topical only), ashwaganda, Baical skullcap, bilberry, Bupleurum, Calendula, chamomile, cat's claw, celery seed, Crataeva, devil's claw, dong quai, Echinacea root, eyebright, fenugreek, feverfew, ginger, golden rod, golden seal, gotu kola, greater celandine, horsechestnut, licorice, meadowsweet, myrrh, neem leaf, Oregon grape, poke root, Rehmannia, sarsaparilla, saw palmetto, Tienchi ginseng, turmeric, Tylophora, uva ursi, white peony, wild yam, yarrow
Antilithic	corn silk, Crataeva, Hydrangea
Antimicrobial (see also Antibacterial, Antifungal, Antiparasitic, Antiseptic, Antiviral)	Albizia, Arnica (topically only), barberry, Calendula, fennel, golden seal, Indian barberry, myrrh, neem leaf, Oregon grape, peppermint (internally and topically), rosemary, sage, St. John's wort, Thuja, thyme, turmeric, yarrow
Antioxidant	Andrographis, Astragalus, bilberry, cat's claw, Ginkgo, hawthorn (leaf & berry), milk thistle, olive leaf, rosemary, sage, Schisandra, thyme, turmeric
Anti-PAF	Ginkgo
Antiparasitic	Euphorbia, pau d'arco, wormwood
Antiplatelet	Andrographis, Coleus, dong quai, ginger, turmeric
Antiprostatic	nettle root, saw palmetto, willow herb

Continued

APPENDIX **D**

Herb Listing by Actions—cont'd

Antiprotozoal	*See Antiparasitic*
Antipruritic	kava (topically), peppermint (topically), neem leaf
Antipsoriatic	Oregon grape
Antipyretic	Andrographis, Baptisia, neem leaf, Rehmannia, yarrow
Antirheumatic	black cohosh, celery seed, chamomile, dandelion, devil's claw, nettle leaf, prickly ash, sarsaparilla, wild yam
Antiseptic	*See Antibacterial, Antimicrobial, Urinary antiseptic*
Antispasmodic	*See Spasmolytic*
Antithyroid	bugleweed, motherwort
Antitumor	Aloe juice concentrate, pau d'arco, red clover (traditional use)
Antitussive	Bupleurum, licorice, neem leaf, peppermint, Schisandra, wild cherry
Antiulcer (peptic)	chamomile, chickweed, licorice
Antiviral	Aloe juice concentrate, Calendula (topically), greater celandine (topically), lemon balm (topically), neem leaf, St. John's wort, Thuja
Anxiolytic	Bacopa, California poppy, green oats, kava, lavender, Mexican valerian, neem leaf, passion flower, spiny jujube, valerian
Aphrodisiac	shatavari
Appetite stimulating	fennel, fenugreek
Aromatic digestive	cinnamon, Coleus
Astringent (see also Antidiarrheal and Vulnerary)	black haw, chickweed, cinnamon, cramp bark, cranesbill root, eyebright, hawthorn (leaf & berry) (mild), horsetail, meadowsweet, myrrh, raspberry leaf, sage, uva ursi, vervain, wild cherry
Bitter tonic (also known as a Bitter; see also Digestive stimulant, Gastric stimulant)	Andrographis, barberry, dandelion, devil's claw, feverfew, gentian, globe artichoke, golden seal, hops, Indian barberry, olive leaf, white horehound, wormwood, yarrow
Bladder tonic	Crataeva
Bronchospasmolytic	black haw, Coleus, elecampane, Grindelia
Cancer preventative (see also Antitumor)	Korean ginseng
Cardioprotective	hawthorn (leaf & berry), Tienchi ginseng
Cardiotonic	Astragalus, Coleus, hawthorn (leaf & berry) (mild), Korean ginseng, motherwort
Carminative	chamomile, cinnamon, fennel, ginger, lavender, lemon balm, peppermint, rosemary, turmeric
Cholagogue	barberry, blue flag, fringe tree, gentian, globe artichoke, greater celandine, Indian barberry, peppermint, yellow dock
Choleretic	Andrographis, barberry, dandelion, fringe tree, globe artichoke, golden seal, greater celandine, Indian barberry, milk thistle, turmeric
Circulatory stimulant	ginger (peripheral), Ginkgo, prickly ash, rosemary
Cognition enhancing	Bacopa, Ginkgo, Korean ginseng, white peony
Collagen stabilizing	hawthorn (leaf & berry)
Demulcent (see also Urinary demulcent)	bladderwrack, chickweed, fenugreek, licorice, marshmallow (root & leaf), mullein
Depurative	Baptisia, blue flag, burdock, cleavers, Echinacea root, fringe tree, globe artichoke, golden seal, gotu kola, Hemidesmus, neem leaf, nettle leaf, Oregon grape, pau d'arco, poke root, red clover, sarsaparilla, Thuja, turmeric, yellow dock
Diaphoretic	Bupleurum, chamomile, elder flower, elecampane, ginger, golden rod, Hemidesmus, lemon balm, lime flowers, peppermint, pleurisy root, prickly ash, vervain (mild), yarrow

APPENDIX D

Herb Listing by Actions—cont'd

Digestive stimulant (see also Bitter tonic)	Coleus, ginger
Diuretic	Astragalus, blue flag, buchu (mild), burdock (mild), celery seed, cleavers, corn silk, couch grass (soothing), dandelion (especially leaf), globe artichoke, golden rod, horsetail, Hydrangea, shatavari
Dopaminergic agonist	chaste tree
Emmenagogue	blue cohosh, feverfew (in high doses), motherwort, neem leaf
Emollient (see Demulcent)	marshmallow (root & leaf)
Estrogen modulating	black cohosh, fennel, false unicorn root, wild yam
Expectorant	elecampane, fennel, Grindelia, licorice, mullein, pleurisy root, thyme, white horehound
Female tonic	dong quai
Galactagogue	chaste tree, fennel, fenugreek, goat's rue, shatavari
Gastric stimulant (see also Bitter tonic, Digestive stimulant, Aromatic digestive)	gentian
Hepatoprotective	Andrographis, Bupleurum, globe artichoke, milk thistle, rosemary, Schisandra
Hepatotrophorestorative	globe artichoke, milk thistle
Hypnotic	California poppy, hops, kava, Mexican valerian, passion flower, spiny jujube, valerian
Hypocholesterolemic (see also Hypolipidemic)	Albizia, fenugreek, globe artichoke, Gymnema, Tienchi ginseng
Hypoglycemic	fenugreek, goat's rue, Gymnema, neem leaf
Hypolipidemic	turmeric
Hypotensive (see also Peripheral vasodilator)	Astragalus, black haw, Coleus, cramp bark, hawthorn (leaf & berry), mistletoe, motherwort, olive leaf, spiny jujube
Immune depressant	Hemidesmus, Tylophora
Immune enhancing	Aloe juice concentrate, Andrographis, Astragalus, Baptisia, cat's claw, Echinacea root, neem leaf, pau d'arco, poke root
Immune modulating	ashwaganda, Echinacea root, Eleutherococcus, Korean ginseng
Laxative	barberry (mild), blue flag, burdock (mild), cascara, damiana (mild), dandelion (mild), dong quai (mild), fringe tree (mild), greater celandine (mild), Indian barberry (mild), licorice (mild), yellow dock (mild)
Local anesthetic	kava
Lymphatic	blue flag, Calendula, Echinacea root, poke root
Male tonic	Korean ginseng, saw palmetto
Mucoprotective	licorice
Mucous membrane tonic	eyebright
Mucous membrane trophorestorative	golden seal
Nervine tonic	Bacopa, damiana, gotu kola, green oats, motherwort, oats seed, pasque flower, Schisandra, skullcap, St. John's wort, vervain
Neuroprotective	Ginkgo
Ovarian tonic	blue cohosh, false unicorn root
Oxytocic	blue cohosh, golden seal (reputed), Schisandra
Parturifacient (see also Oxytocic)	raspberry leaf

Continued

Herb Listing by Actions—cont'd

Partus preparator	raspberry leaf
Peripheral vasodilator	cramp bark, hawthorn (leaf & berry), lime flowers, mistletoe, yarrow
Progesterogenic	chaste tree (indirectly)
Prolactin inhibitor	chaste tree
Pungent	ginger
Refrigerant	chickweed
Rubefacient	thyme
Sedative (mild)	ashwaganda, Bacopa, bugleweed, California poppy, chamomile, cramp bark, hops, Jamaica dogwood, kava, lemon balm, lime flowers, Mexican valerian, mistletoe, passion flower, peppermint, skullcap, spiny jujube, valerian, wild cherry
Sexual tonic	shatavari
Sialagogue	Echinacea root, gentian, prickly ash
Skeletal muscle relaxant	kava, white peony (mild)
Spasmolytic	black cohosh, blue cohosh, chamomile, Coleus, cramp bark, elecampane, fennel, ginger, greater celandine, Grindelia, hops, Jamaica dogwood, kava, lavender, lemon balm, lime flowers, Mexican valerian, motherwort, pasque flower, passion flower, peppermint, rosemary, sage, saw palmetto, shatavari, skullcap, thyme, valerian, white horehound, white peony, wild yam, yarrow
Styptic (hemostatic) (see also Vulnerary)	Calendula, horsetail, nettle leaf, yarrow
Thymoleptic	oats seed
Thyroid stimulant	bladderwrack
Tissue perfusion enhancing	Ginkgo
Tonic (also known as General body tonic; see also other specific body tonics)	ashwaganda, Astragalus, Codonopsis, damiana, Eleutherococcus, Korean ginseng, oats seed, shatavari
TSH antagonist	bugleweed, lemon balm
Urinary antiseptic	buchu, meadowsweet (mild), shepherd's purse, uva ursi
Urinary demulcent	corn silk, couch grass, marshmallow (root & leaf)
Uterine sedative	black haw
Uterine tonic	black cohosh, blue cohosh, false unicorn root
Vasoprotective	bilberry
Venotonic	horsechestnut
Vulnerary (see also Antiulcer, Astringent, Demulcent)	Aloe juice concentrate, Calendula, chamomile, Echinacea root, golden seal, gotu kola, greater celandine (topical), mullein, myrrh, St. John's wort, yarrow
Weight reducing	bladderwrack, Gymnema

APPENDIX E

Action Listing by Herbs

Herb	Actions
Albizia	Antiallergic, hypocholesterolemic, antimicrobial.
Aloe juice concentrate	Immune enhancing, antiviral, vulnerary, antiinflammatory, antitumor.
Andrographis	Bitter tonic, choleretic, immune enhancing, hepatoprotective, antipyretic, antiinflammatory, antiplatelet, antioxidant, anthelmintic.
Arnica	Topical only: Antiinflammatory, antiecchymotic (against bruises), analgesic, antimicrobial.
Ashwaganda	Tonic, adaptogenic, mild sedative, antiinflammatory, immunomodulator, antianemic.
Astragalus	Immune enhancing, tonic, adaptogenic, cardiotonic, diuretic, hypotensive, antioxidant.
Bacopa	Cognition enhancing, nervine tonic, mild sedative, mild anticonvulsant, anxiolytic, possibly adaptogenic.
Baical skullcap	Antiinflammatory, antiallergic, antibacterial.
Baptisia	Depurative, antipyretic, immune enhancing.
Barberry	Antimicrobial, cholagogue, choleretic, antiemetic, mild laxative, bitter tonic.
Bilberry	Vasoprotective, antiedema, antioxidant, antiinflammatory.
Black cohosh	Antirheumatic, spasmolytic, estrogen modulating, uterine tonic.
Black haw	Uterine sedative, bronchospasmolytic, antiasthmatic, hypotensive, astringent.
Bladderwrack	Weight reducing, thyroid stimulant, demulcent.
Blue cohosh	Spasmolytic, uterine and ovarian tonic, emmenagogue, oxytocic.
Blue flag	Depurative, laxative, cholagogue, lymphatic, diuretic.
Buchu	Urinary antiseptic, mild diuretic.
Bugleweed	TSH antagonist, antithyroid, reduces heart rate, mild sedative.
Bupleurum	Antiinflammatory, hepatoprotective, diaphoretic, antitussive.
Burdock	Depurative, mild diuretic, mild laxative.
Calendula	Vulnerary, antiinflammatory, lymphatic, styptic (hemostatic), antimicrobial, antiviral (topically), antifungal (topically).
California poppy	Anxiolytic, mild sedative, analgesic, hypnotic.
Cascara	Laxative.
Cat's claw	Immune enhancing, antiinflammatory, antioxidant.
Celery seed	Diuretic, antiinflammatory, antirheumatic.
Chamomile	Antiinflammatory, spasmolytic, carminative, mild sedative, antiulcer, vulnerary, diaphoretic.
Chaste tree	Prolactin inhibitor, dopaminergic agonist, indirectly progesterogenic, galactagogue.
Chickweed	Demulcent, astringent, refrigerant, antiulcer (peptic).
Cinnamon	Carminative, aromatic digestive, astringent.
Cleavers	Diuretic, depurative.
Codonopsis	Tonic.
Coleus	Hypotensive, antiplatelet, bronchospasmolytic, spasmolytic, cardiotonic, digestive stimulant, aromatic digestive.
Corn silk	Diuretic, antilithic, urinary demulcent.
Couch grass	Soothing diuretic, urinary demulcent.
Cramp bark	Spasmolytic, mild sedative, astringent, hypotensive, peripheral vasodilator.
Cranesbill root	Astringent, antidiarrheal, antihemorrhagic.
Crataeva	Antilithic, bladder tonic, antiinflammatory.
Damiana	Nervine tonic, tonic, mild laxative.
Dandelion (root & leaf)	Bitter tonic, choleretic, diuretic (especially leaf), mild laxative, antirheumatic.
Devil's claw	Antiinflammatory, antirheumatic, analgesic, bitter tonic.
Dong quai	Antiinflammatory, antianemic, antiplatelet, female tonic, mild laxative, antiarrhythmic.

Continued

APPENDIX E

Action Listing by Herbs—cont'd

Echinacea root	Immune modulator, immune enhancing, depurative, antiinflammatory, vulnerary, lymphatic, sialagogue.
Elder flower	Diaphoretic, anticatarrhal.
Elecampane	Expectorant, diaphoretic, antibacterial, spasmolytic, bronchospasmolytic.
Eleutherococcus	Adaptogenic, immunomodulator, tonic.
Euphorbia	Expectorant, antiasthmatic, spasmolytic, antiprotozoal.
Eyebright	Astringent, anticatarrhal, mucous membrane tonic, antiinflammatory.
False unicorn root	Uterine tonic, ovarian tonic, estrogen modulating.
Fennel	Carminative, appetite stimulating, spasmolytic, galactagogue, estrogen modulating, antimicrobial, expectorant.
Fenugreek	Appetite stimulating, galactagogue, antiinflammatory, demulcent, hypoglycemic, hypocholesterolemic.
Feverfew	Antiinflammatory, antiallergic, bitter tonic, emmenagogue (in high doses), anthelmintic.
Fringe tree	Cholagogue, choleretic, mild laxative, antiemetic, depurative.
Gentian	Bitter tonic, gastric stimulant, sialagogue, cholagogue.
Ginger	Carminative, antiemetic, peripheral circulatory stimulant, spasmolytic, antiinflammatory, antiplatelet, diaphoretic, digestive stimulant, pungent.
Ginkgo	Antioxidant, anti-PAF (anti-platelet-activating factor) activity, tissue perfusion enhancing, circulatory stimulant, cognition enhancing, neuroprotective.
Globe artichoke	Hepatoprotective, hepatic trophorestorative, choleretic, cholagogue, bitter tonic, hypocholesterolemic, antiemetic, diuretic, depurative.
Goat's rue	Hypoglycemic, antidiabetic, galactagogue.
Golden rod	Antiinflammatory, diaphoretic, diuretic, anticatarrhal.
Golden seal	Antihemorrhagic, anticatarrhal, trophorestorative for mucous membranes, antibacterial, bitter tonic, antiinflammatory, depurative, vulnerary, choleretic, reputed oxytocic.
Gotu kola	Vulnerary, antiinflammatory, depurative, adaptogenic, nervine tonic.
Greater celandine	Choleretic, cholagogue, spasmolytic, mild laxative, antiinflammatory, antiviral (topically), vulnerary (topical).
Green oats	Nervine tonic, anxiolytic.
Grindelia	Expectorant, spasmolytic, bronchospasmolytic.
Gymnema	Antidiabetic, hypoglycemic, hypocholesterolemic, weight reducing.
Hawthorn berry	Cardioprotective, mild cardiotonic, hypotensive, peripheral vasodilator, antiarrhythmic, antioxidant, mild astringent, collagen stabilizing.
Hawthorn leaf	Cardioprotective, mild cardiotonic, hypotensive, peripheral vasodilator, antiarrhythmic, antioxidant, mild astringent, collagen stabilizing.
Hemidesmus	Depurative, diaphoretic, immune depressant.
Hops	Hypnotic, mild sedative, spasmolytic, bitter tonic.
Horsechestnut	Venotonic, antiedematous, antiinflammatory, antiecchymotic (against bruises).
Horsetail	Diuretic, astringent, styptic (hemostatic).
Hydrangea	Diuretic, antilithic.
Indian barberry	as for barberry: Antimicrobial, cholagogue, choleretic, antiemetic, mild laxative, bitter tonic.
Jamaica dogwood	Analgesic, spasmolytic, mild sedative.
Kava	Anxiolytic, hypnotic, anticonvulsant, mild sedative, skeletal muscle relaxant, spasmolytic, local anesthetic, mild analgesic, antipruritic (topically).
Korean ginseng	Adaptogenic, tonic, immune modulator, cardiotonic, male tonic, cancer preventative, cognition enhancing.

Action Listing by Herbs—cont'd

Lavender	Carminative, spasmolytic, antidepressant, anxiolytic.
Lemon balm	Carminative, spasmolytic, mild sedative, diaphoretic, TSH antagonist, antiviral (topically).
Licorice	Antiinflammatory, mucoprotective, demulcent, antiulcer (peptic), adrenal tonic, expectorant, antitussive, mild laxative, anticariogenic.
Lime flowers	Spasmolytic, peripheral vasodilator, mild sedative, diaphoretic.
Marshmallow leaf	Demulcent, urinary demulcent, emollient.
Marshmallow root	Demulcent, urinary demulcent, emollient.
Meadowsweet	Antacid, antiinflammatory, mild urinary antiseptic, astringent.
Mexican valerian	Anxiolytic, mild sedative, hypnotic, spasmolytic.
Milk thistle	Hepatoprotective, hepatic trophorestorative, antioxidant, choleretic.
Mistletoe	Hypotensive, peripheral vasodilator, mild sedative.
Motherwort	Nervine tonic, cardiotonic, hypotensive, antiarrhythmic, antithyroid, spasmolytic, emmenagogue.
Mullein	Expectorant, demulcent, anticatarrhal, vulnerary.
Myrrh	Astringent, antimicrobial, antibacterial, antiinflammatory, vulnerary.
Neem leaf	Antimicrobial, antifungal, antiviral, antipyretic, adaptogenic, antipruritic, antitussive, depurative, antiinflammatory, anxiolytic, emmenagogue, hypoglycemic, immune enhancing.
Nettle leaf	Antirheumatic, antiallergic, depurative, styptic (hemostatic).
Nettle root	Antiprostatic.
Oats seed	Nervine tonic, tonic, thymoleptic.
Olive leaf	Hypotensive, antioxidant, bitter tonic.
Oregon grape	Antipsoriatic, antiinflammatory, depurative, antimicrobial.
Pasque flower	Spasmolytic, analgesic.
Passion flower	Anxiolytic, spasmolytic, mild sedative, hypnotic.
Pau d'arco	Immune enhancing, antitumor, antibacterial, antifungal, antiparasitic, depurative.
Peppermint	Spasmolytic, carminative, cholagogue, antiemetic, antitussive, antimicrobial (internally and topically), mild sedative, diaphoretic, analgesic (topically), antipruritic (topically).
Pleurisy root	Diaphoretic, expectorant.
Poke root	Antiinflammatory, lymphatic, depurative, immune enhancing.
Prickly ash	Circulatory stimulant, diaphoretic, antirheumatic, sialagogue.
Raspberry leaf	Astringent, partus preparator, parturifacient, antidiarrheal.
Red clover	Depurative, antitumor (traditional use).
Rehmannia	Antipyretic, adrenal tonic, antihemorrhagic, antiinflammatory.
Rosemary	Carminative, spasmolytic, antioxidant, antimicrobial, circulatory stimulant, hepatoprotective.
Sage	Spasmolytic, antioxidant, astringent, antihyperhidrotic, antimicrobial.
Sarsaparilla	Antirheumatic, depurative, antiinflammatory.
Saw palmetto	Antiinflammatory, male tonic, antiprostatic, spasmolytic, possibly antiandrogenic.
Schisandra	Hepatoprotective, antioxidant, adaptogenic, nervine tonic, antitussive, oxytocic, mild antidepressant.
Shatavari	Tonic, galactagogue, sexual tonic, aphrodisiac, adaptogenic, antispasmodic, antidiarrheal, diuretic.
Shepherd's purse	Antihemorrhagic, urinary antiseptic.
Skullcap	Nervine tonic, spasmolytic, mild sedative.
Spiny jujube	Hypnotic, mild sedative, hypotensive, anxiolytic.
St. John's wort	Antiviral, nervine tonic, antidepressant, vulnerary, antimicrobial.
Thuja	Antimicrobial, depurative, antiviral, antifungal.

Continued

Action Listing by Herbs—cont'd

Thyme	Expectorant, spasmolytic, antibacterial, antifungal, antioxidant, rubefacient (topically), antimicrobial.
Tienchi ginseng	Antihemorrhagic, cardioprotective, antiinflammatory, antiarrhythmic, hypocholesterolemic.
Turmeric	Antiinflammatory, antiplatelet, antioxidant, hypolipidemic, choleretic, antimicrobial, carminative, depurative.
Tylophora	Antiasthmatic, antiinflammatory, immune depressant, antiallergic.
Uva ursi	Urinary antiseptic, astringent, antiinflammatory.
Valerian	Anxiolytic, mild sedative, hypnotic, spasmolytic.
Vervain	Nervine tonic, mild depressant, mild diaphoretic, astringent.
White horehound	Expectorant, spasmolytic, bitter tonic.
White peony	Spasmolytic, mild skeletal muscle relaxant, anticonvulsant, antiinflammatory, cognition enhancing.
Wild cherry	Antitussive, mild sedative, astringent.
Wild yam	Spasmolytic, antiinflammatory, antirheumatic, estrogen modulating.
Willow herb	Antiprostatic.
Wormwood	Bitter tonic, anthelmintic, antiparasitic.
Yarrow	Diaphoretic, antipyretic, peripheral vasodilator, antiinflammatory, spasmolytic, bitter tonic, styptic (hemostatic), antimicrobial, antihemorrhagic, vulnerary.
Yellow dock	Mild laxative, cholagogue, depurative.

APPENDIX F

Herbs Possibly Contraindicated in Pregnancy

Herb	Notes
Andrographis	The antifertility effect in female mice (albeit at high doses) suggests that Andrographis should not be used during human pregnancy, especially in the first trimester.
Arnica	Not for internal use, for topical use only.
Barberry	Contraindicated in pregnancy.
Black cohosh	Contraindicated in pregnancy and lactation, except for assisting birth during the last month.
Bladderwrack	Contraindicated in pregnancy and lactation.
Blue cohosh	Contraindicated in pregnancy and lactation.
Bugleweed	Contraindicated in pregnancy and lactation because of potential antigonadotropic activity.
Cascara	According to the *British Herbal Compendium* cascara is contraindicated in pregnancy and lactation. However, this caution seems excessive provided the recommended therapeutic dosage is observed. Doses which cause an excessively loose stool should not be used during pregnancy.
Cat's claw	Use with caution in pregnancy and lactation.
Chaste tree	Use cautiously in pregnancy and only in the early stages for treatment of insufficient corpus luteal function. Although the dopaminergic activity might suggest that chaste tree is best avoided during lactation, clinical trials have demonstrated its positive activity on milk production, albeit at low doses.
Dong quai	Contraindicated in the first trimester of pregnancy, especially in higher doses.
Elecampane	According to the *British Herbal Compendium* elecampane is contraindicated in pregnancy and lactation. However there appears to be no substantial basis for this concern.
Feverfew	Doses during pregnancy should be kept to a minimum (no more than 1.5 mL of a 1:5 tincture per day). No adverse effects expected during lactation as long as the recommended dosage levels are observed.
Ginger	No adverse effects are expected within the recommended dosage (0.7 to 2 mL of 1:2 liquid extract). A daily dose of 2 g of dried ginger should not be exceeded in pregnancy. Ginger has been successfully utilized in clinical trials to treat pregnant women with nausea.
Golden seal	Contraindicated in pregnancy.
Indian barberry	Contraindicated in pregnancy.
Jamaica dogwood	Contraindicated in pregnancy.
Licorice	Doses up to 3 g per day (i.e., up to 3 mL of 1:1 liquid extract or 3 mL of 1:1 high glycyrrhizin liquid extract) are likely to be safe.
Motherwort	Contraindicated in pregnancy.
Myrrh	Contraindicated in pregnancy.
Neem leaf	Avoid use during pregnancy, especially in the first trimester.
Oregon grape	Contraindicated in pregnancy.
Pasque flower	Contraindicated in pregnancy and lactation.
Pau d'arco	Caution in pregnancy due to possible abortive and teratogenic actions.
Poke root	Contraindicated in pregnancy and lactation.
Raspberry leaf	No adverse effects expected in pregnancy or lactation, but it is more appropriate to confine use to the second and third trimesters.
Sage	Contraindicated in pregnancy and lactation. However, sage has been used traditionally to stop milk flow.
Schisandra	Contraindicated in pregnancy, except to assist childbirth.

Continued

Herbs Possibly Contraindicated in Pregnancy—cont'd

Tienchi ginseng	Contraindicated in pregnancy, according to TCM.
Tylophora	Contraindicated in pregnancy and lactation.
Uva ursi	Contraindicated in pregnancy and lactation.
Wormwood	Contraindicated in pregnancy and lactation.
Yarrow	No adverse effects expected. However thujone-containing varieties should be avoided.
Yellow dock	Use with caution during pregnancy.

Index